AF709600

Color Atlas of Cerebral Revascularization

Anatomy, Techniques, Clinical Cases

Thieme

Color Atlas of Cerebral Revascularization

Anatomy, Techniques, Clinical Cases

Robert F. Spetzler, MD
Director, Barrow Neurological Institute
J. N. Harber Chairman and Professor of Neurological Surgery
Division of Neurological Surgery
Barrow Neurological Institute
Phoenix, Arizona

Albert L. Rhoton Jr., MD
R. D. Keene Family Professor and Chairman Emeritus
Department of Neurosurgery
University of Florida
Gainesville, Florida

Peter Nakaji, MD, FACS, FAANS
Professor of Neurosurgery
Director, Neurosurgery Residency Program
Director, Minimally Invasive Neurosurgery
Division of Neurological Surgery
Barrow Neurological Institute
Phoenix, Arizona

Masatou Kawashima, MD, PhD
Associate Professor
Department of Neurosurgery
Faculty of Medicine
Saga University
Saga, Japan

Thieme
New York • Stuttgart

Thieme Medical Publishers, Inc.
333 Seventh Ave.
New York, New York 10001

Executive Editor: Kay Conerly
Managing Editor: Judith Tomat
Senior Vice President, Editorial and Electronic Product Development: Cornelia Schulze
Production Editor: Teresa Exley, Maryland Composition
International Production Director: Andreas Schabert
Vice President, Finance and Accounts: Sarah Vanderbilt
President: Brian D. Scanlan
Compositor: Maryland Composition
Printer: Everbest Printing Co.
Cover art by Kristen Larson, MS, CMI
Digital presentation designed and produced by Marie Clarkson

Copyright © 2013 by Thieme Medical Publishers, Inc. This book, including all parts thereof, is legally protected by copyright. Any use, exploitation, or commercialization outside the narrow limits set by copyright legislation without the publisher's consent is illegal and liable to prosecution. This applies in particular to photostat reproduction, copying, mimeographing or duplication of any kind, translating, preparation of microfilms, and electronic data processing and storage.

Barrow Neurological Institute holds copyright to all diagnostic images, photographs, videos, the video presentation, and art, including the cover art, used in this work and the accompanying digital content, unless otherwise stated. Used with permission from Barrow Neurological Institute.

Thieme holds copyright to Fig. 1.3 b–h; 2.0 c (photograph); 2.6 a, e, g, h, and m; 2.7 a–f and h–k; 2.8 a–f; 2.9 a–d; 2.10 a–d, e (photograph), f–j; 4.1 b, c, d (photograph), e, and f; 4.4 b–d, e (photograph), f (photograph), g (photograph), and i; 6.1 a–c, e–o; 7.0 a (photograph), b (photograph), c (photograph), and d (photograph); 7.8 a–f, g (photograph), h–k; 9.0 h (photograph), i (photograph), and j (photograph); 9.1 a–c, d (photograph), f, g (photograph), h, and k; 9.2 a–g, i–p; 9.3 a–l, m (photograph), n (photograph), o (photograph), p–s; 10.1 c–k, l (photograph), m–o; 11.1 a–e, f (photograph), g (photograph), h–p; 11.2 a–e, f (photograph), g–k; 12.1 a–d; 12.2 a, b, c (photograph), d, f–h; 12.4 a–i, j (photograph), and k; 13.1 a, c, e, f, h, and i; 14.1 a, b, and f; 16.1 a, d–g, and i; and 16.3 b–f, g (photograph), h (photograph), i, and k.

Library of Congress Cataloging-in-Publication Data

Color atlas of cerebral revascularization / by Robert F. Spetzler ... [et al.].
p. ; cm.
ISBN 978-1-60406-822-1 (alk. paper)
I. Spetzler, Robert F. (Robert Friedrich), 1944-
[DNLM: 1. Cerebral Revascularization--Atlases. WL 17]

616.8'100222--dc23

2012043136

Important note: Medical knowledge is ever changing. As new research and clinical experience broaden our knowledge, changes in treatment and drug therapy may be required. The authors and editors of the material herein have consulted sources believed to be reliable in their efforts to provide information that is complete and in accord with the standards accepted at the time of publication. However, in view of the possibility of human error by the authors, editors, or publisher of the work herein or changes in medical knowledge, neither the authors, editors, nor publisher, nor any other party who has been involved in the preparation of this work, warrants that the information contained herein is in every respect accurate or complete, and they are not responsible for any errors or omissions or for the results obtained from use of such information. Readers are encouraged to confirm the information contained herein with other sources. For example, readers are advised to check the product information sheet included in the package of each drug they plan to administer to be certain that the information contained in this publication is accurate and that changes have not been made in the recommended dose or in the contraindications for administration. This recommendation is of particular importance in connection with new or infrequently used drugs.

Some of the product names, patents, and registered designs referred to in this book are in fact registered trademarks or proprietary names even though specific reference to this fact is not always made in the text. Therefore, the appearance of a name without designation as proprietary is not to be construed as a representation by the publisher that it is in the public domain.

Printed in China

5 4 3 2 1

ISBN 978-1-60406-822-1
eISBN 978-1-60406-823-8

To our patients who continue to instruct and inspire us.

Contents

Preface

Dedicated to the memory of Wolfgang T. Koos, master surgeon, mentor, colleague, friend

More than 20 years ago, an older, generous, and more experienced neurosurgeon than I invited me to help him translate a volume, subsequently entitled *Color Atlas of Neurosurgery*, from German into English. That collaboration was one of the defining moments of both my academic career and my personal life. It led to a lifelong friendship with Dr. Wolfgang Koos, who built and presided over modern neurosurgery in Vienna until his death in the year 2000. That collaboration also led to a second edition and several subsequent volumes of the *Color Atlas*, the last of which was also published in 2000.

Not surprisingly, then, readers of this new surgical atlas, which is devoted to cerebral revascularization, will find a fresh look albeit a familiar format and focus: intraoperative photographs with accompanying illustrations intended to highlight surgical technique. The clinical cases are placed in microsurgical context by the exquisite anatomical photographs from the laboratory of that incomparably meticulous anatomist and my primary co-author, Dr. Albert L. Rhoton, Jr., who was assisted by his talented colleague, Dr. Masatou Kawashima. Readers will also find included with this volume a DVD of more than 30 related surgical cases narrated by my colleague Dr. Peter Nakaji and by me. Each case on the surgical video DVD is noted in the corresponding text for ease of reference. Animations are also included to help clarify technical nuances of procedures.

Cerebral revascularization refers to a set of techniques used to overcome the presence of or potential for ischemia in the brain. The ischemia can develop from a myriad of causes: moyamoya disease, aneurysms that recur after coiling, giant aneurysms, vascular tears, vertebral artery insufficiency, severe vascular stenosis, and radiation-induced occlusion. These are among the clinical cases whose treatment is showcased in this atlas.

Foremost among revascularization techniques, of course, is the surgical bypass. In 1967, when I was completing my undergraduate degree at Knox College in Illinois, still a long way from pursuing my dream of becoming a neurosurgeon, Donagy and Yasargil performed the first extracranial-to-intracranial (EC-to-IC) bypass using the superficial temporal artery (STA) and middle cerebral artery (MCA). Use of this bypass spread rapidly until publication of the results of the EC-to-IC bypass trial in 1985 called the efficacy of the technique into question. Although aspects of this important issue are still debated more than 25 years later, most neurosurgeons would agree that bypasses are an integral part of the neurosurgical armamentarium. In fact, the STA-to-MCA bypass became and remains the most widely used of all bypasses for cerebral revascularization. Indeed, STA-to-MCA bypasses represent the largest number of cases in this volume. As in past volumes, however, related controversies, including the inseparable issues of diagnosis, indications, and outcomes, have been excluded. All are amply discussed elsewhere in the literature. The overarching goal of this volume was to concentrate solely on techniques as taught and performed at the Barrow Neurological Institute, which currently has the largest neurosurgical residency program in the United States. Readers will also find less common bypasses, such as the bonnet bypass, middle meningeal artery–to–MCA bypass, onlay bypass, and facial artery–to–vertebral artery bypass, represented in this text.

Across my career I have been fortunate to witness and participate in many advances that have driven changes in how neurosurgery is conducted. One of the most wide-sweeping developments has been the advent of endovascular procedures. As a neurovascular surgeon, my bias is for definitive surgical treatment. Nonetheless, endovascular procedures are important surgical adjuncts and two such cases are included. Even newer treatments are also represented. Dr. Albert van der Zwan generously provided a case treated by excimer laser-assisted nonocclusive anastomosis (ELANA), a procedure developed to create a bypass without the need to interrupt the blood supply in the recipient blood vessels. Compared to traditional bypass techniques, this subtle difference is intended to decrease the risk of stroke or rupture of aneurysm related to the temporary ischemia induced in regions supplied by the artery receiving the bypass. The volume also includes an example of the internal maxillary artery–to–MCA bypass known as the Abdulrauf bypass after its developer, Dr. Saleem Abdulrauf, who kindly provided the case. Finally, cases showing vertebral artery reconstruction and transposition for the treatment of occlusive disease are also presented. My hope is that the diversity of treatment and cases will be of interest to practicing neurosurgeons, neurosurgical fellows and residents, and interventional neuroradiologists and that the volume, which spans my career, will serve as a valuable resource for years to come.

As with previous volumes of the *Color Atlas*, it took a village to produce this book devoted exclusively to cerebral revascularization. The members of the Neuroscience Publications Office of Barrow Neurological Institute again worked tirelessly to produce this book under the guidance of our long-suffering editor, Shelley Kick, PhD. The enormous task of translating the complex spatial relationships into understandable illustrations was accomplished by our talented medical illustrators, Mark Schornak, MS, and Kristen Larson,

MS. Mark Schornak directed the visual media team and created many of the side-by-side illustrations; his profound understanding of neuroanatomy, coupled with a strong commitment to didactic excellence, continually challenges us all to live up to his expectations. Throughout the project, Kristen Larson displayed her skill and untiring persistence in creating not only many of the side-by-side illustrations, but also the orientation diagrams, section art, and exquisite cover illustration. Marie Clarkson showed her talent and creativity by single-handedly designing and producing the exceptional video presentation on the DVD. Jaime-Lynn Canales, our production editor, kept us organized, while also devoting herself to the task of processing and cataloging all of the more than 1,300 images included in the book and providing countless revisions as the text was assembled. Dawn Mutchler carefully perused each page to ensure accuracy and consistency. Clare Prendergast, Mandi Leite, Talisa Umfress, and Diantha Leavitt worked assiduously in their roles as editorial assistants at different times during the project.

Our friends at Thieme also need to be recognized for their unfailing patience and continued commitment to quality publishing. It is clear why the company has become the premier publisher of neurosurgical texts. Kay Conerly, Executive Editor, was a delight to work with and handled all issues with both alacrity and aplomb. Judith Tomat, Managing Editor, faultlessly helped keep this large project organized and on track. Torsten Scheihagen, Associate Manager, Book Production, oversaw production. Finally, Teresa Exley and her team at Absolute Service showed exceptional professionalism and attention to detail in producing this beautiful volume.

My expression of gratitude would be sorely incomplete and inadequate if I did not acknowledge the loving support of my wife and family, both while working on this book and over the long years of my career, which too often demanded long hours away from them. I have been blessed with their understanding and generosity of spirit.

And last but certainly far from least, I thank the countless patients who have been my most profound instructors over my career. Their courage, humor, and selflessness when confronted with sometimes dire diagnoses and frightening treatments have been beyond inspirational. The lessons that I have learned—sometimes even at their expense—ultimately have served to raise the bar of knowledge so that others have happier outcomes. Any legacy my own fleeting efforts may earn, I offer to them in tribute.

Robert F. Spetzler, MD
Phoenix, Arizona
September 2012

Abbreviations

Abbreviations used in this volume

General Anatomy Terms
a., aa = artery, arteries
anast. = anastomosis
ant. = anterior
arach. = arachnoid
br. = branch
cap. = capitis
f. = foramen
g. = gland
gr. = greater
inf. = inferior
int. = internal
L = left
lat. = lateral
m. = muscle
maj. = major
n., nn. = nerve, nerves
obl. = oblique
post. = posterior
R = ribs, right
rec. = rectus
sup. = superior
temp. = temporal
tent. = tentorium
v. = vein

Cranial Nerves
CN I = olfactory nerve
CN II = optic nerve
CN III = oculomotor nerve
CN IV = trochlear nerve
CN V = trigeminal nerve
V1 = ophthalmic branch of trigeminal nerve
V2 = maxillary branch of trigeminal nerve
V3 = mandibular branch of trigeminal nerve
CN VI = abducent nerve
CN VII = facial nerve
CN VIII = vestibulocochlear nerve
CN IX = glossopharyngeal nerve
CN X = vagus nerve
CN XI = spinal accessory nerve
CN XII = hypoglossal nerve

Vessels
A1 = first segment of the anterior cerebral artery
A2 = second segment of the anterior cerebral artery
A3 = third segment of the anterior cerebral artery
ACA = anterior cerebral artery
ACAS = asymptomatic carotid artery stenosis
AChoA = anterior choroidal artery
ACoA = anterior communicating artery
AICA = anterior inferior cerebellar artery
ATA = anterior temporal artery
BA = basilar artery
CCA = common carotid artery
Cerv. ICA = cervical internal carotid artery
ECA = external carotid artery
FA = facial artery
ICA = internal carotid artery
IJV / Int. jugular v. = internal jugular vein
IMA = internal maxillary artery
M1 = the sphenoidal segment of the middle cerebral artery
M2 = an insular segment of the middle cerebral artery
M3 = an opercular segment of the middle cerebral artery
M4 = a cortical segment of the middle cerebral artery
MCA = middle cerebral artery
MMA = middle meningeal artery
OA = occipital artery
Ophth. A. = ophthalmic artery
P1 = first segment of the posterior cerebral artery
P2 = second segment of the posterior cerebral artery
P1A = anterior division of first segment of the posterior cerebral artery
P1P = posterior division of the first segment of the posterior cerebral artery
P4 = fourth segment of the posterior cerebral artery
PCA = posterior cerebral artery
PCoA = posterior communicating artery
Pet. Car. A. = petrous carotid artery
Pet. ICA = petrous internal carotid artery
PICA = posterior inferior cerebellar artery
Saph. v. = saphenous vein
SCA = superior cerebellar artery
STA = superficial temporal artery
VA = vertebral artery

Other
AVM = arteriovenous malformation
BTO = balloon test occlusion
C1, C2, C3 = nerve roots of the first, second, and third cervical vertebrae
CBF = cerebral blood flow
CMRO2 = cerebral metabolic rate of oxygen
CNS = central nervous system
COSS = Carotid Occlusion Surgery Study
CT = computed tomography
EC-IC = extracranial-intracranial
EEG = electroencephalography
ELANA = excimer laser-assisted nonocclusive anastomosis
GSPN = greater superficial petrosal nerve
ICG = indocyanine green
ICP = intracranial pressure
ICU = intensive care unit
infund. = infundibulum
MR = magnetic resonance
NASCET = North American Symptomatic Carotid Endarterectomy Trial

OEF = oxygen extraction fraction
PET = positron emission tomography
SAH = subarachnoid hemorrhage
SCM = sternocleidomastoid muscle
SPECT = single photon emission computed tomography
SSEP = somatosensory evoked potential
Sup. pet. sinus = superior petrosal sinus
T1, T2, T3 = nerve roots of the first, second, and third thoracic vertebrae
TIA = transient ischemic attack

1 ACA Bypass

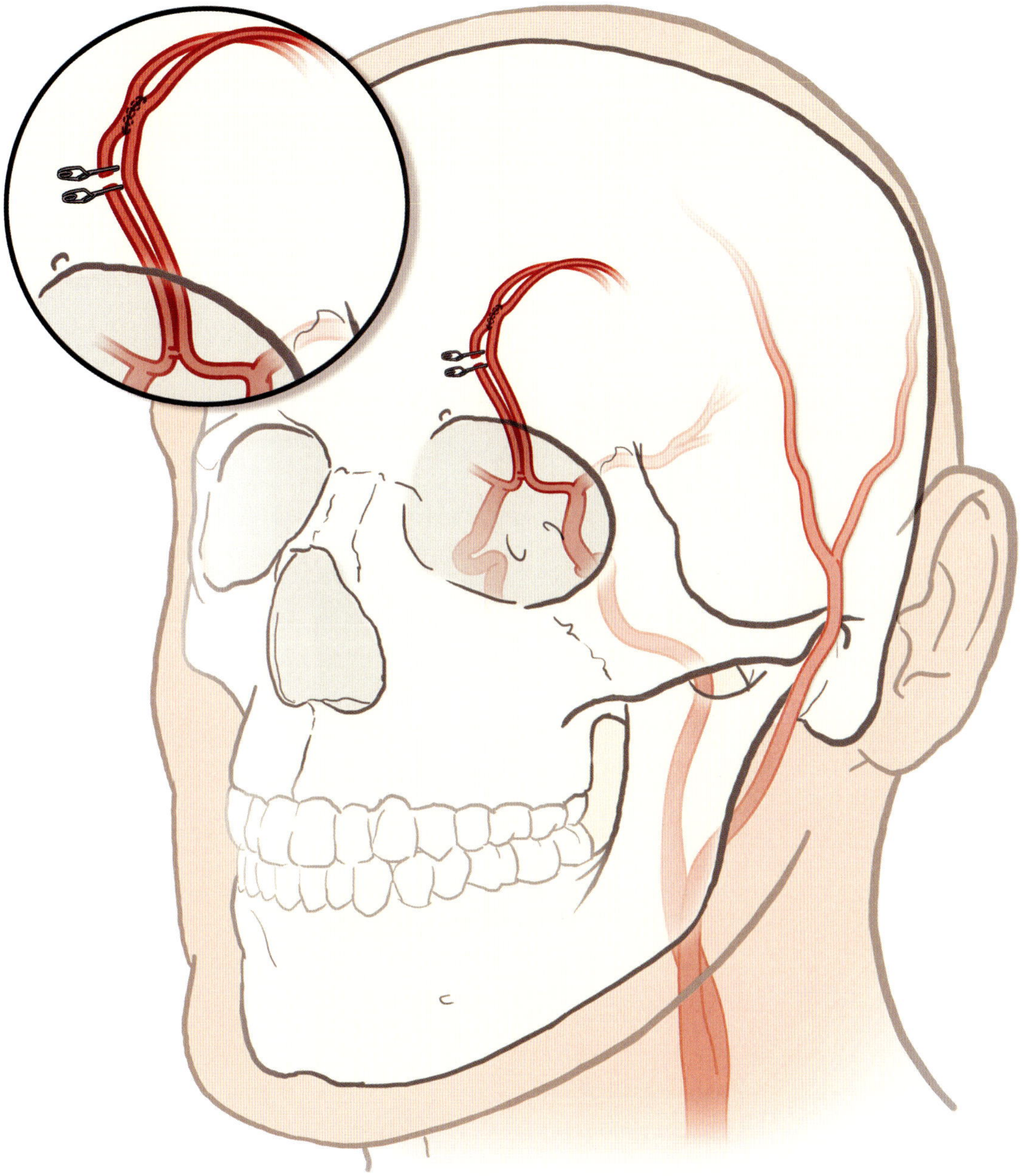

When an A2 segment of the ACA has to be sacrificed, as may be required for the treatment of a giant A2 aneurysm, the parallel anatomy of the distal A2 and A3 branches creates the opportunity to preserve blood flow in both ACA territories by forming a side-to-side bypass distal to the aneurysm in the A3 segment.

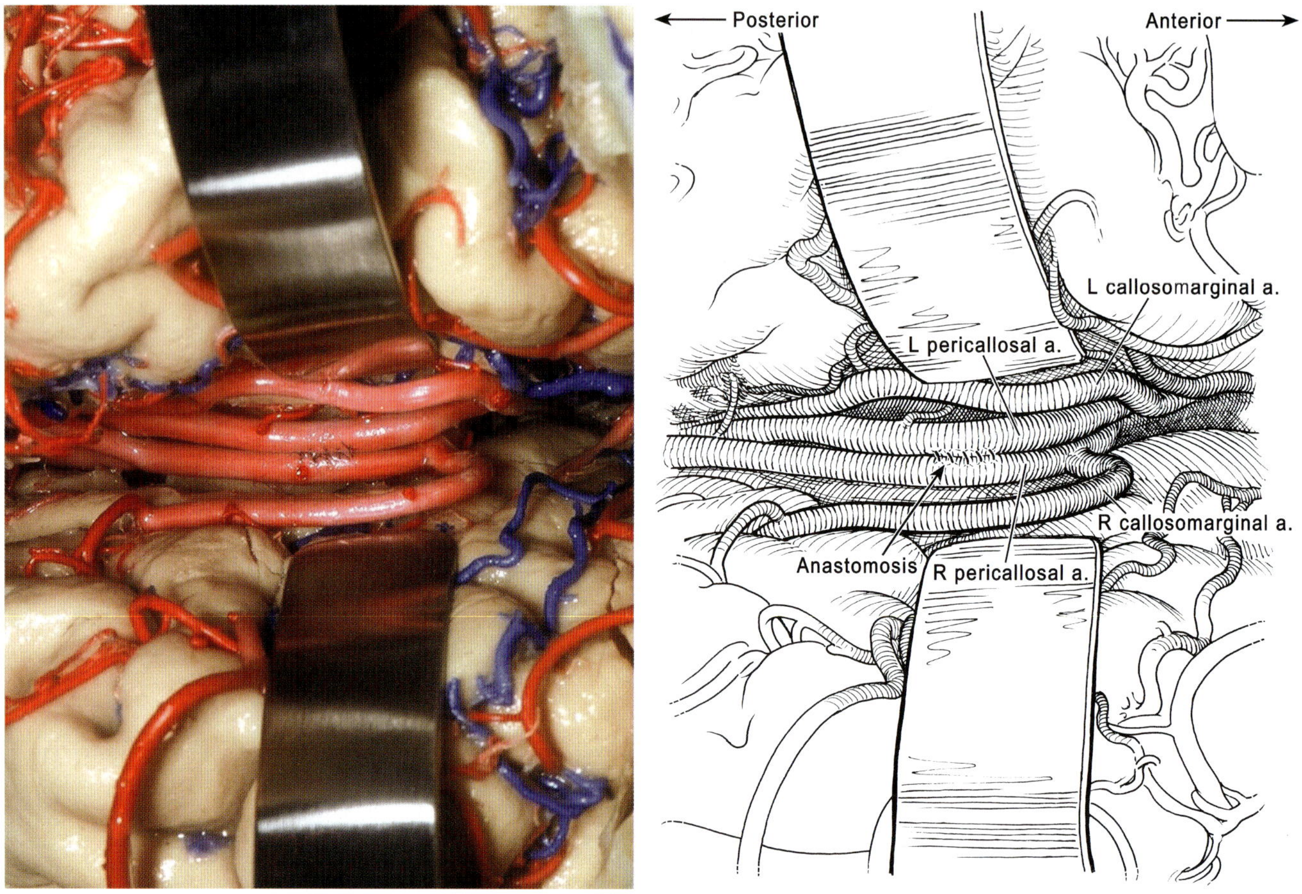

Fig. 1.0a In this anatomical specimen, the ACAs have been exposed in the interhemispheric fissure. A side-to-side anastomosis has been performed. (Photograph used with permission from *Journal of Neurosurgery*.)

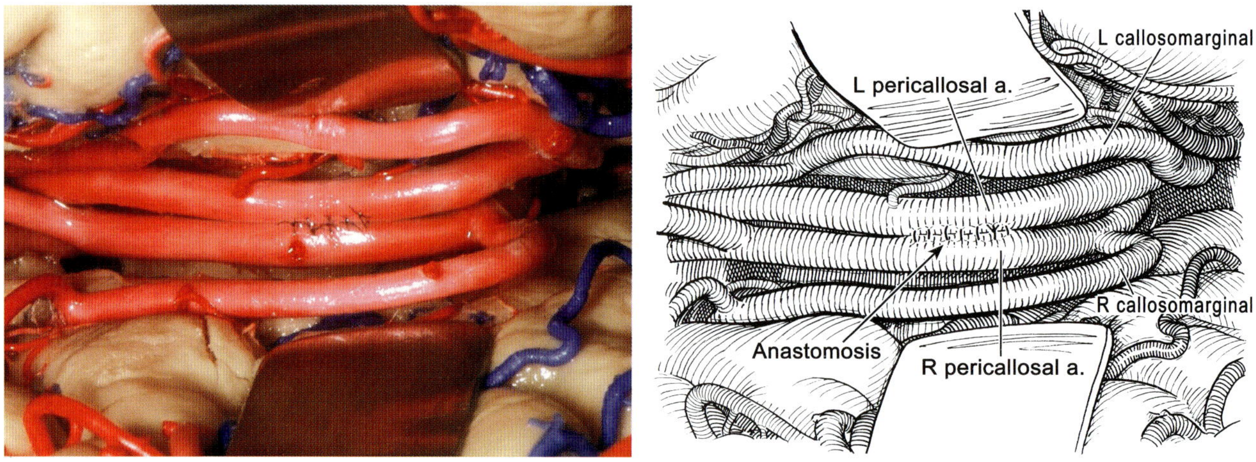

Fig. 1.0b A higher magnification view of the side-to-side ACA-to-ACA bypass. (Photograph used with permission from *Journal of Neurosurgery*.)

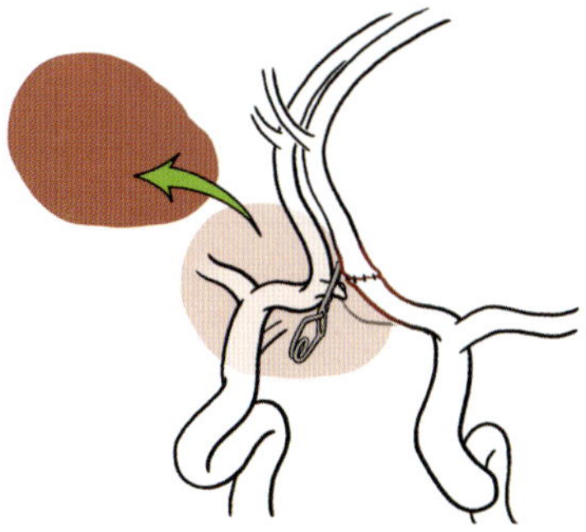

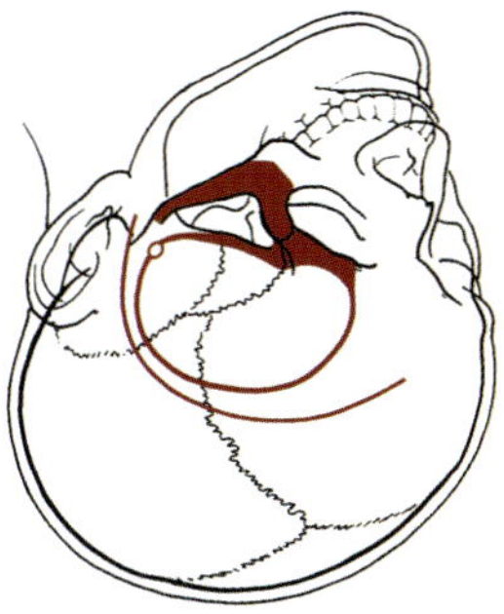

Case 1-1

Diagnosis: Recurrent giant ACA aneurysm after previous coiling

Bypass: Direct ACA-to-ACA

Approach: Left orbitozygomatic

Video

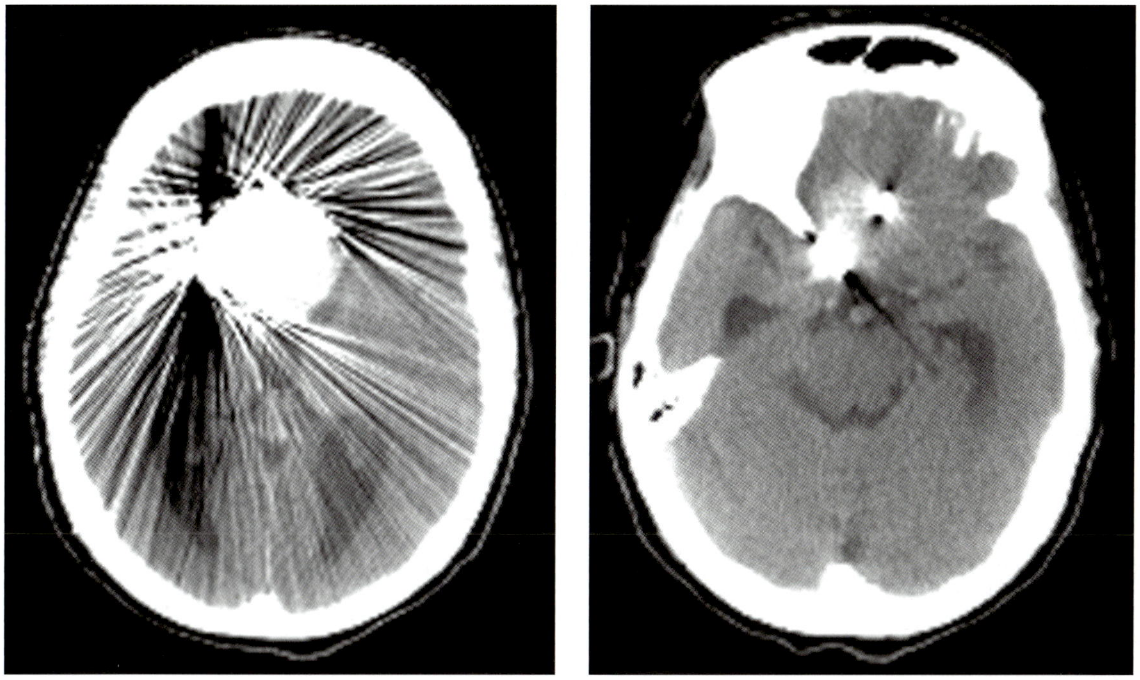

a b

Fig. 1.1a, b CT scans demonstrate coil artifact and large ventricles from cerebrospinal fluid outflow obstruction.

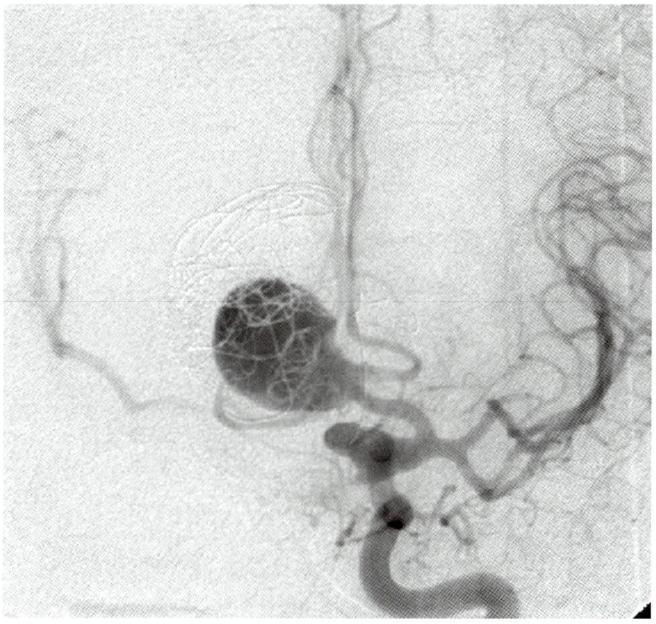

Fig. 1.1c Anteroposterior angiogram shows the left ICA, A1, and A2; the large mass of coils; and the recurrent aneurysm. Note the decreased filling of the right A2.

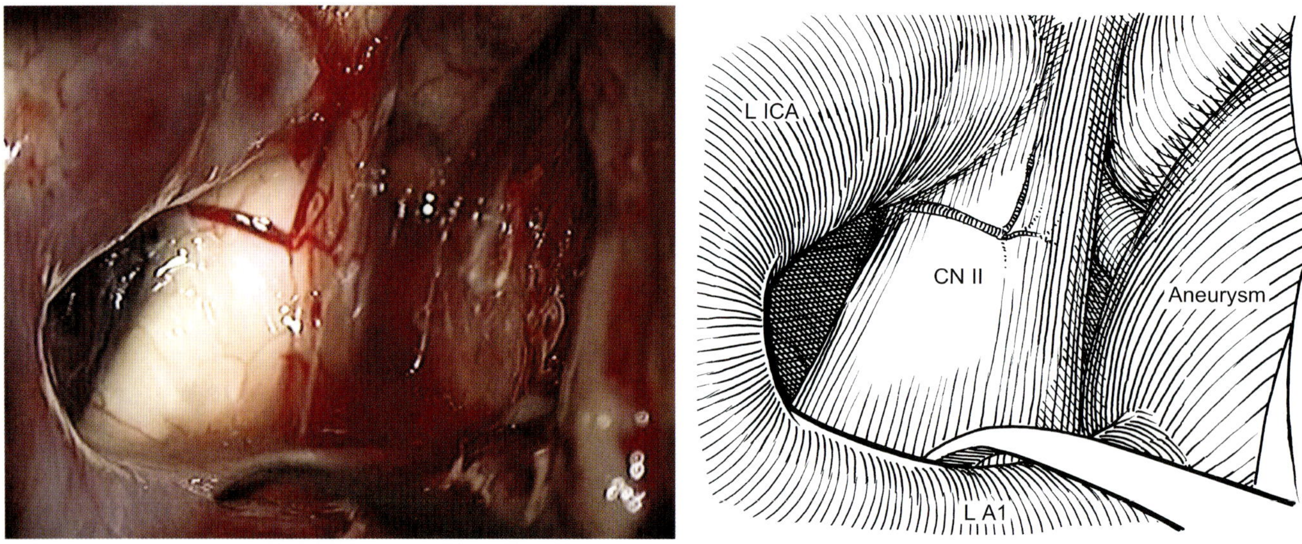

Fig. 1.1d The left ACA is exposed through a left orbitozygomatic approach.

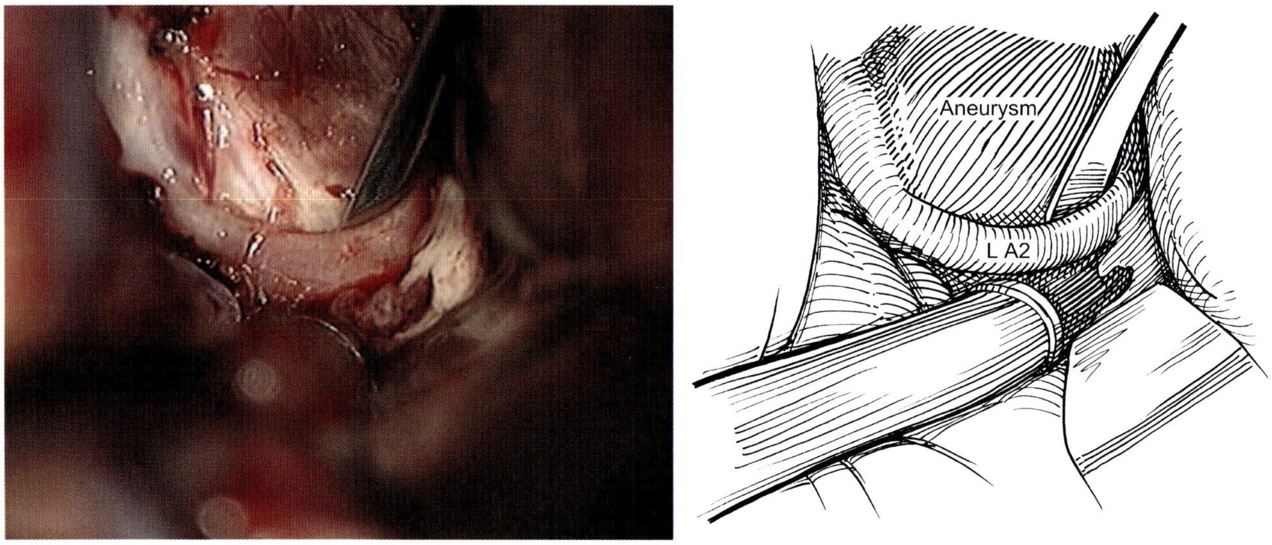

Fig. 1.1e The left A2 is mobilized.

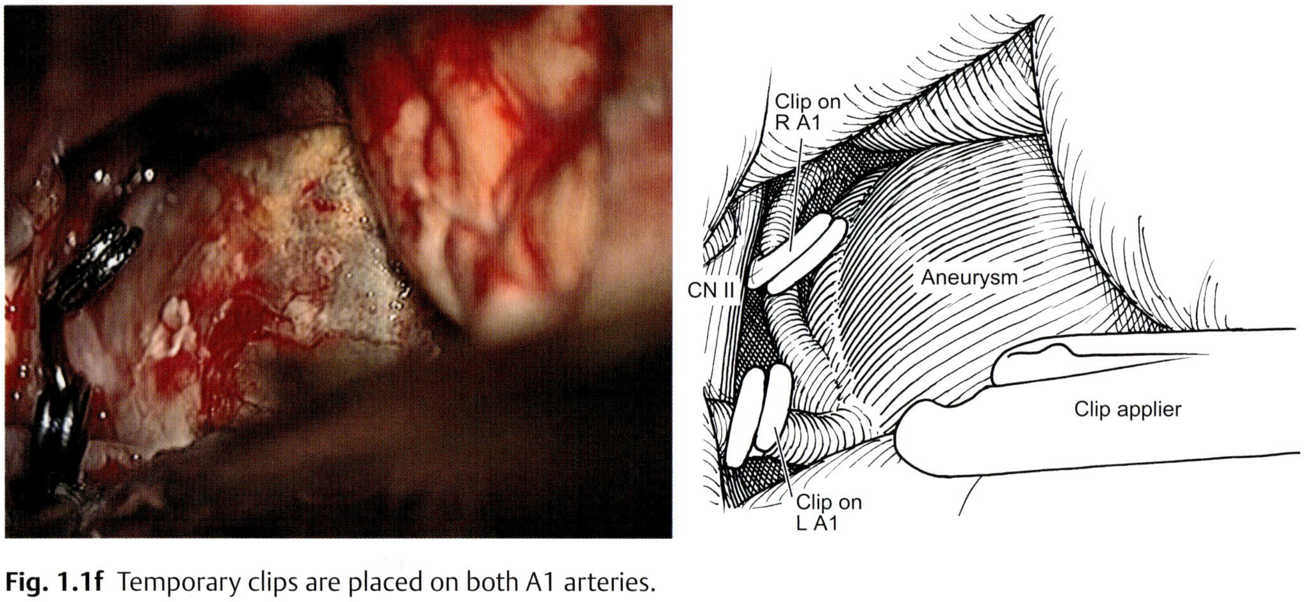

Fig. 1.1f Temporary clips are placed on both A1 arteries.

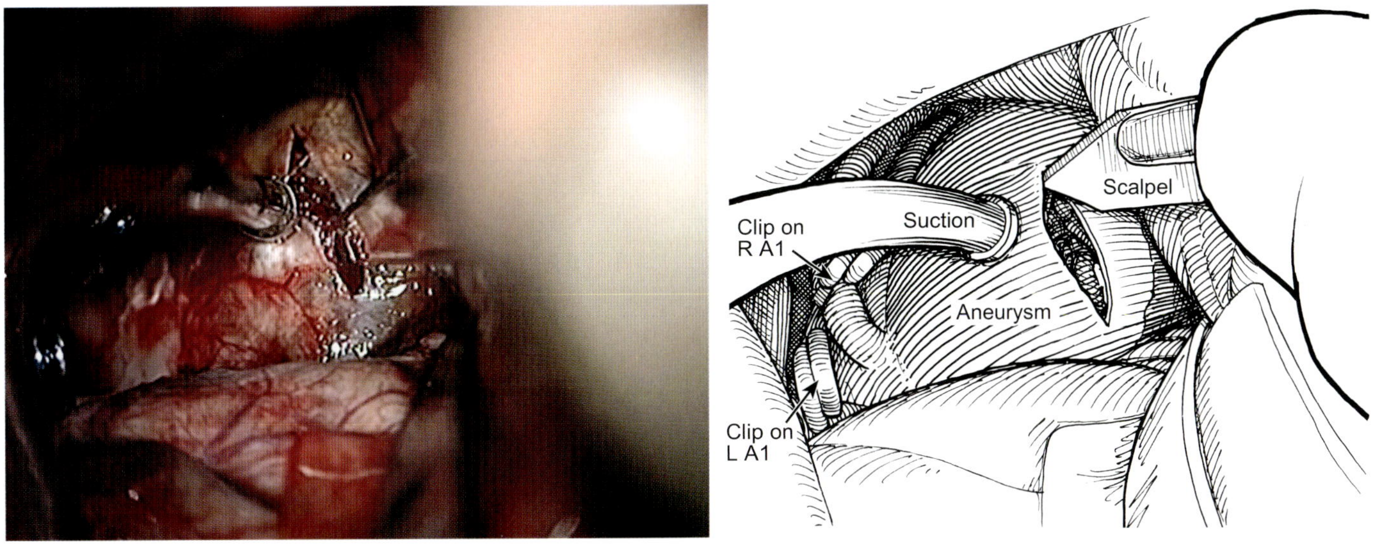

Fig. 1.1g The dome of the aneurysm is incised a distance away from the neck.

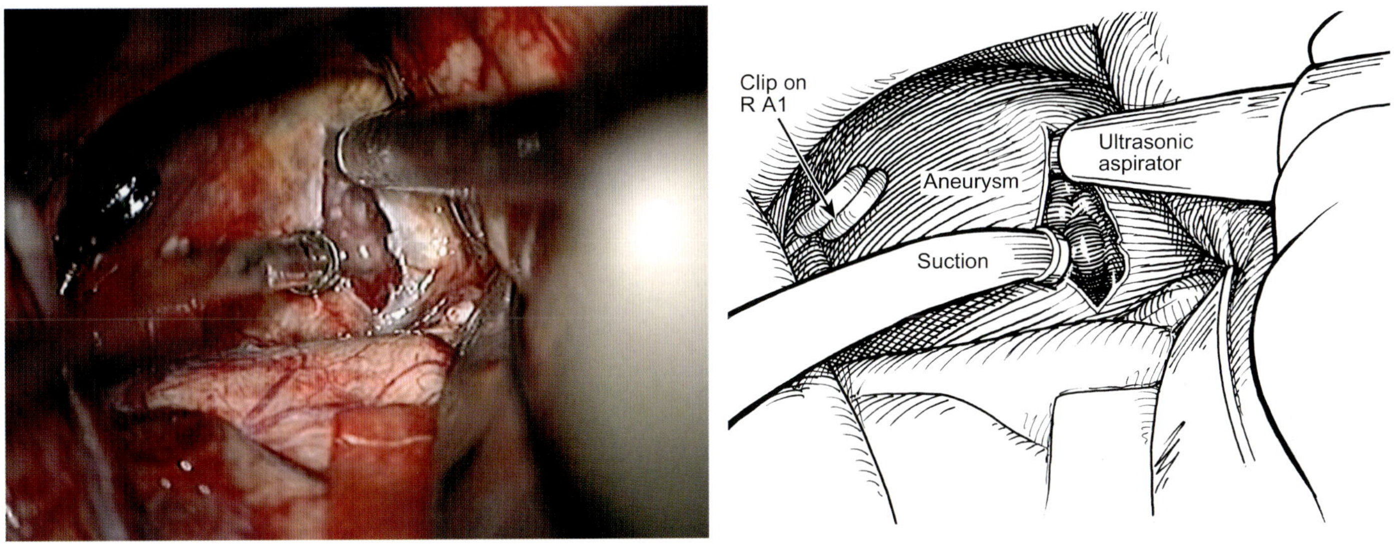

Fig. 1.1h An ultrasonic aspirator is used to remove thrombosis.

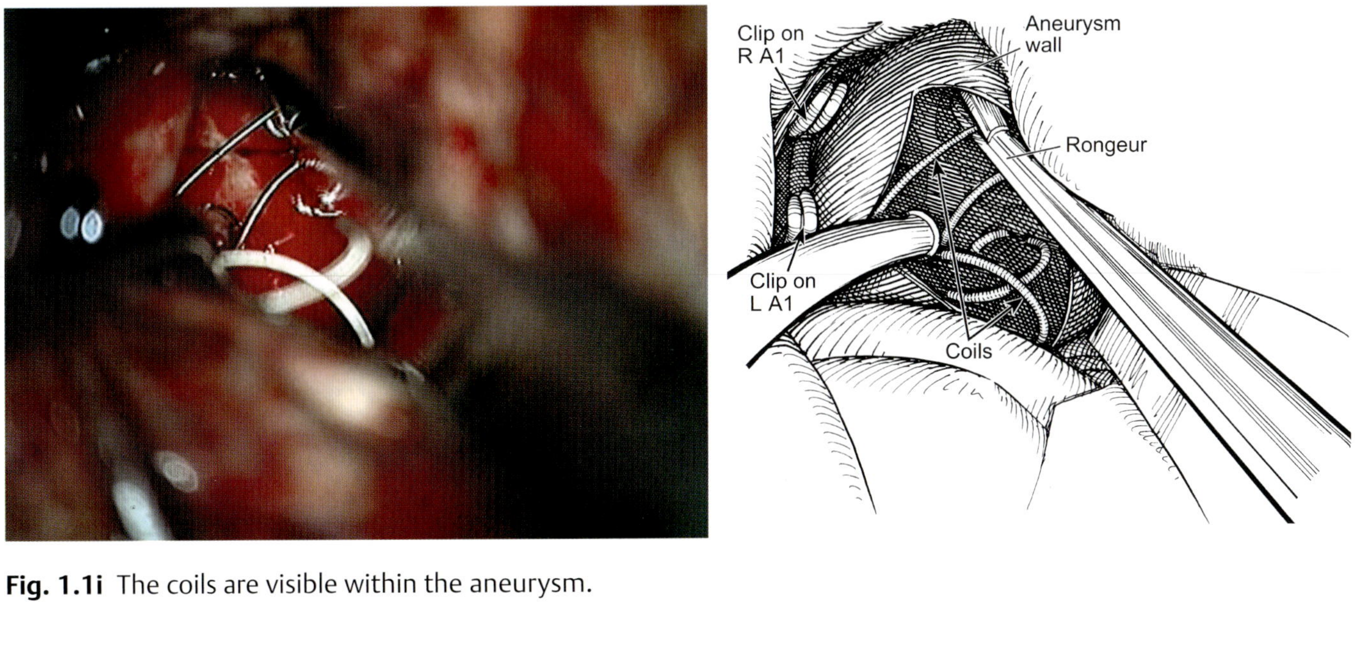

Fig. 1.1i The coils are visible within the aneurysm.

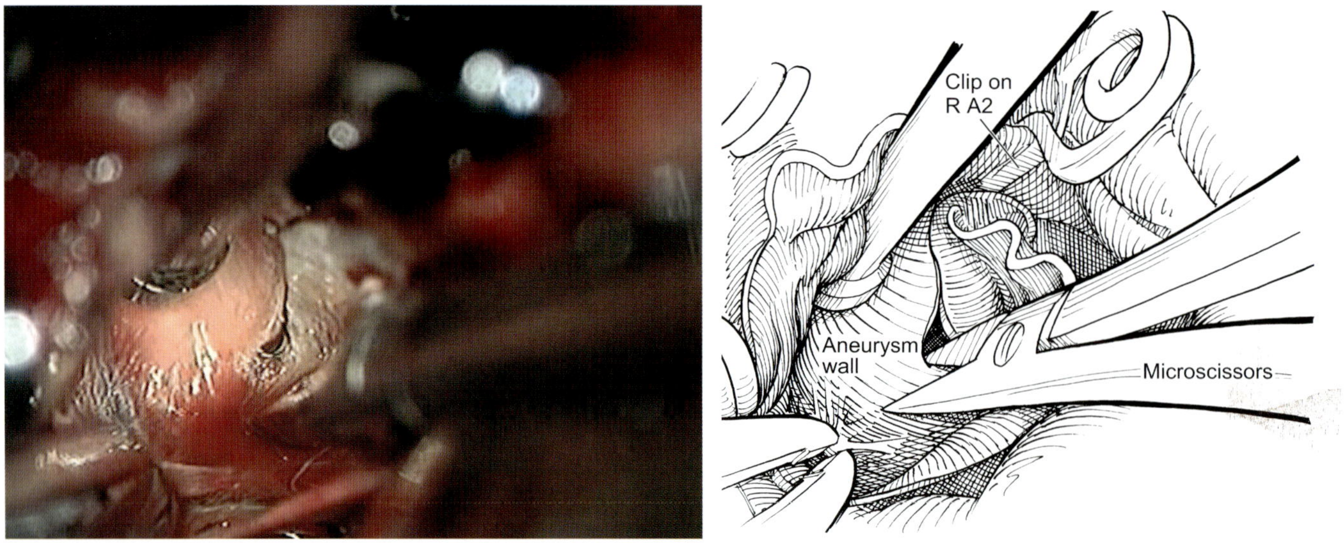

Fig. 1.1j The A2 arteries are exposed.

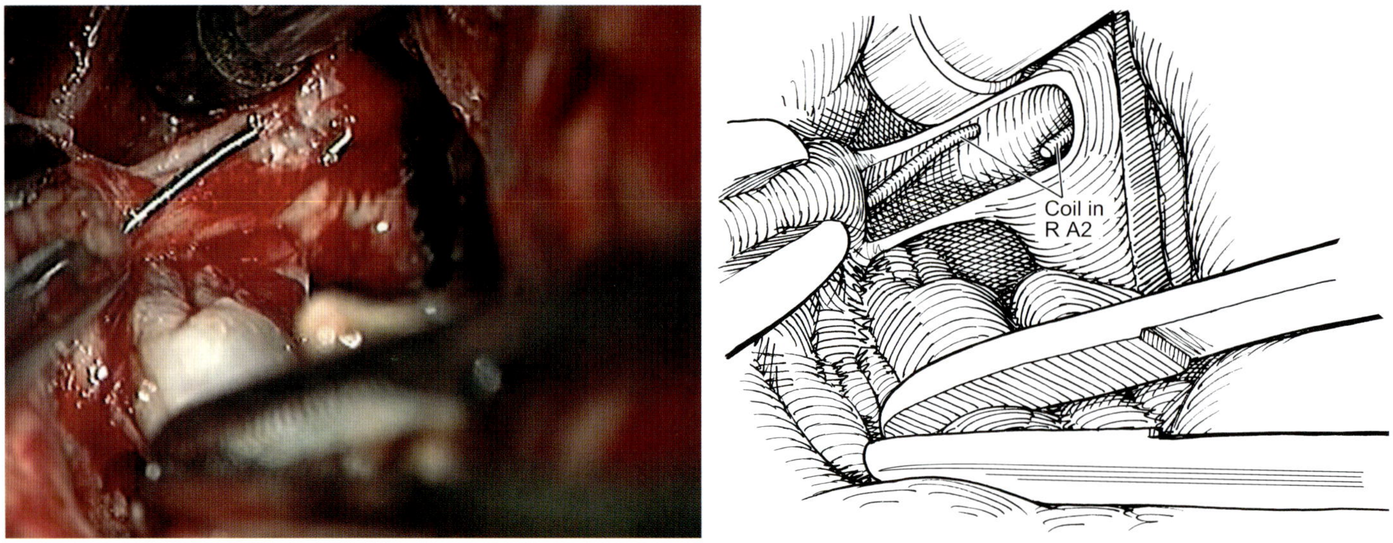

Fig. 1.1k A coil is discovered in the right A2.

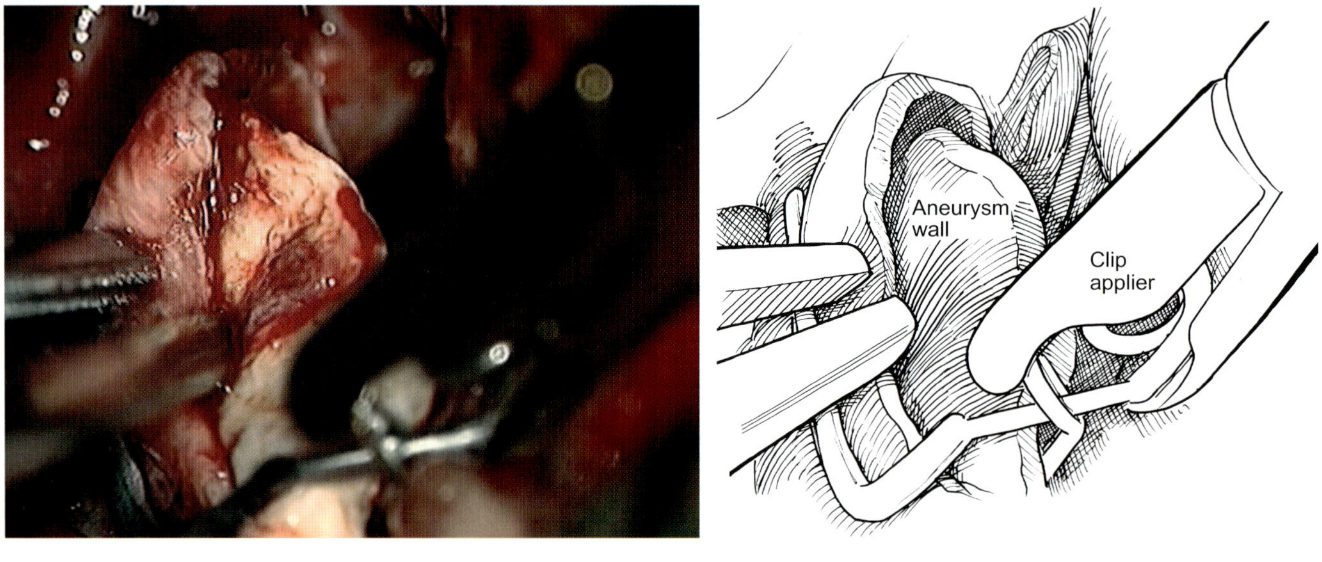

Fig. 1.1l The aneurysm is clipped.

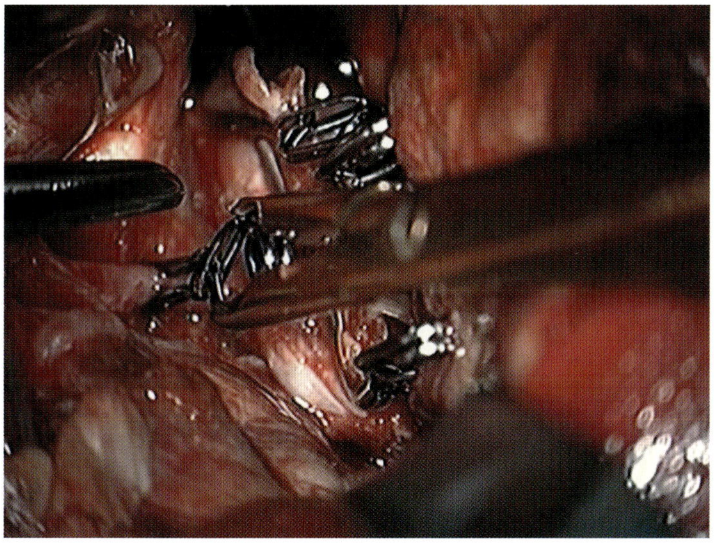

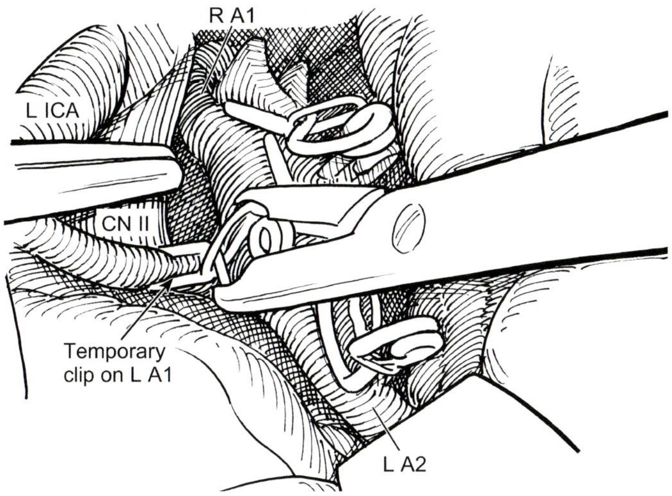

Fig. 1.1m The temporary clips are removed.

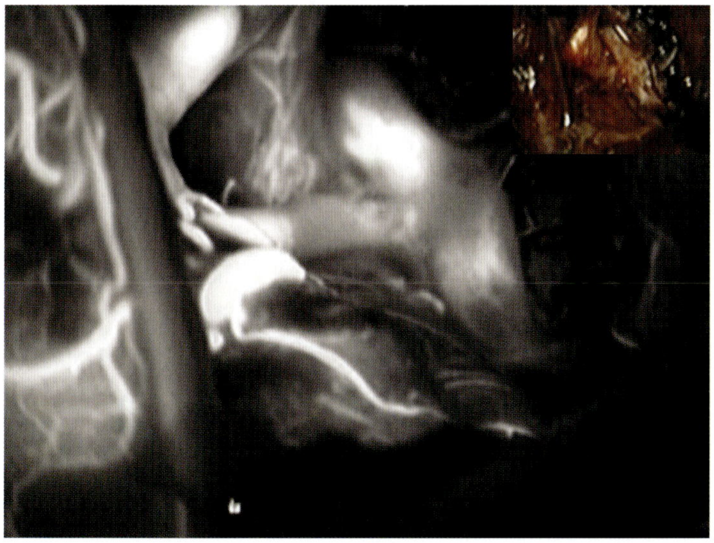

Fig. 1.1n Intraoperative ICG angiogram demonstrates obstruction of both A2 arteries.

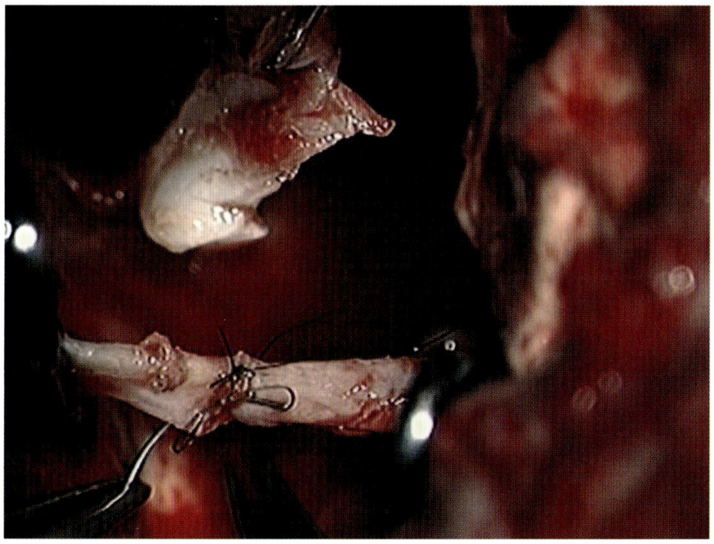

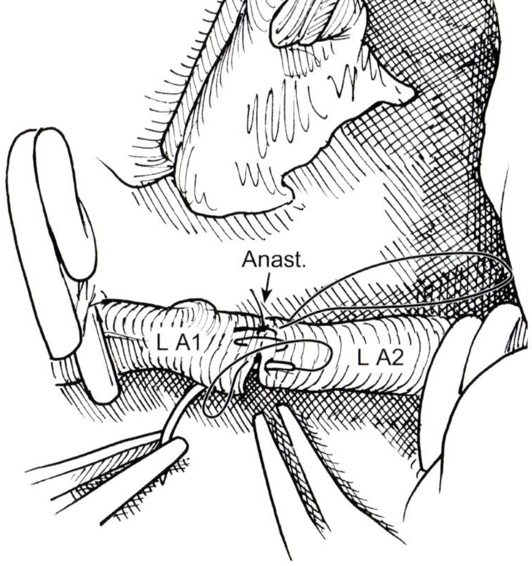

Fig. 1.1o A direct anastomosis between the left A1 and A2 is performed.

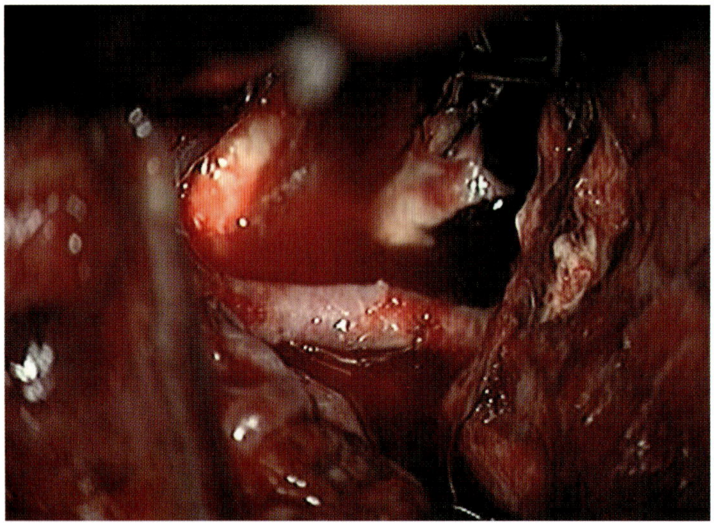

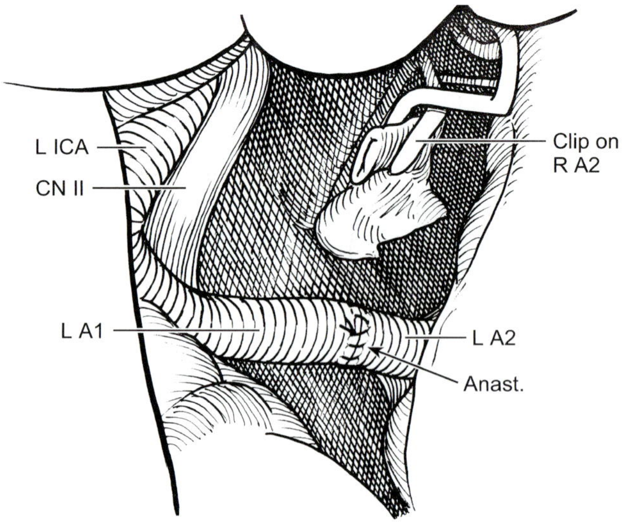

Fig. 1.1p The anastomosis of A1 to A2 is completed.

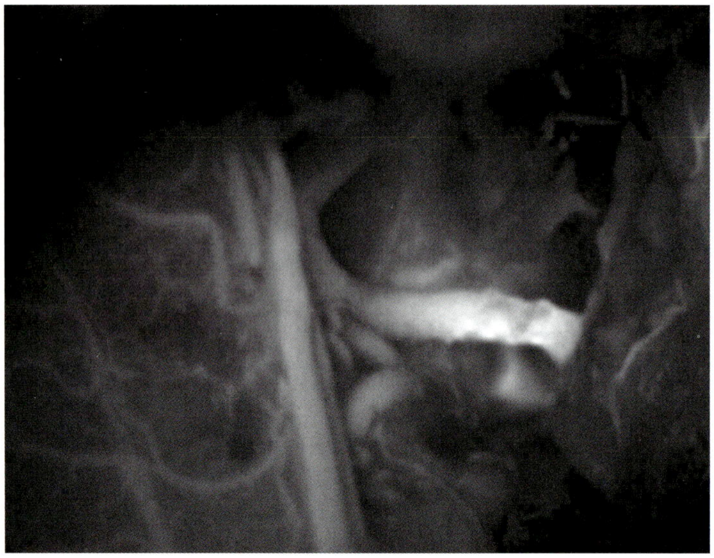

Fig. 1.1q An ICG angiogram demonstrates patency of the anastomosis.

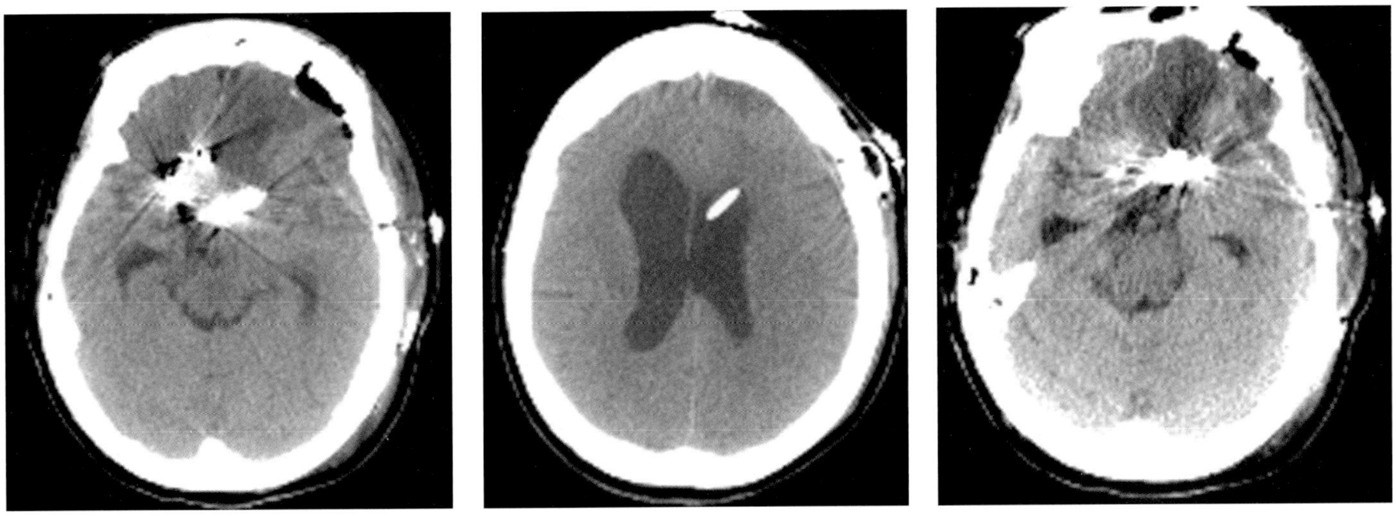

Fig. 1.1r Axial CT scans show the postoperative result.

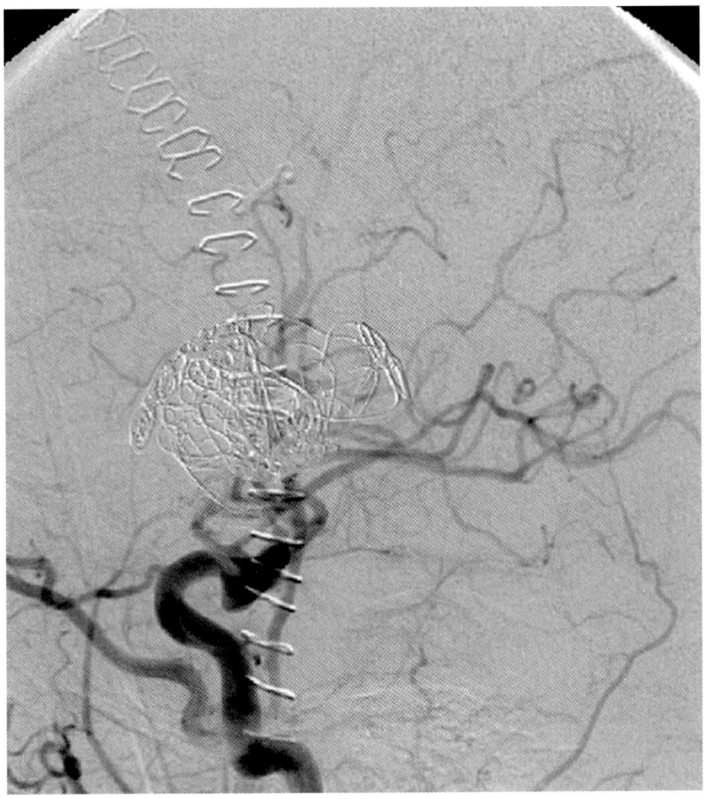

Fig. 1.1s Postoperative angiography shows good patency. This patient had no ischemic event and made an excellent recovery.

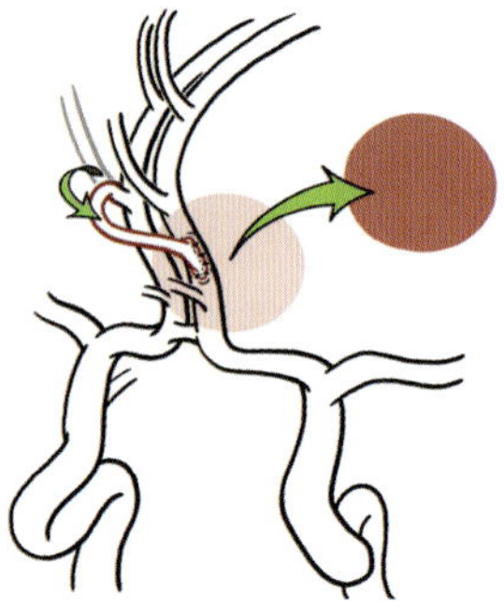

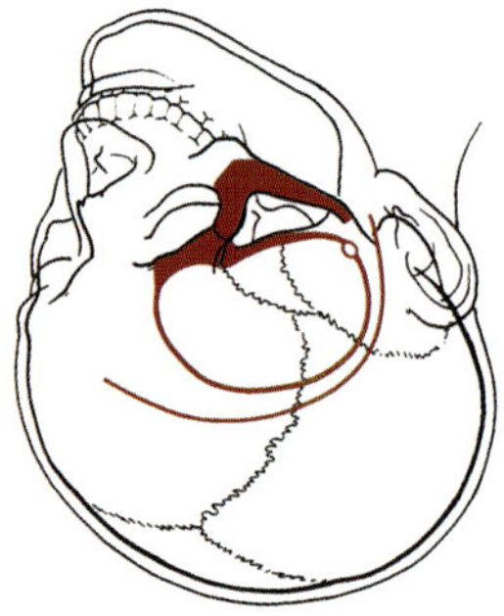

Case 1-2

Diagnosis: Complex dissecting aneurysm of the left A2

Bypass: Right frontopolar artery–to–left A2

Approach: Right orbitozygomatic

▶ Video

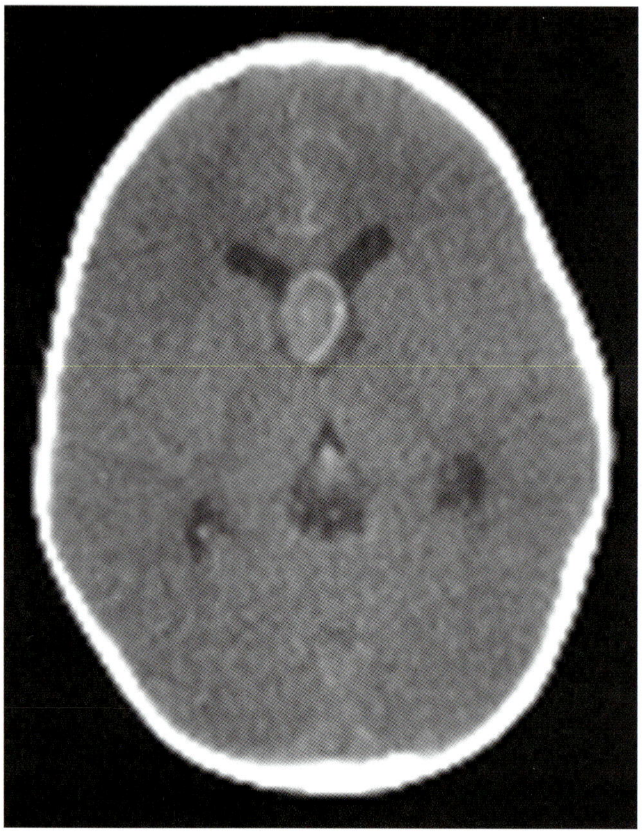

Fig. 1.2a CT scan of an 18-month-old child with lethargy shows diffuse SAH and a clot in the region of the third ventricle.

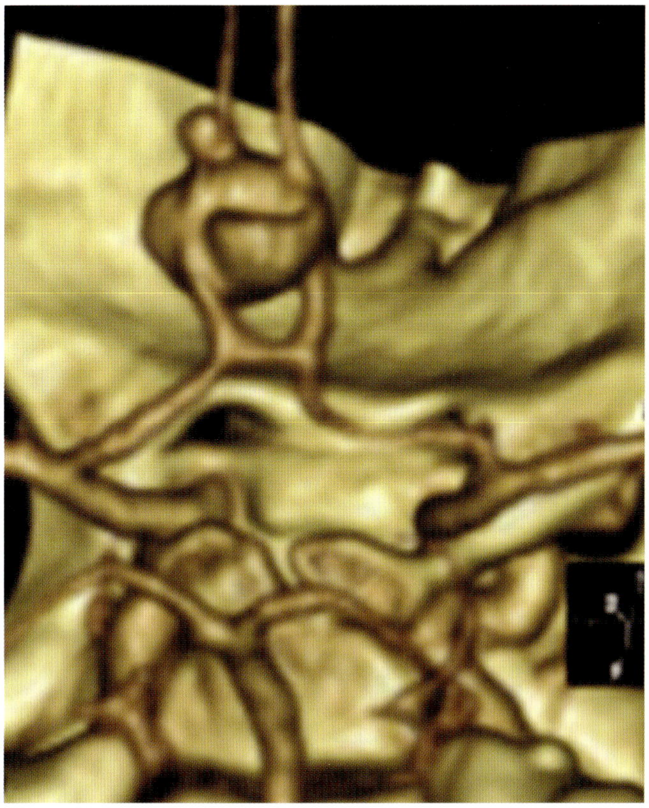

Fig. 1.2b Three-dimensional angiographic reconstruction shows a complex dissecting aneurysm arising from the A2 segment a few millimeters beyond ACoA.

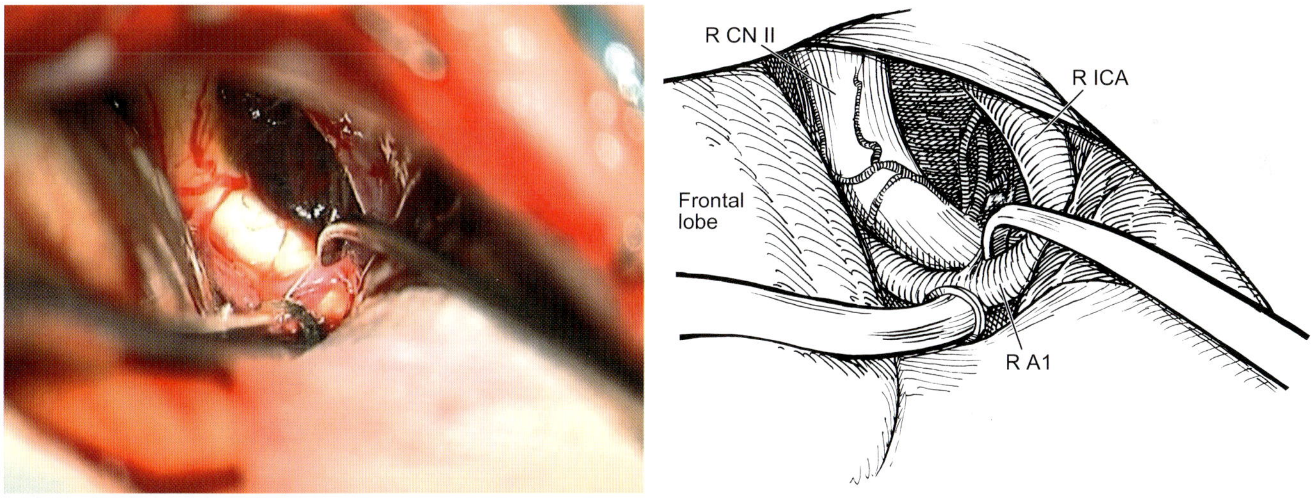

Fig. 1.2c Through a right orbitozygomatic approach, the CN II, the ACA, and the ICA are visible.

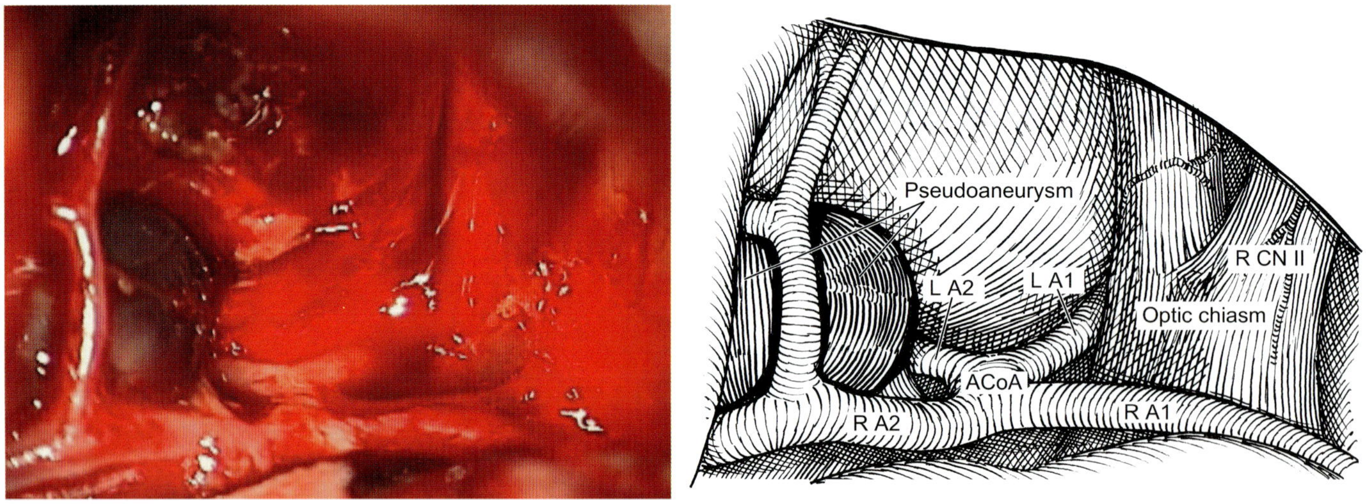

Fig. 1.2d The pseudoaneurysm is visible from the left A2 segment above the ACoA with surrounding hematoma.

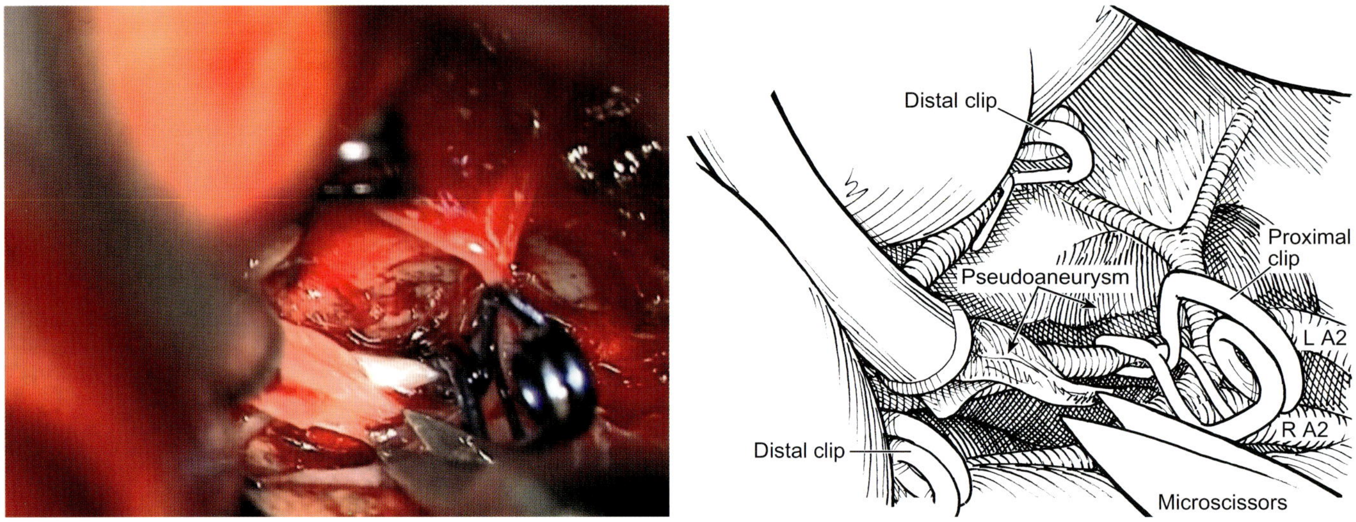

Fig. 1.2e The pseudoaneurysm is opened and temporary clips have been applied to the proximal and distal portions of the left A2, trapping the aneurysm.

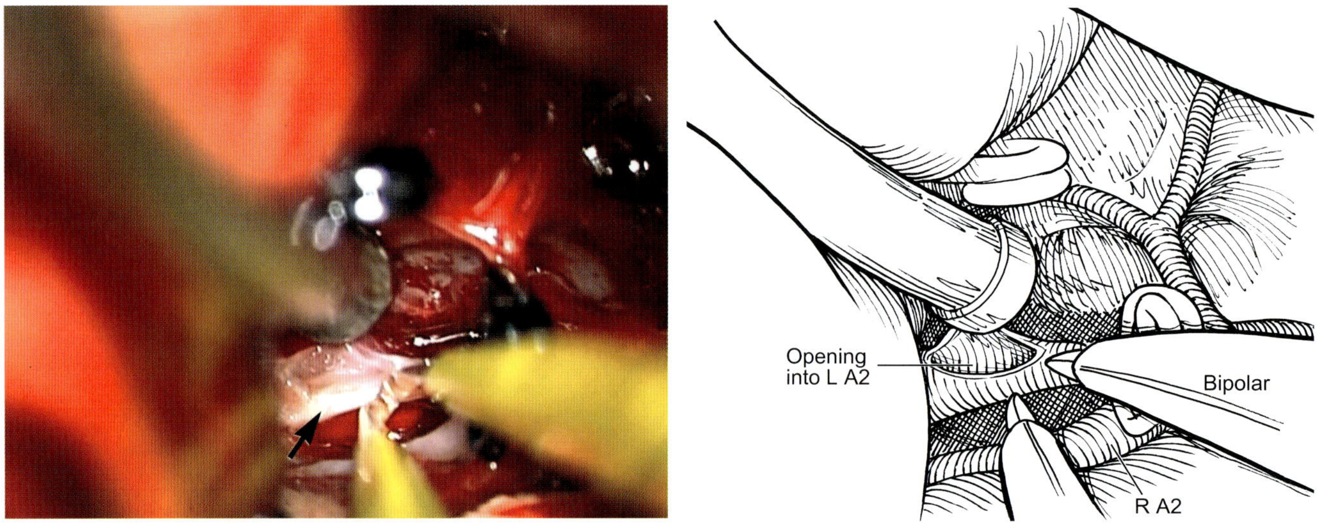

Fig. 1.2f The pseudoaneurysm is resected. The opening into the left A2 (*arrow*) is visible.

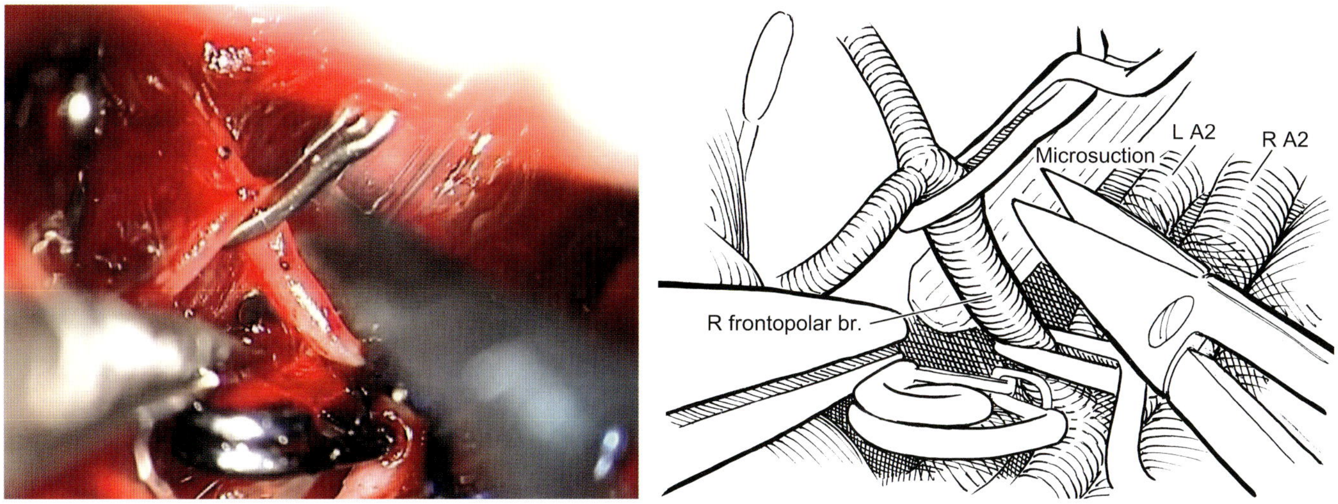

Fig. 1.2g The right frontopolar branch is clipped in preparation for the bypass.

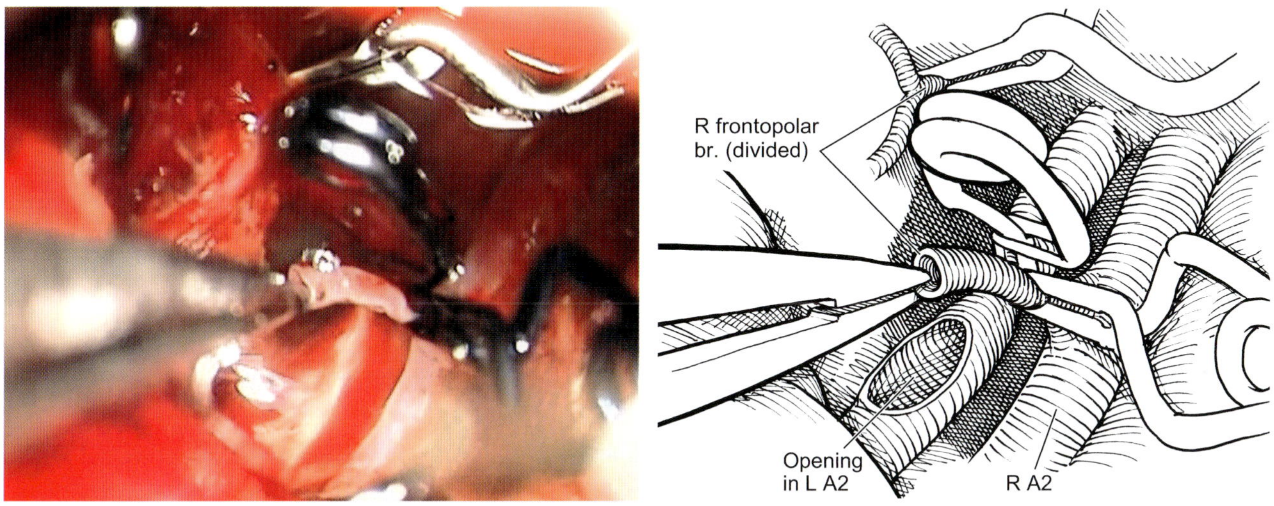

Fig. 1.2h The right frontopolar branch is divided, positioned near the left A2 defect, and fishmouthed.

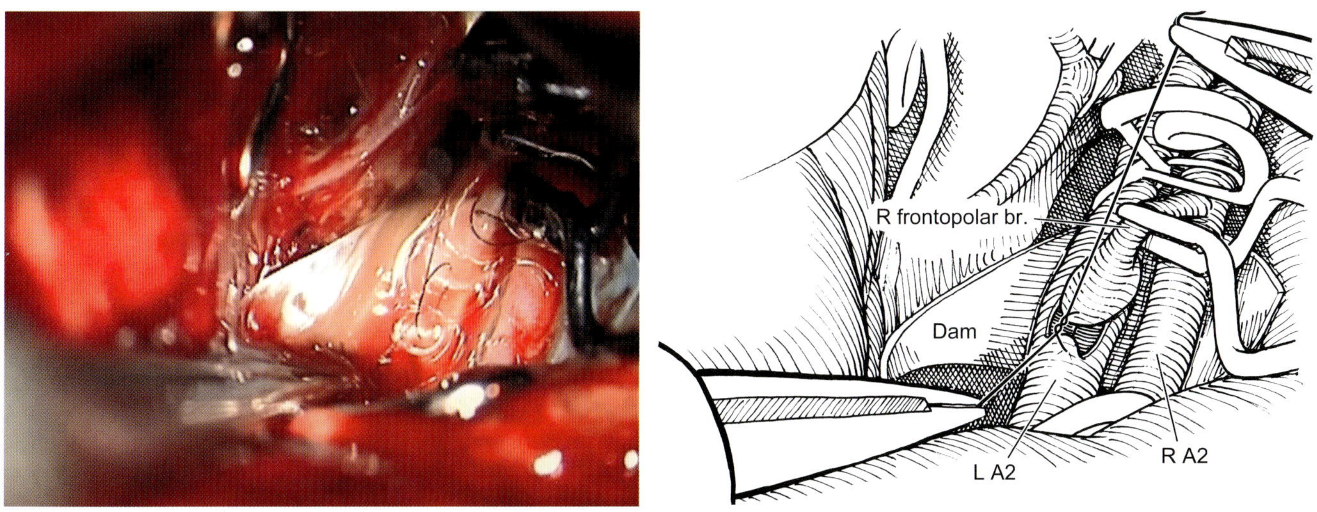

Fig. 1.2i The frontopolar branch is used to close the opening that produced the pseudoaneurysm and to provide another avenue of anastomotic blood flow to the left A2.

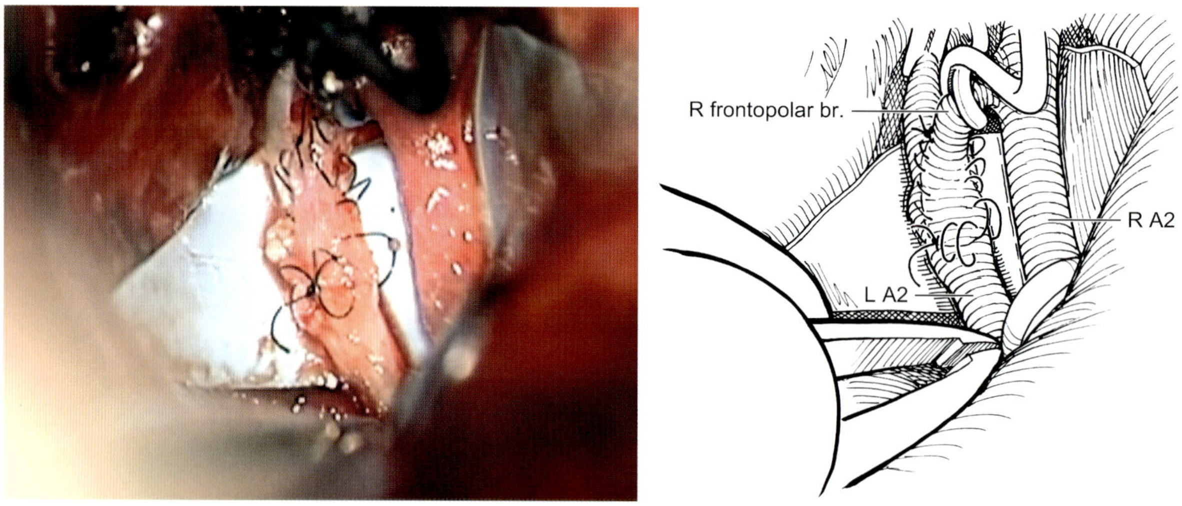

Fig. 1.2j The bypass is completed and the 11-0 sutures are tightened.

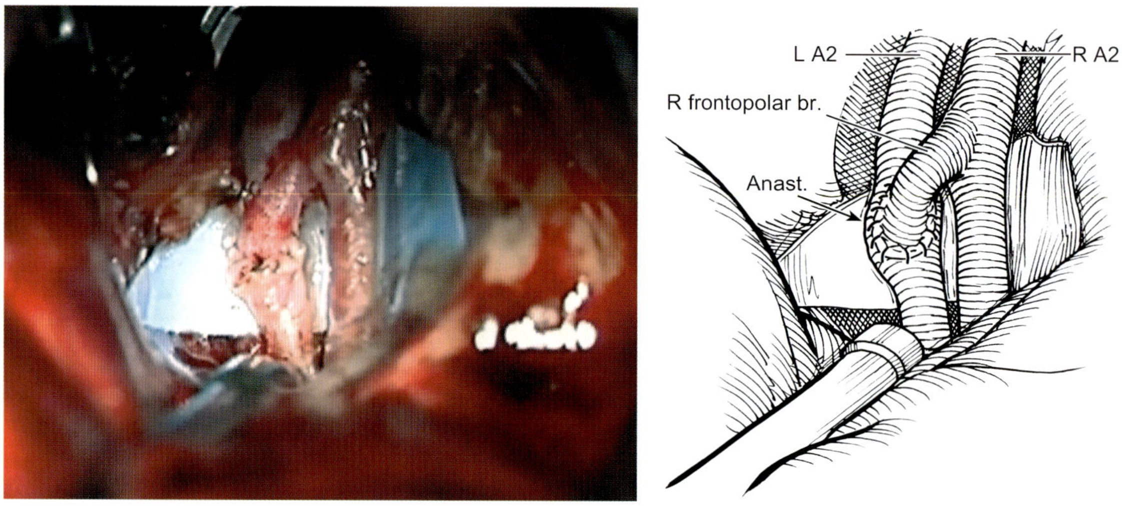

Fig. 1.2k The bypass is completed.

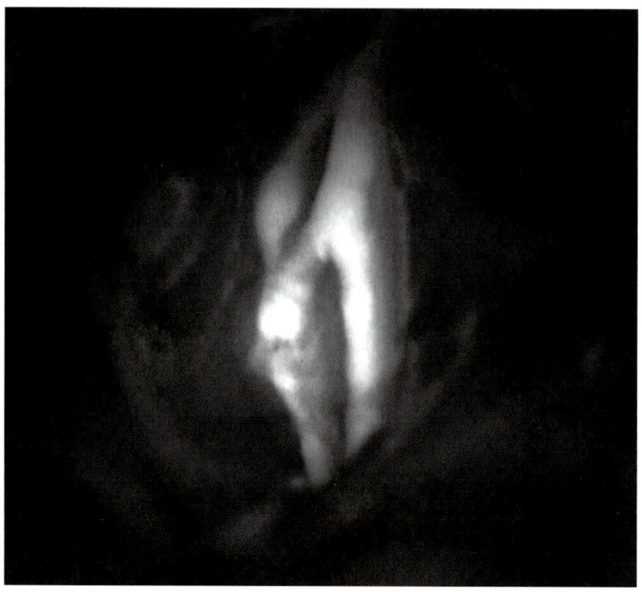

Fig. 1.2l ICG angiogram confirms good filling of both A2 arteries and patency of the frontopolar bypass.

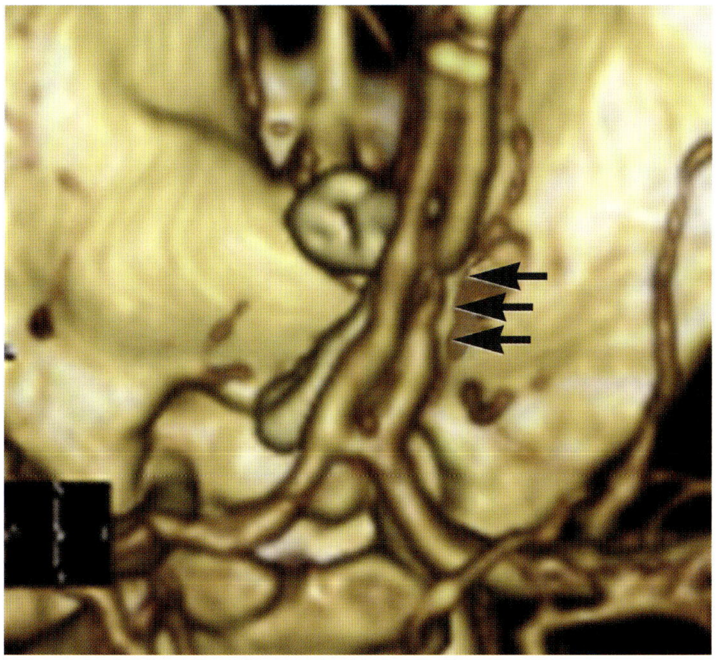

Fig. 1.2m Postoperative three-dimensional CT angiogram confirms patency of the direct anastomosis (*arrows*).

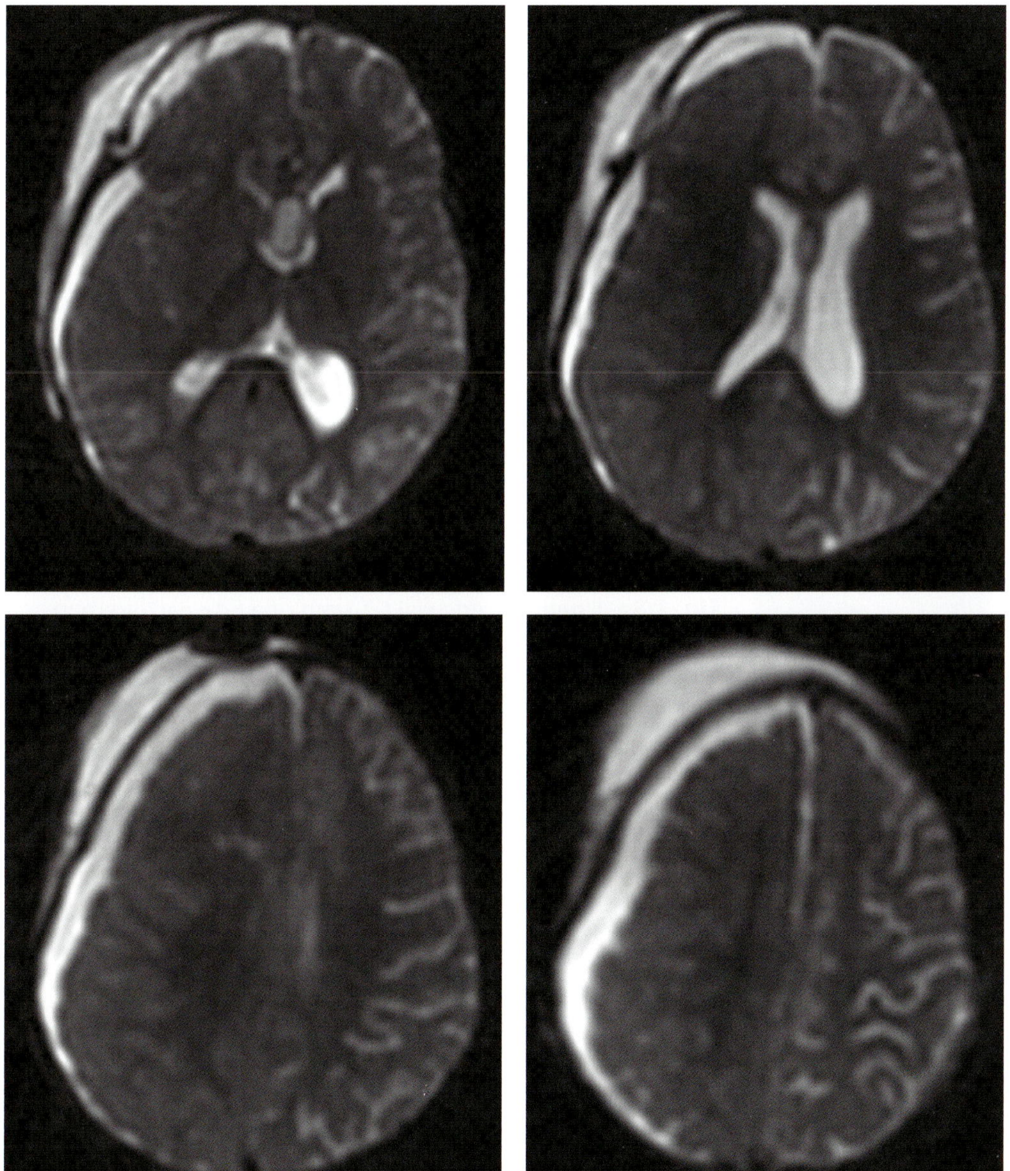

Fig. 1.2n Postoperative MR images show no ischemic region. The patient was normal at 3 years old.

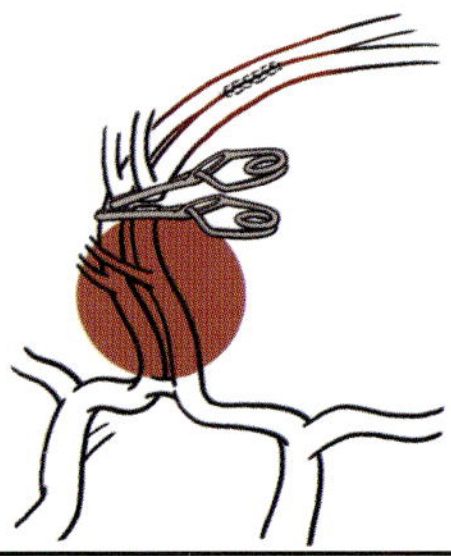

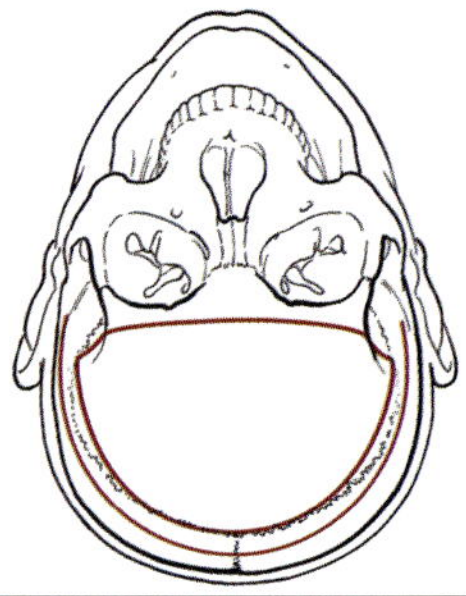

Case 1-3

Diagnosis: Left A2 giant aneurysm

Bypass: A3-to-A3

Approach: Bifrontal hemispheric with trapping of aneurysm and side-to-side anastomosis of pericallosal arteries

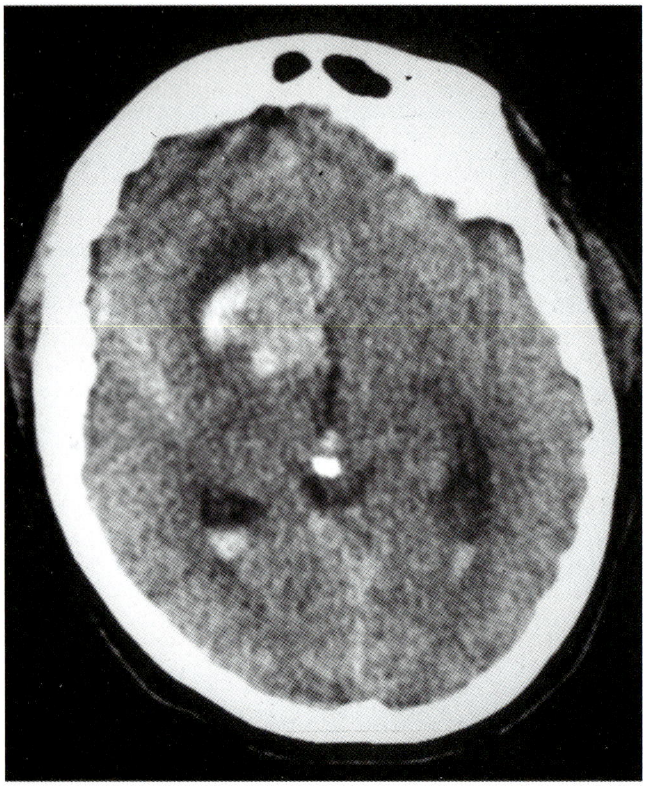

Fig. 1.3a Unenhanced axial CT scan of a 64-year-old man with thromboembolic symptoms shows a hyperdense interhemispheric mass with intraventricular hemorrhage in the occipital horns.

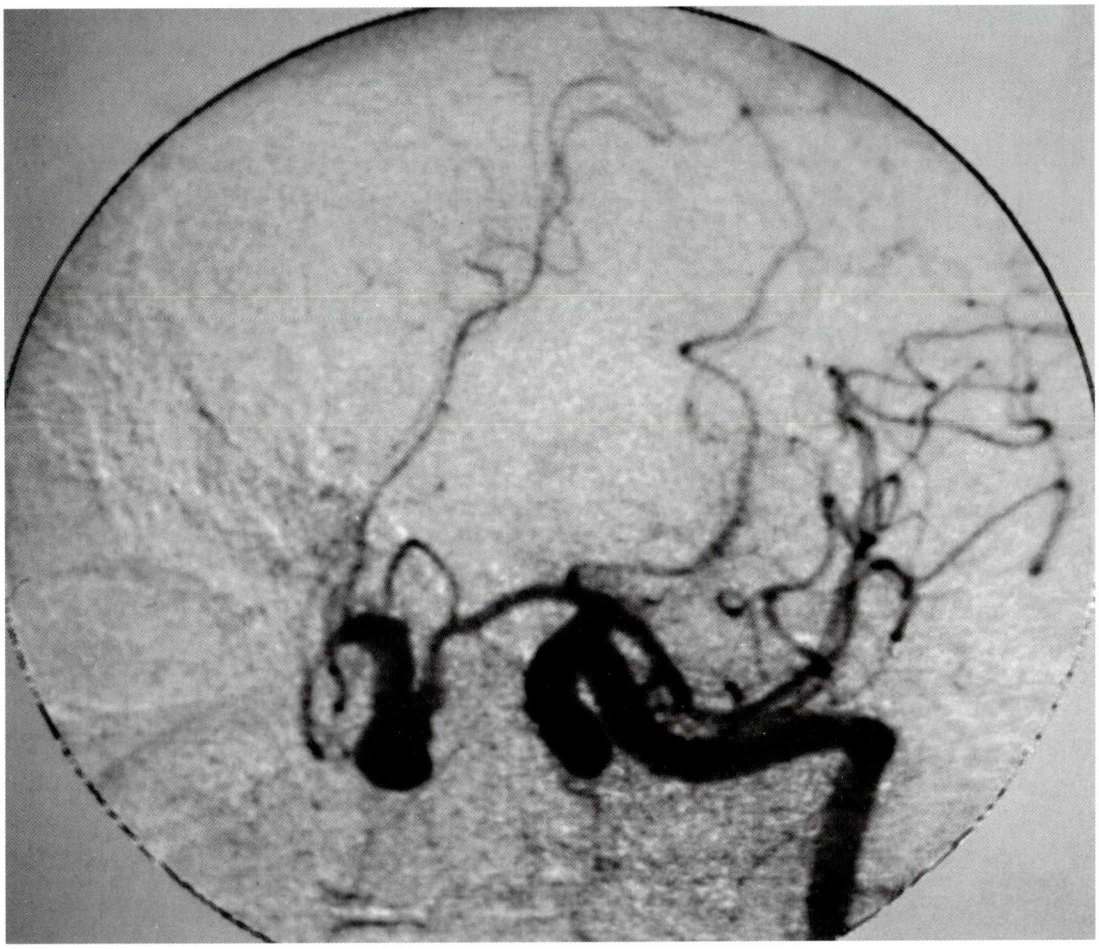

Fig. 1.3b Anteroposterior angiogram shows a complex serpiginous channel traversing the aneurysm, implying that most of the aneurysm is thrombosed. These aneurysms are not amenable to direct reconstruction.

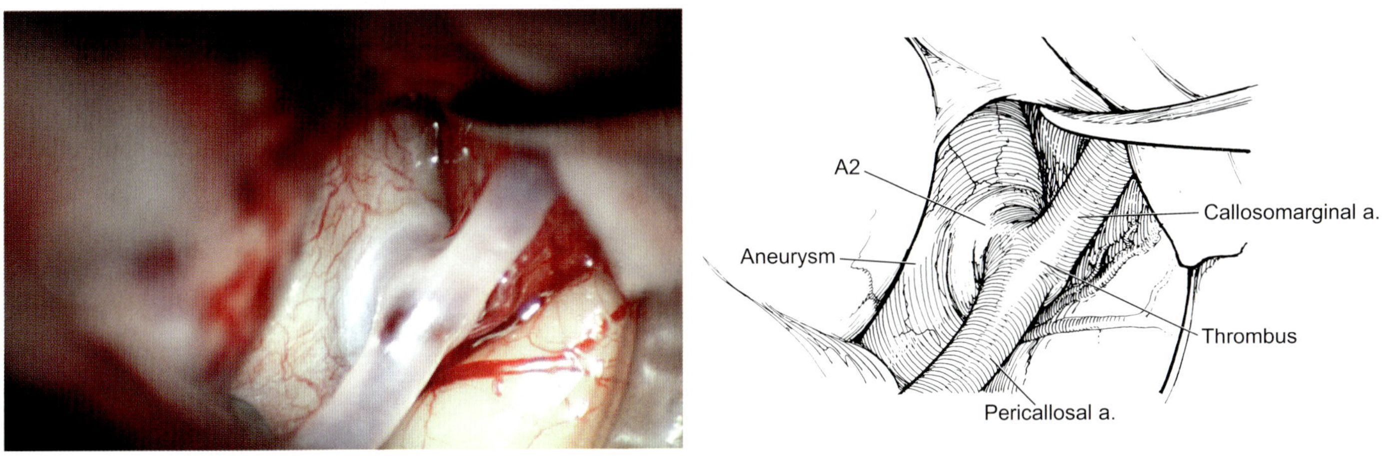

Fig. 1.3c The distal segment of A2 is visible as it emerges from the aneurysm and divides into pericallosal and callosomarginal branches. Thrombus can be seen within the lumen of the artery.

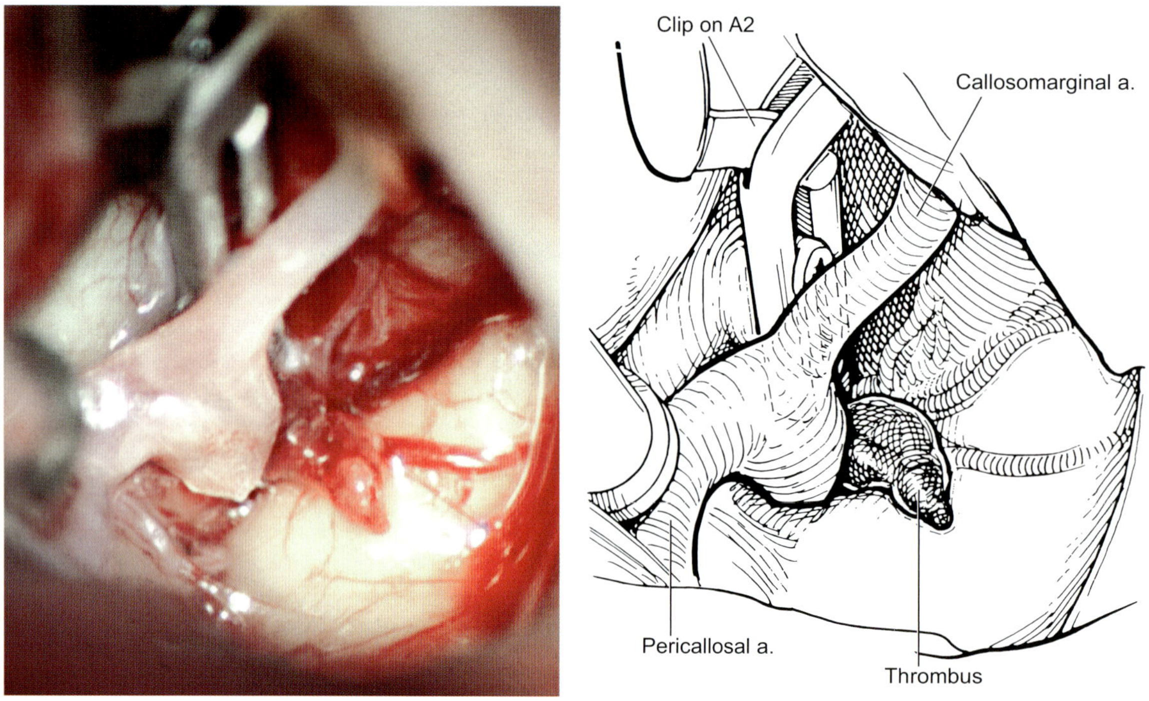

Fig. 1.3d A clip applied on the distal A2 stops flow through the aneurysm. A2 is divided and the extruding thrombus is visible.

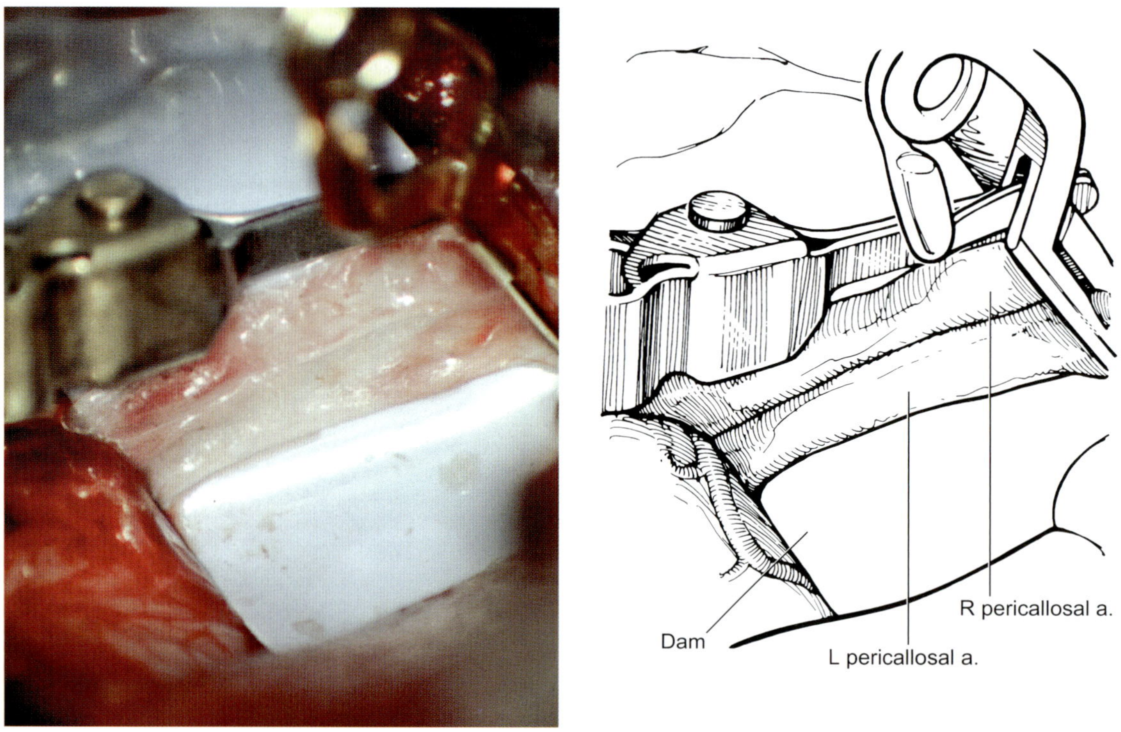

Fig. 1.3e The two pericallosal arteries are placed side by side over a dam and temporarily occluded while barbiturates are administered to the patient.

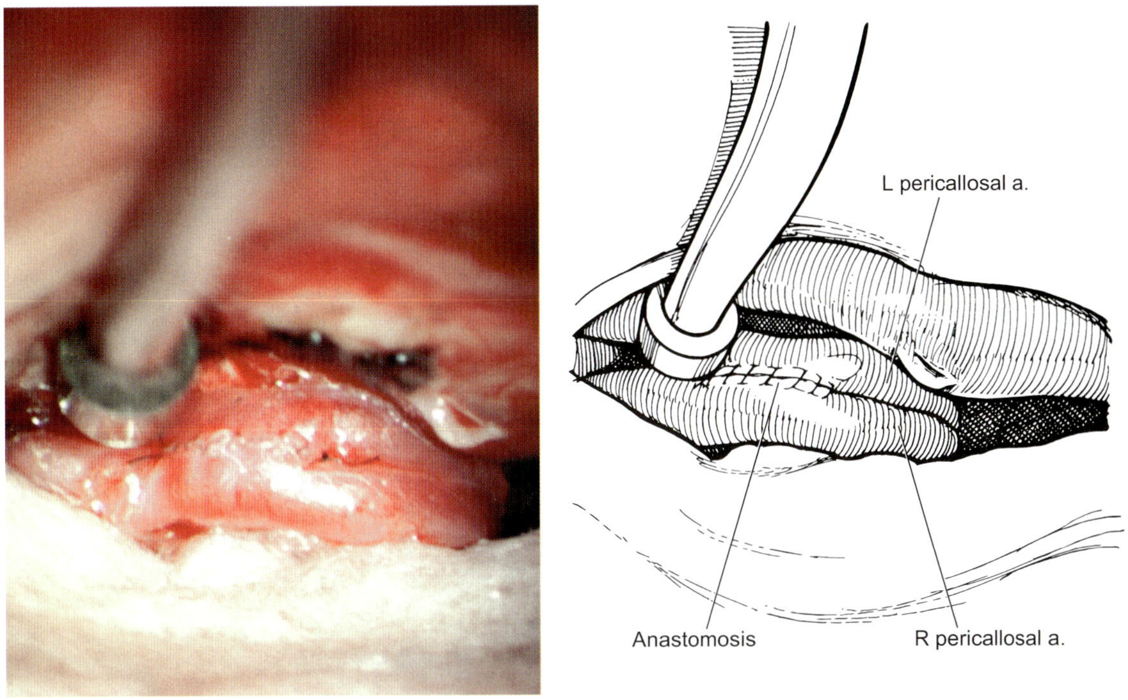

Fig. 1.3f A side-to-side A3-to-A3 anastomosis is completed interhemispherically distal to the aneurysm.

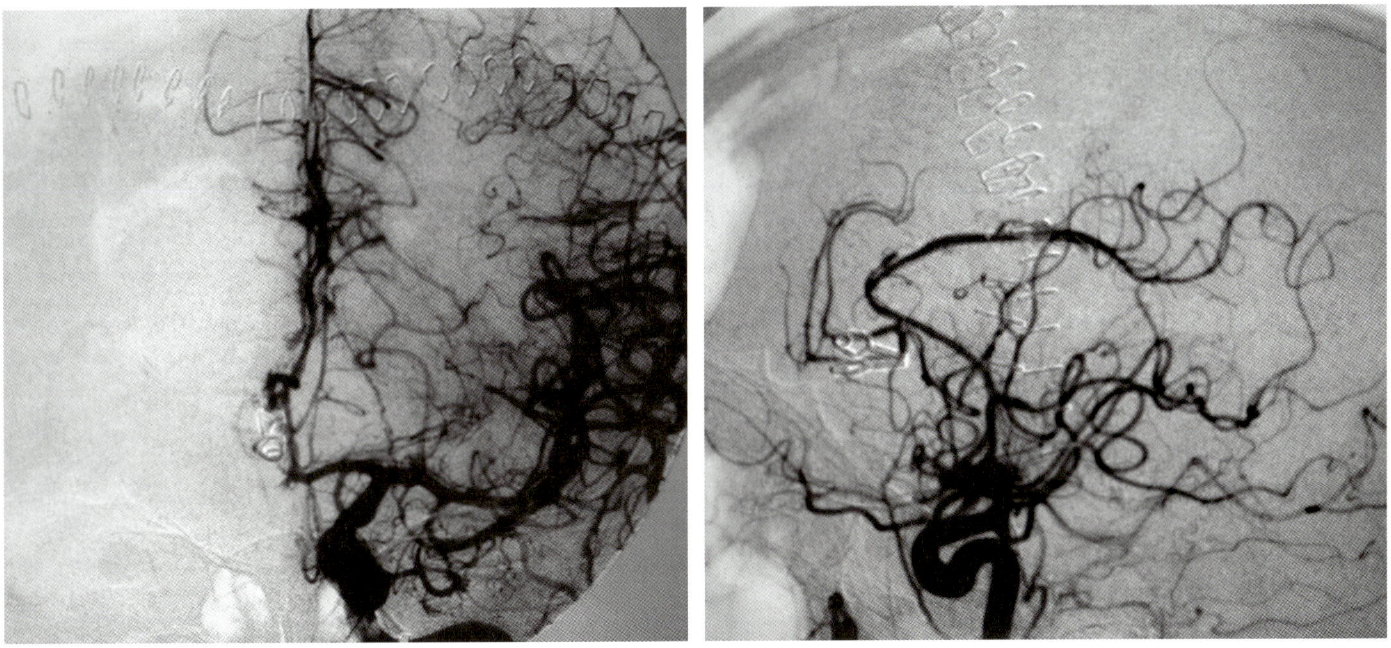

Fig. 1.3g, h Postoperative anteroposterior (**g**) and lateral (**h**) left ICA angiograms confirm obliteration of the aneurysm and filling of the territories of both distal ACAs through the bypass.

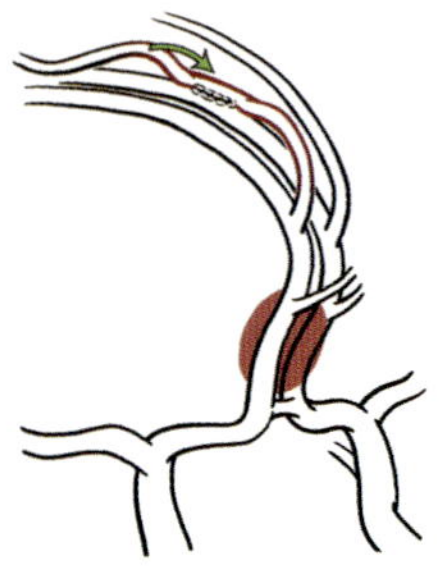

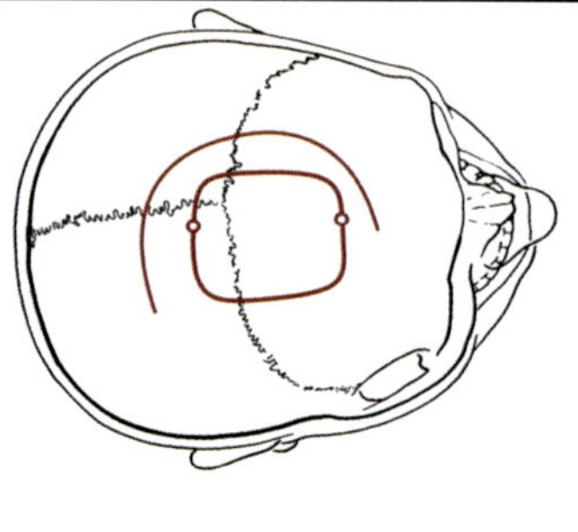

Case 1-4

Diagnosis: Left fusiform A2 aneurysm

Bypass: A3-to-A3

Approach: Interhemispheric

Video

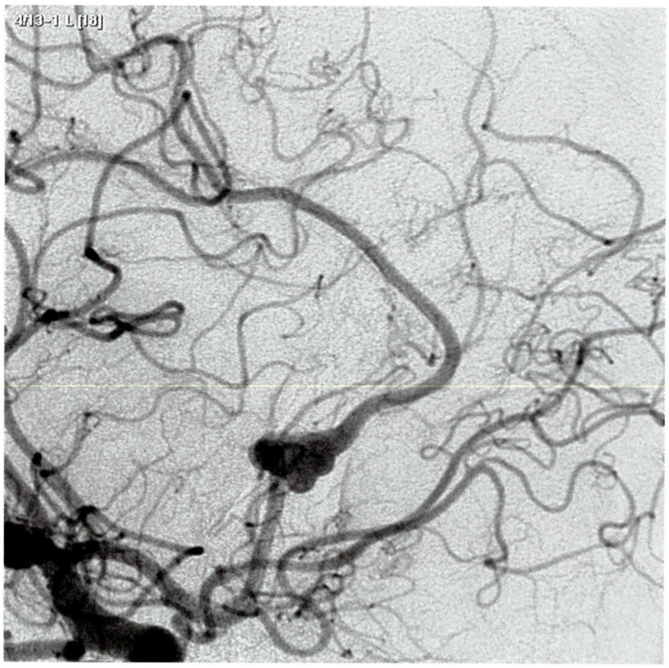

Fig. 1.4a The left ICA lateral angiogram shows a fusiform aneurysm involving the left A2.

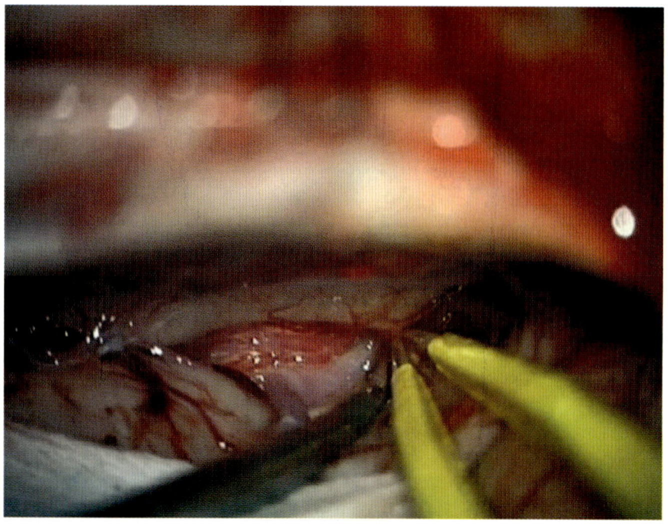

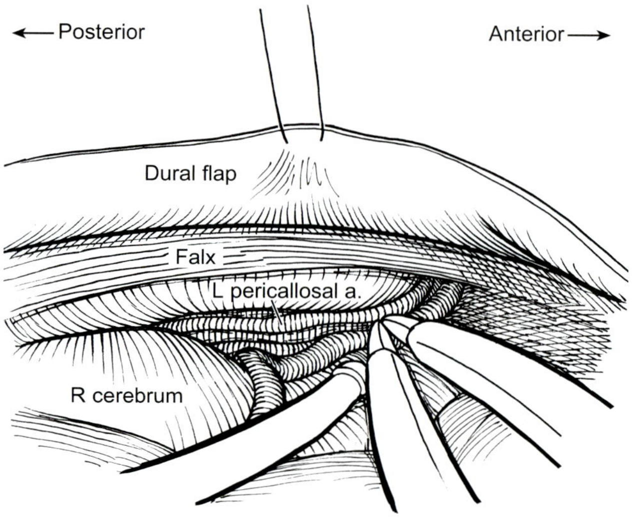

Fig. 1.4b Through a right interhemispheric approach, the A3 to be sacrificed is located at the bottom of the interhemispheric fissure. The front of the head is to the right and the right side of the patient is down.

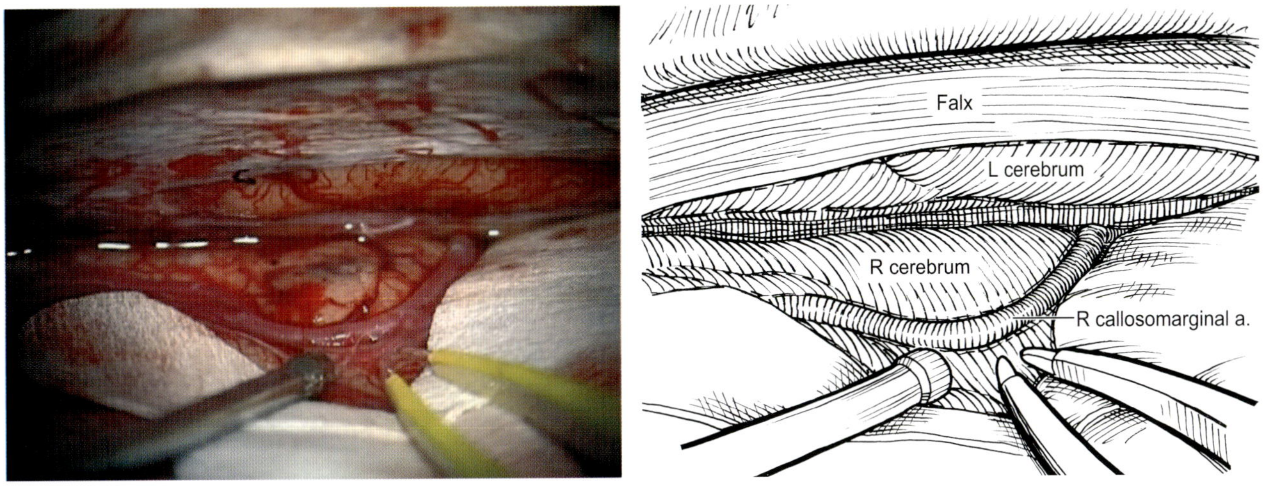

Fig. 1.4c No adjacent pericallosal branch is available, so a callosomarginal branch is freed from the gyrus above.

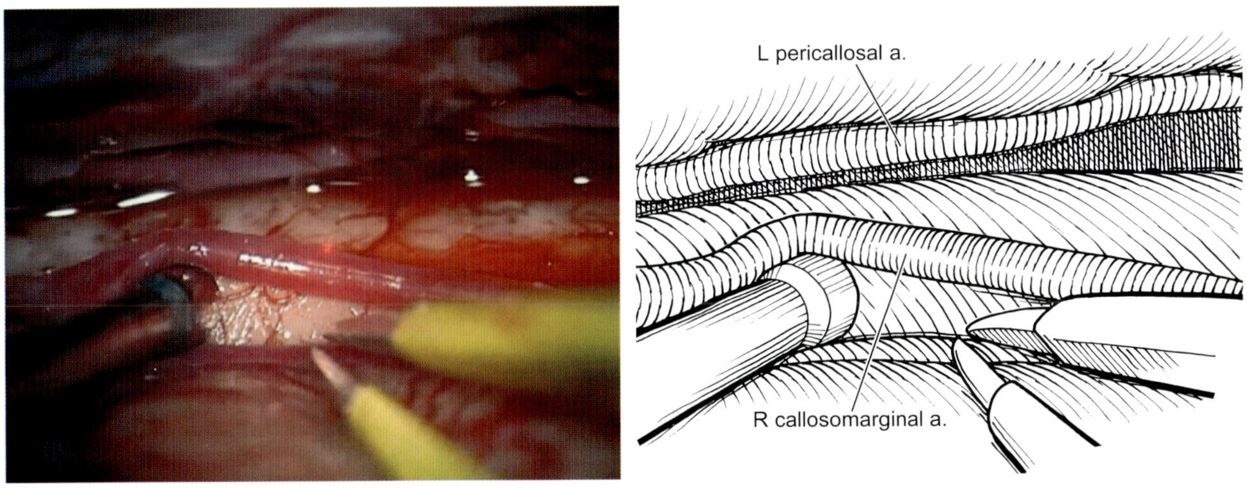

Fig. 1.4d The callosomarginal branch is gradually mobilized to bring it close to the pericallosal artery deep to it.

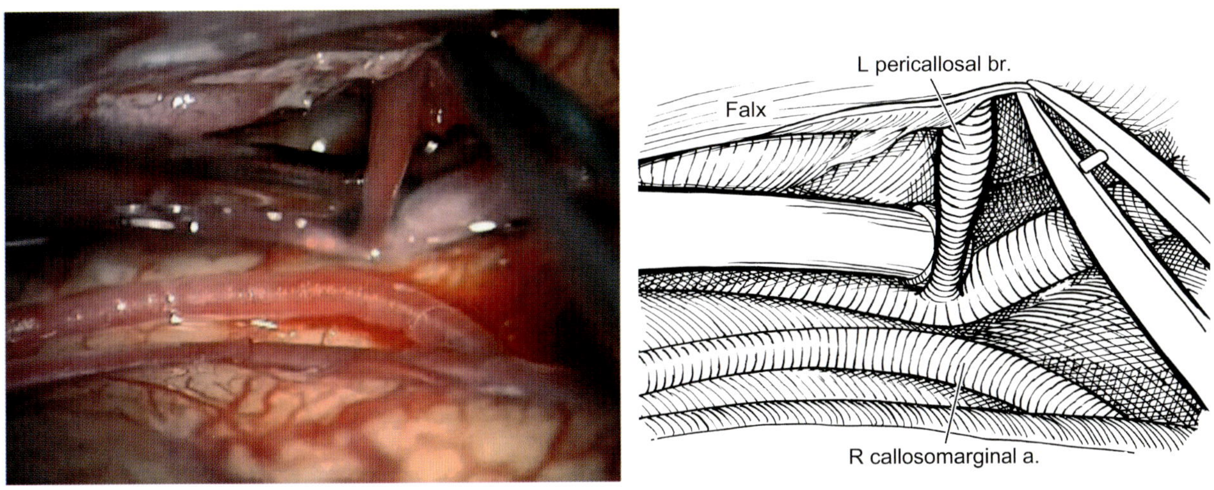

Fig. 1.4e The falx is slit and a branch from the pericallosal artery is mobilized from its sulcus to allow the pericallosal artery to be further mobilized.

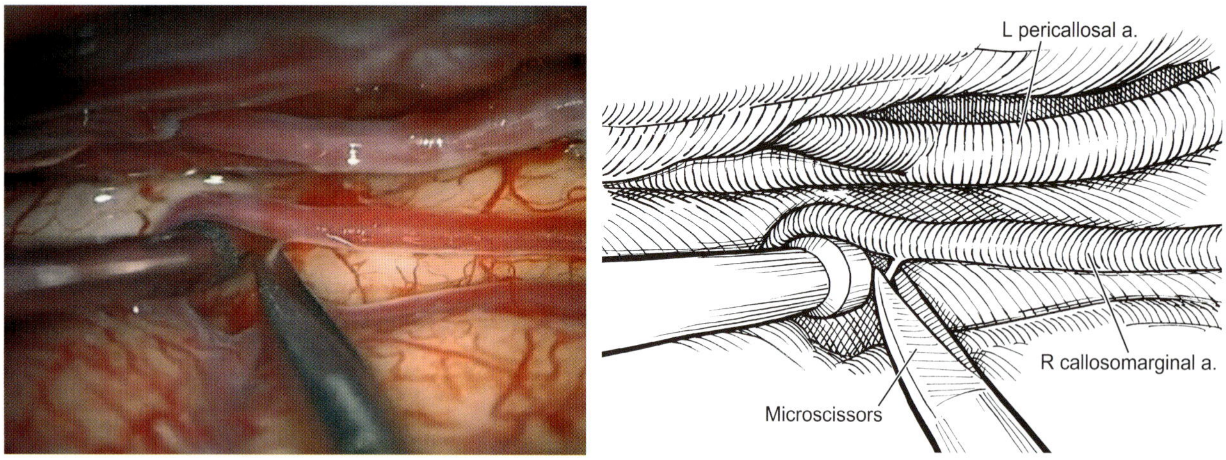

Fig. 1.4f One small branch on the callosomarginal artery must be sacrificed to permit the arteries to be apposed without tension.

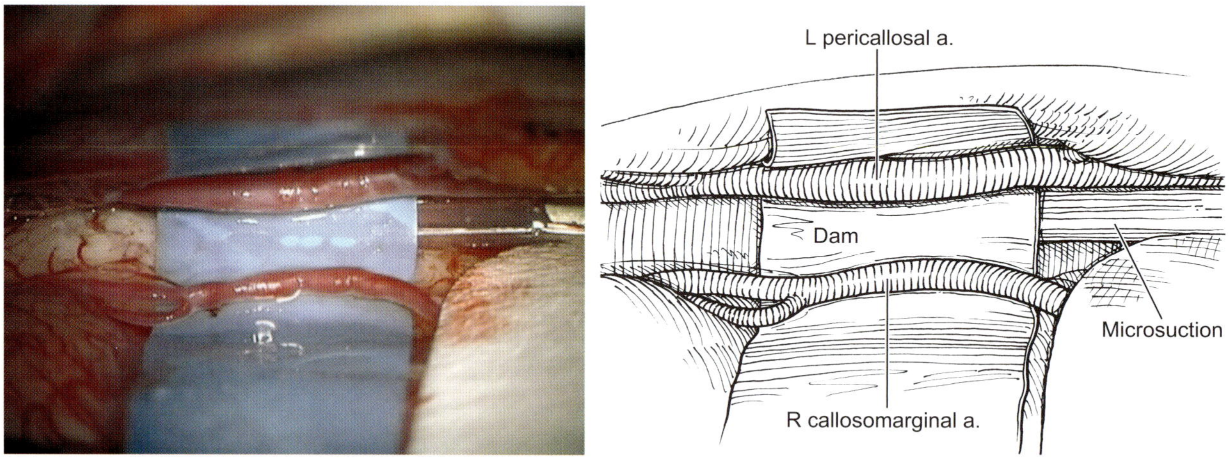

Fig. 1.4g The two vessels lie parallel on a blue dam.

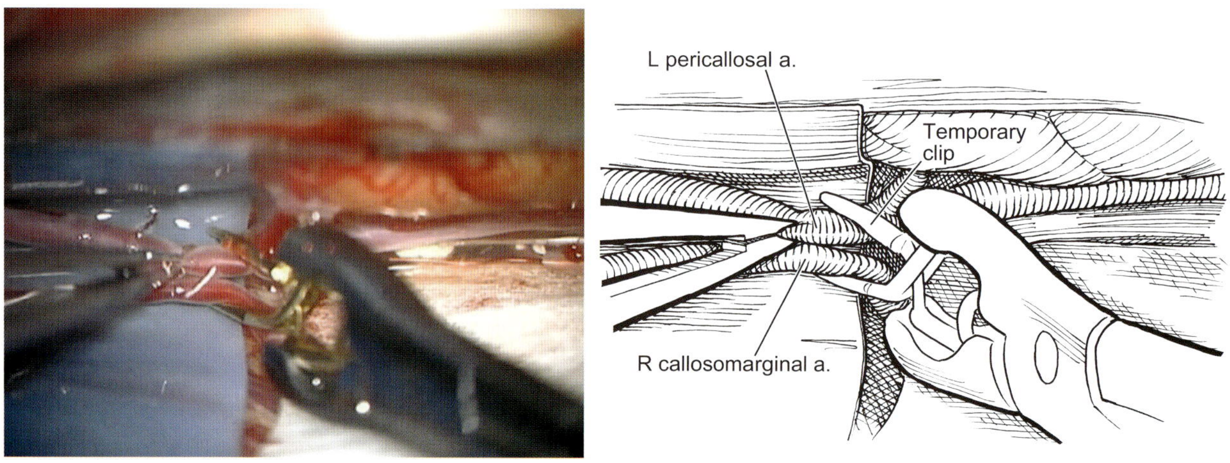

Fig. 1.4h A temporary clip is applied across both vessels.

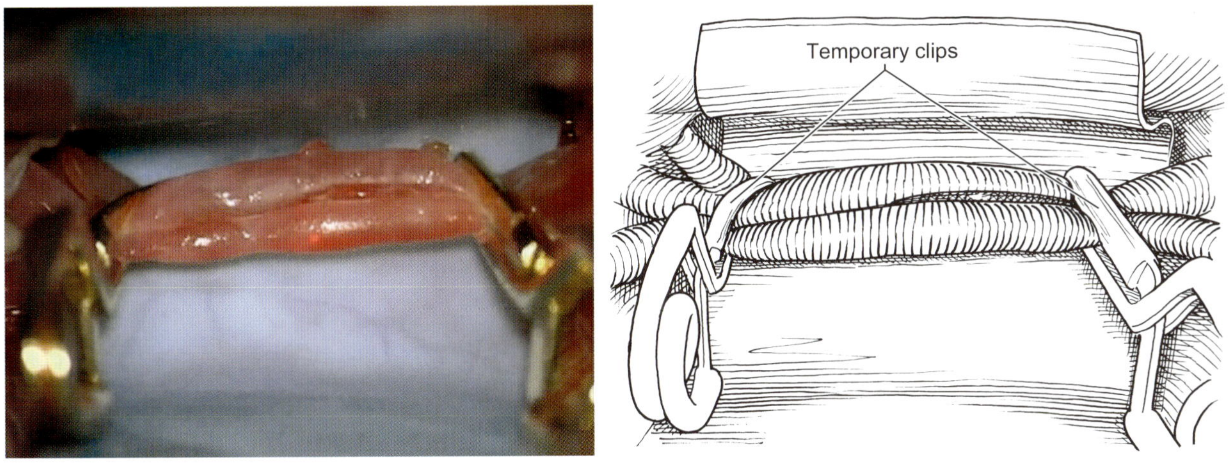

Fig. 1.4i A second clip is applied distally in the same fashion.

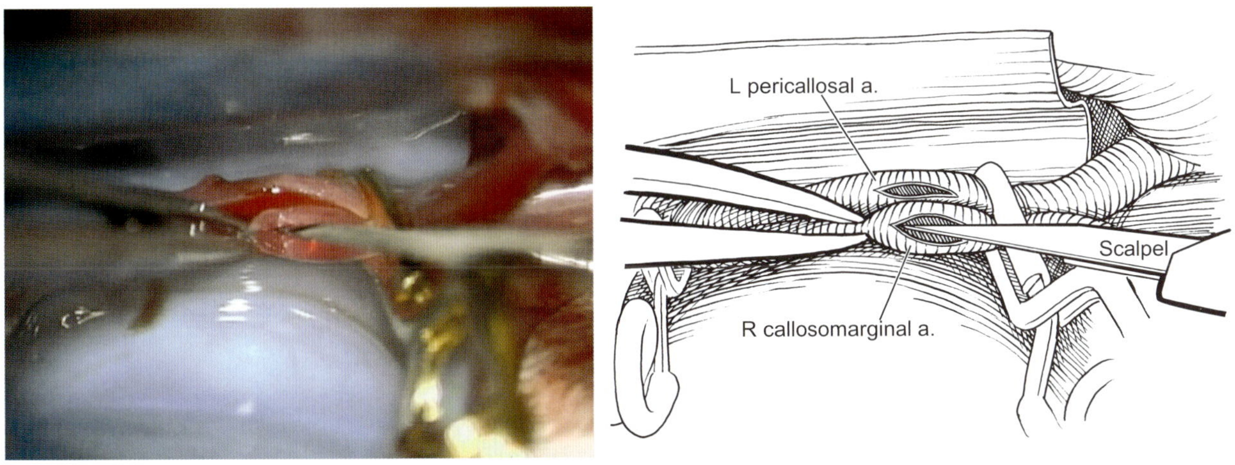

Fig. 1.4j Each vessel is incised.

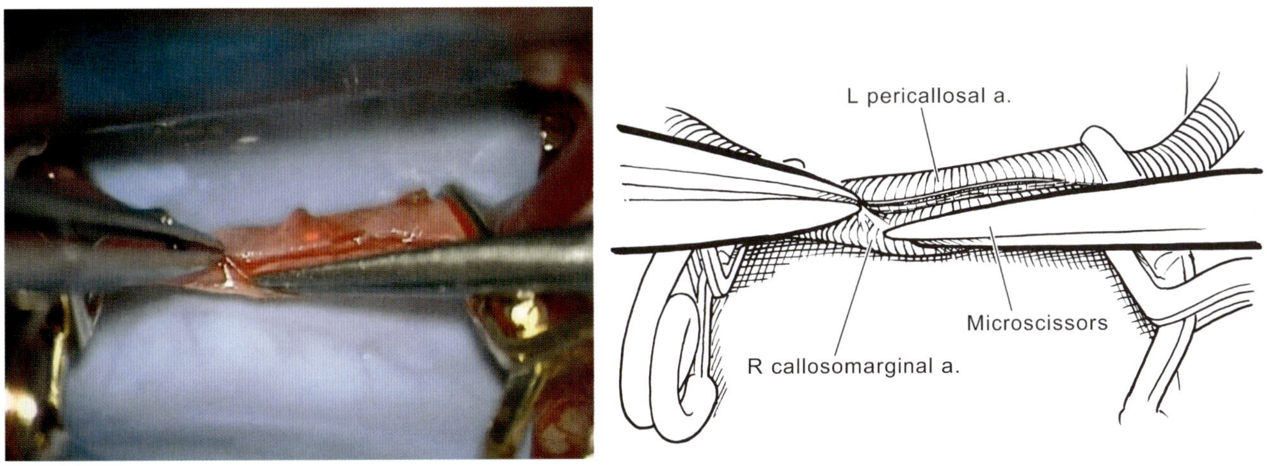

Fig. 1.4k Fine microscissors are used to extend the cuts and make them equal in length in both vessels.

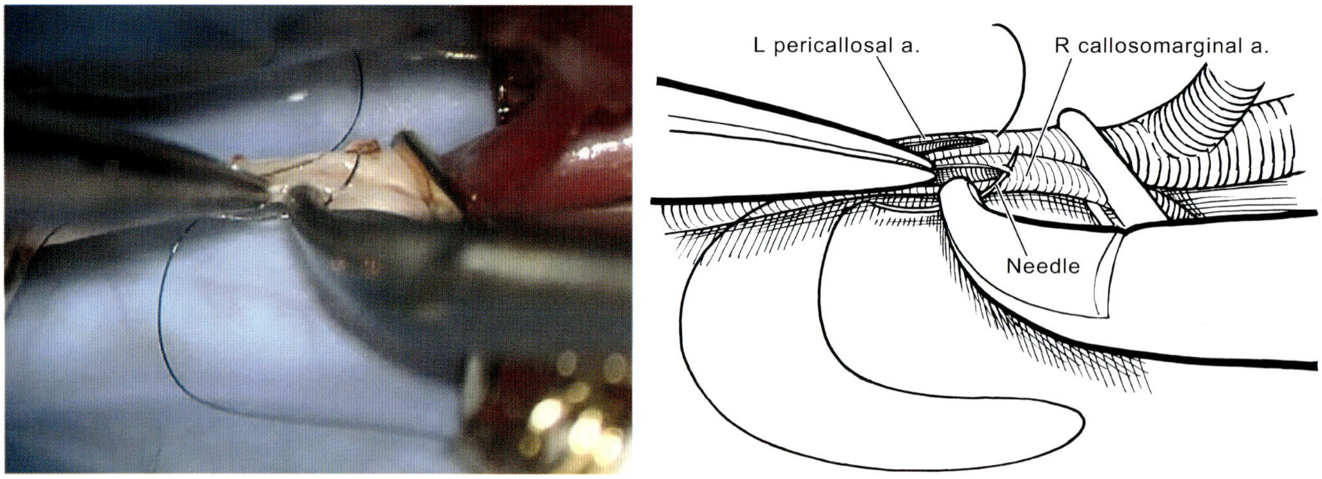

Fig. 1.4l A suture is placed outside to inside at one apex, then reversed and passed from inside the lumen to the outside of the other vessel and knotted.

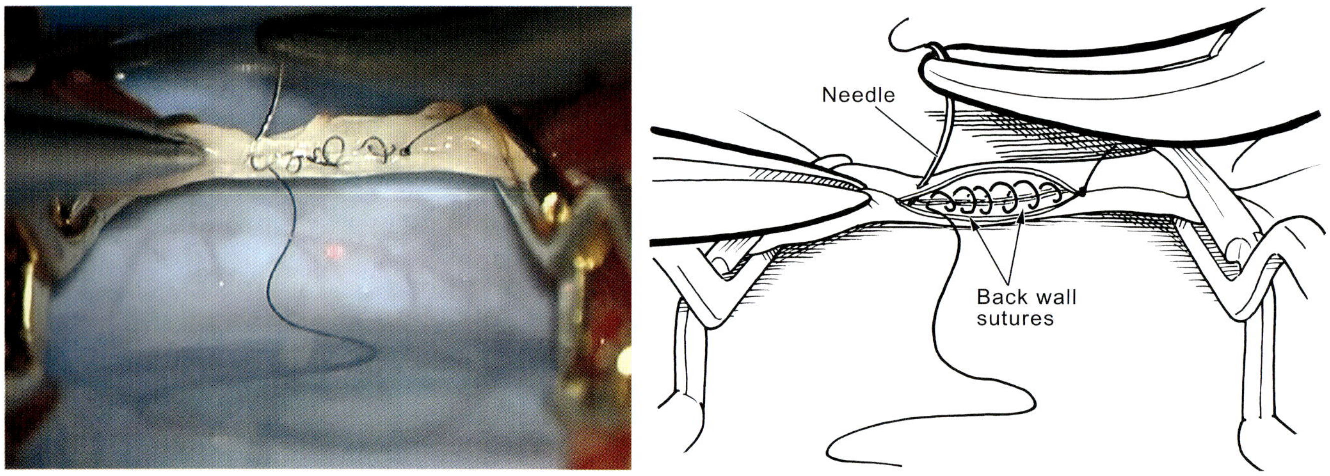

Fig. 1.4m A suture is placed at the other apex with the knot on the outside. The needle is then placed from the outside to the inside of the lumen, and the anastomosis of the back wall is performed on the inside of the vessels. The last stitch is then passed again to the outside.

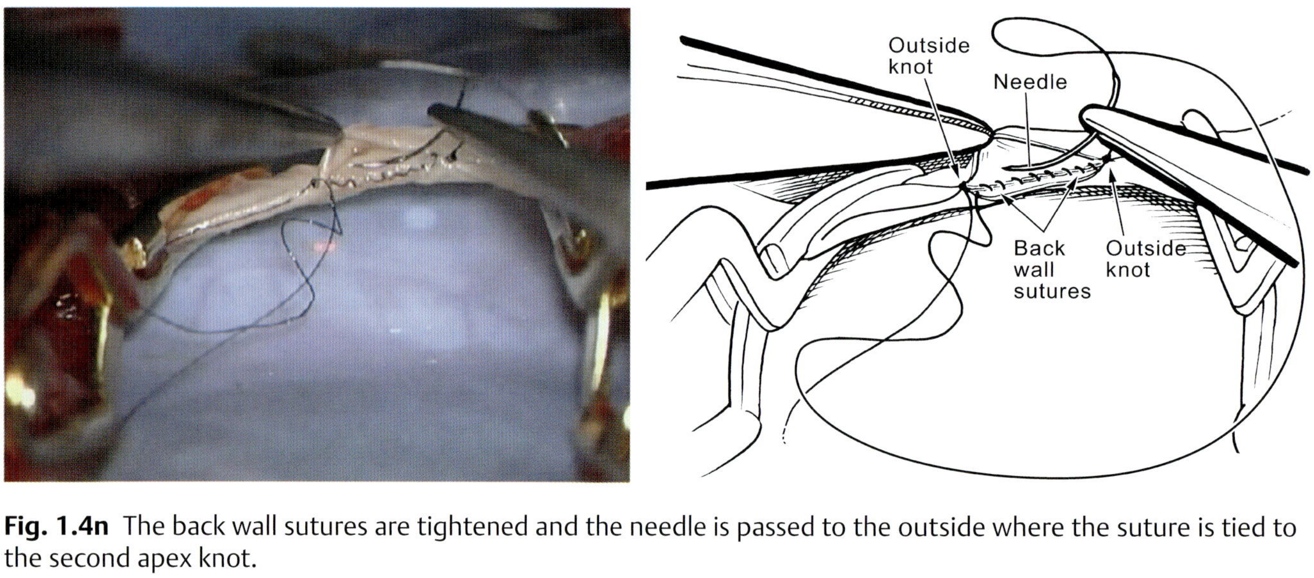

Fig. 1.4n The back wall sutures are tightened and the needle is passed to the outside where the suture is tied to the second apex knot.

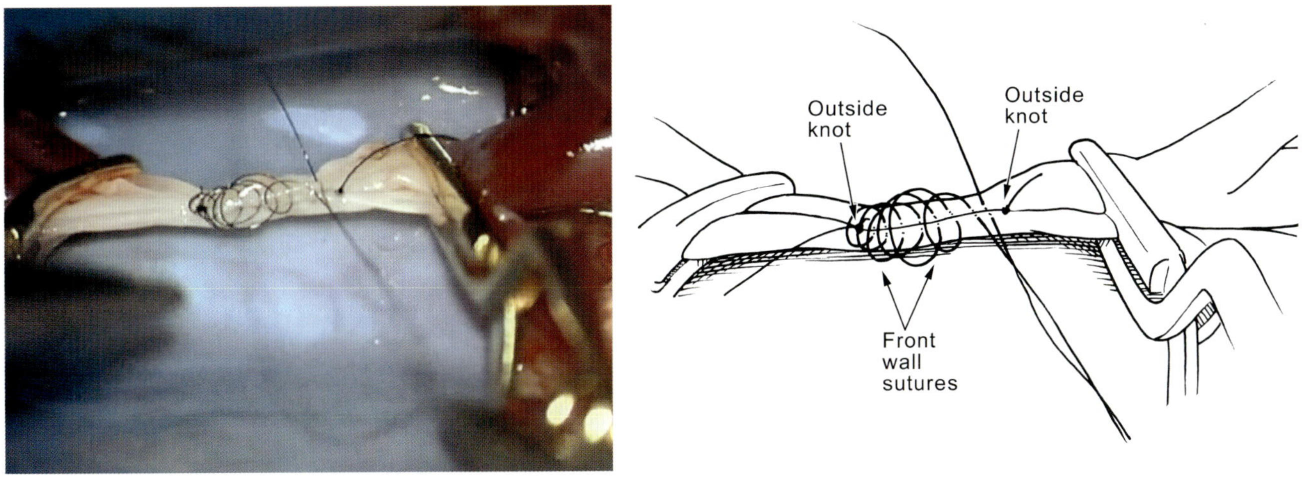

Fig. 1.4o The front walls are joined with loose running loops, tightened, and tied to the first knot.

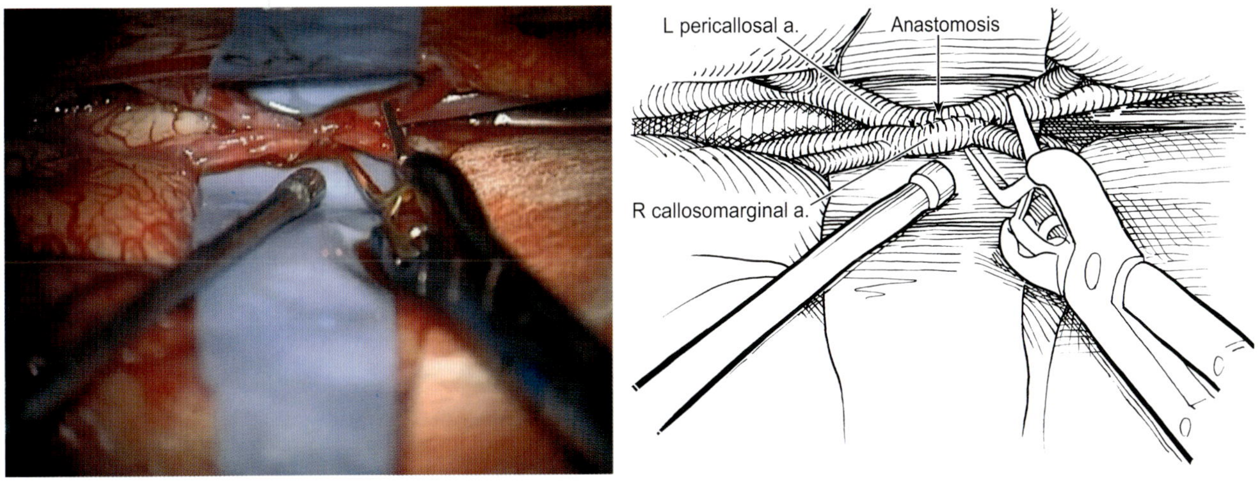

Fig. 1.4p The temporary clips are removed, restoring blood flow.

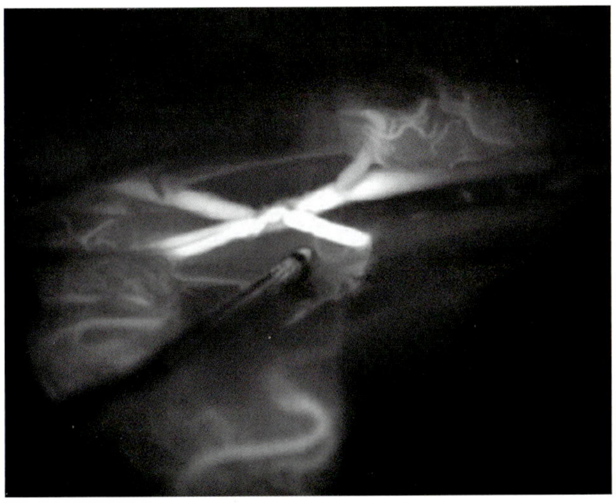

Fig. 1.4q After a temporary clip has been placed on the vessel to be sacrificed, ICG angiography shows the patency of the bypass.

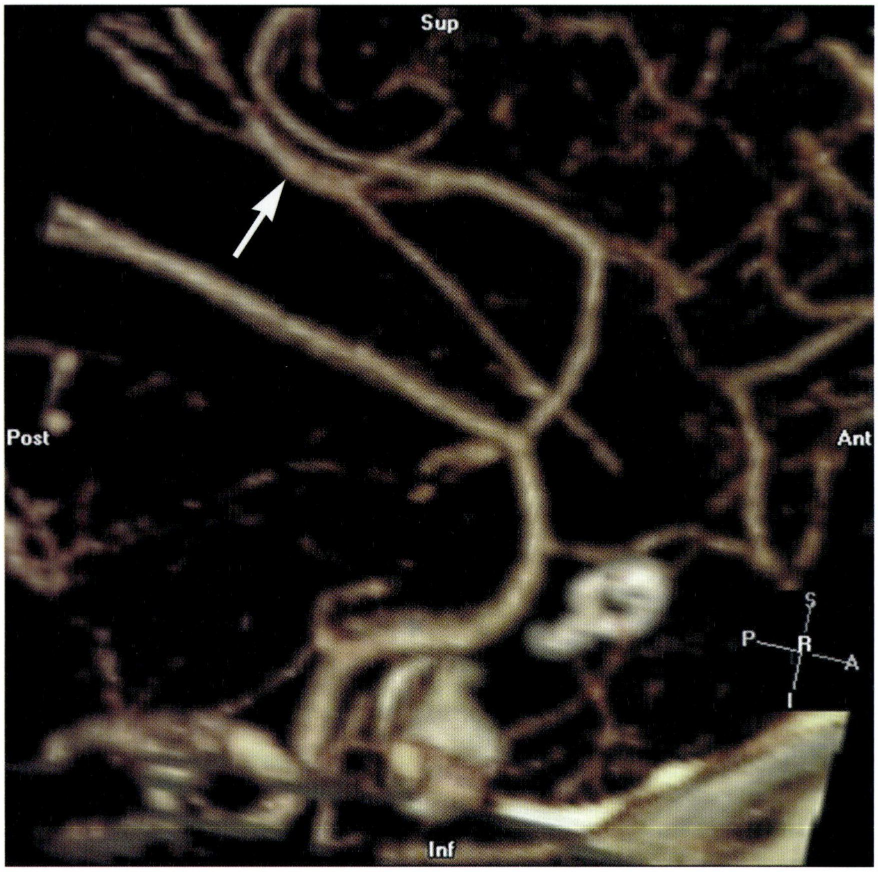

Fig. 1.4r Postoperative three-dimensional reconstructed CT angiogram shows the clip in place with no filling of the aneurysm. The distal bypass (*arrow*) is open.

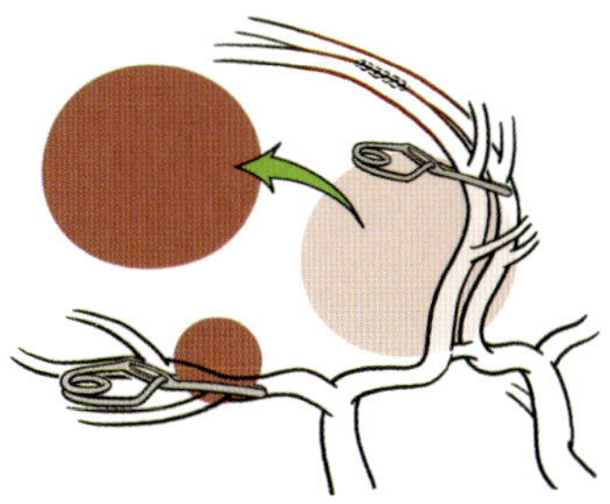

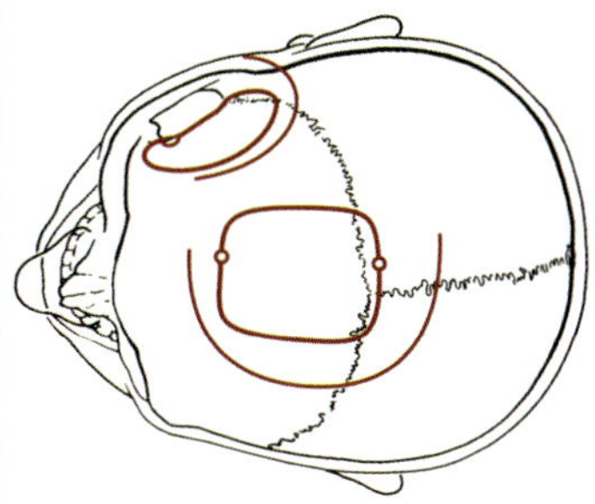

Case 1-5

Diagnosis: Right A2 giant aneurysm

Bypass: A3-to-A3 side-to-side

Approach: Interhemispheric, and right pterional for clipping second right MCA bifurcation aneurysm and endovascular sacrifice of right A2

Video

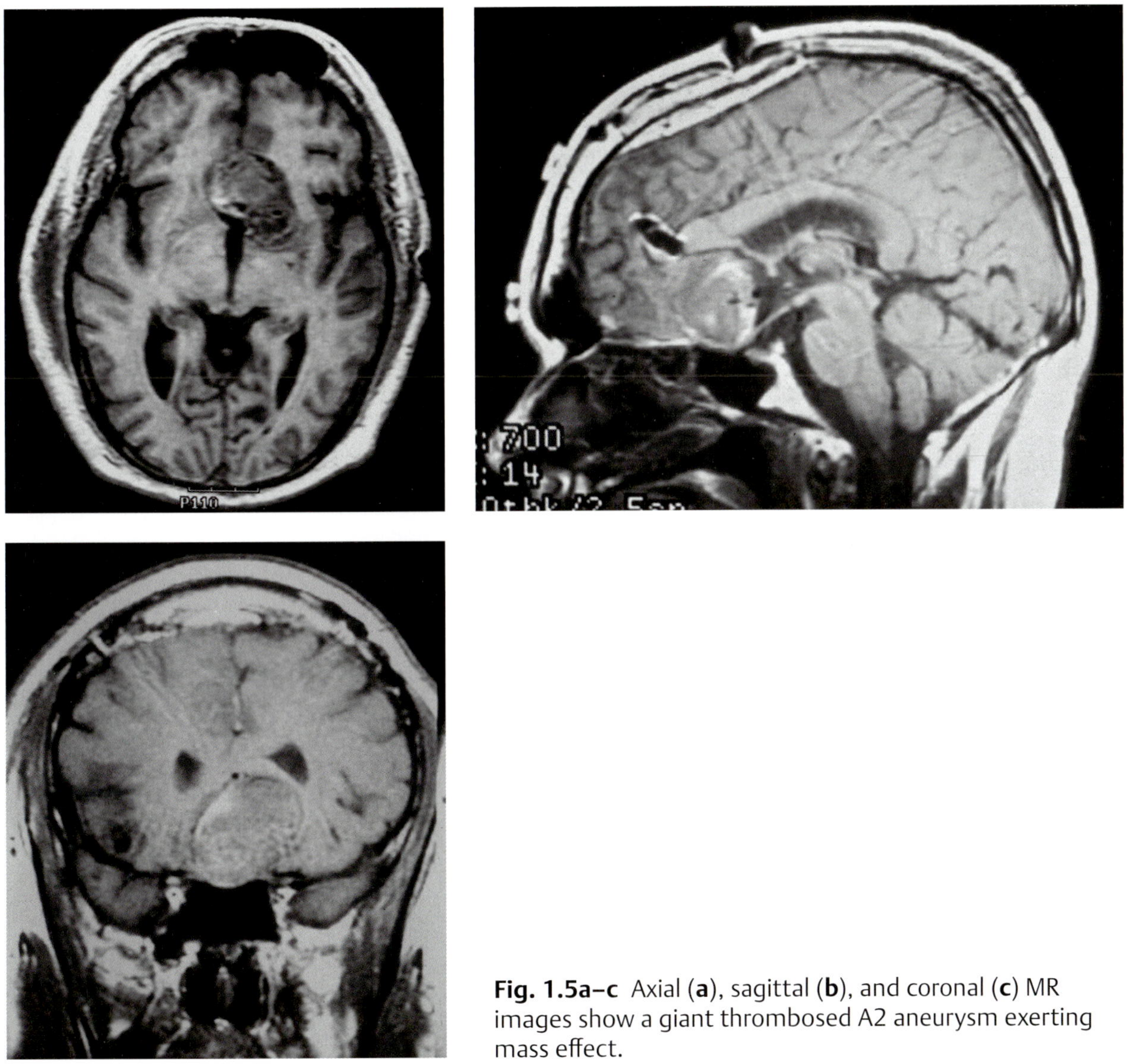

Fig. 1.5a–c Axial (**a**), sagittal (**b**), and coronal (**c**) MR images show a giant thrombosed A2 aneurysm exerting mass effect.

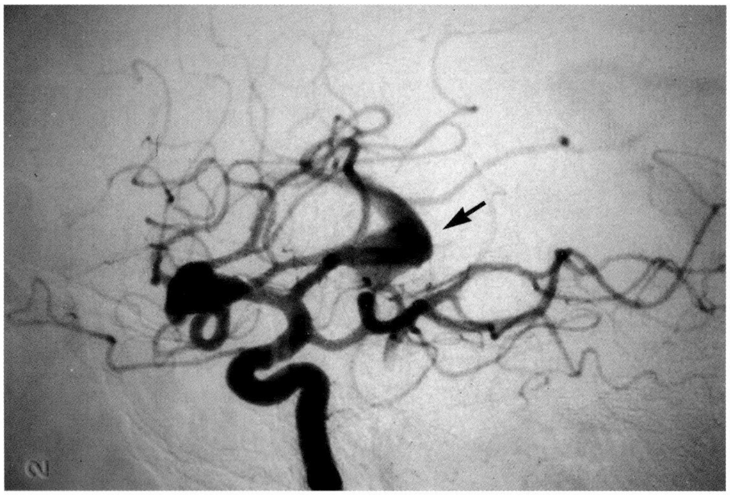

Fig. 1.5d Lateral angiogram shows the serpiginous channel through the thrombosed aneurysm (*arrow*).

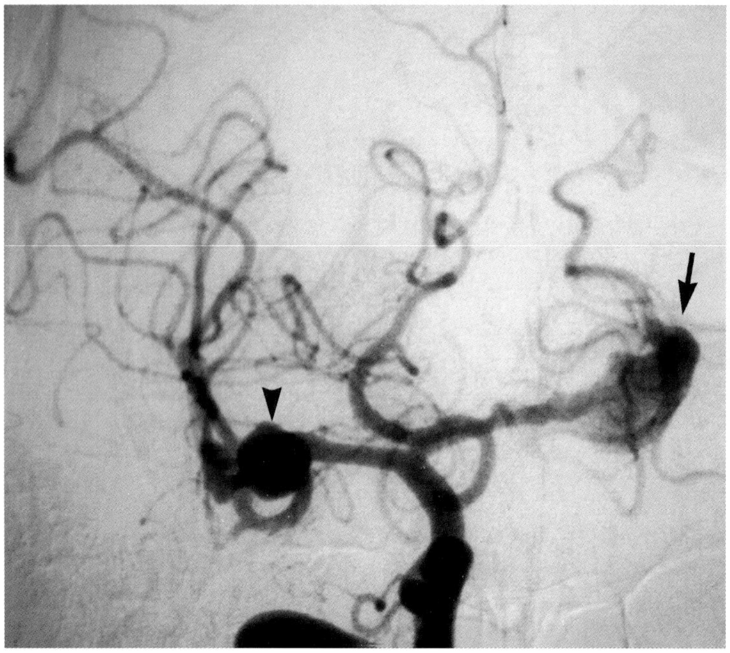

Fig. 1.5e Anteroposterior angiogram shows the complex ACA aneurysm (*arrow*) as well as an MCA aneurysm (*arrowhead*).

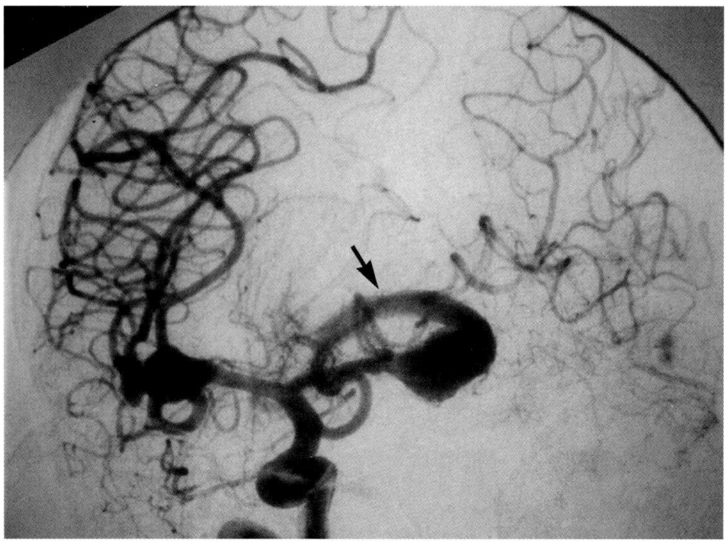

Fig. 1.5f Later phase anteroposterior angiogram shows the serpiginous vessel (*arrow*) and the intact contralateral ACA.

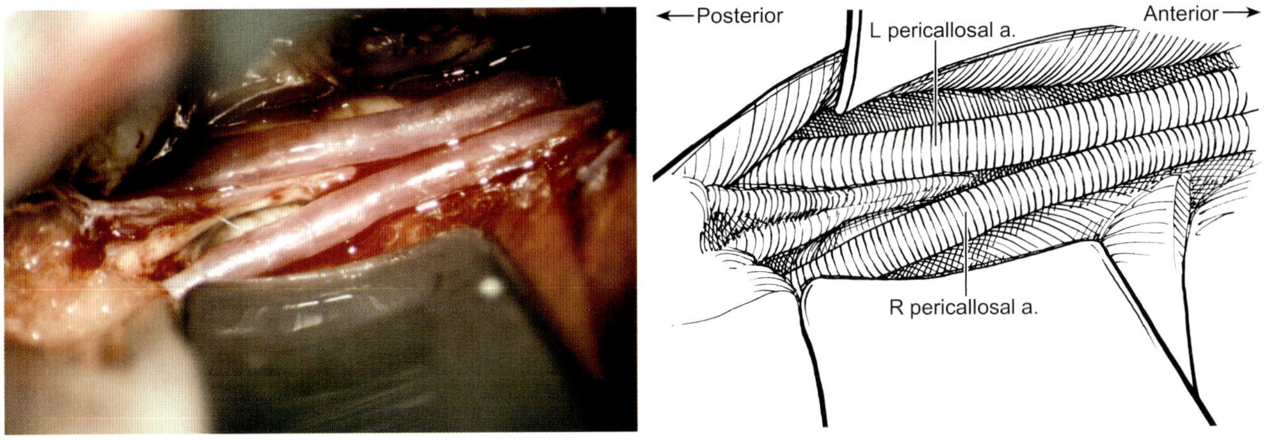

Fig. 1.5g With the patient's head in a horizontal position, the two pericallosal arteries are exposed through an interhemispheric approach.

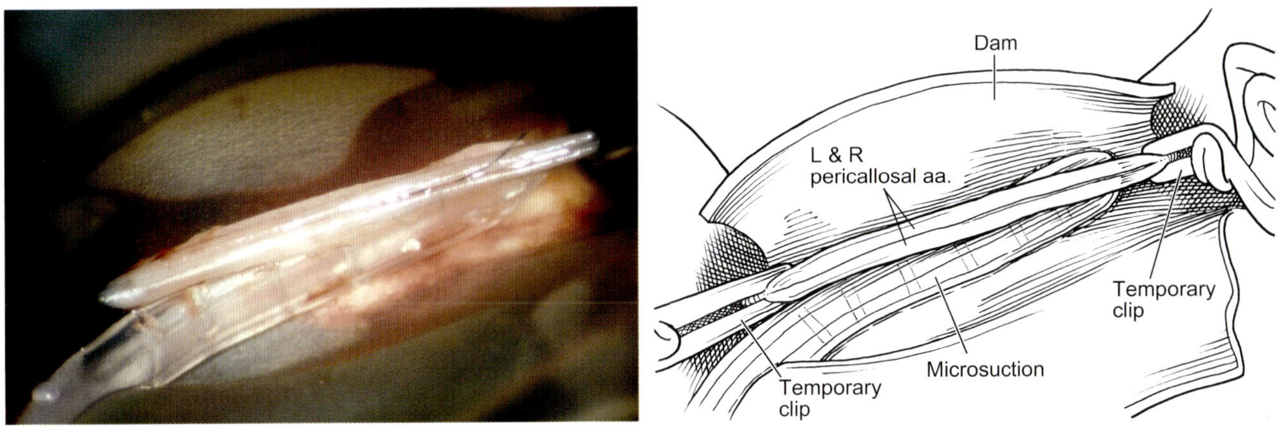

Fig. 1.5h The two pericallosal arteries are placed side by side over a dam and temporarily occluded in preparation for the bypass.

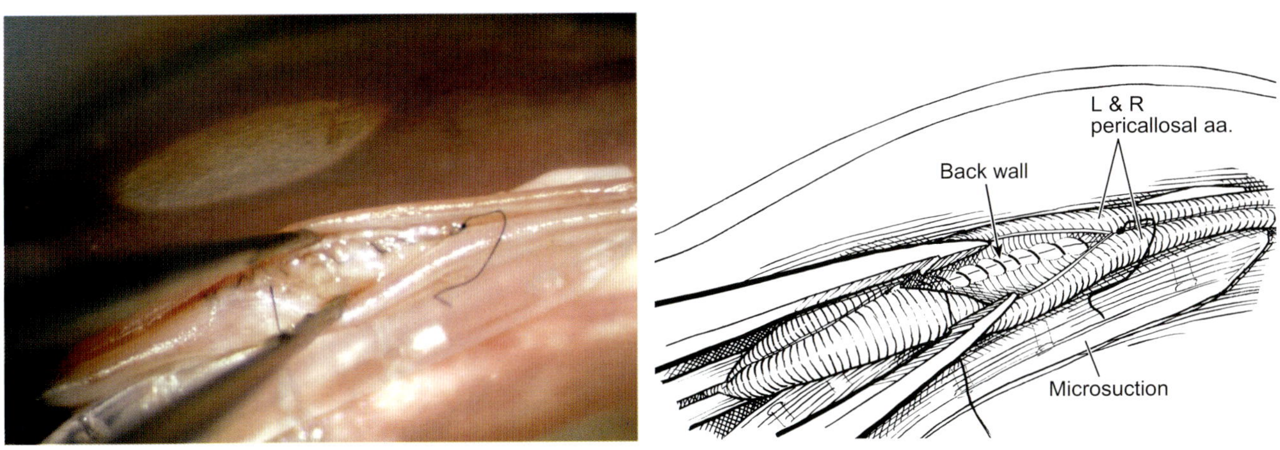

Fig. 1.5i The back wall of the anastomosis is completed.

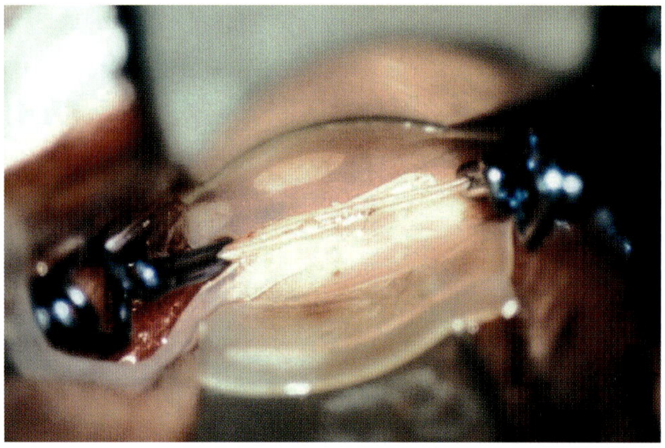

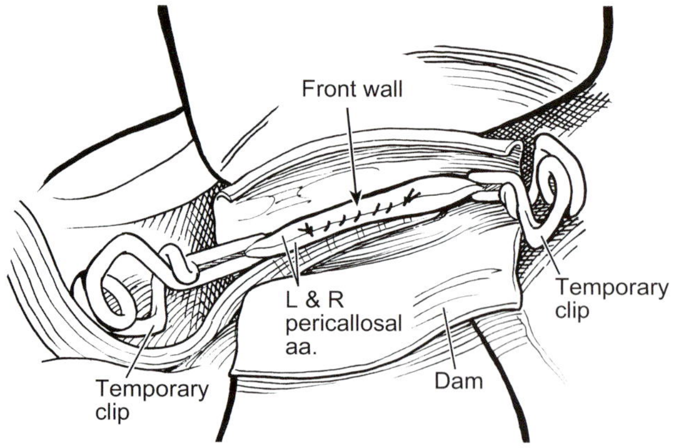

Fig. 1.5j The front wall of the bypass is completed.

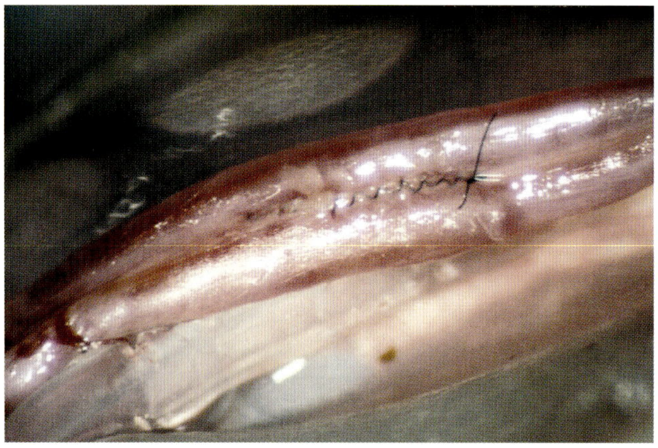

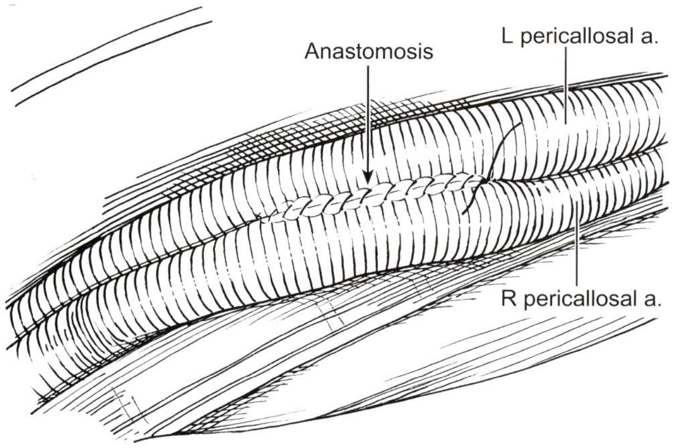

Fig. 1.5k The clips are removed, showing the side-to-side anastomosis.

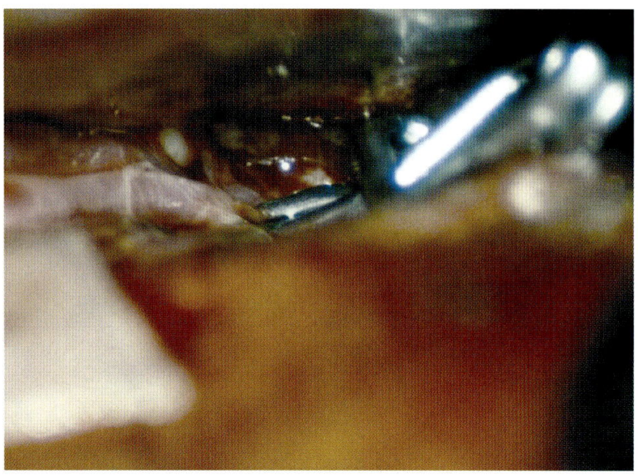

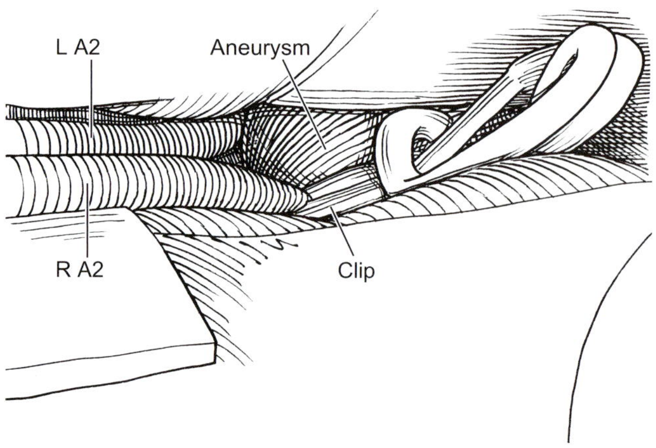

Fig. 1.5l The distal clip on the right ACA, as it exits the giant aneurysm, is visible.

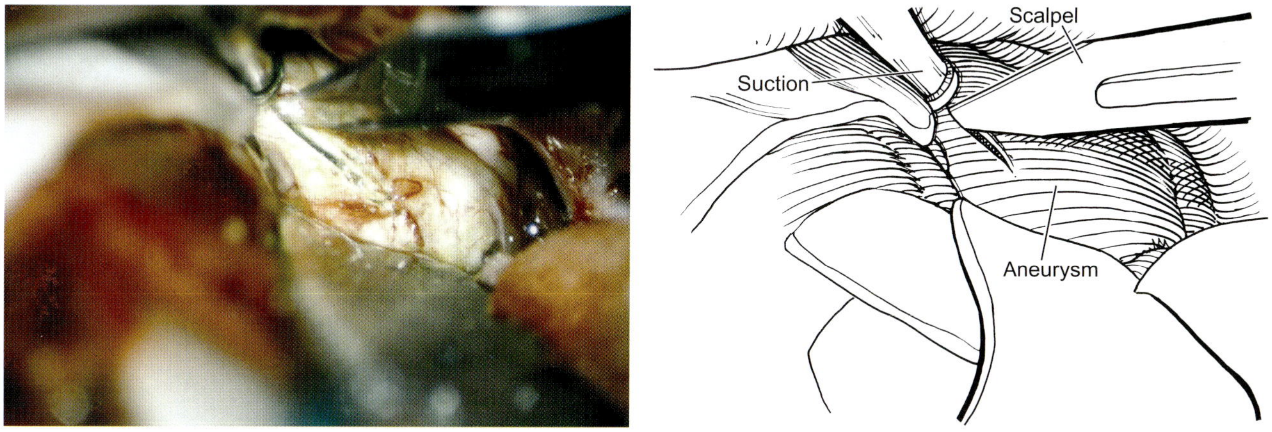

Fig. 1.5m The aneurysm is incised so that some of the thrombosis can be debulked to minimize the mass effect.

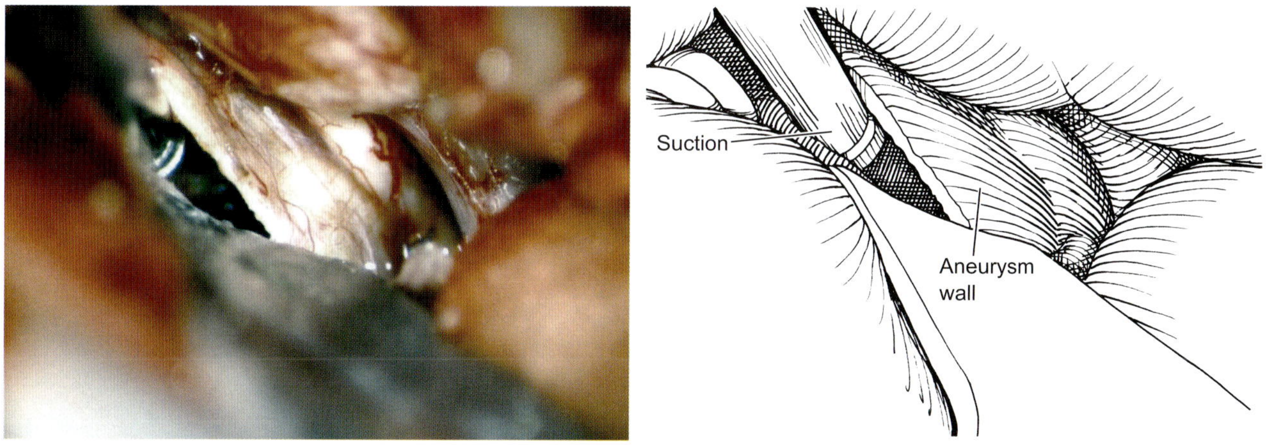

Fig. 1.5n After debulking is completed, an opening is visible in the aneurysm.

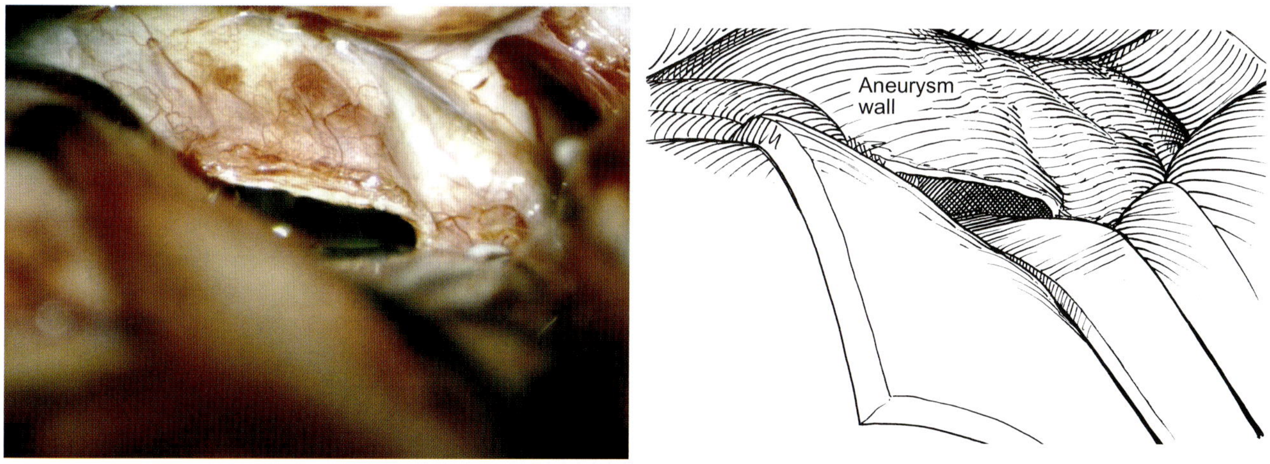

Fig. 1.5o The thrombosis has been evacuated.

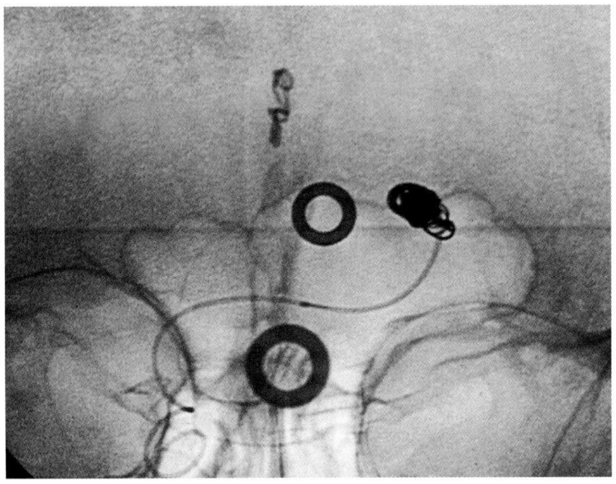

Fig. 1.5p Anteroposterior angiographic projection shows the clip on the distal portion of the aneurysm.

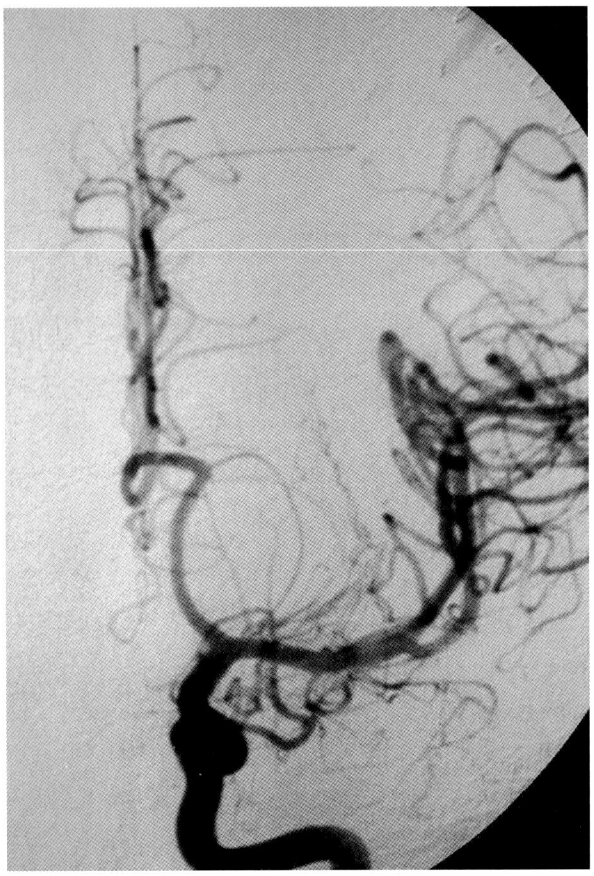

Fig. 1.5q Anteroposterior angiographic projection shows no further filling of the aneurysm and good patency of the side-to-side anastomosis.

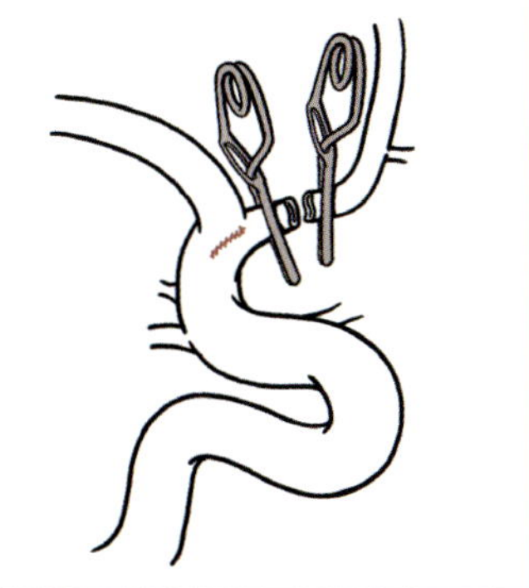

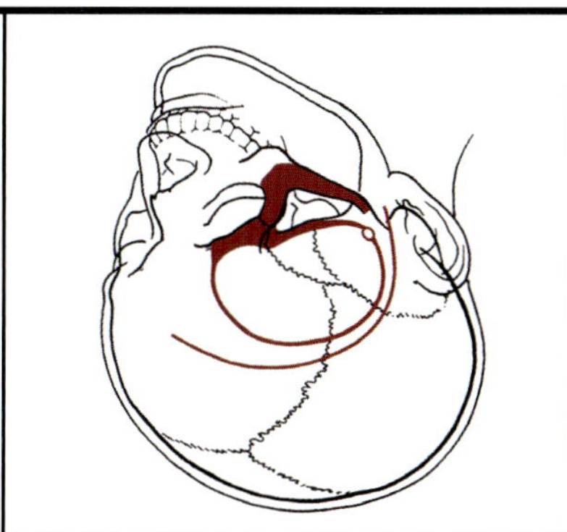

Case 1-6

Diagnosis: Giant suprasellar tumor with ICA tear

Bypass: ICA repair

Approach: Right orbitozygomatic with sacrifice of right A1

Video

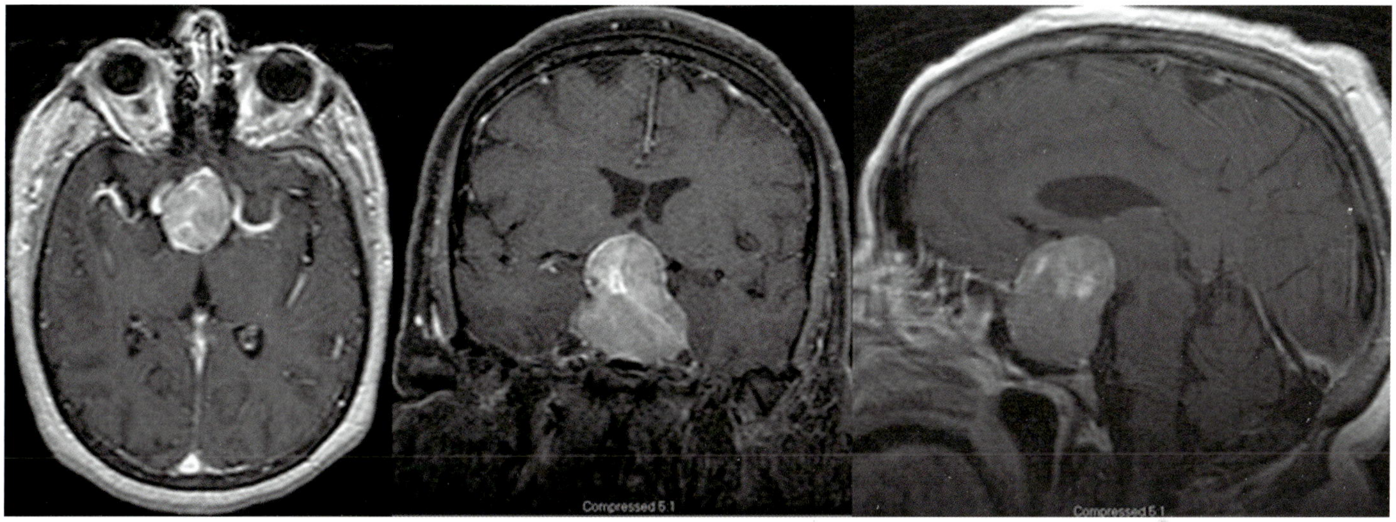

Fig. 1.6a MR images show a large pituitary tumor.

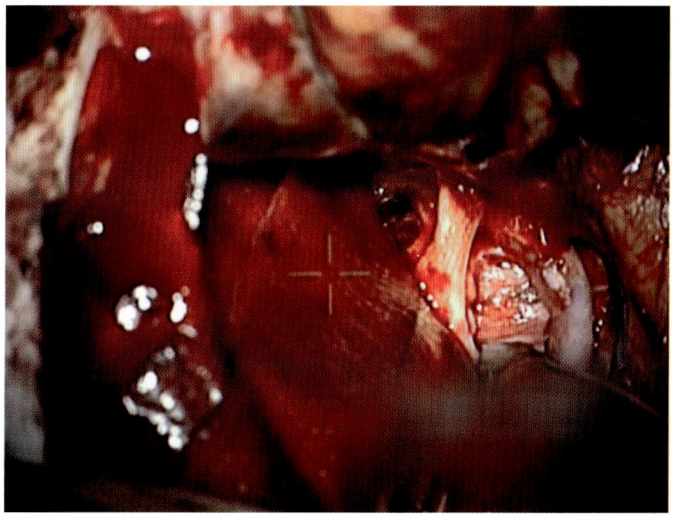

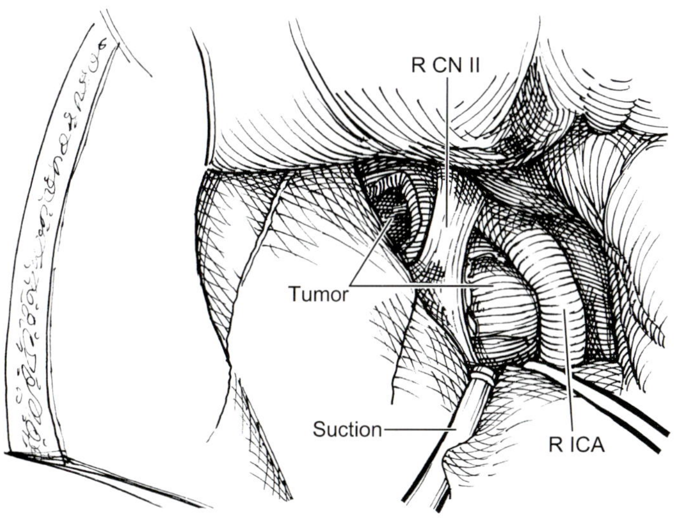

Fig. 1.6b The tumor is being resected. The right CN II is visible.

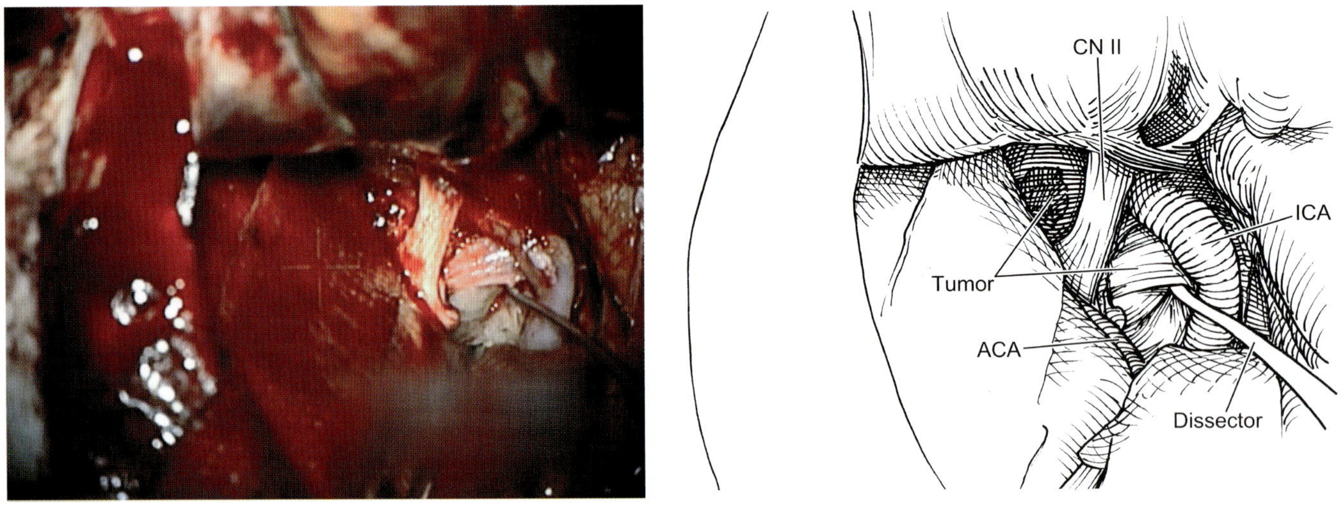

Fig. 1.6c As tumor resection progresses, the ICA is mobilized.

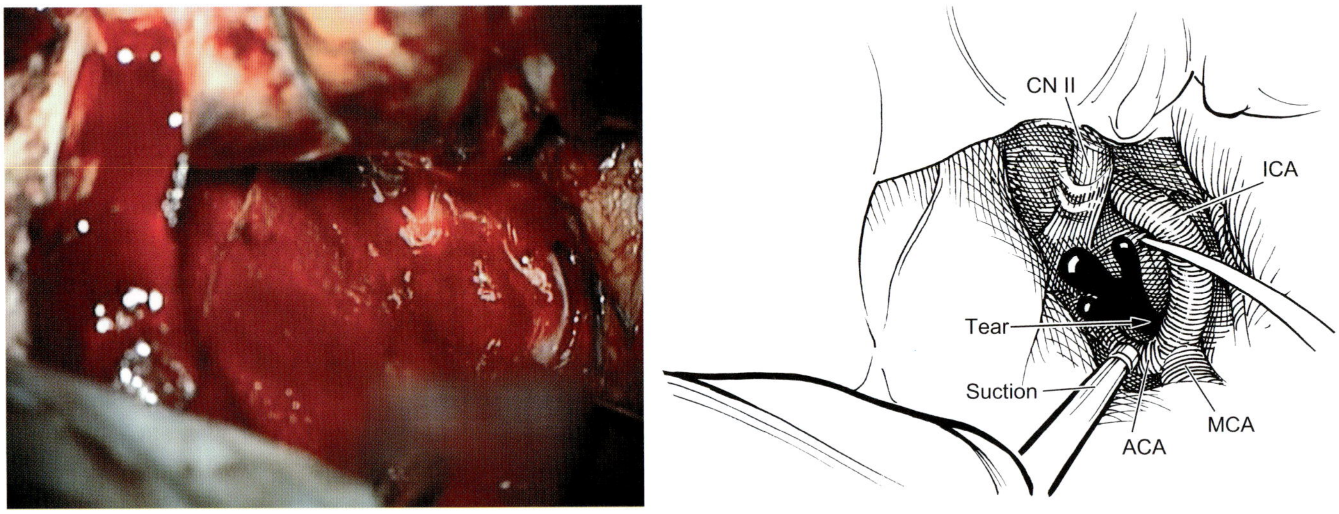

Fig. 1.6d During tumor resection, a tear in the ICA occurs and tamponade is applied.

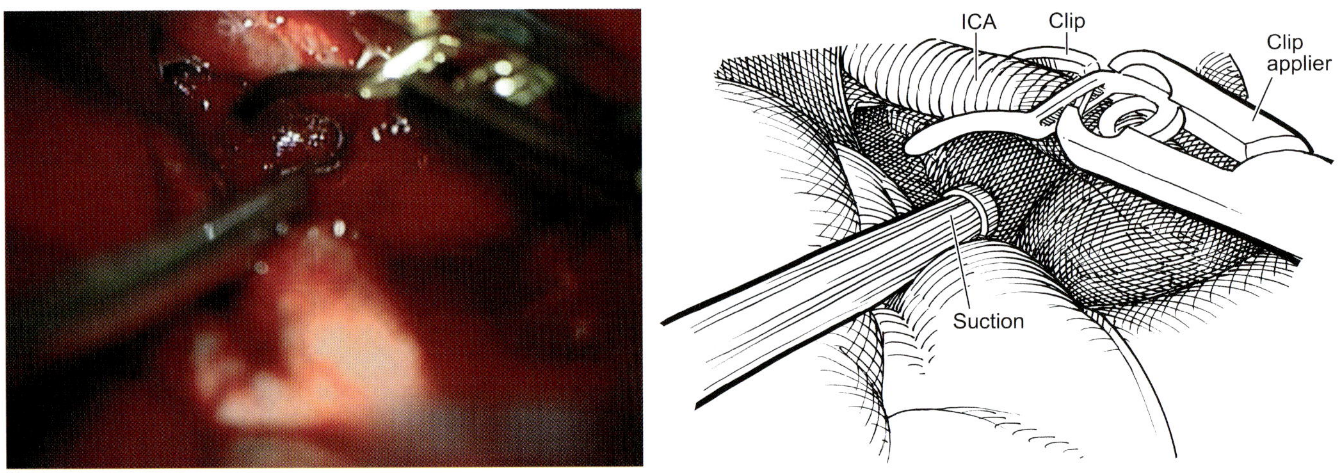

Fig. 1.6e The vascular neurosurgeon has been called and temporary clips are applied.

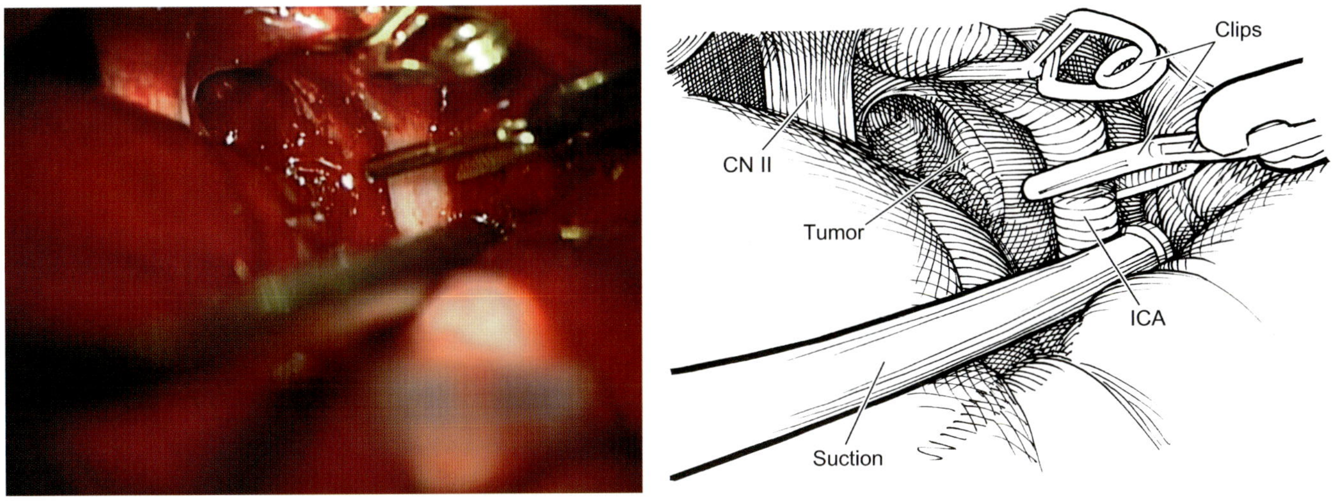

Fig. 1.6f Application of the clips provides hemostasis.

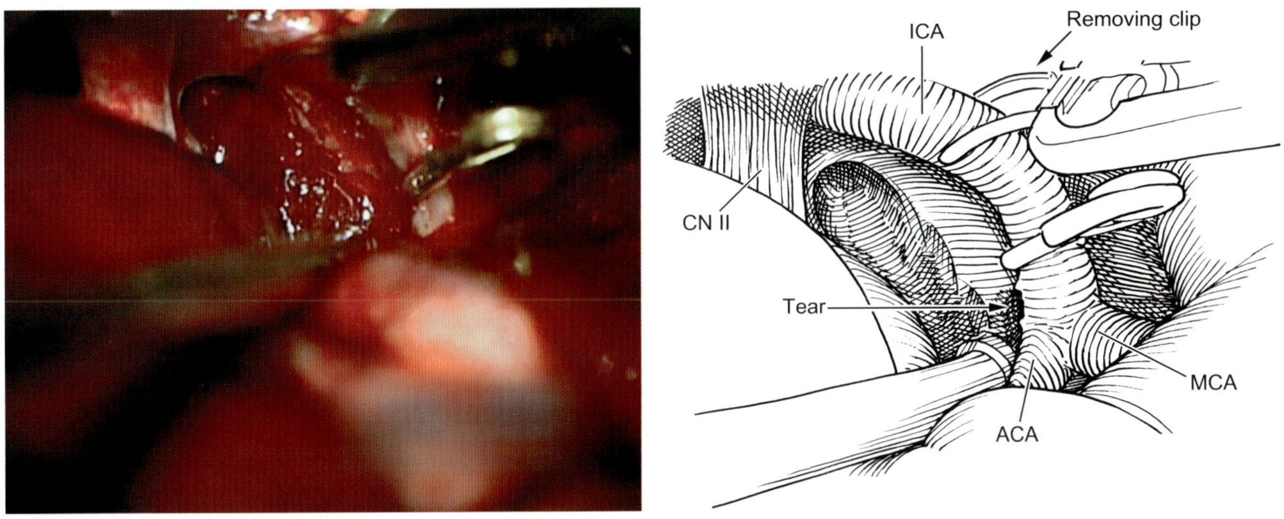

Fig. 1.6g The clips are reapplied to gain better exposure of the damaged part of the ICA. The large tear in the back wall of the ICA, which is opposite the MCA, is visible but not accessible for direct repair.

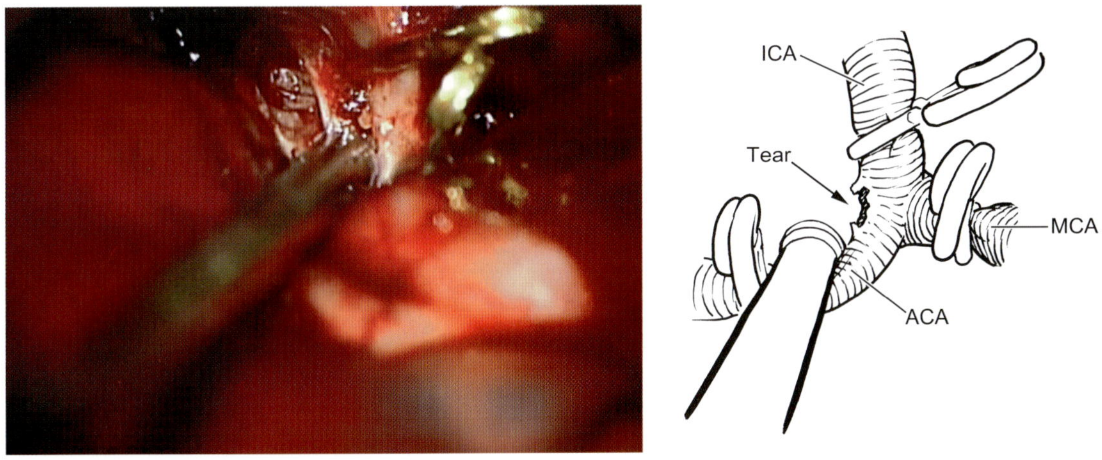

Fig. 1.6h Temporary clips are placed on the ICA, MCA, and ACA.

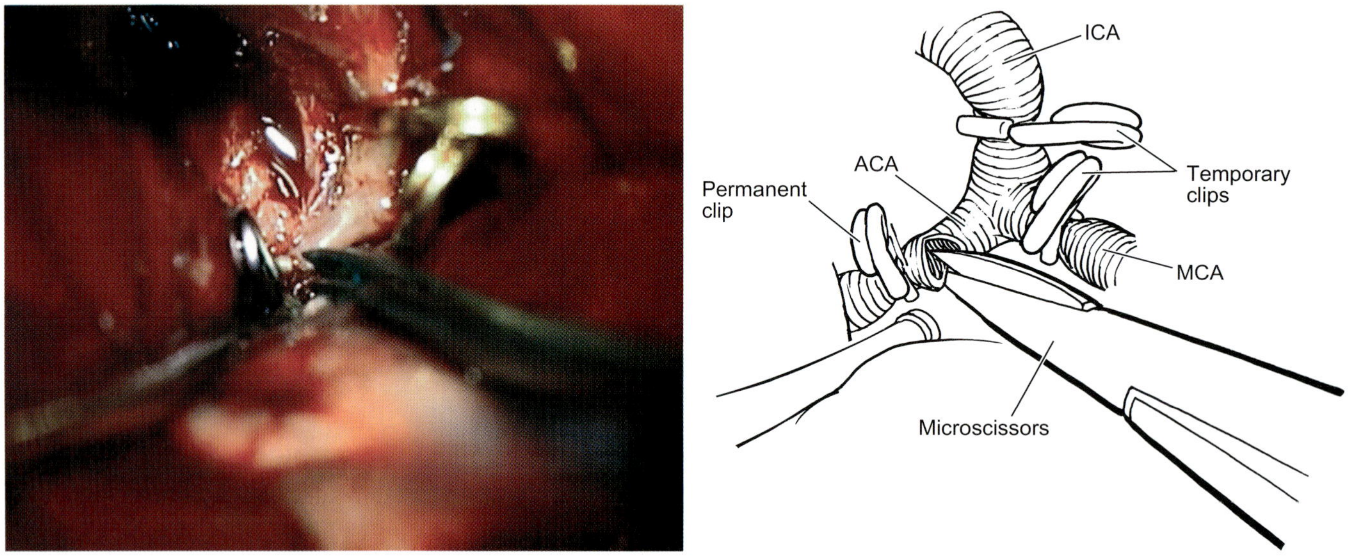

Fig. 1.6i After good backflow from the contralateral ACA is demonstrated, the right ACA is cut in preparation for mobilization.

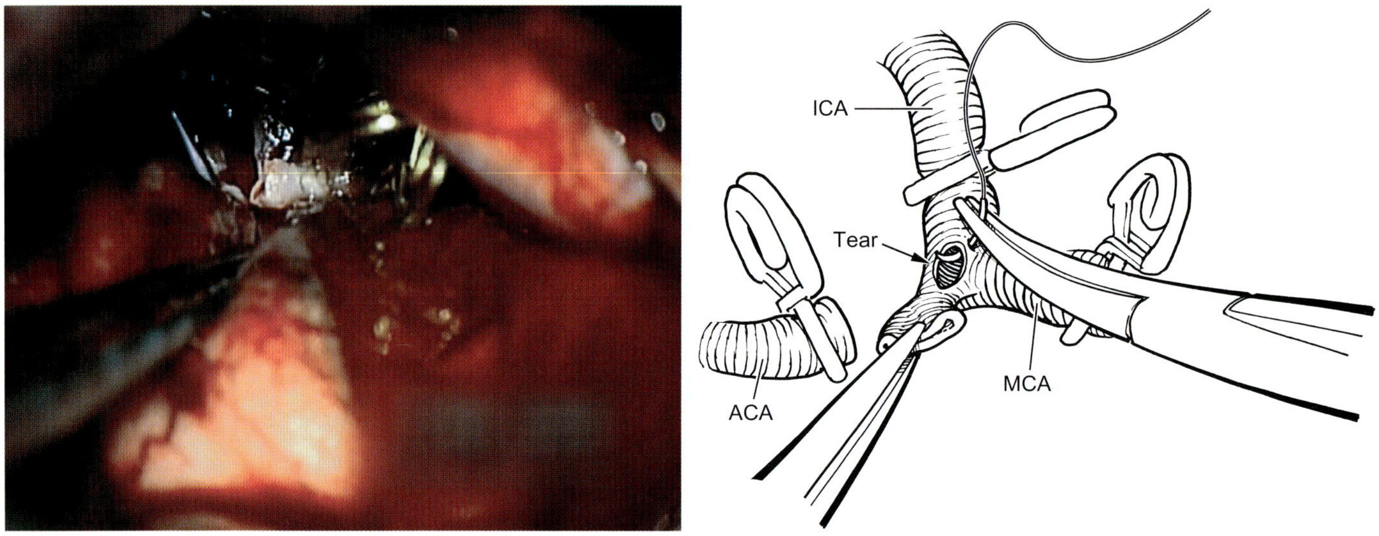

Fig. 1.6j After the ACA is mobilized, the edges of the tear in the back wall of the ICA are apposed for direct closure.

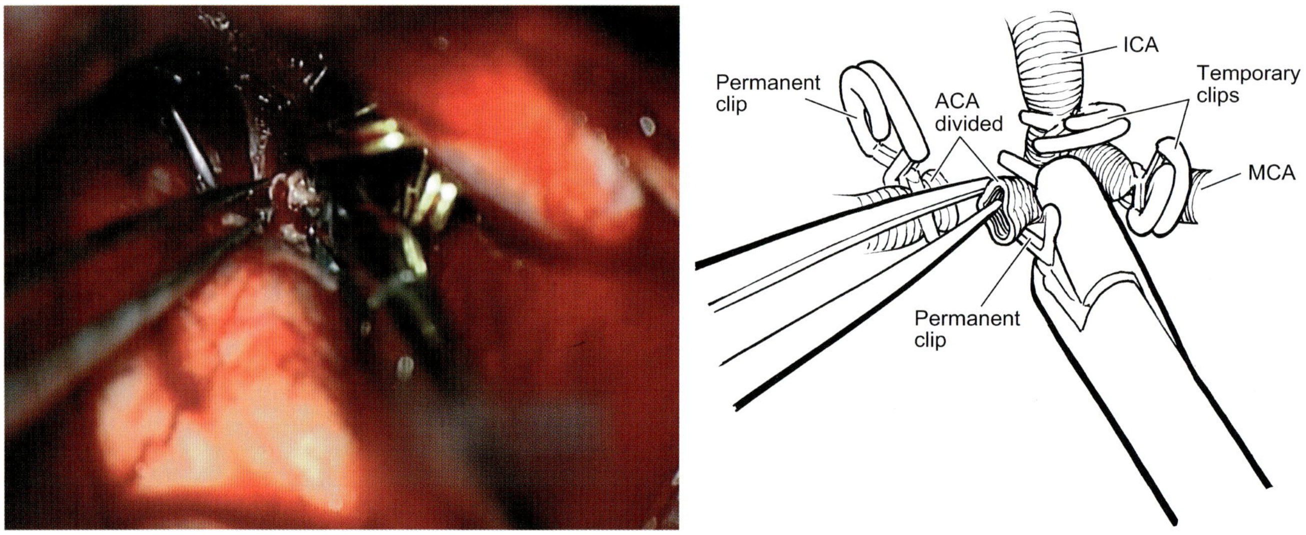

Fig. 1.6k After the tear is closed, the ACA opening is closed with a permanent clip.

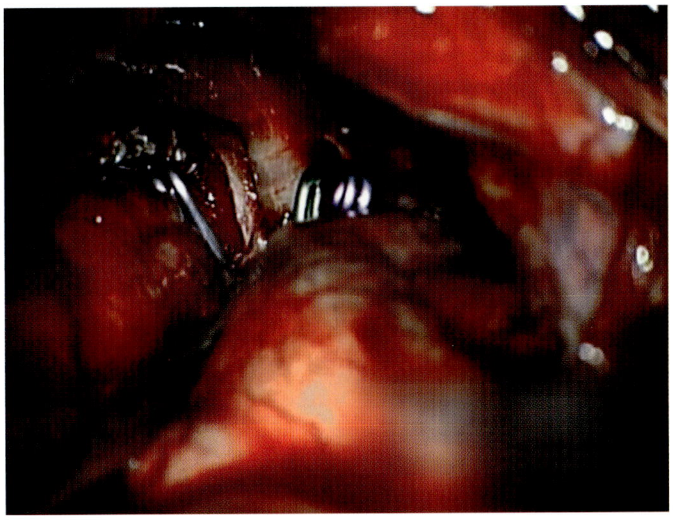
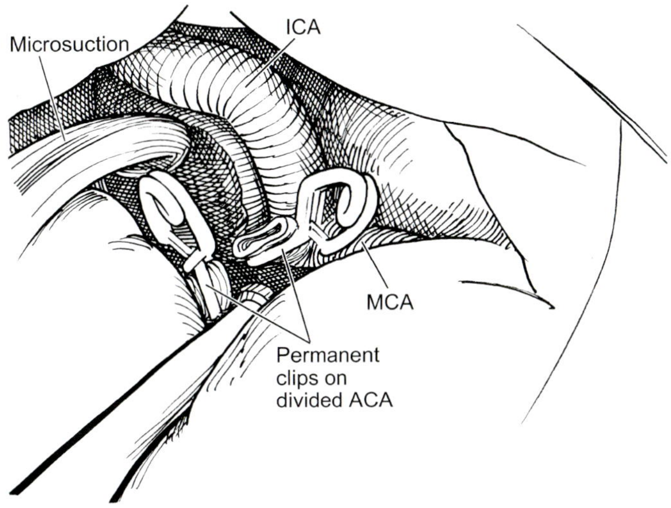

Fig. 1.6l Hemostasis is achieved.

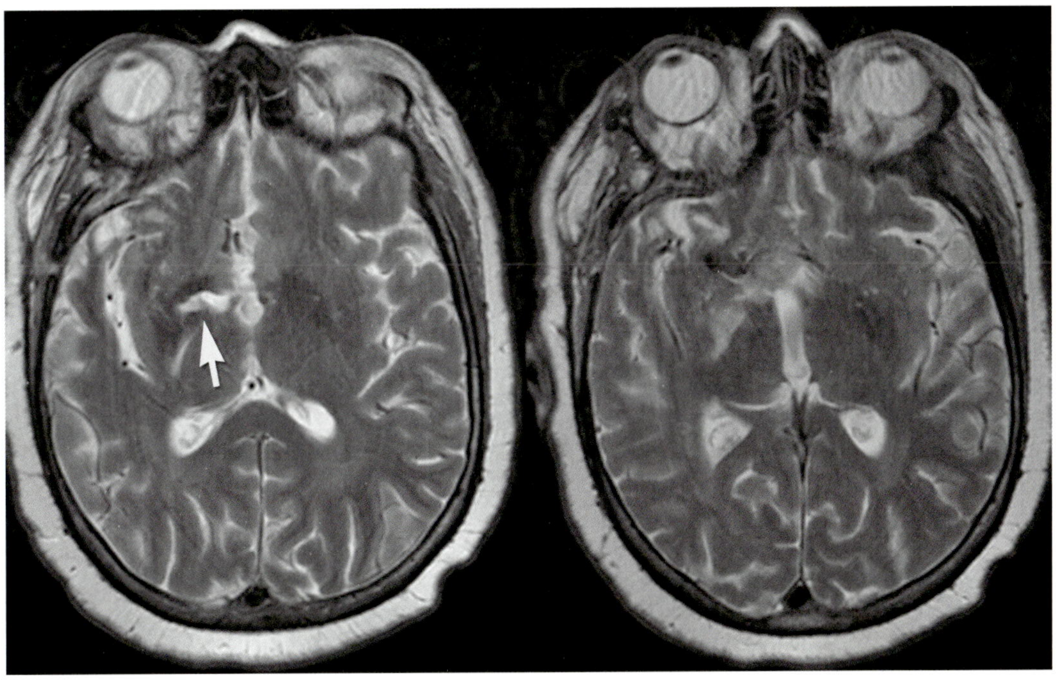

Fig. 1.6m Postoperative MR images show a small infarction (*arrow*) that was probably related to damage of a thalamoperforating artery or AChoA and good patency of the MCA. Postoperatively, the patient had temporary weakness that resolved.

2 STA-to-MCA Bypass

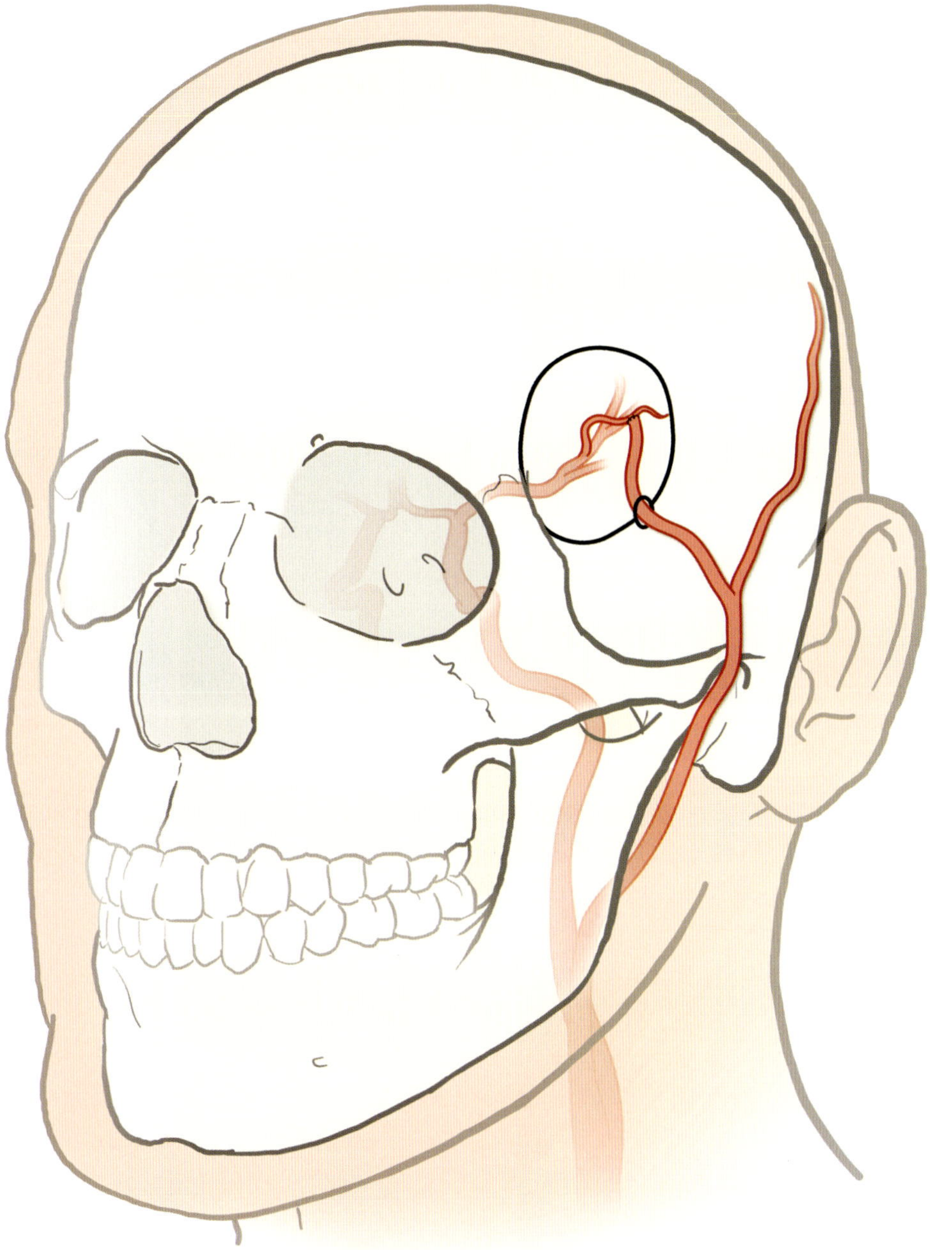

The most commonly performed low-flow bypass is from the STA to the MCA. This bypass, which was first introduced to the neurosurgical community by Drs. Yasargil and Donaghy, has the ability to revascularize the MCA. The STA branch under consideration—either the frontal or parietal branch—can usually be identified with a Doppler probe. For the basic bypass, the branch is outlined and the incision is made directly over the artery. The artery is gently dissected free and left intact until the time of the anastomosis.

An appropriate recipient MCA branch can be located 6 cm above the external auditory canal perpendicular to a line that runs from the external auditory canal to the zygomatic prominence. When a 3-cm opening is made at that point, an appropriate MCA branch can be identified and freed of its arachnoid adhesions. Either running or interrupted 10–0 or 11–0 sutures are used to perform a bypass between these two vessels.

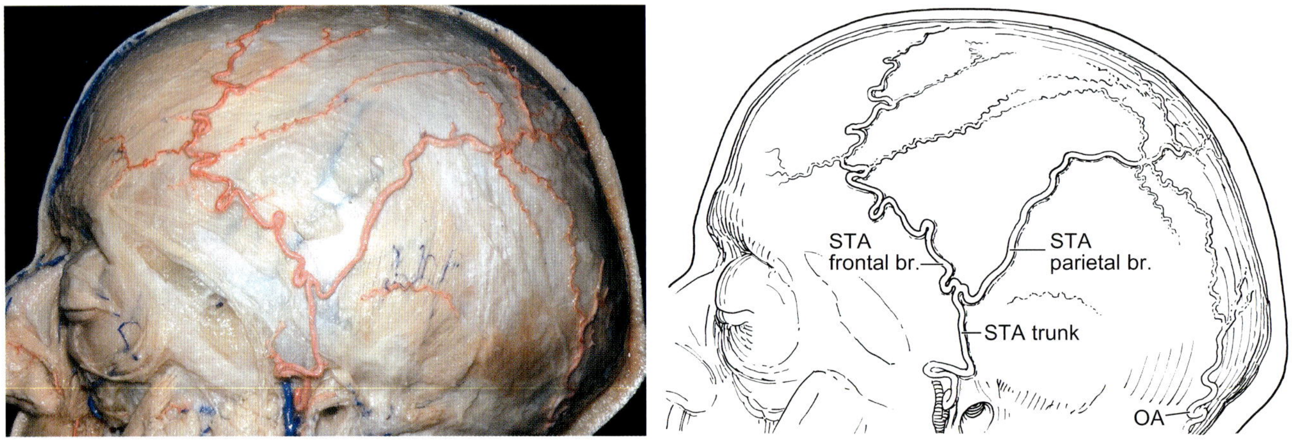

Fig. 2.0a Exposure of the scalp vessels shows the frontal and parietal branches of the STA. The anastomotic connections between the various scalp vessels, which are beautifully demonstrated, are clearly a reason that one of these vessels can be harvested without the risk of scalp necrosis. (Photograph used with permission from *Journal of Neurosurgery*.)

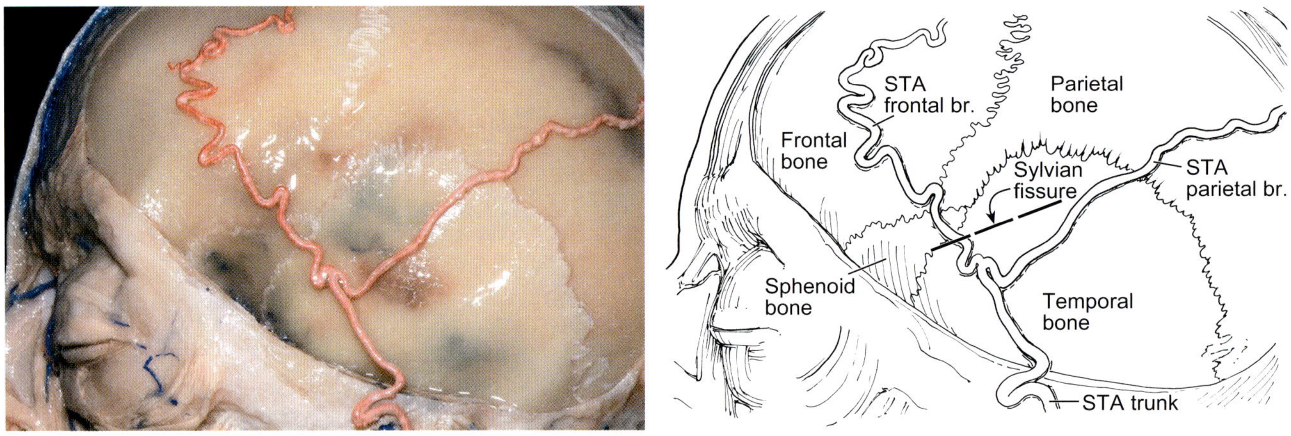

Fig. 2.0b After the subcutaneous tissues and muscles have been removed, the STA and its two branches are visible. The *dashed line* demonstrates the sylvian fissure below the skull. (Photograph used with permission from *Journal of Neurosurgery*.)

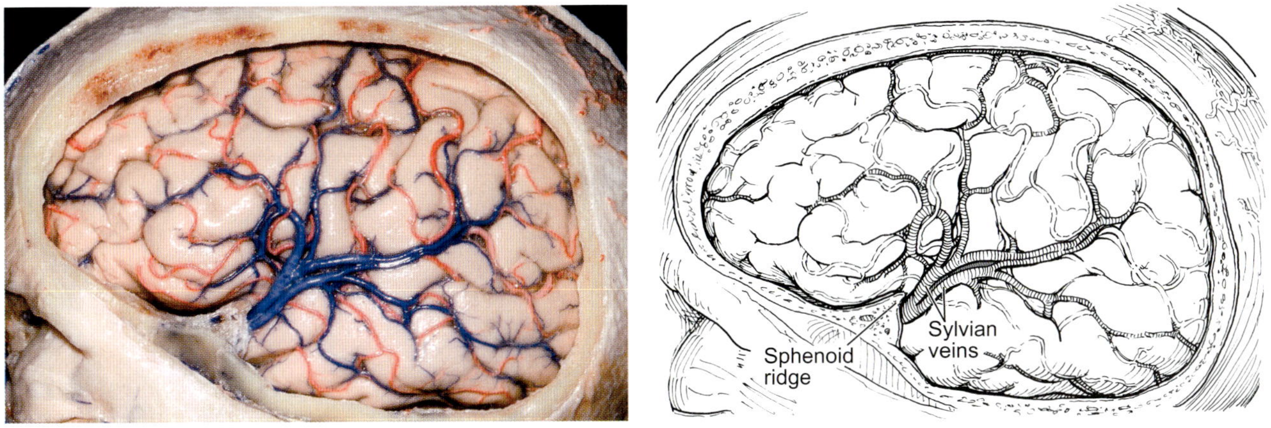

Fig. 2.0c With the skull flap removed, the sylvian fissure and the branches of the arteries and veins on the surface of the cerebrum are visible.

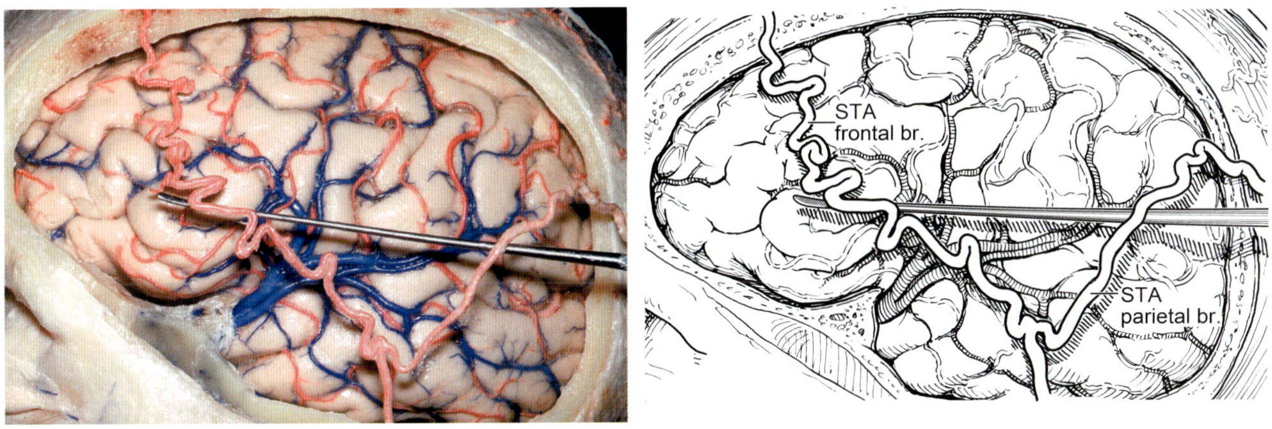

Fig. 2.0d The STA and its two branches are laid over the exposed cortical surface. (Photograph used with permission from *Journal of Neurosurgery*.)

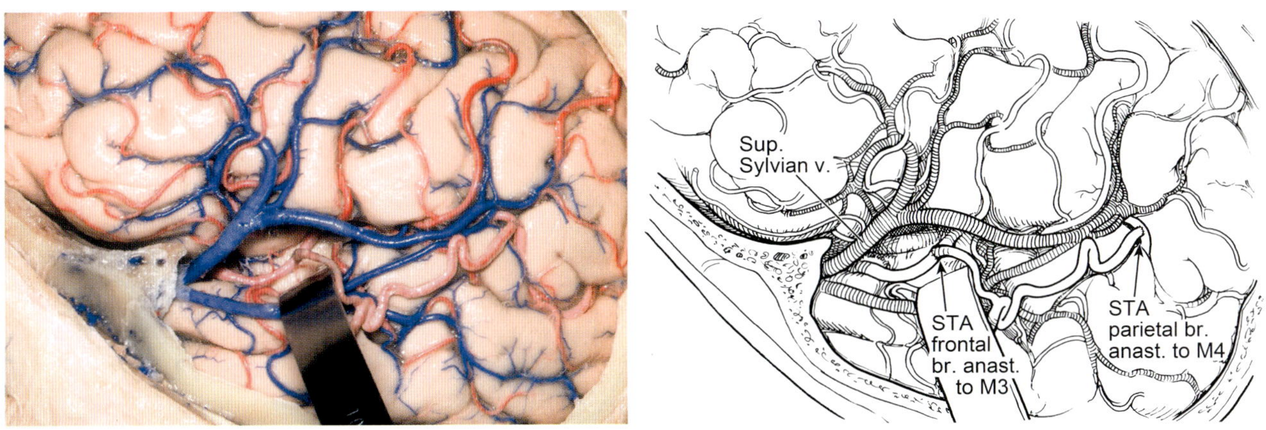

Fig. 2.0e The sylvian fissure is opened, and the frontal branch of the STA is anastomosed to an M3 branch of the MCA within the fissure. The parietal branch of the STA is anastomosed to an M4 branch. (Photograph used with permission from *Journal of Neurosurgery*.)

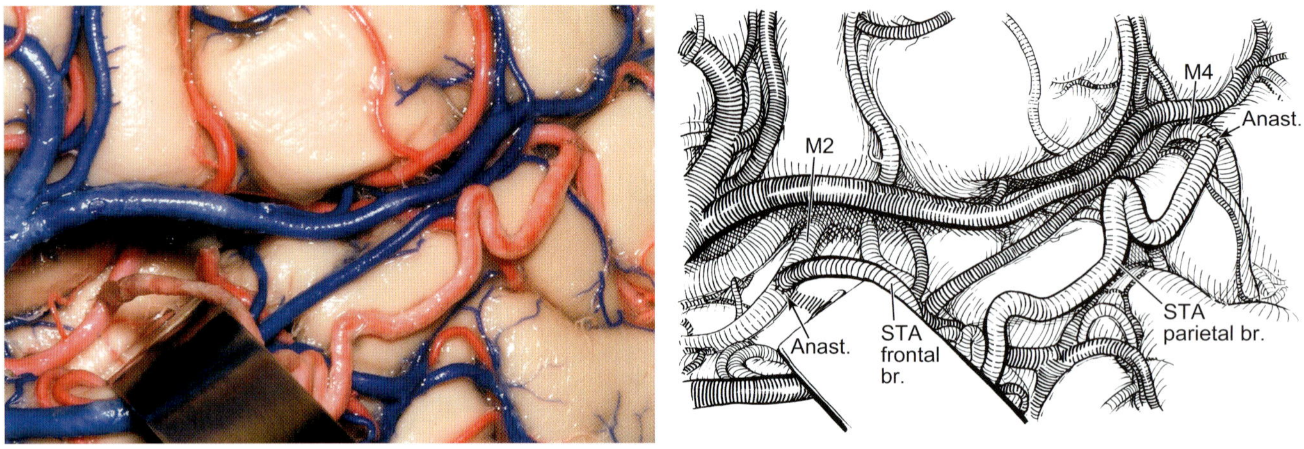

Fig. 2.0f A high-power view shows the frontal and parietal branches of the STA anastomosed to the MCA branches. (Photograph used with permission from *Journal of Neurosurgery*.)

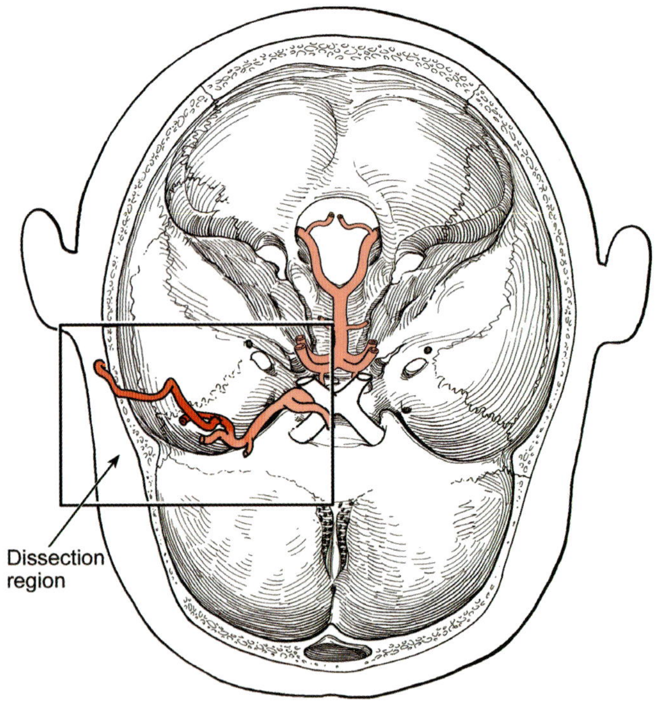

Fig. 2.0g Inset shows orientation overview. After the brain has been removed, the anastomosis of the STA to an M2 branch of the MCA is visible from a superior view. (Photograph used with permission from *Journal of Neurosurgery*.)

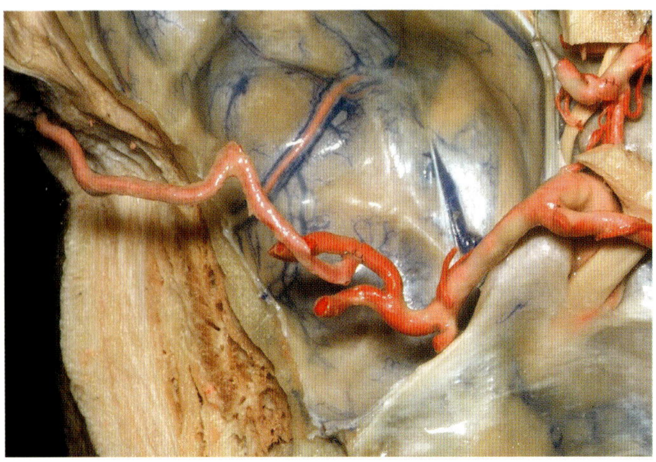

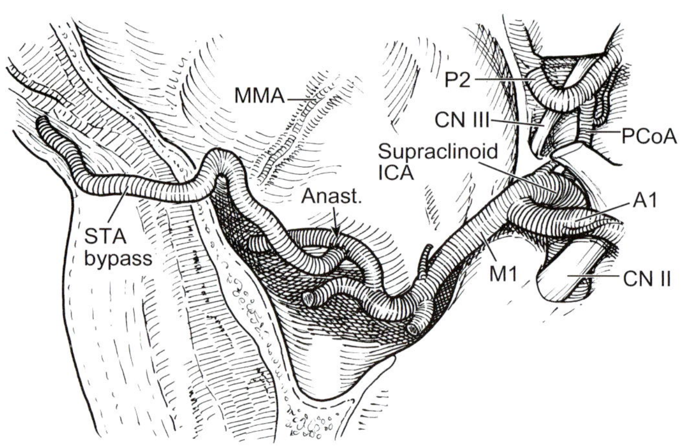

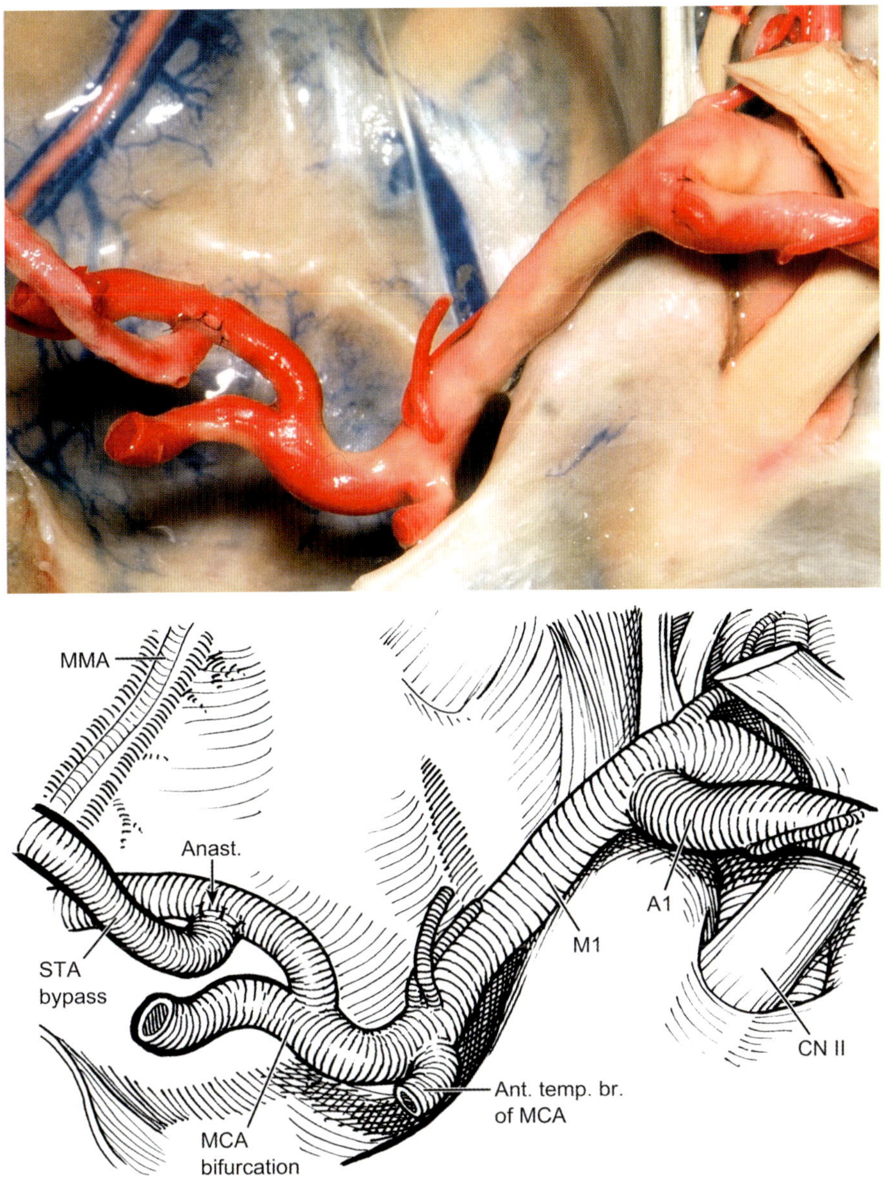

Fig. 2.0h Close-up view shows the anastomosis of the STA to the M2 branch of the MCA. (Photograph used with permission from *Journal of Neurosurgery*.)

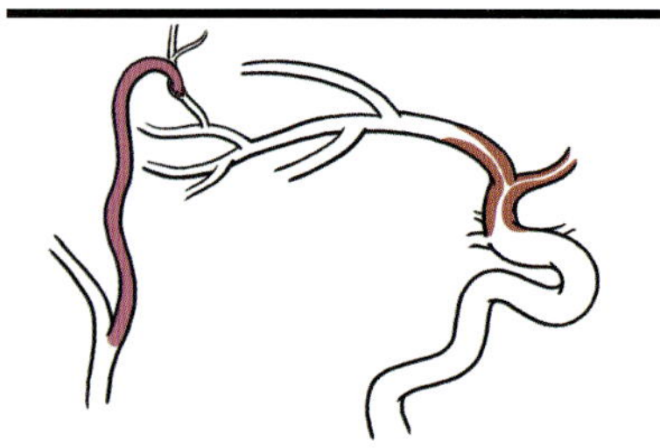

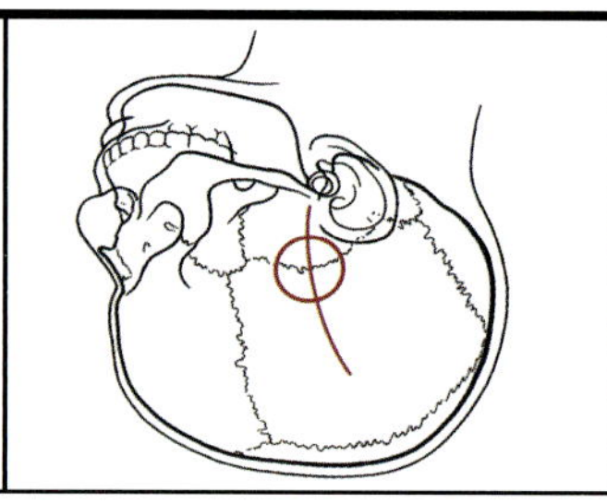

Case 2-1

Diagnosis: Moyamoya disease

Bypass: STA-to-MCA

Approach: Right temporal

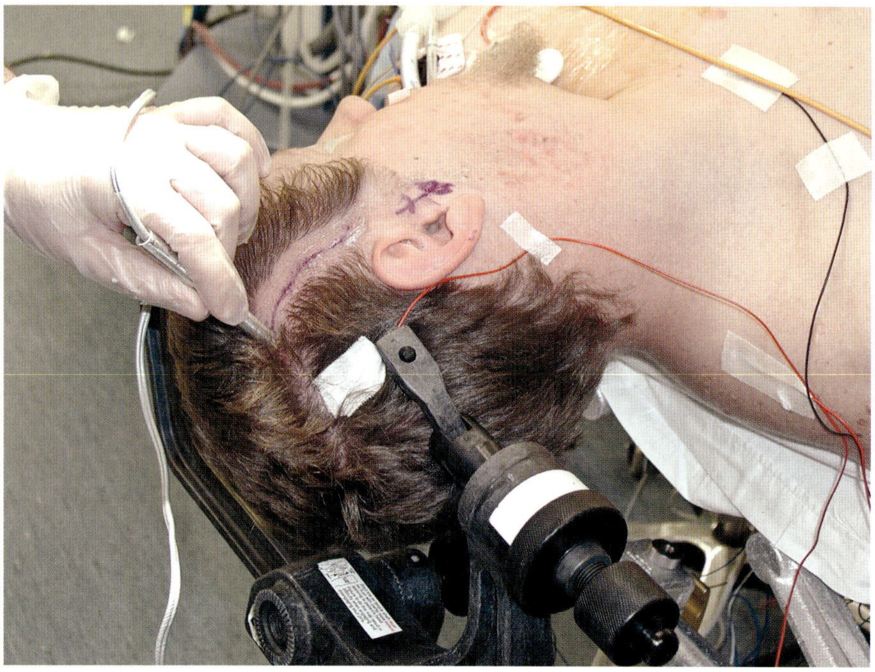

Fig. 2.1a The parietal branch of the STA is insonated and the hair is clipped over the course of the vessel.

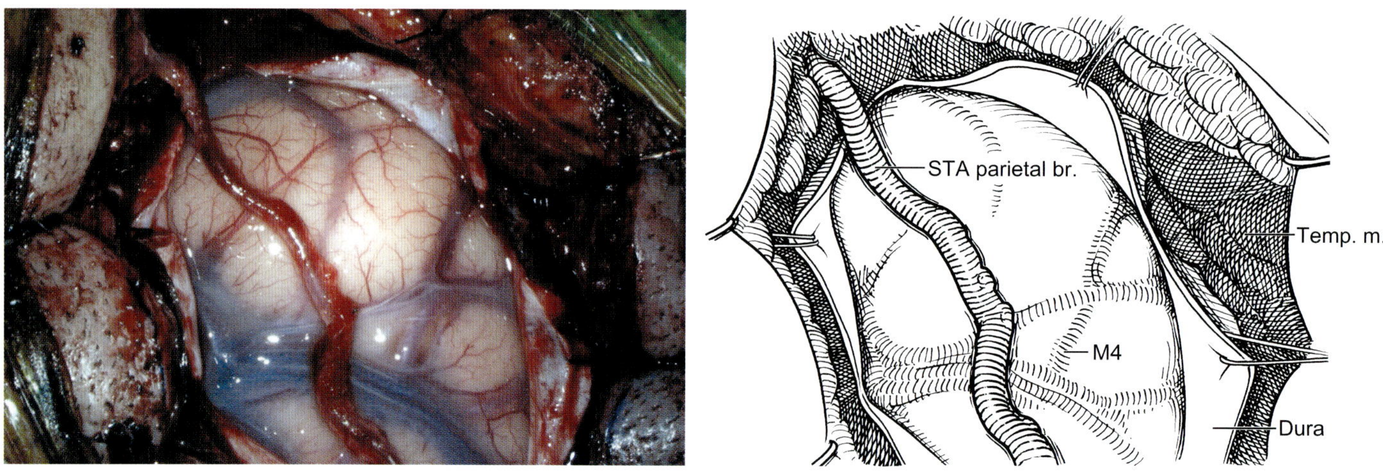

Fig. 2.1b After the STA has been dissected free, a craniotomy with approximately a 3-cm diameter is performed to expose a cortical branch of the MCA.

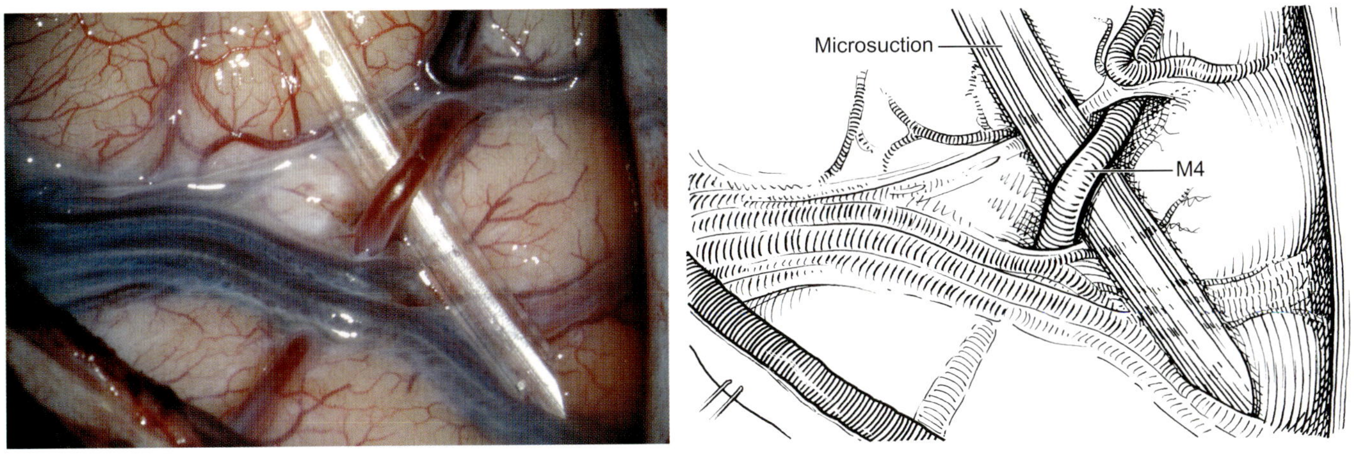

Fig. 2.1c After the superficial MCA branch has been dissected free, Spetzler MicroVac suction tubing (P.M.T. Inc, Hopkins, MN) is placed underneath the vessel to remove the fluid, which is used to irrigate constantly throughout the bypass.

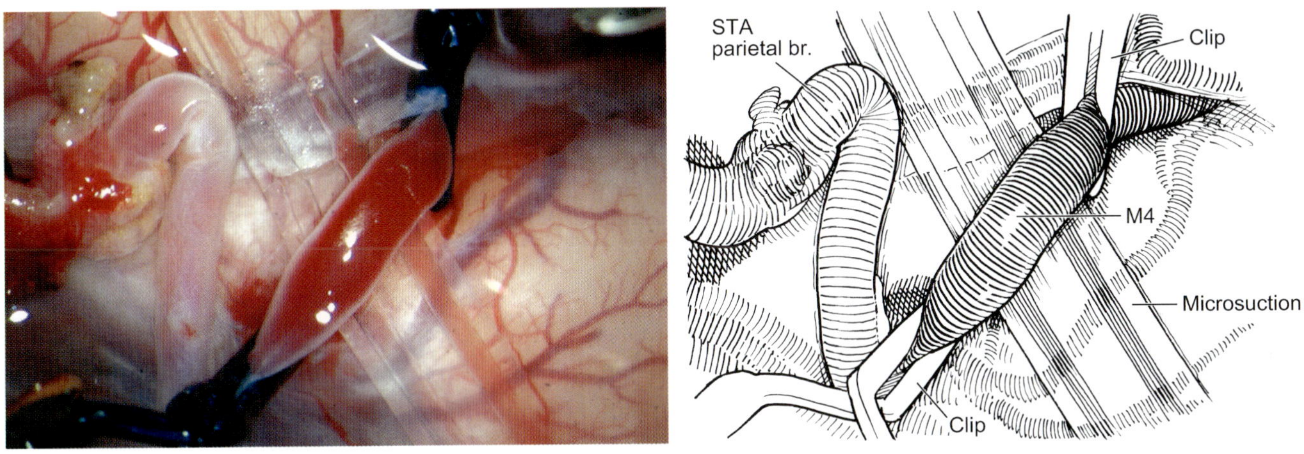

Fig. 2.1d Before the MCA branch is opened, small temporary clips are placed at either end of the vessel.

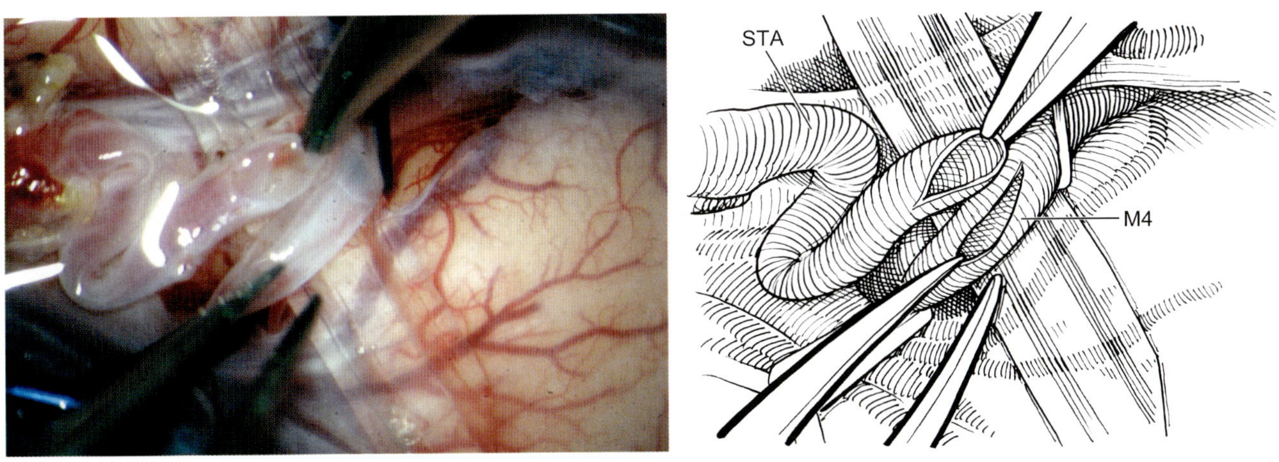

Fig. 2.1e The end of the STA is cut at a bevel and slit at the base until it matches the length of the MCA opening.

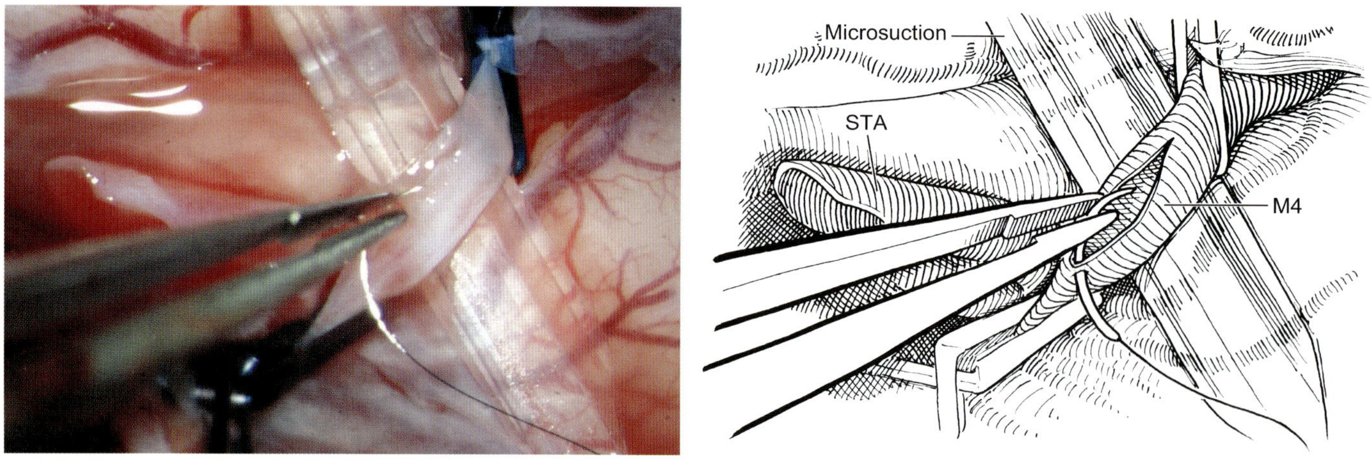

Fig. 2.1f The first suture is placed in the end of the MCA opening and then hooked to the heel of the fishmouthed STA.

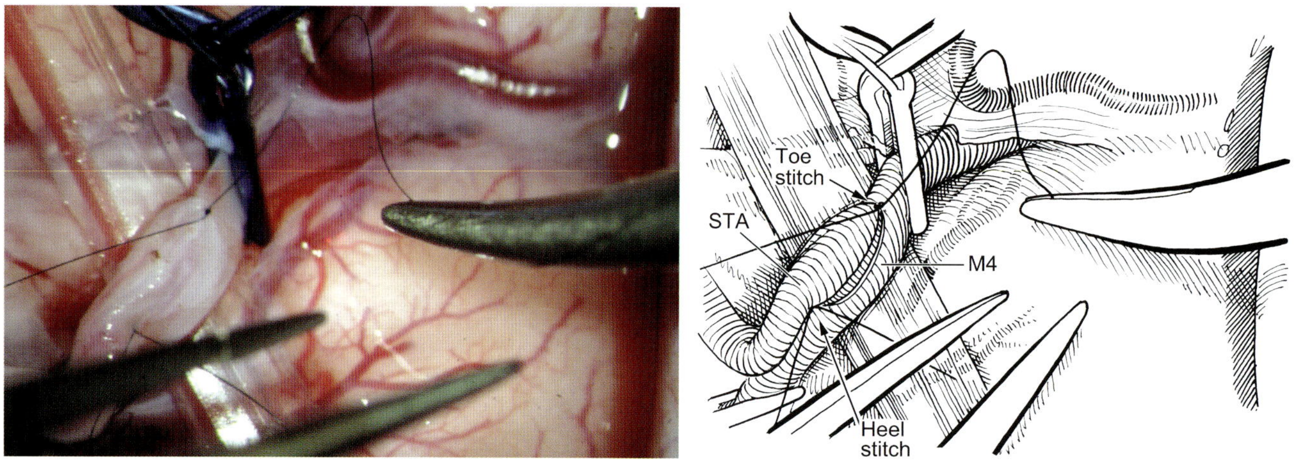

Fig. 2.1g The second suture goes from the other end of the MCA opening to the toe of the fishmouthed STA.

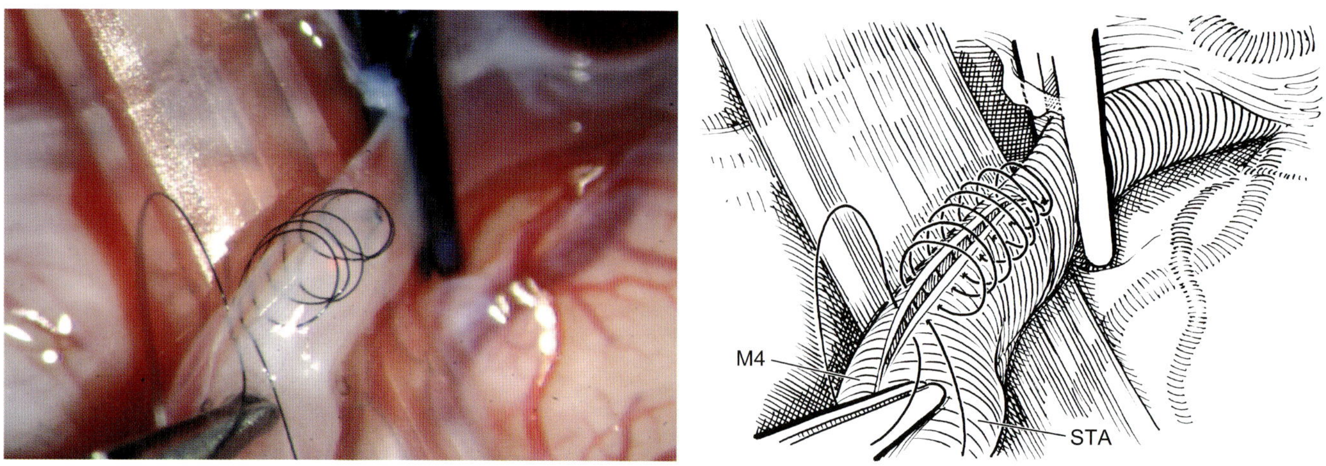

Fig. 2.1h A running suture is performed along one side of the two vessels. Tightening the loops at the end of the bypass keeps the edges of the vessels visible. Alternatively, interrupted sutures can be placed.

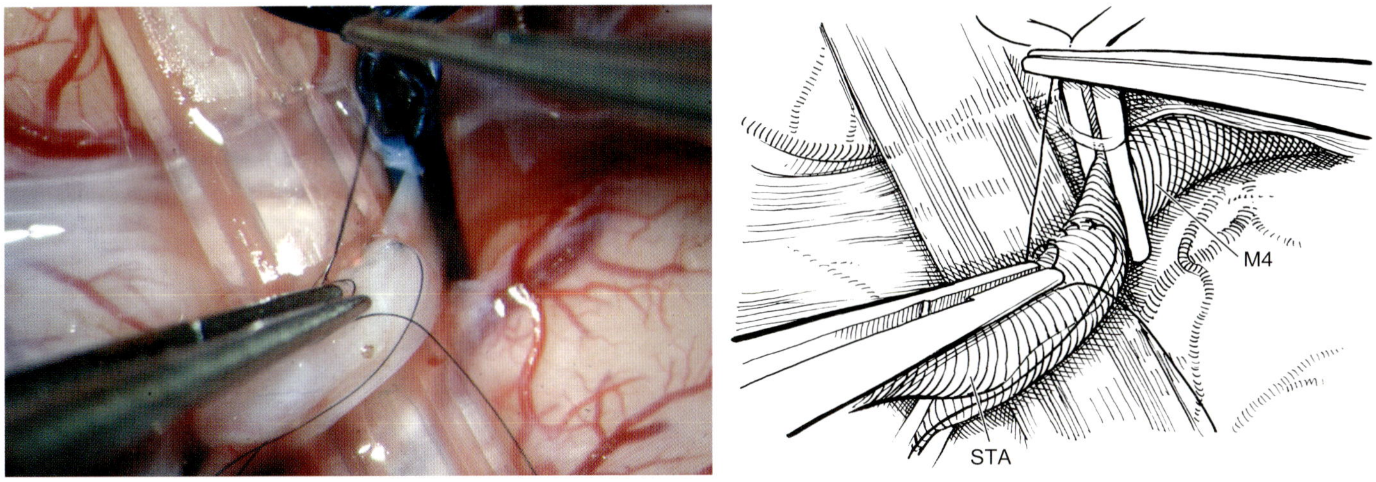

Fig. 2.1i The vessel loops are tightened.

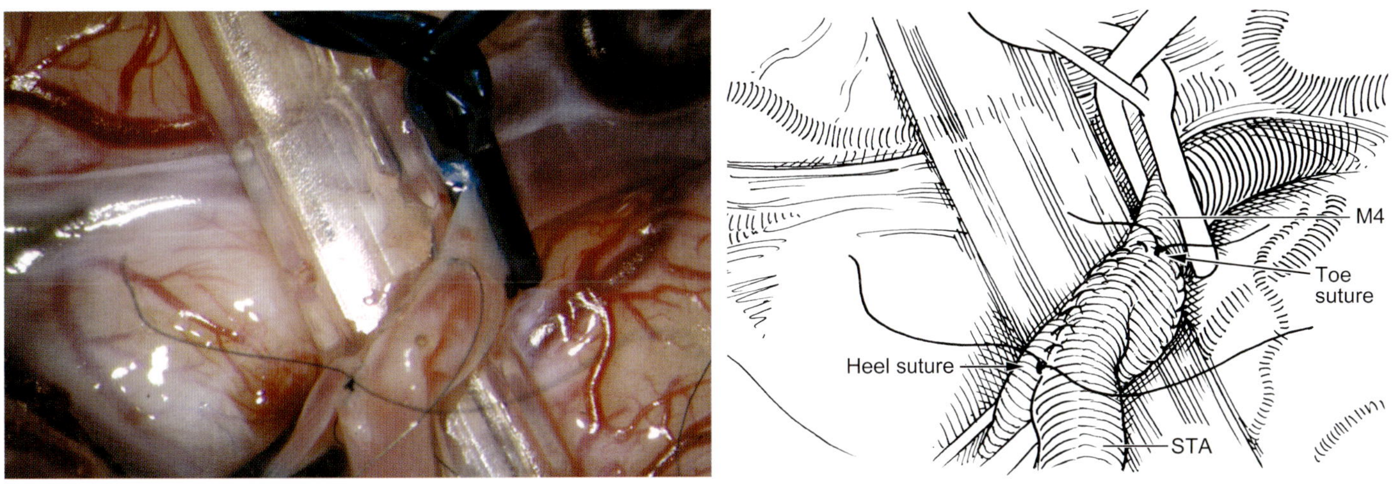

Fig. 2.1j The two sutures are tied to the previously placed heel and toe knots.

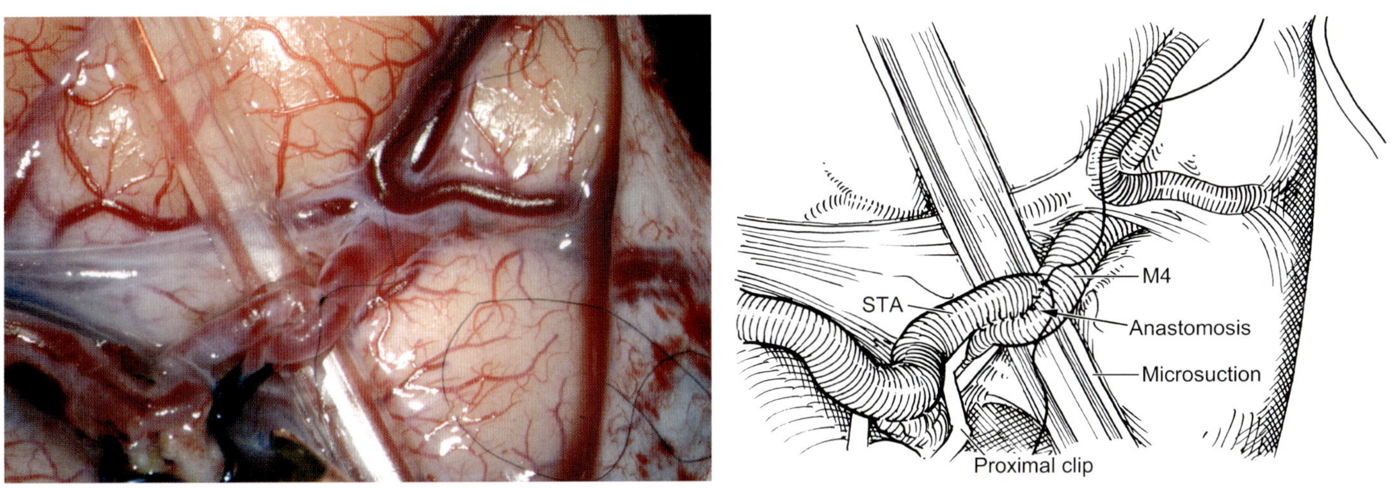

Fig. 2.1k The anastomosis has been completed.

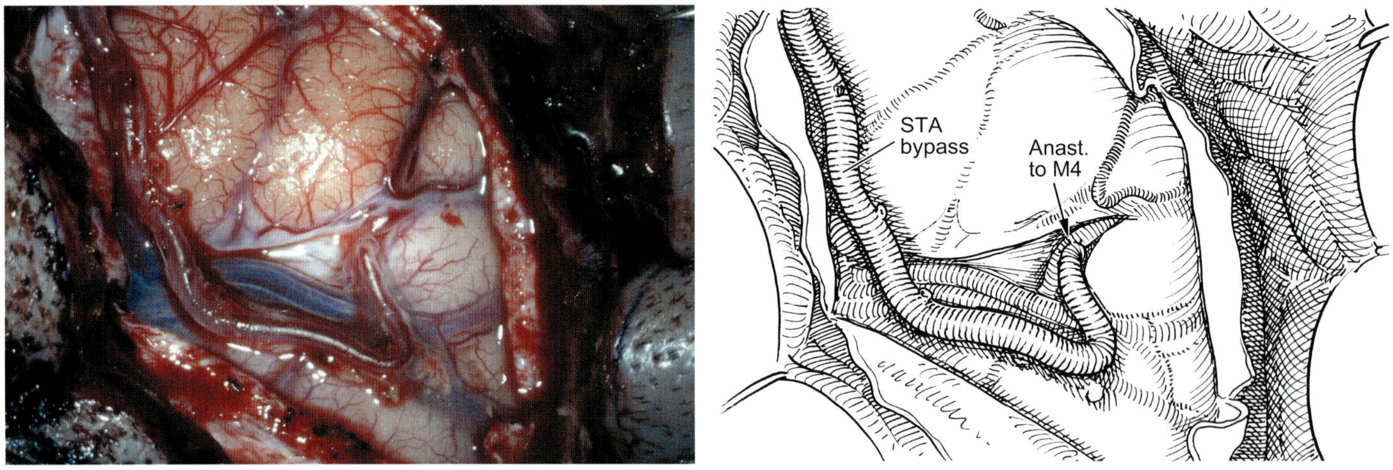

Fig. 2.1l Overview of the anastomosis.

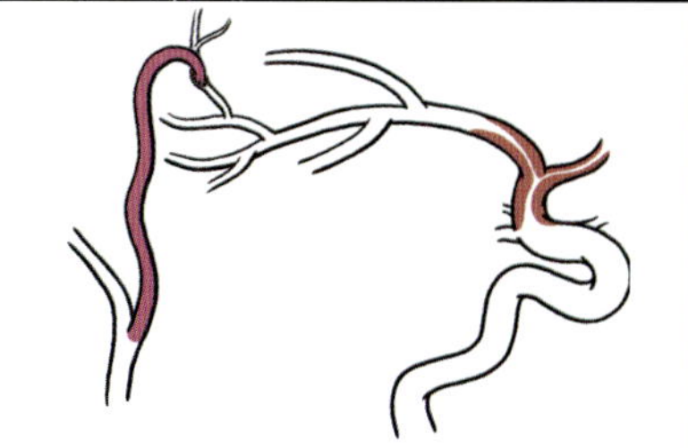

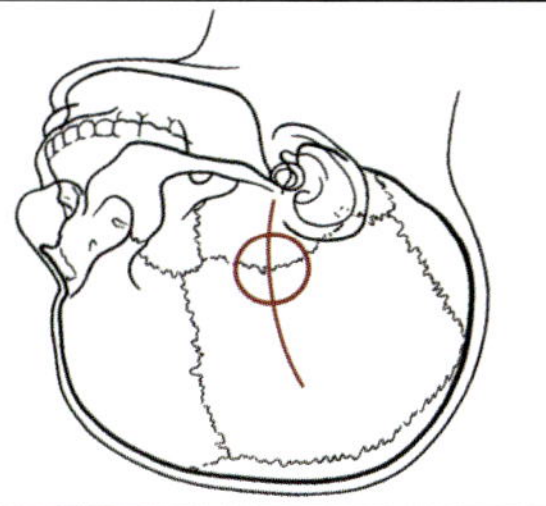

Case 2-2

Diagnosis: Moyamoya disease

Bypass: STA-to-MCA

Approach: Right temporal

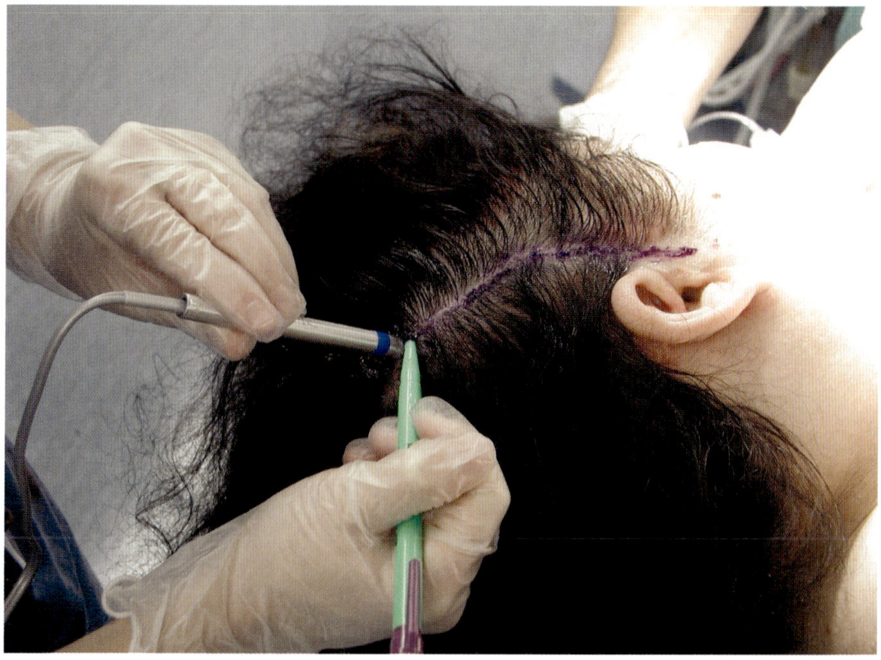

Fig. 2.2a The course of the STA is marked on the skin using a Doppler pen probe.

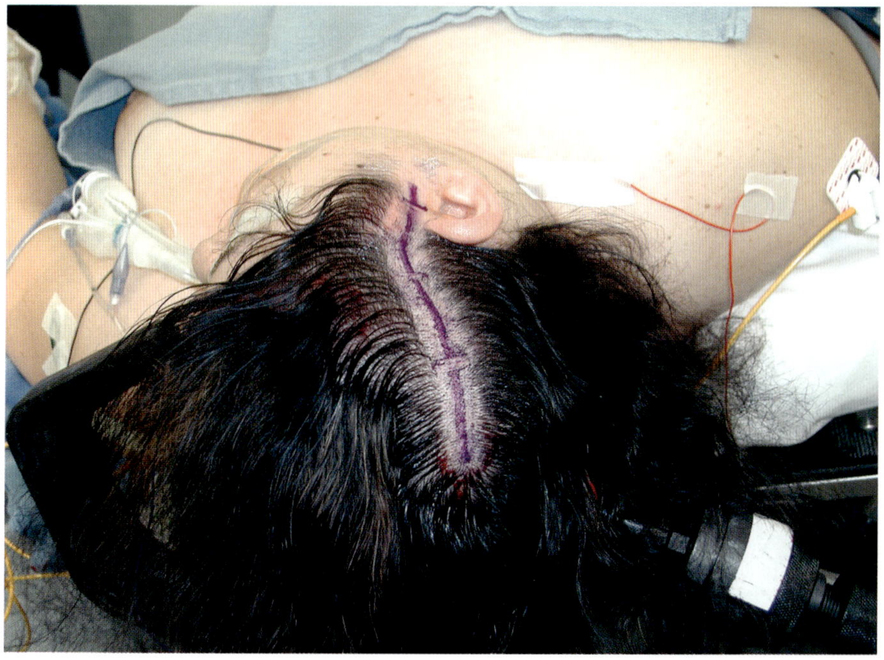

Fig. 2.2b A narrow strip shave is performed. In most cases the parietal division of the STA begins anterior to the ear and courses superiorly and slightly posteriorly.

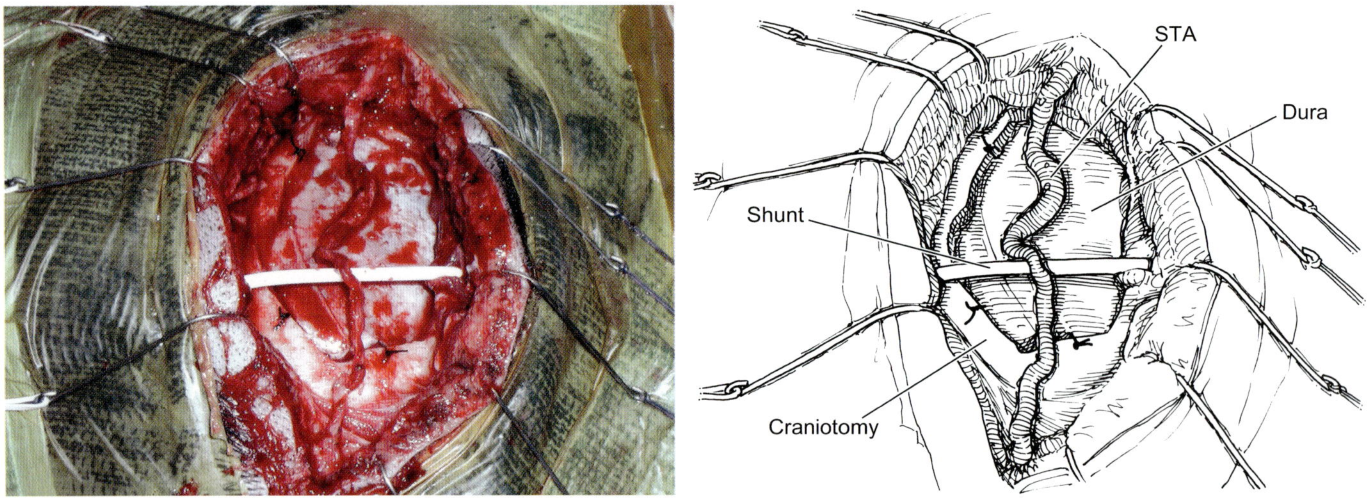

Fig. 2.2c The dissected STA is shown. The patient's shunt crosses the field and has been preserved intact. Fishhooks are used to retract the edges of the scalp incision, flattening the operative field. This technique allows the surgeon's hands to work closer to the anastomosis.

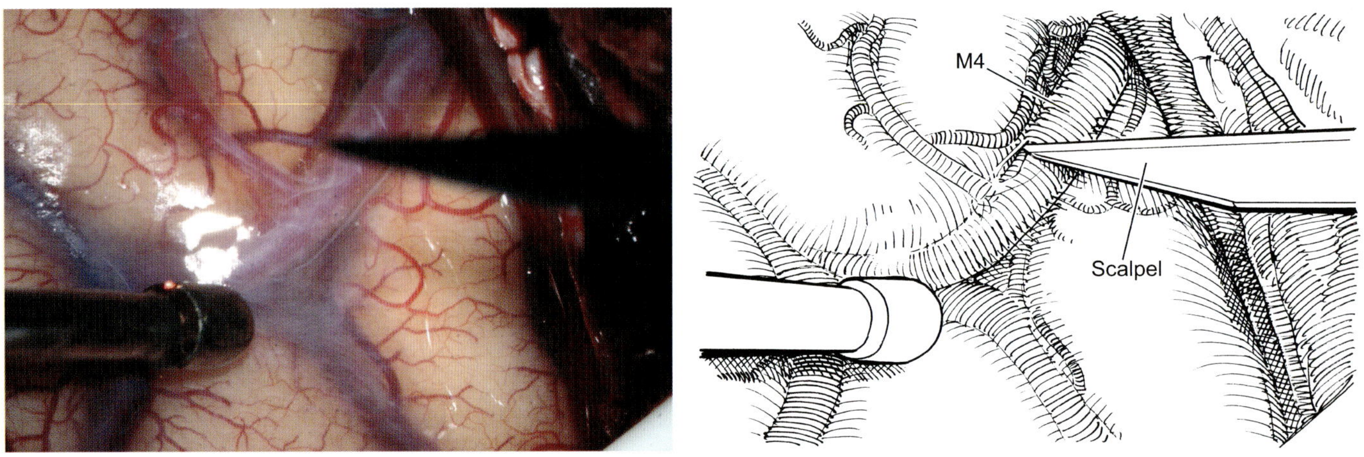

Fig. 2.2d A cortical branch of the MCA is identified under the arachnoid.

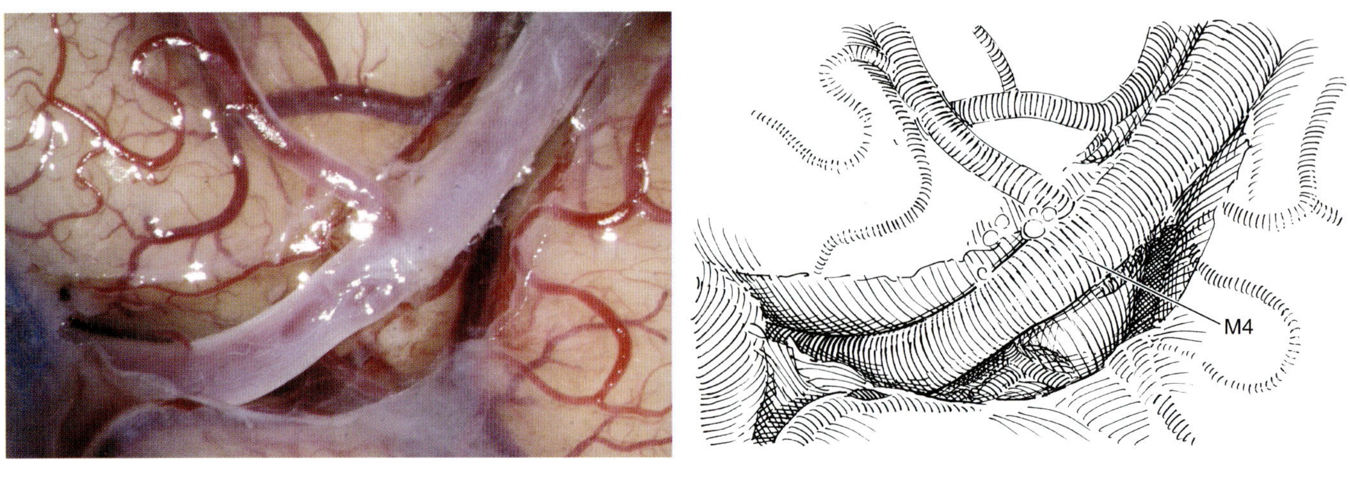

Fig. 2.2e The branch is dissected free.

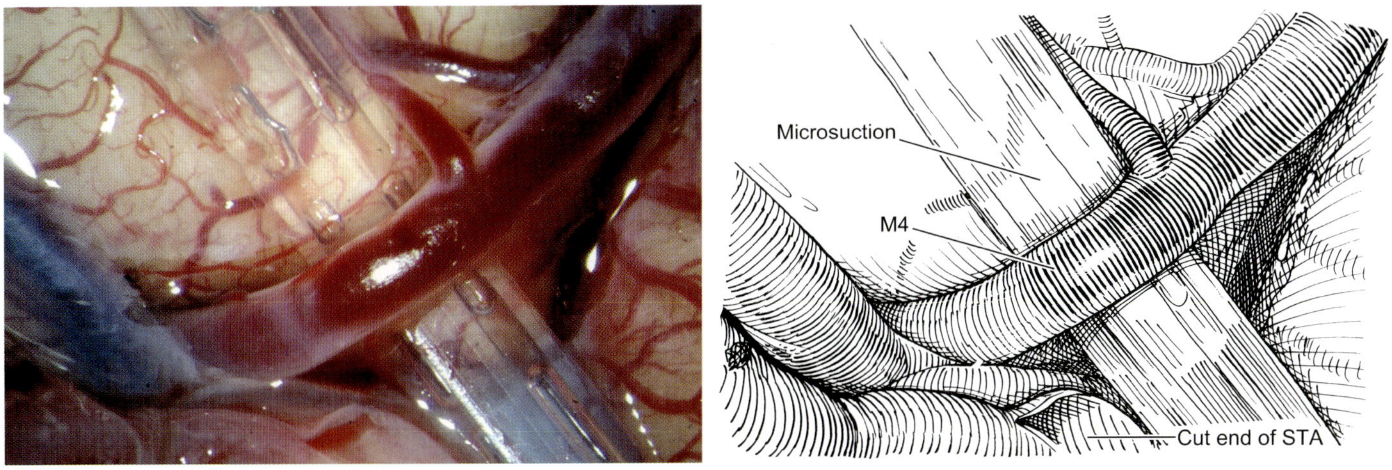

Fig. 2.2f The Spetzler MicroVac suction tubing (P.M.T. Inc, Hopkins, MN) is placed below the branch to clear any blood and cerebrospinal fluid.

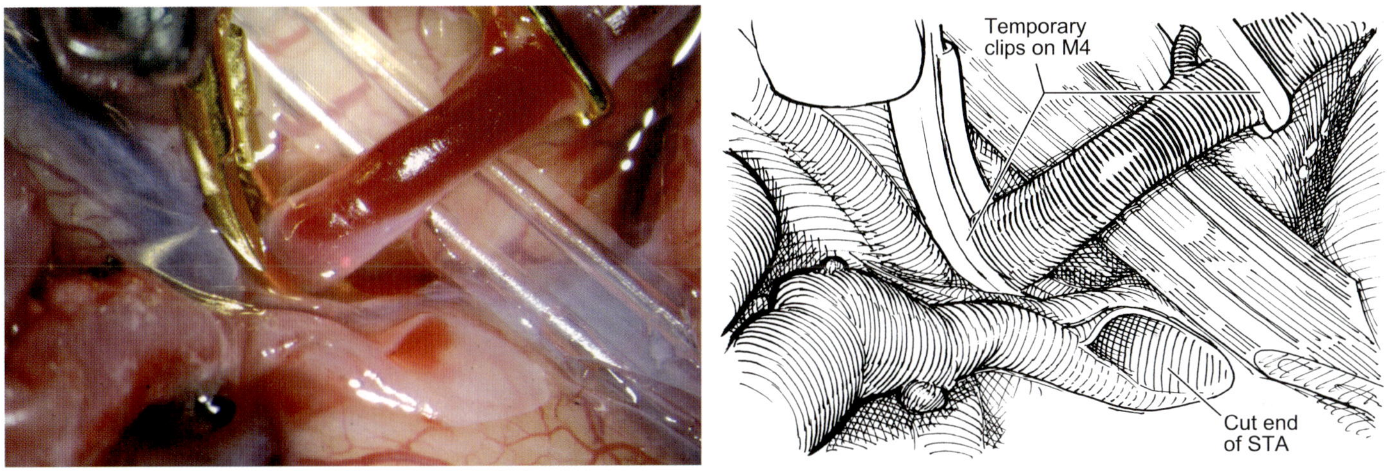

Fig. 2.2g Temporary clips are applied.

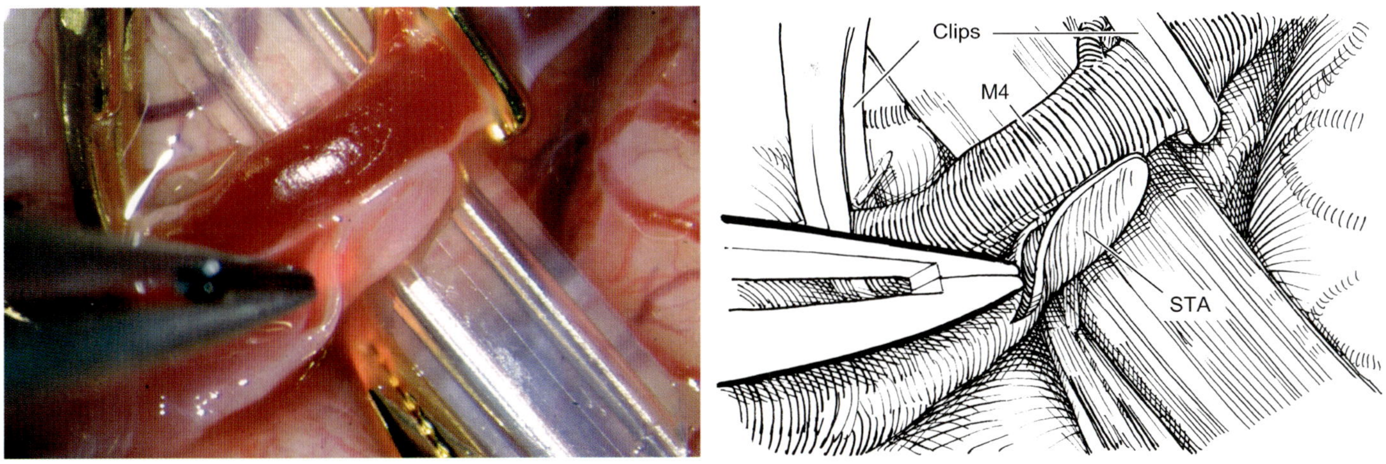

Fig. 2.2h The STA is apposed to the MCA.

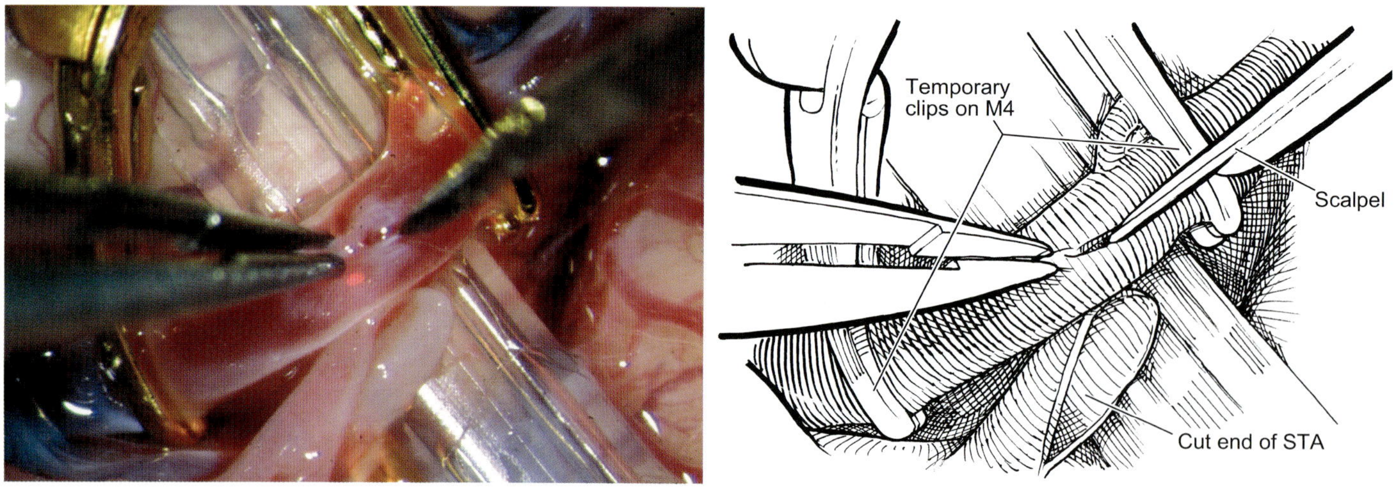

Fig. 2.2i The MCA branch is opened with a no. 11 blade.

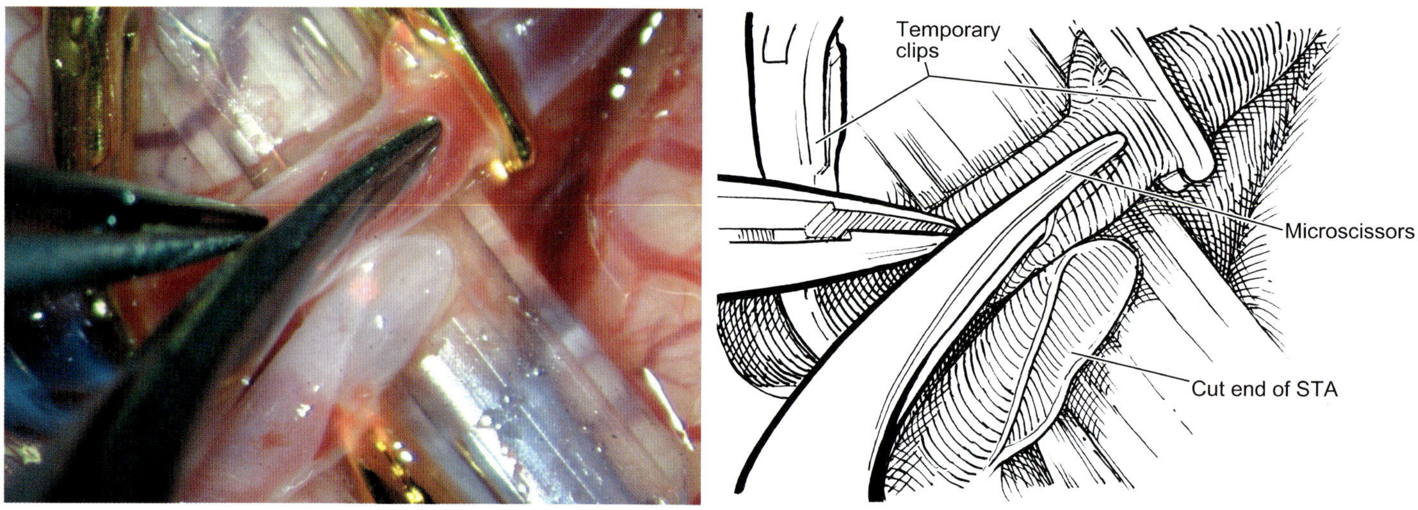

Fig. 2.2j The opening is expanded with a small pair of microscissors.

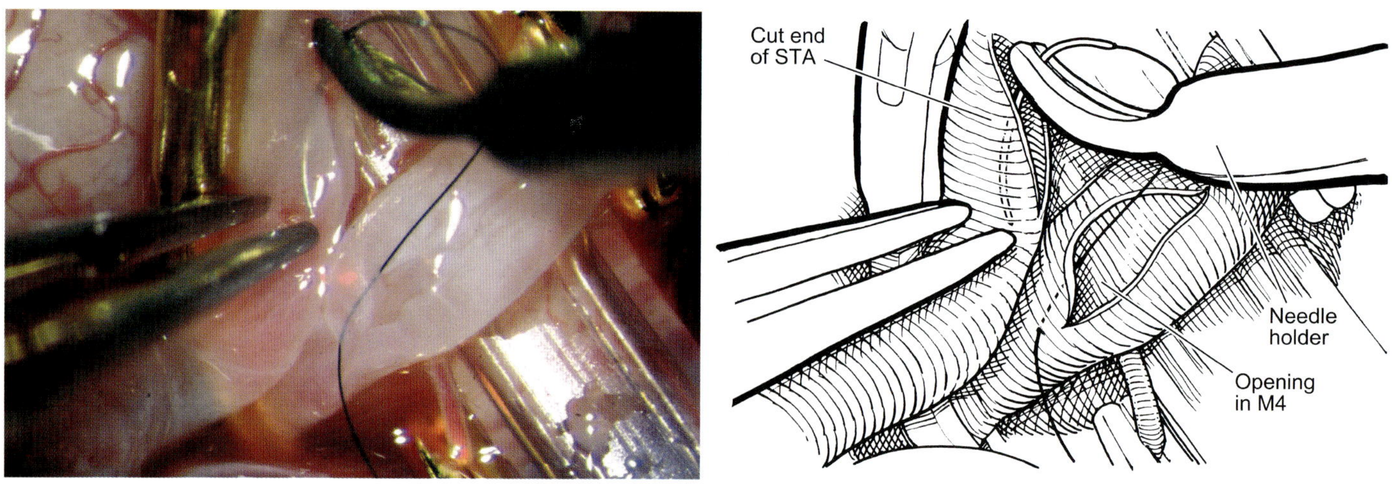

Fig. 2.2k A heel stitch 10–0 suture is placed from outside to inside the lumen of the MCA and then from inside to outside the lumen of the STA so that the knot remains on the outside of the anastomosis.

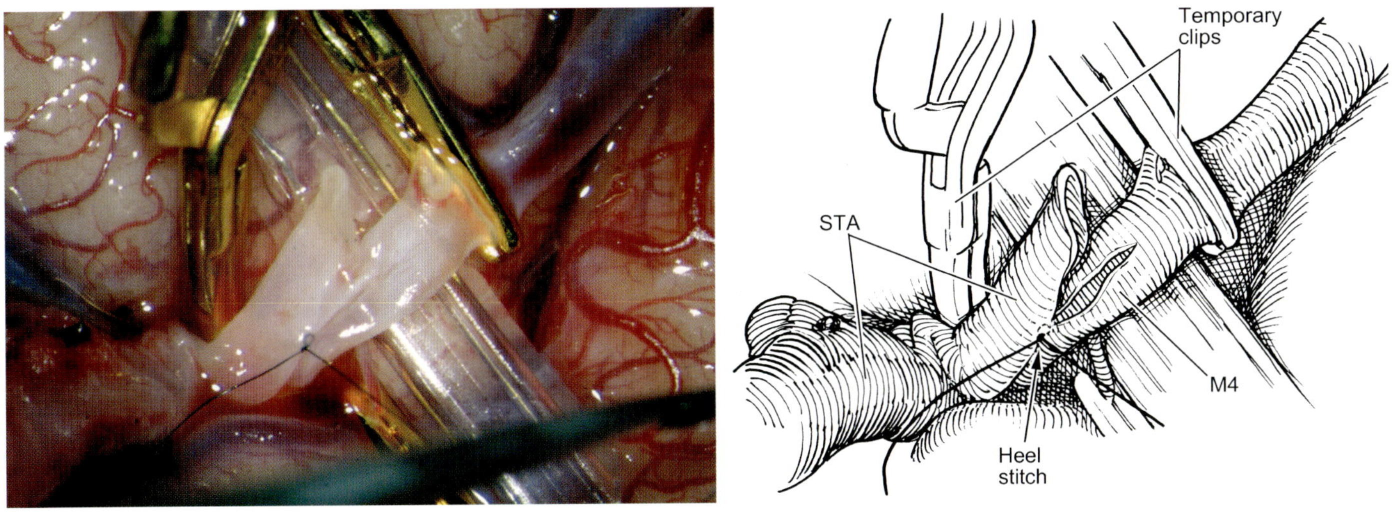

Fig. 2.2l The heel stitch is tightened.

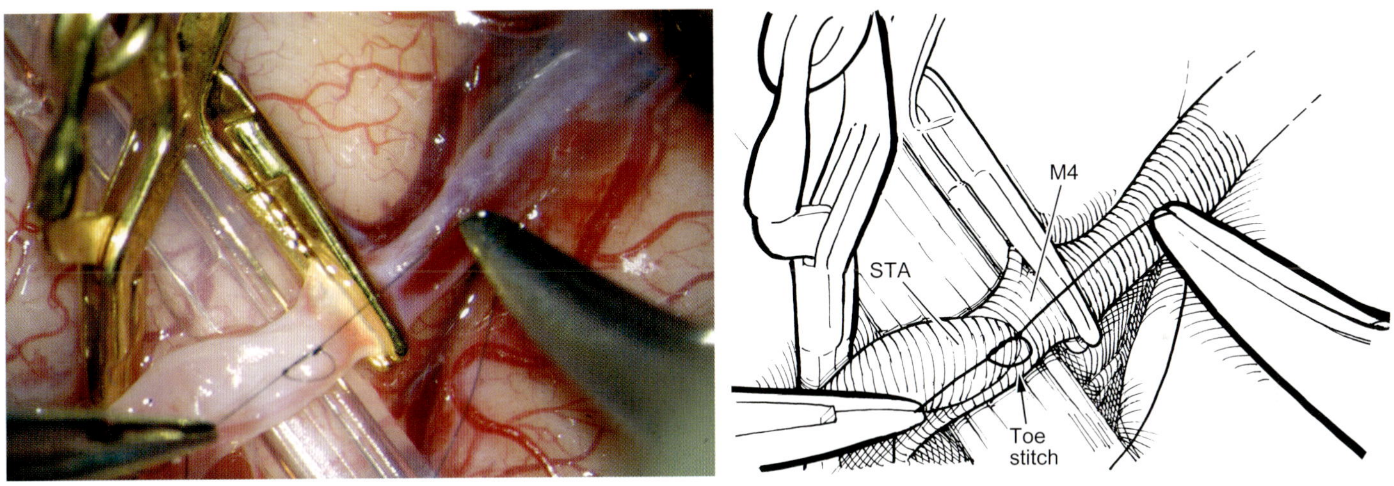

Fig. 2.2m The toe stitch is placed and tightened.

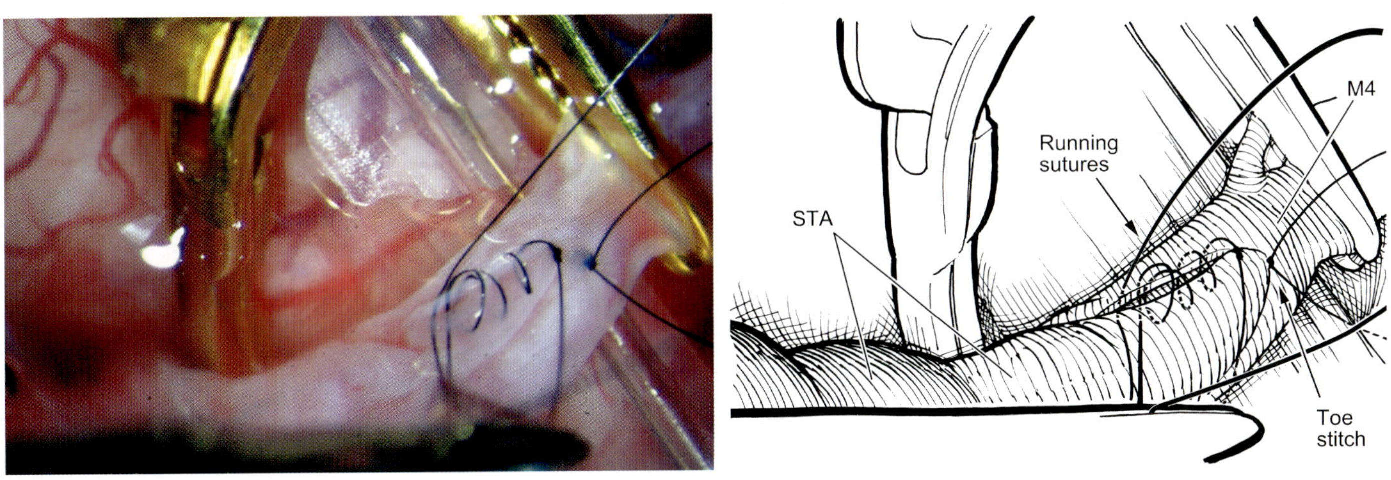

Fig. 2.2n Each stitch is placed loosely as shown, and then each stitch is tightened in turn.

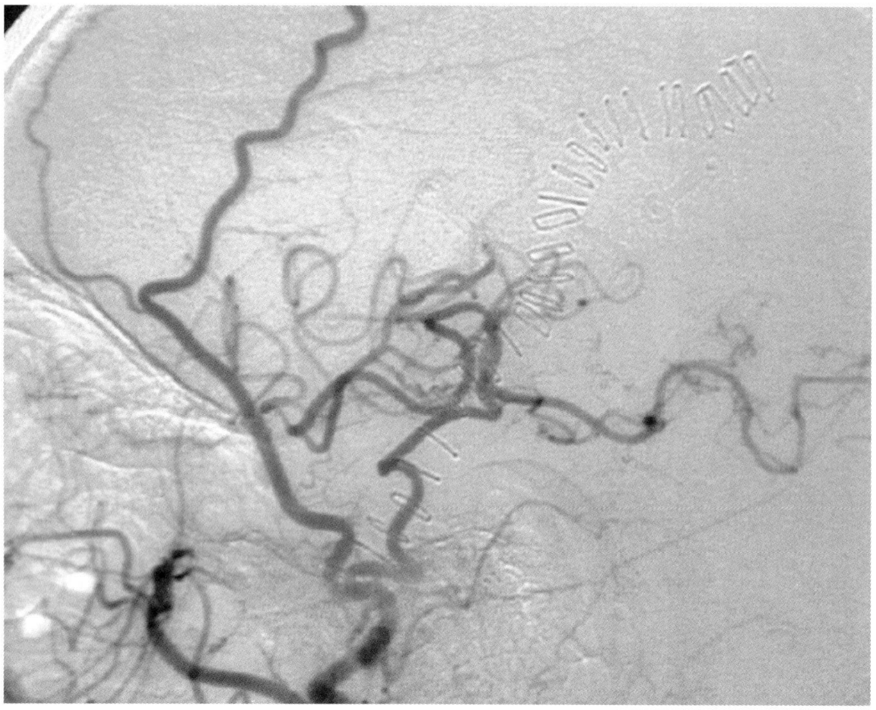

Fig. 2.2o Postoperative angiogram confirms excellent filling of the MCA territory through the bypass.

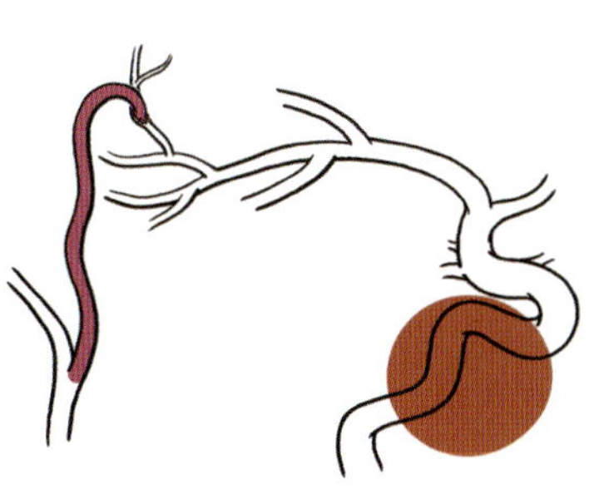

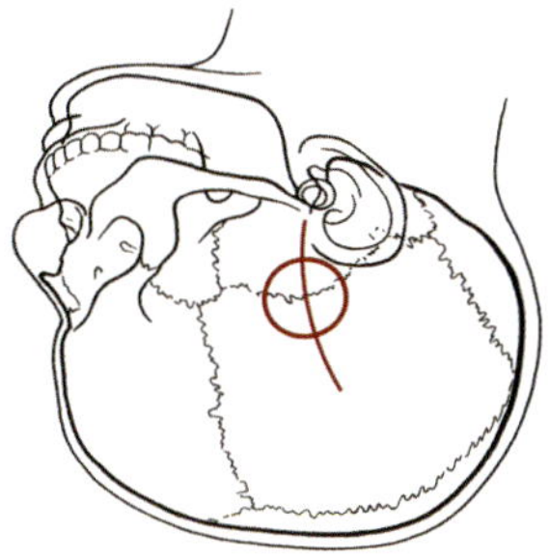

Case 2-3

Diagnosis: Cavernous sinus aneurysm

Bypass: STA-to-MCA

Approach: Right temporal

Video

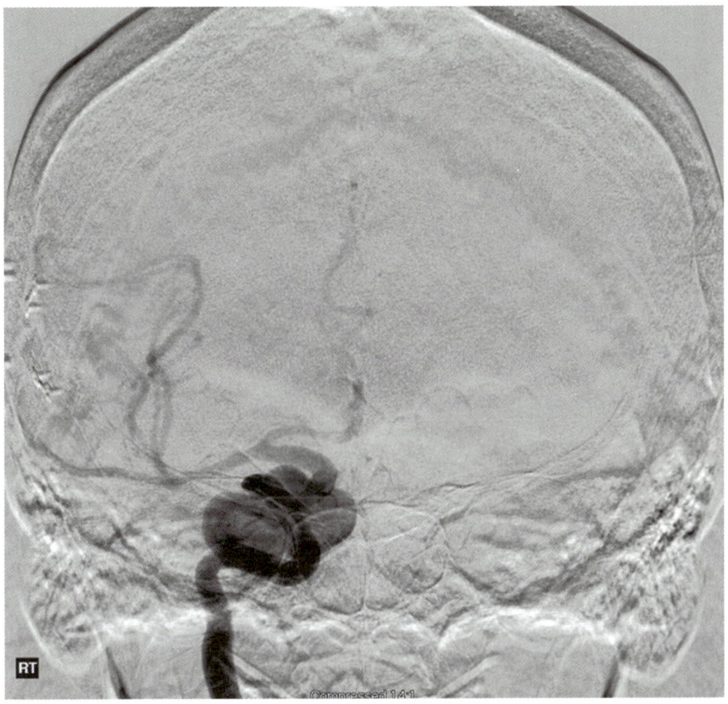

Fig. 2.3a Anteroposterior angiogram of an injection of the right ICA shows a symptomatic giant dysplastic cavernous sinus carotid artery aneurysm.

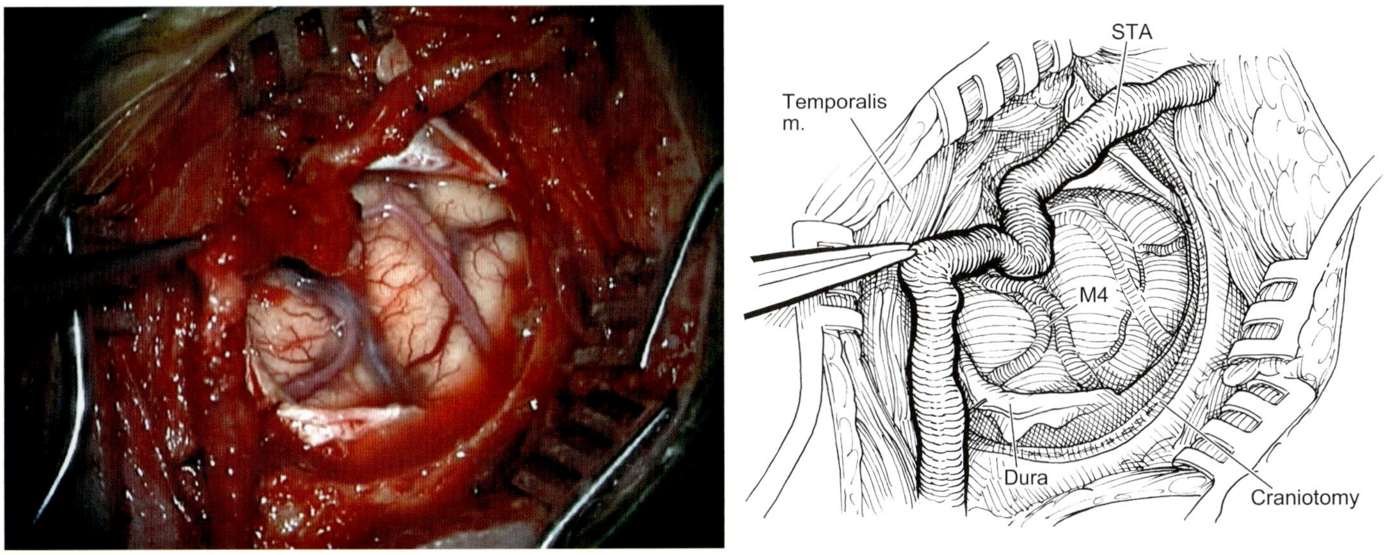

Fig. 2.3b The craniotomy exposes a good recipient MCA vessel on the cortical surface.

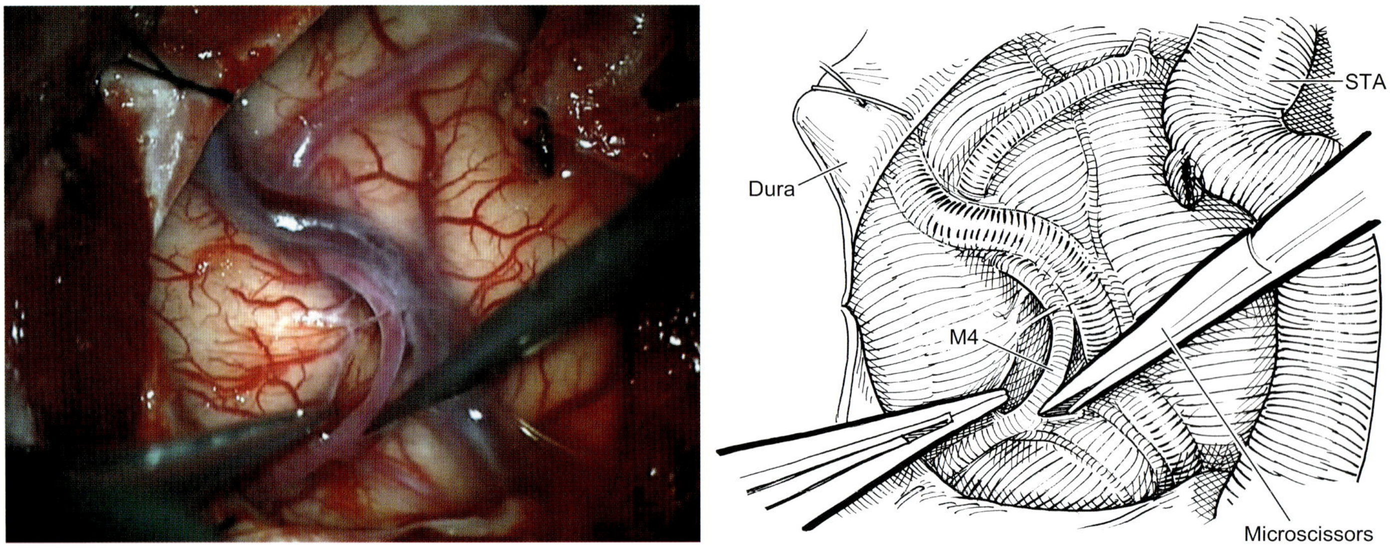

Fig. 2.3c The branch is dissected free of arachnoid.

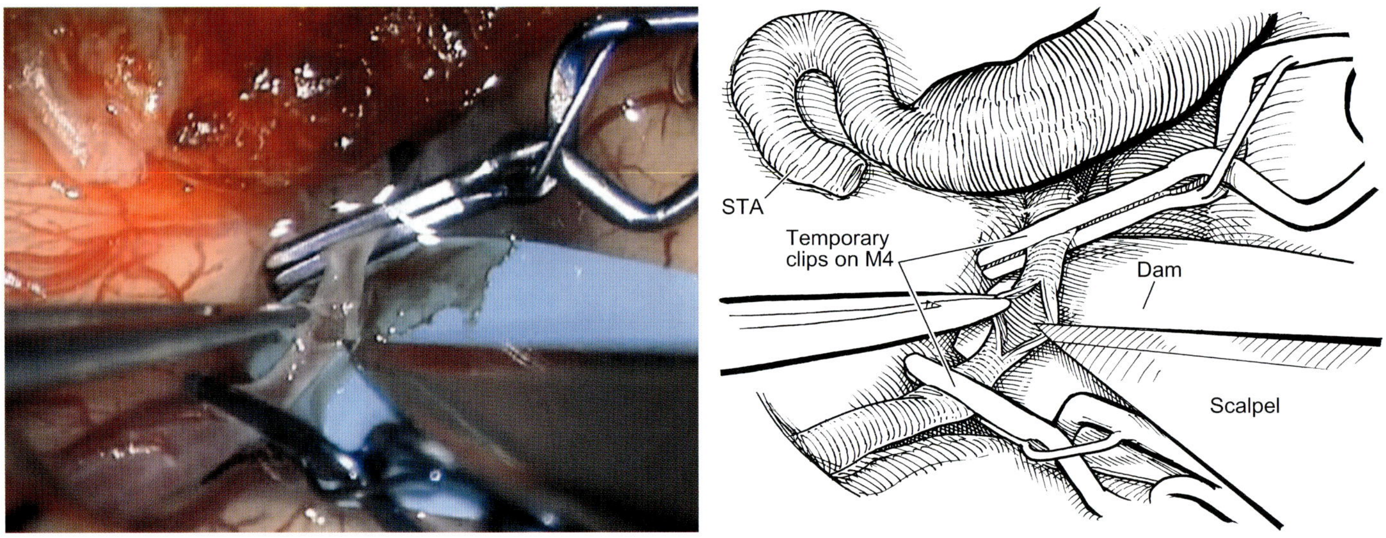

Fig. 2.3d The freed segment of M4 is trapped between temporary clips, and the vessel is incised with the tip of a no. 11 blade.

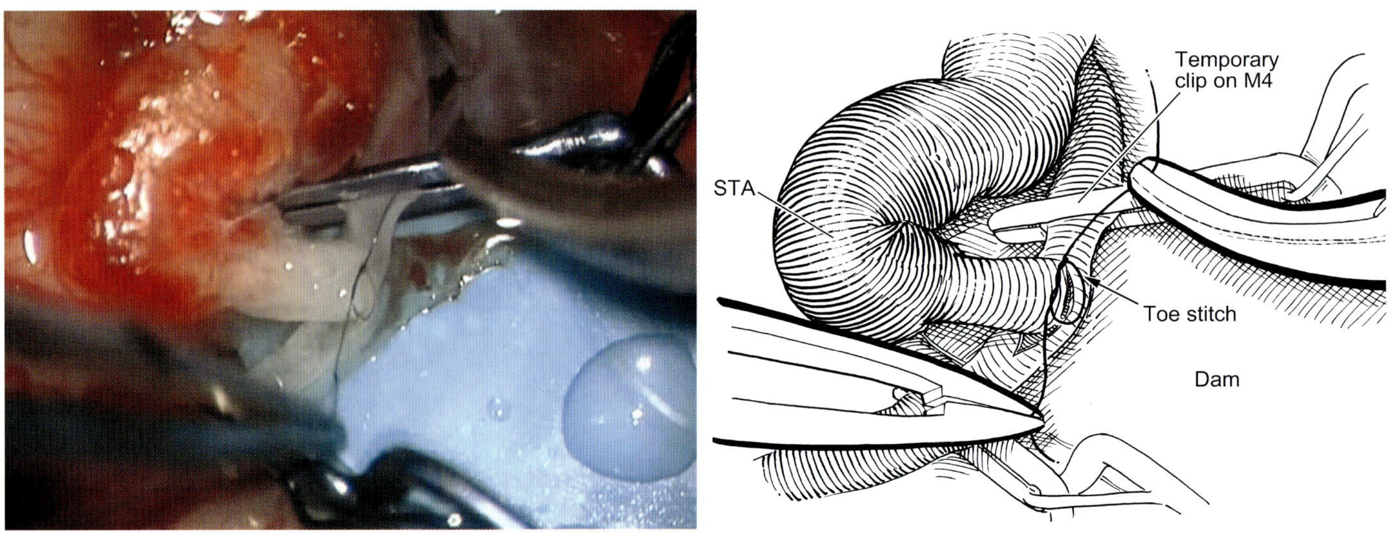

Fig. 2.3e The toe stitch is placed and tied.

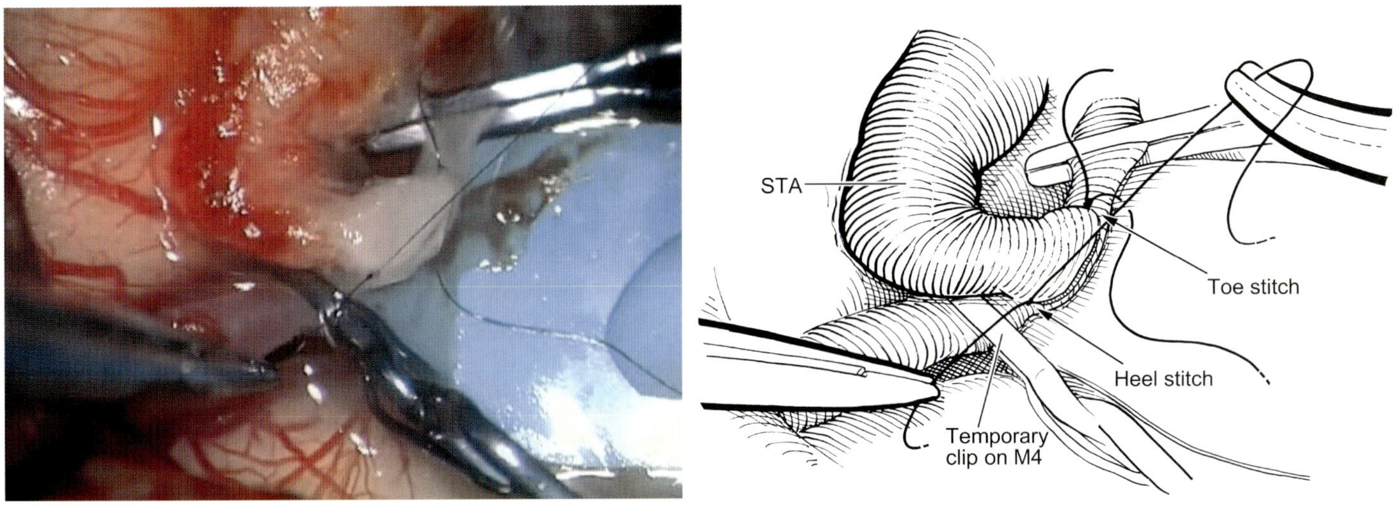

Fig. 2.3f Next, the heel stitch is placed.

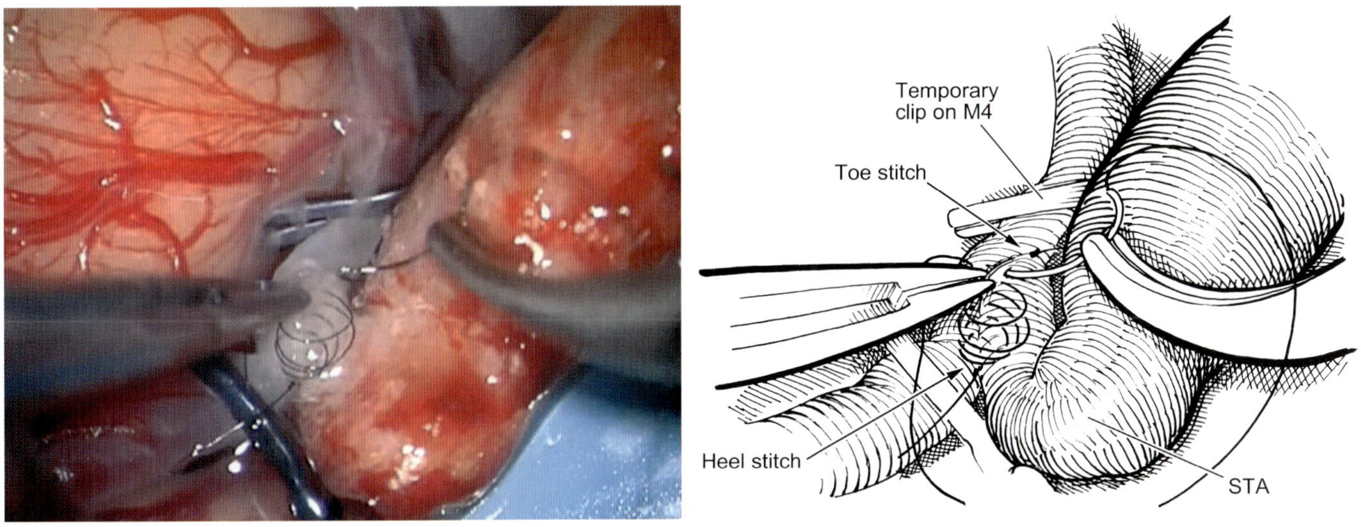

Fig. 2.3g The suture is run back from the heel stitch toward the toe stitch in loose running loops.

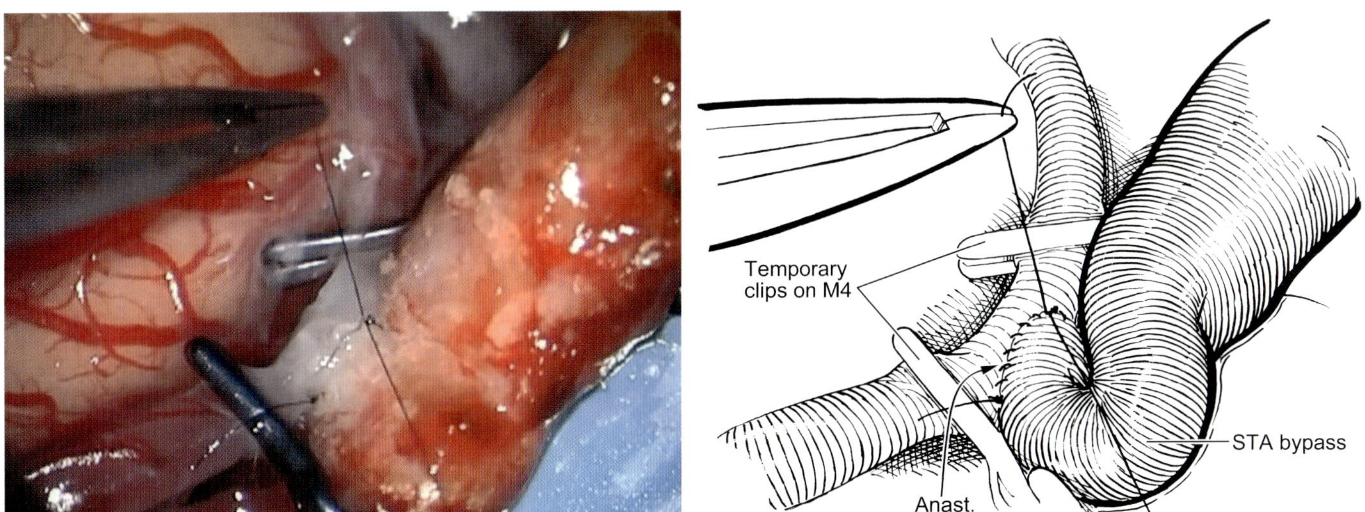

Fig. 2.3h After the loops are drawn and tightened, the first side of the anastomosis is completed and the suture is tied to the free end of the toe stitch.

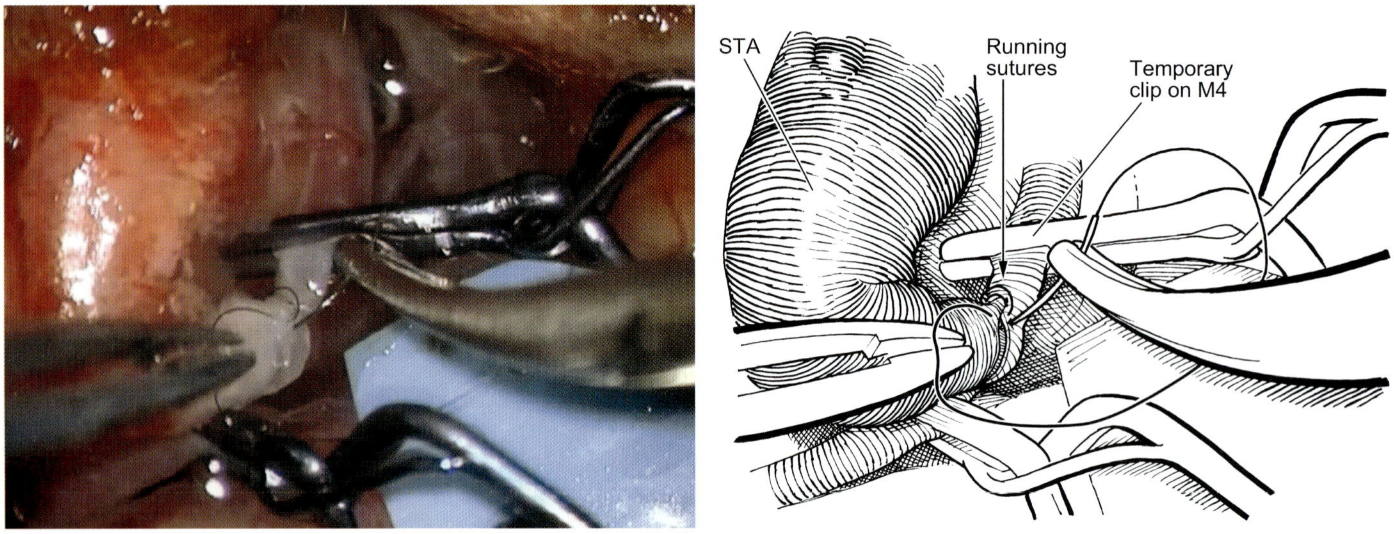

Fig. 2.3i In a similar fashion, the front wall is sutured from the toe toward the heel.

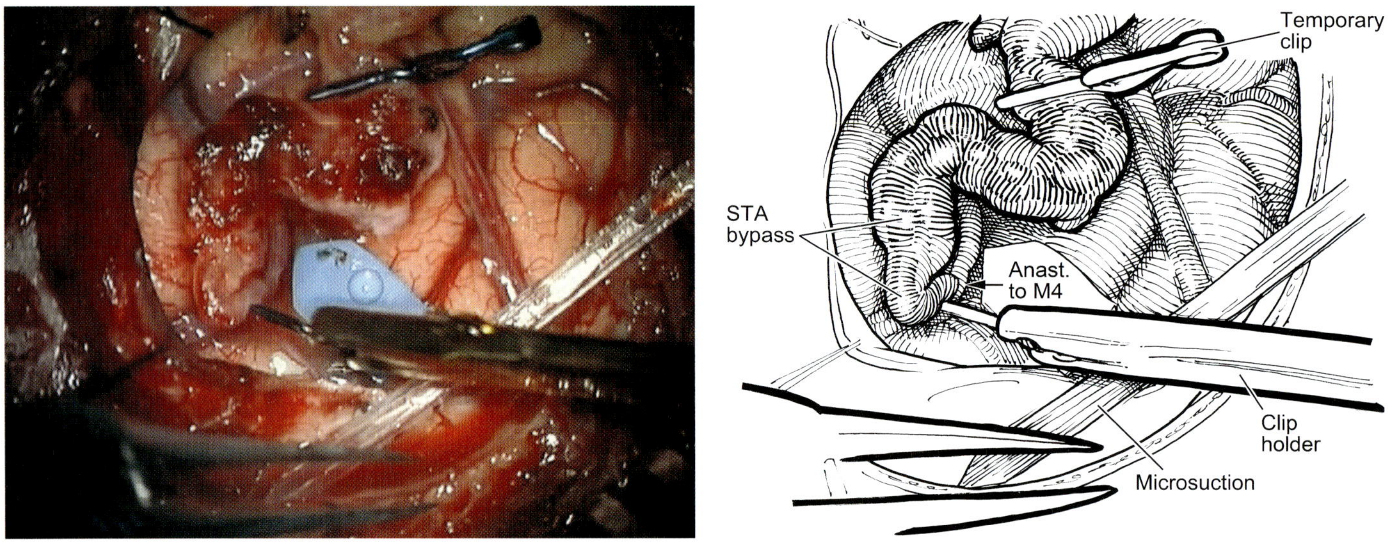

Fig. 2.3j The temporary clips are removed with no bleeding from the anastomosis.

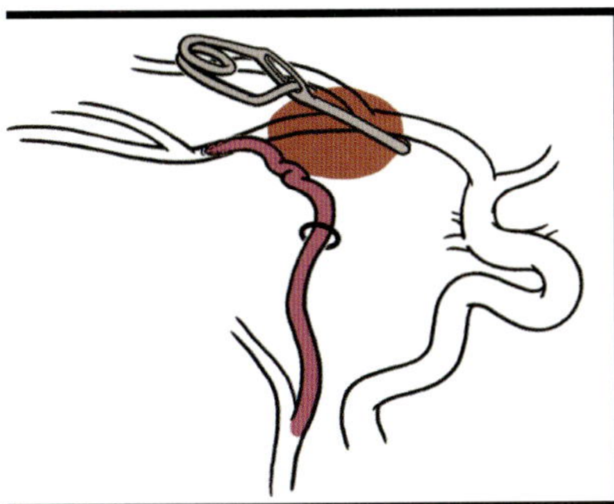

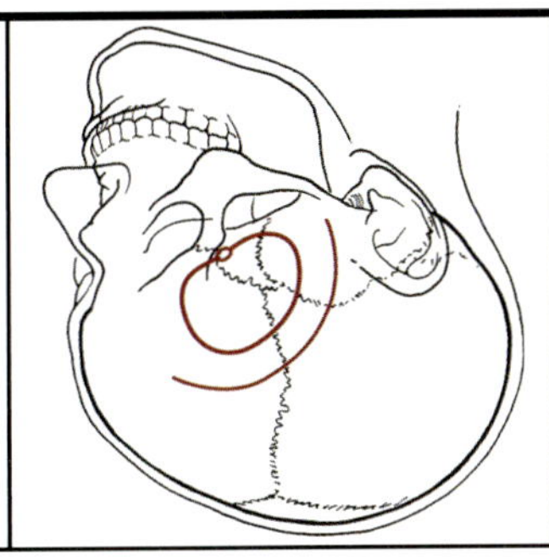

Case 2-4

Diagnosis: Large right MCA fusiform aneurysm

Bypass: STA-to-MCA

Approach: Right pterional

Video

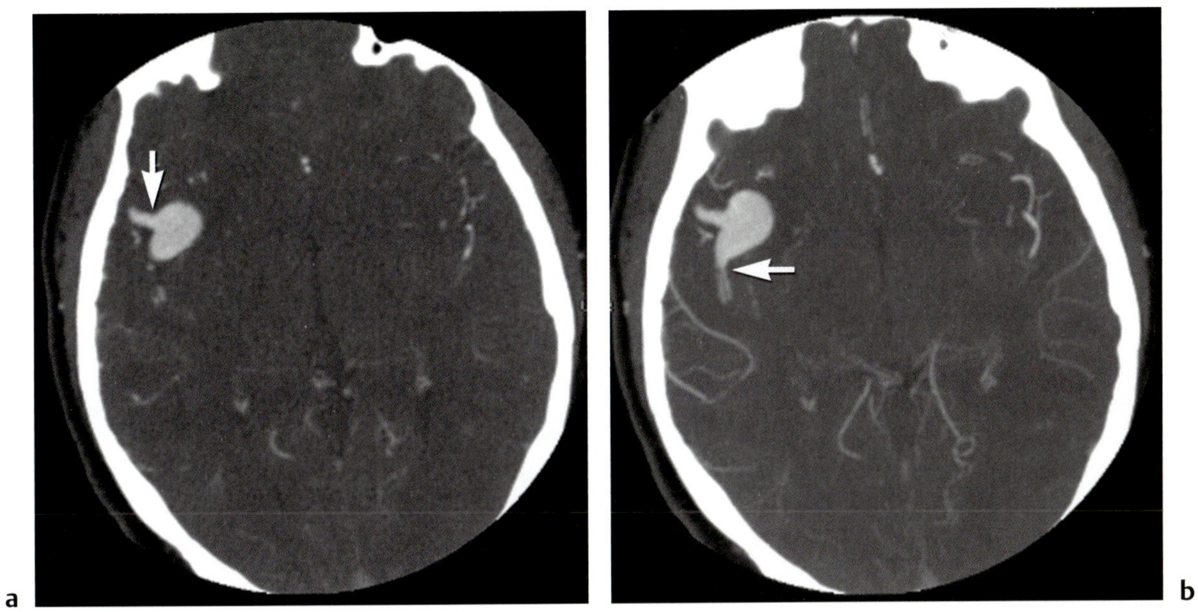

Fig. 2.4a, b Axial CT scans show a large fusiform MCA aneurysm and two outflow branches (*arrows*).

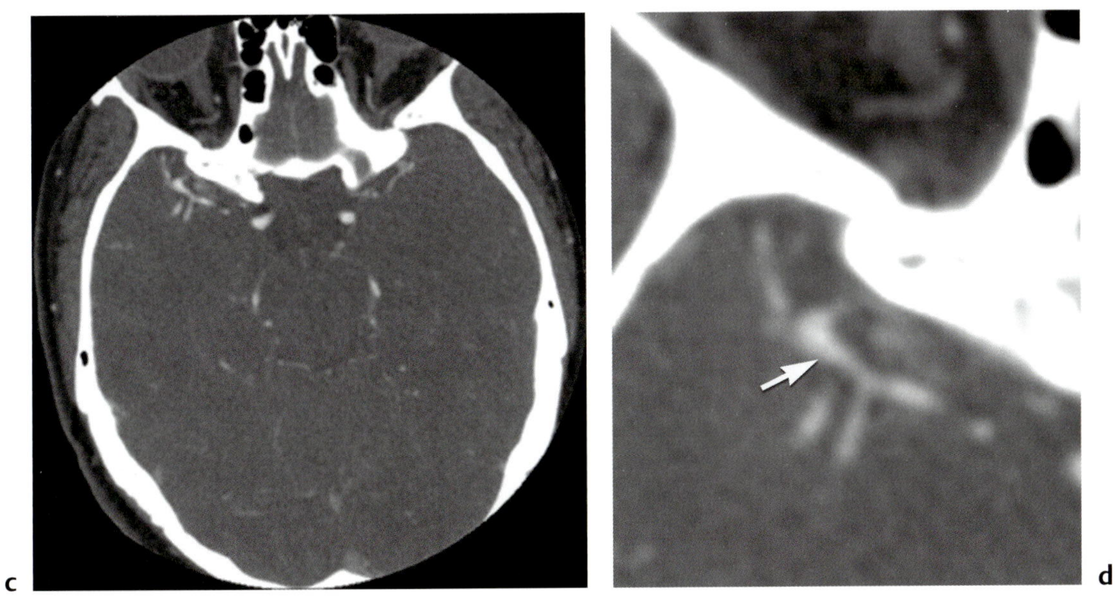

Fig. 2.4c, d Axial CT scan and an enlarged view show the inflow (*arrow*) of the large fusiform MCA aneurysm.

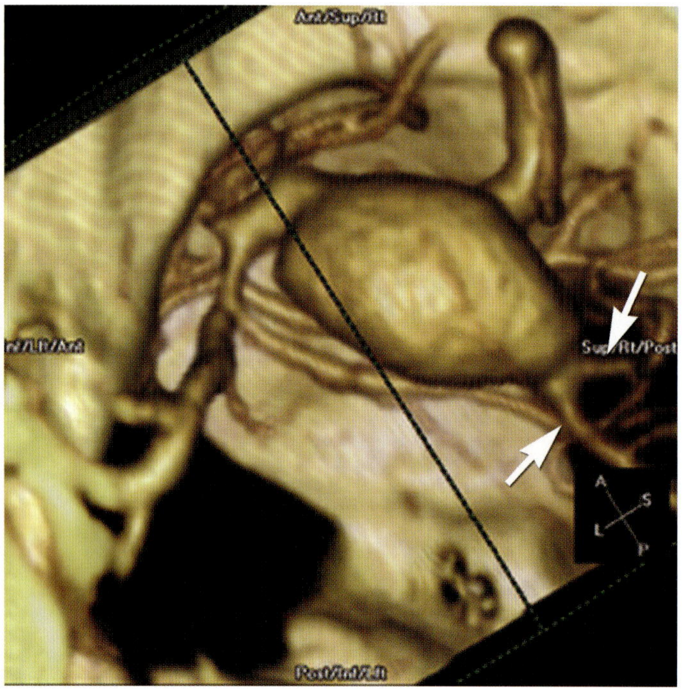

Fig. 2.4e A three-dimensional CT reconstruction shows two outflow vessels (*arrows*) from the aneurysm. MCA branches can be seen proximal to the aneurysm.

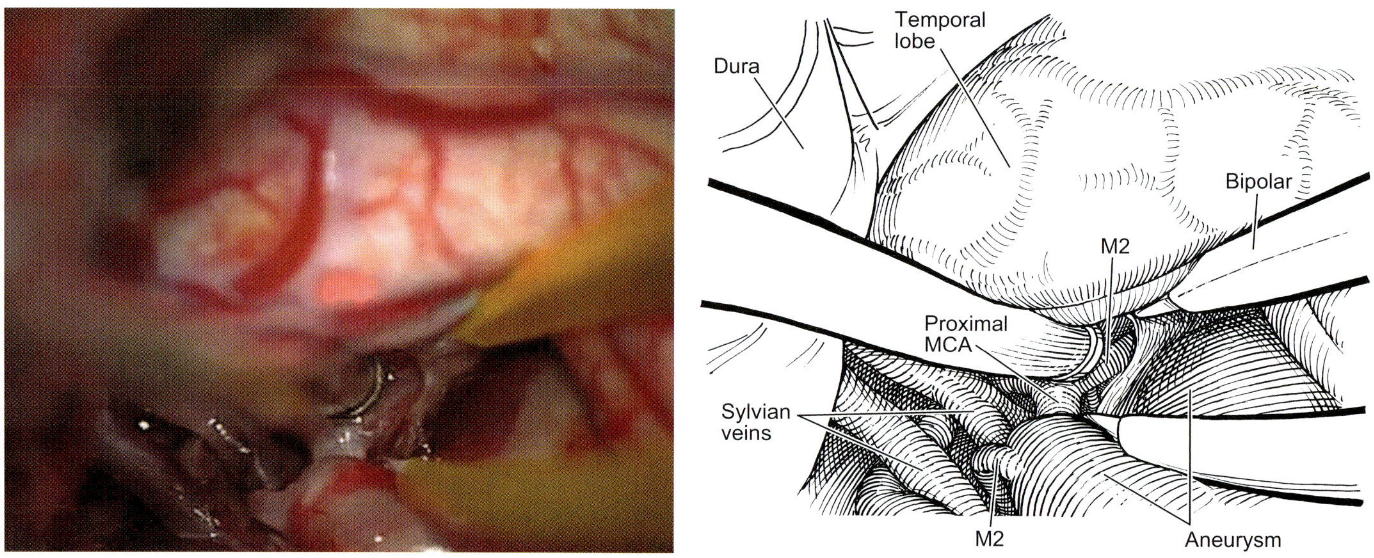

Fig. 2.4f The sylvian fissure has been opened to expose the distal portion of the aneurysm.

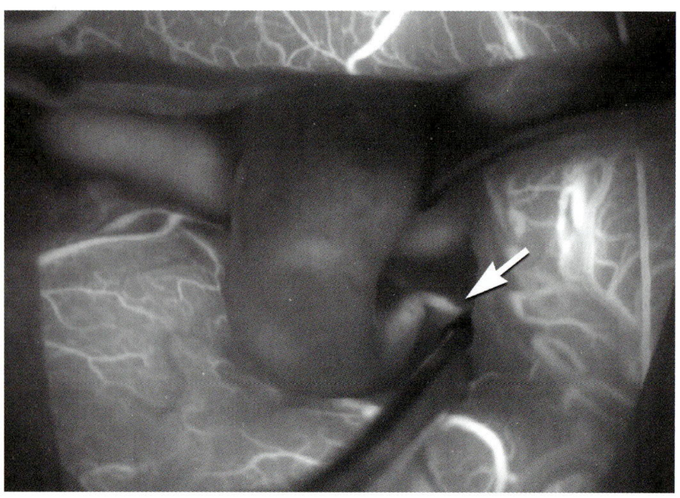

Fig. 2.4g Intraoperative ICG angiogram demonstrates the distal outflow (*arrow*) of the aneurysm.

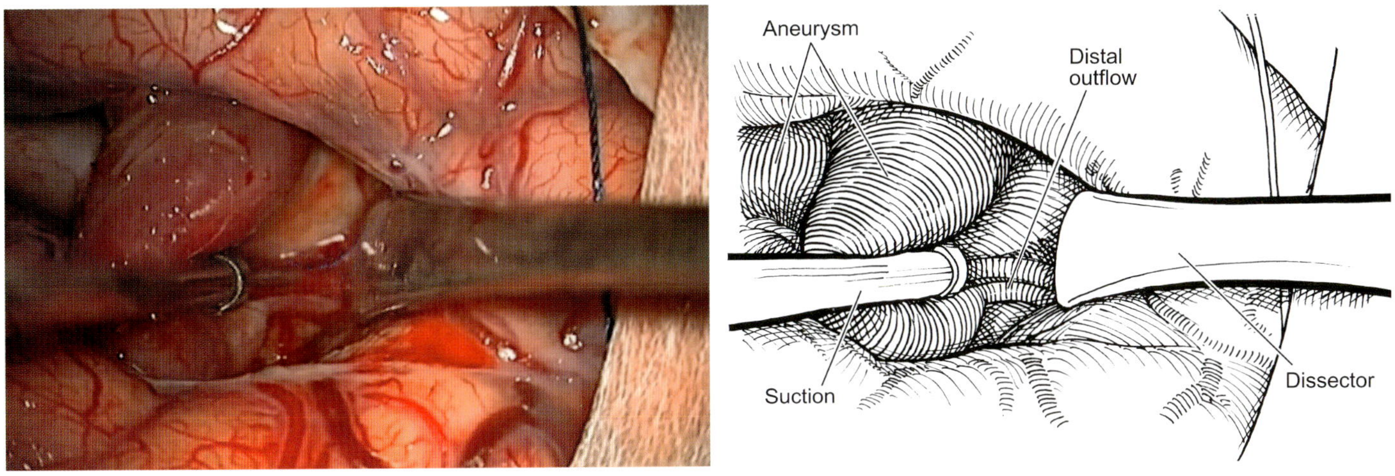

Fig. 2.4h The aneurysm is dissected circumferentially and the outflow vessels are identified.

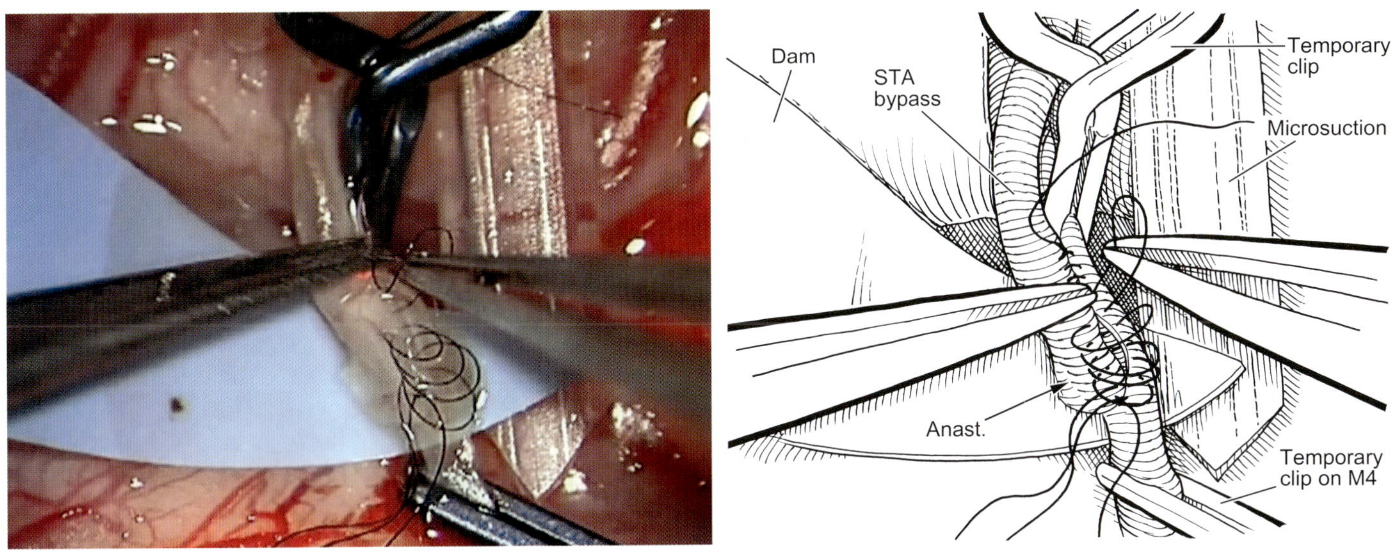

Fig. 2.4i The fishmouthed STA is matched to the size of the arteriotomy in one of the outflow branches of the MCA.

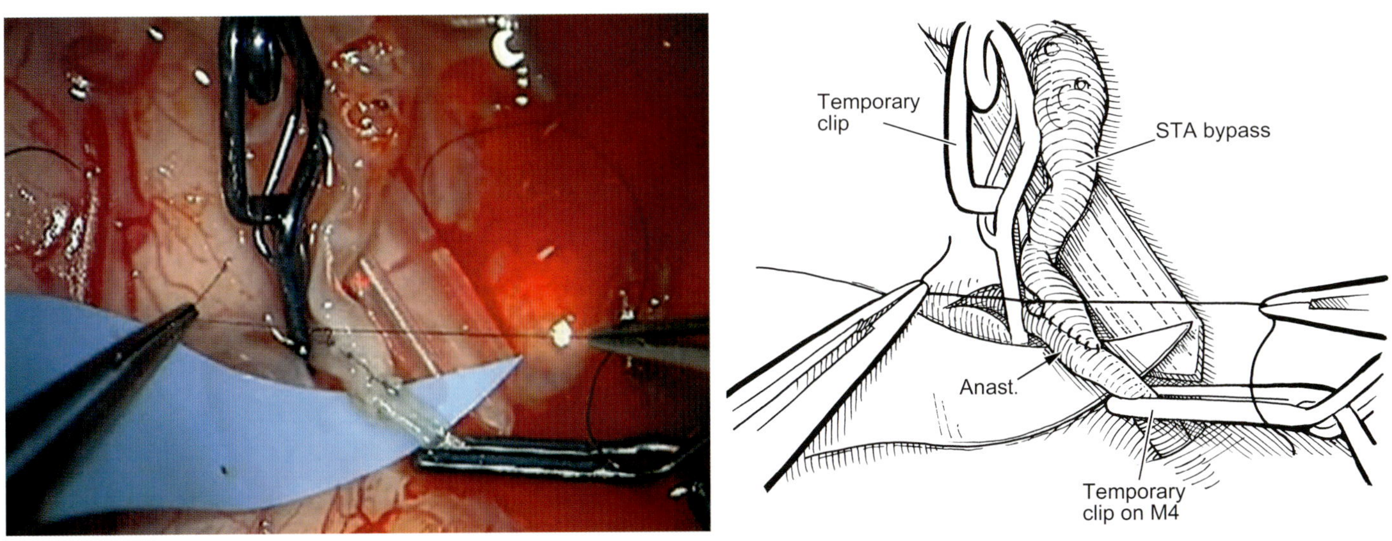

Fig. 2.4j The STA bypass is completed.

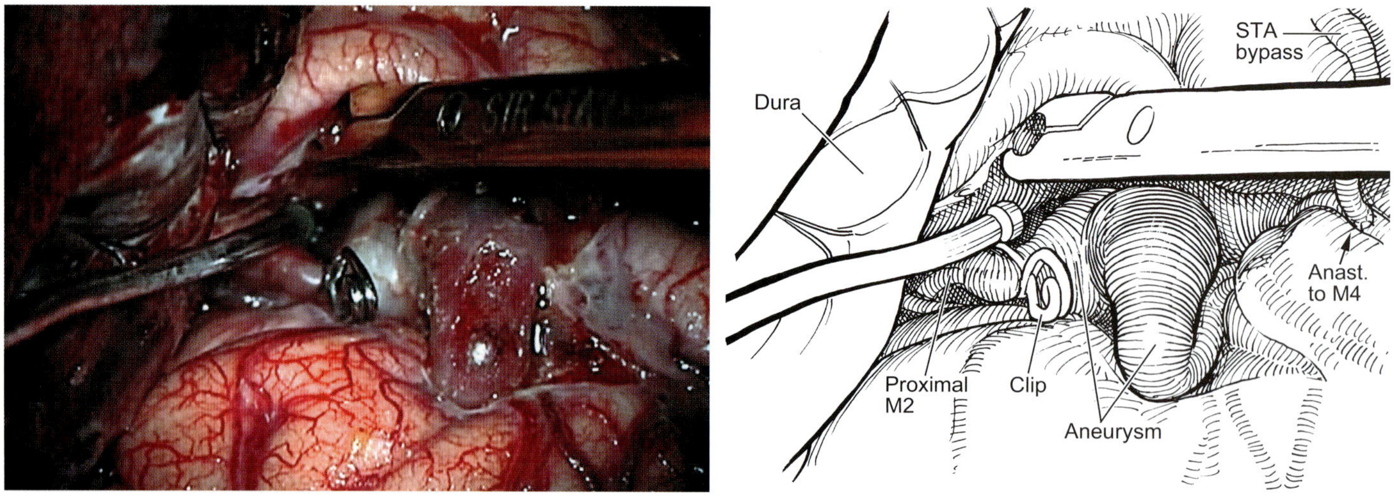

Fig. 2.4k The STA bypass to the distal outflow of the aneurysm is completed, and the proximal portion of the aneurysm is occluded with a clip to preserve flow to the remaining outflow vessel.

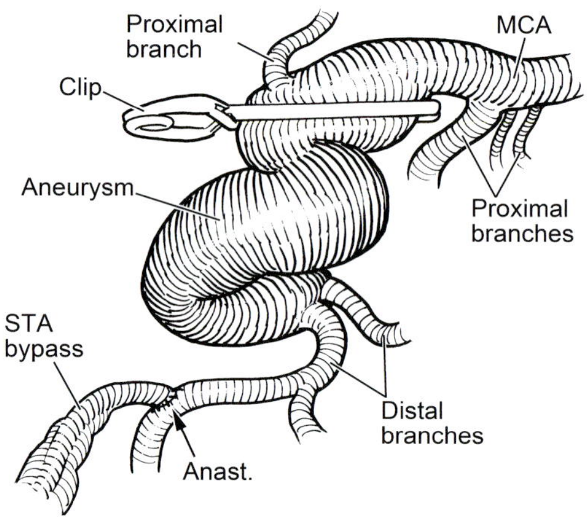

Fig. 2.4l Overview of the clipped aneurysm and STA bypass.

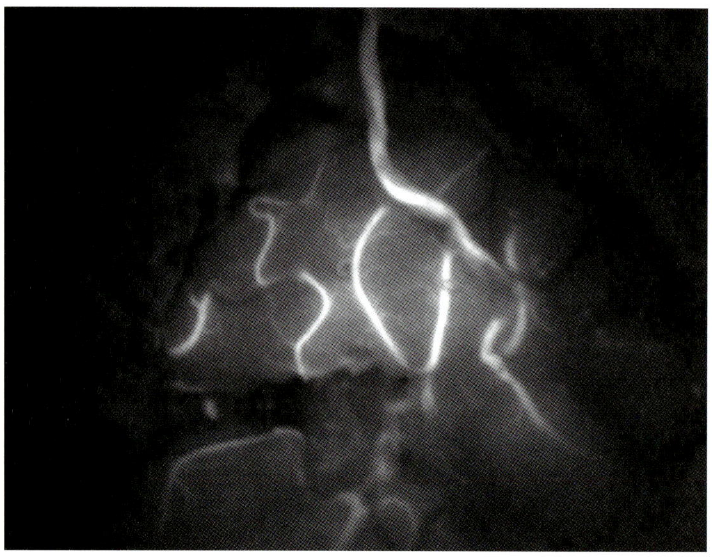

Fig. 2.4m Intraoperative ICG angiogram shows the patency of the bypass.

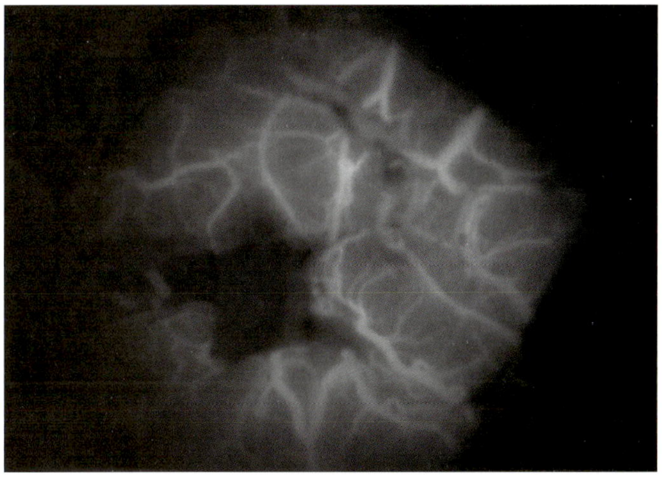

Fig. 2.4n ICG angiogram demonstrates good flow in the exposed hemisphere.

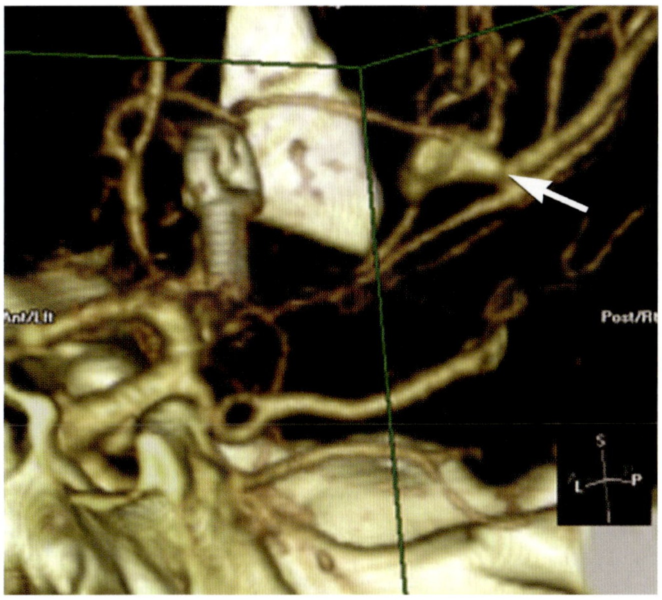

Fig. 2.4o Three-dimensional CT reconstruction shows clipping of the proximal portion of the aneurysm and the distal flow through the STA bypass (*arrow*).

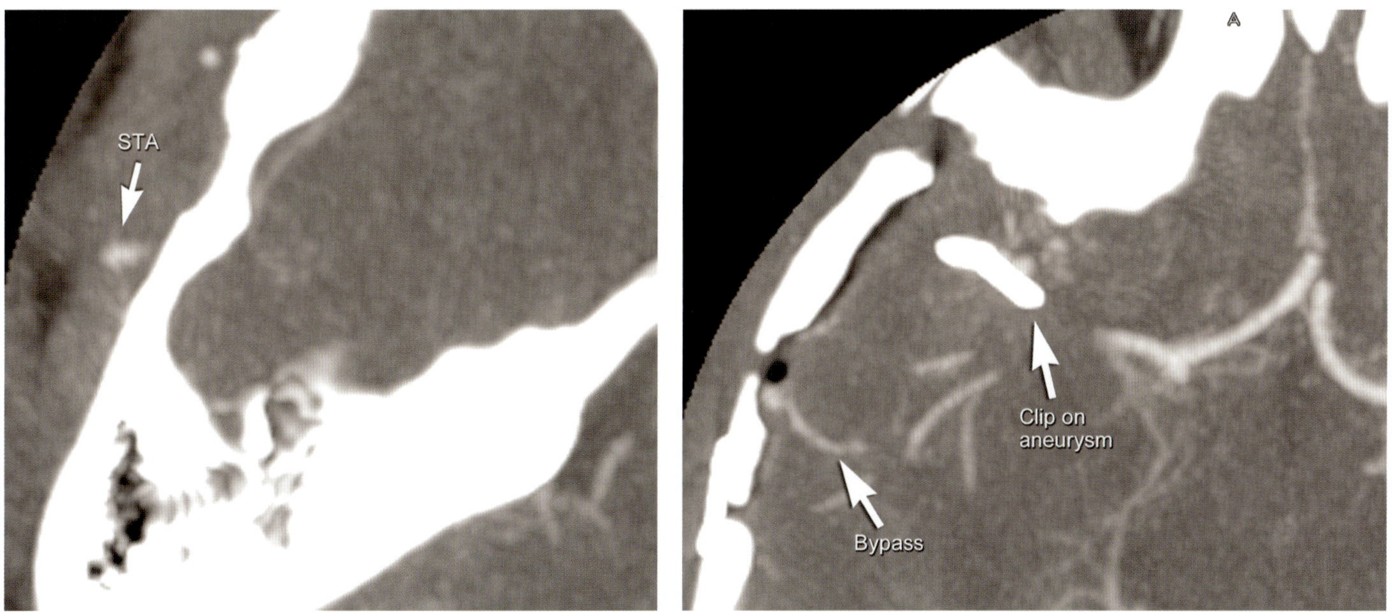

p q

Fig. 2.4p, q Axial CT angiograms demonstrate the occlusion of the MCA aneurysm and the bypass to the distal portion of the aneurysm.

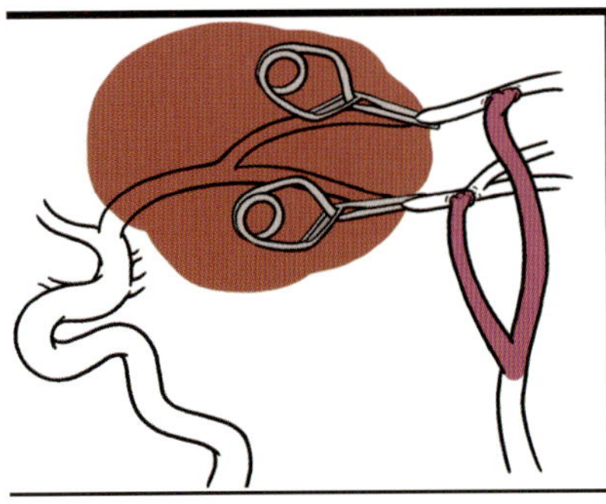

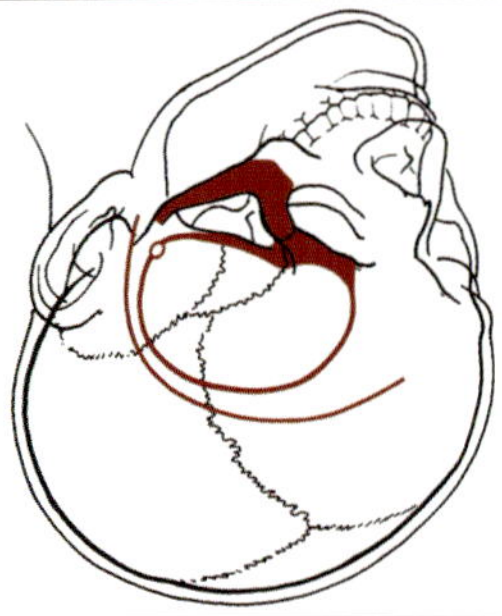

Case 2-5

Diagnosis: Giant left thrombosed MCA aneurysm

Bypass: Double-barrel STA-to-MCA

Approach: Left orbitozygomatic

▶ Video

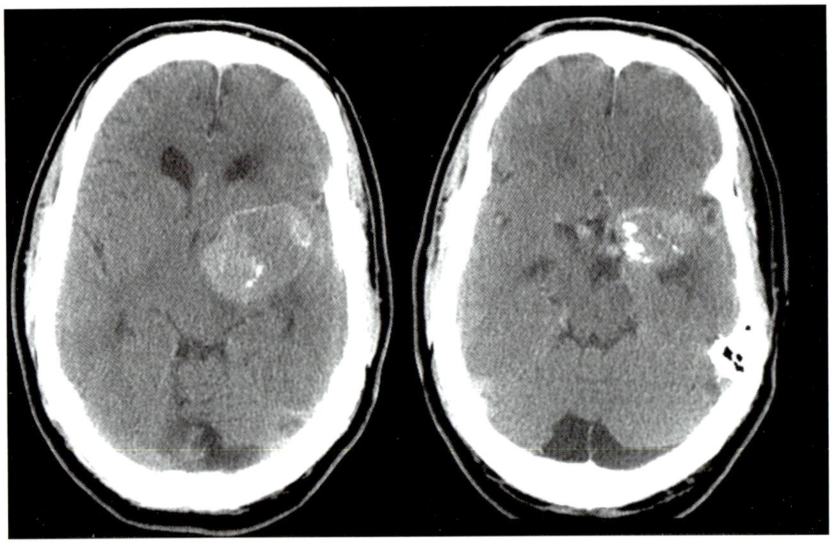

Fig. 2.5a Axial CT scans show giant thrombosed MCA aneurysm in a 51-year-old man with speech arrest and fluctuating aphasia.

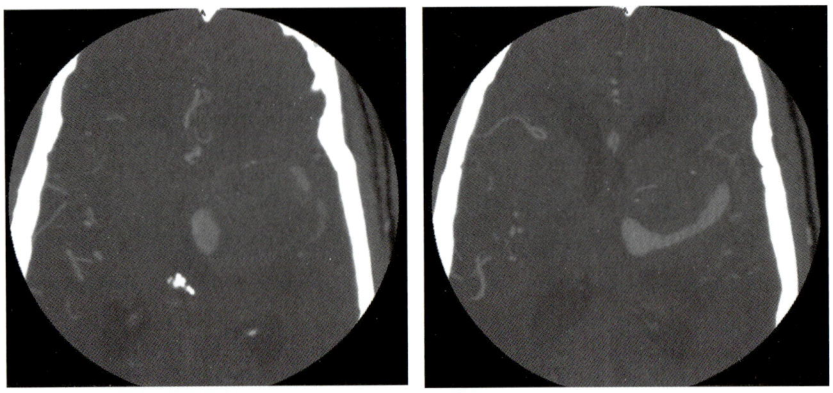

b

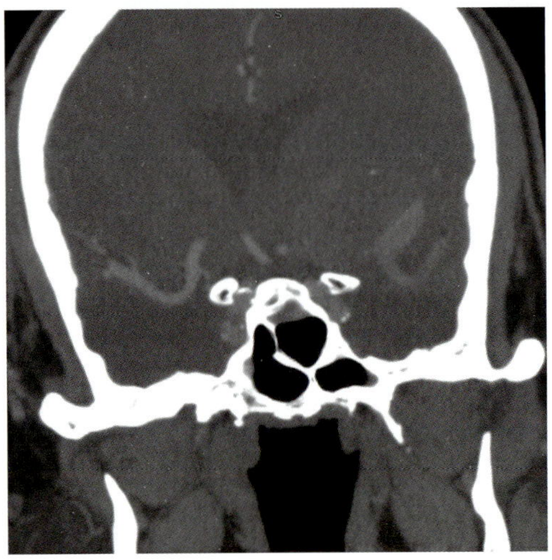

c

Fig. 2.5b, c Axial (**b**) and coronal (**c**) CT angiograms show the flow through a serpiginous channel in the thrombosed left MCA aneurysm.

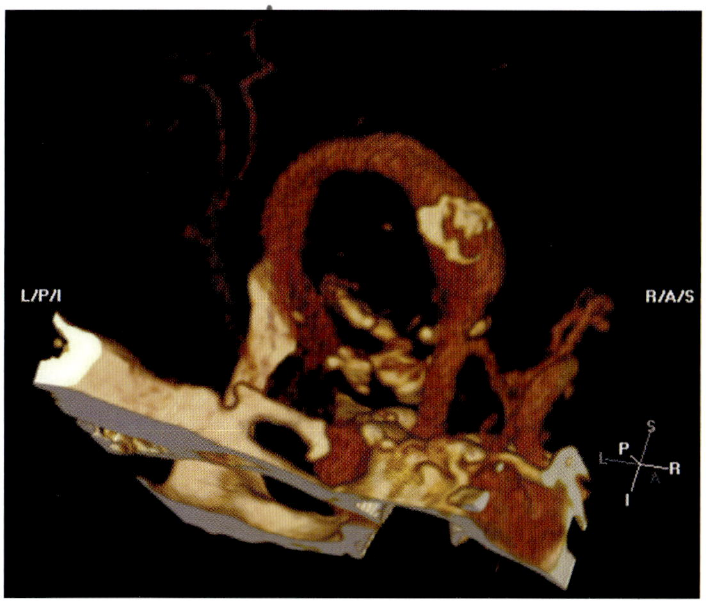

Fig. 2.5d Three-dimensional CT reconstruction demonstrates the serpiginous channel and the residual lumen of the partially thrombosed aneurysm.

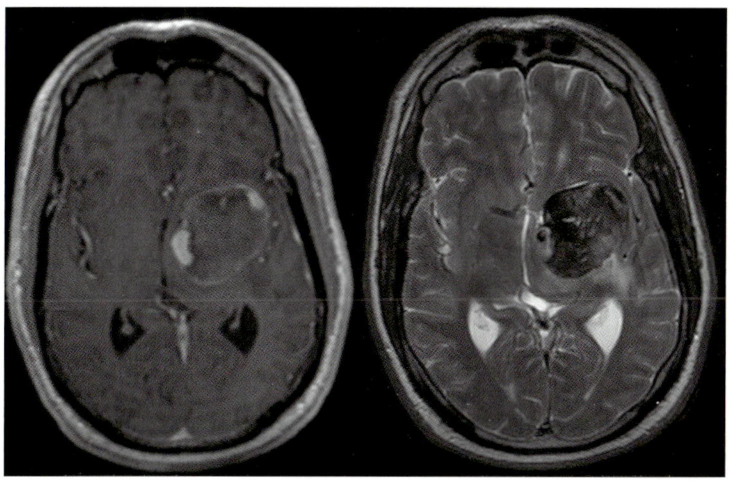

Fig. 2.5e Axial MR images show the large mass with the flow channels in the MCA aneurysm.

f

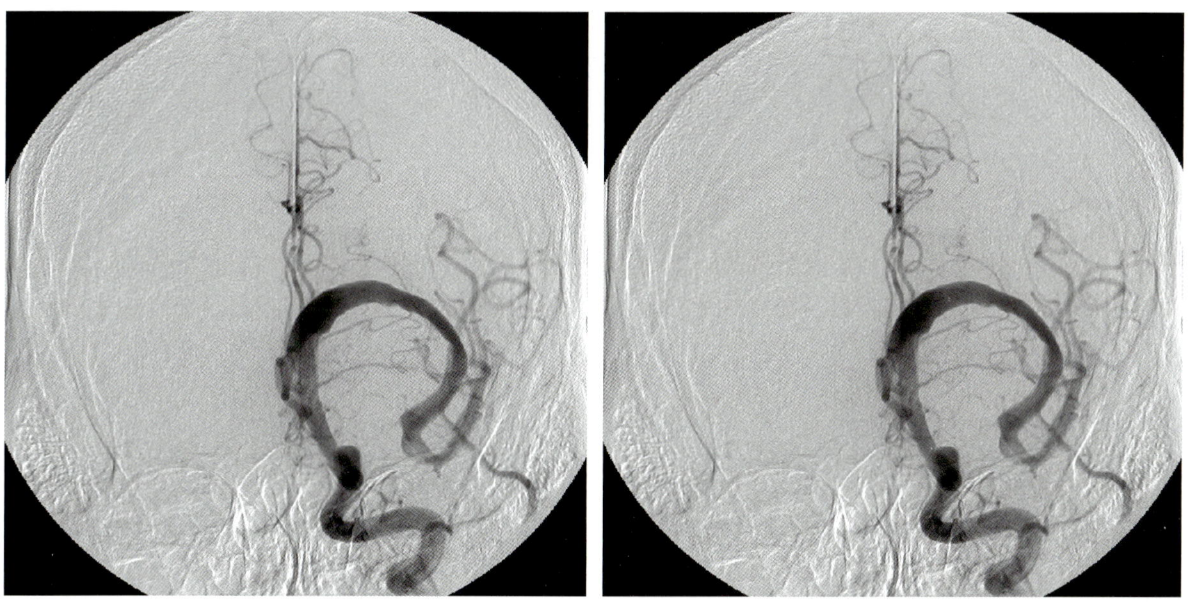

g

Fig. 2.5f, g Anteroposterior and lateral angiograms show the serpiginous channel through the MCA filling the distal left MCA branches.

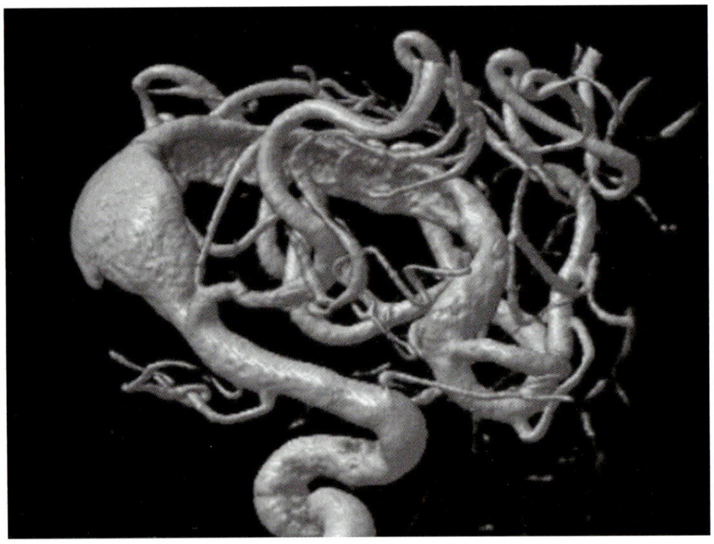

Fig. 2.5h Three-dimensional reconstruction demonstrates the serpiginous vessel ending in two distal MCA branches filling the left hemisphere.

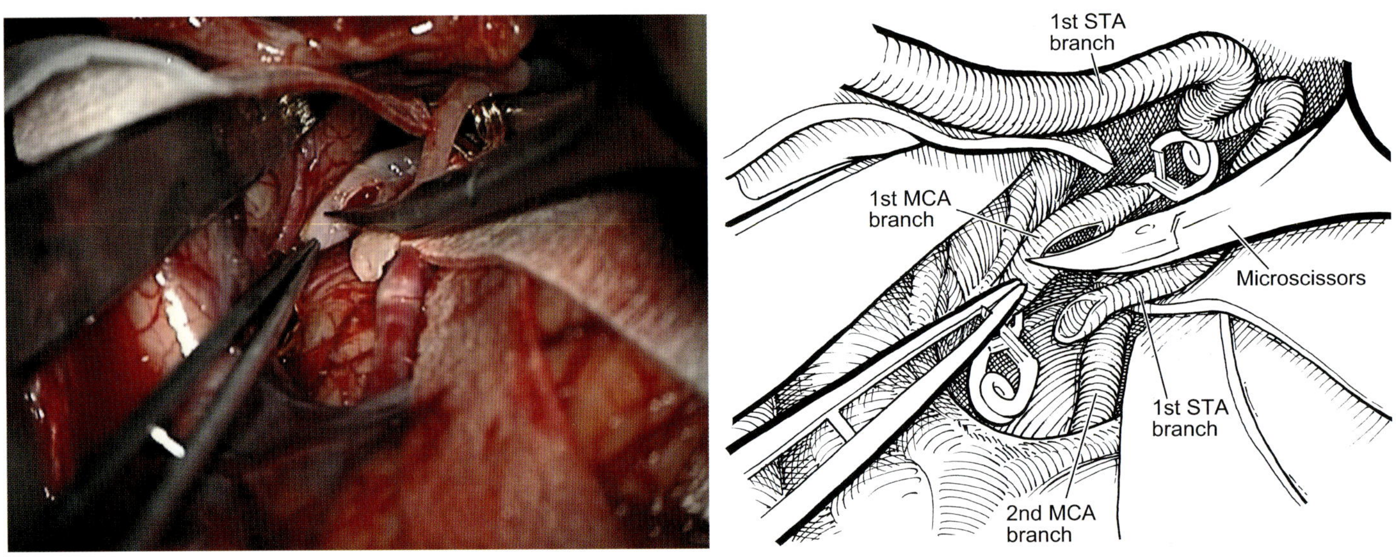

Fig. 2.5i The two branches of the STA are prepared, and the first MCA branch is opened to proceed with the first anastomosis.

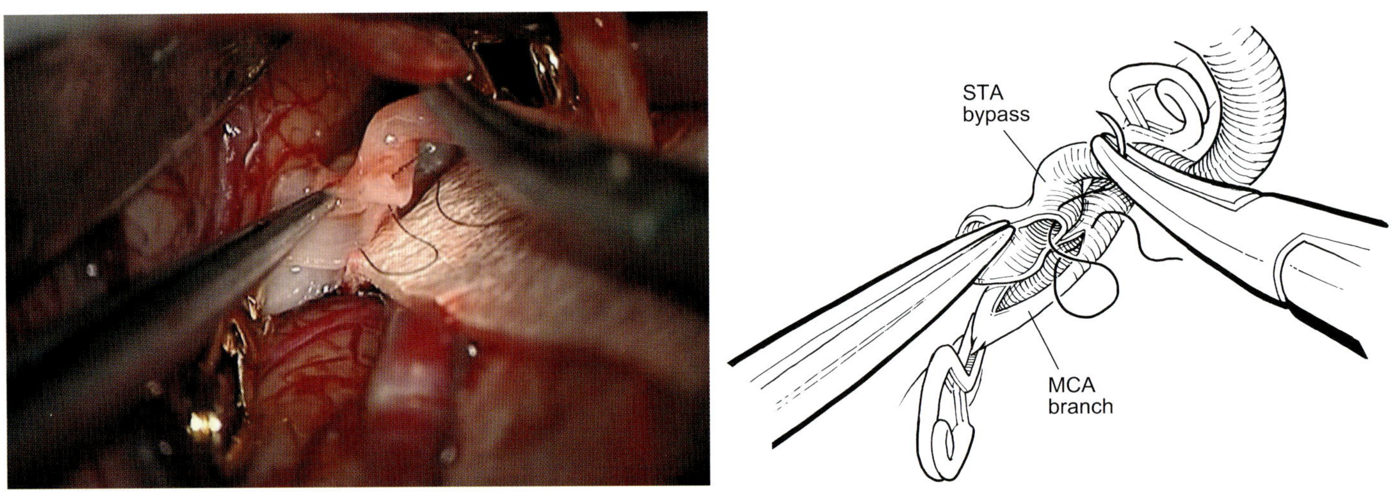

Fig. 2.5j The first stitch is placed at one end of the MCA opening and then through one end of the fishmouthed STA.

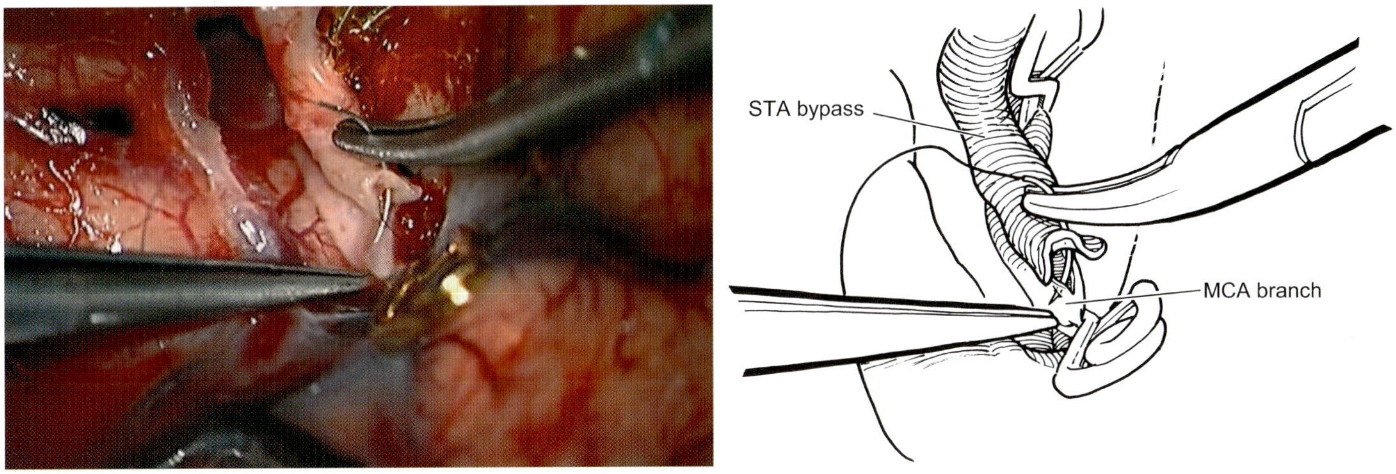

Fig. 2.5k In the second anastomosis, a toe stitch extends from the MCA to the end of the fishmouthed STA.

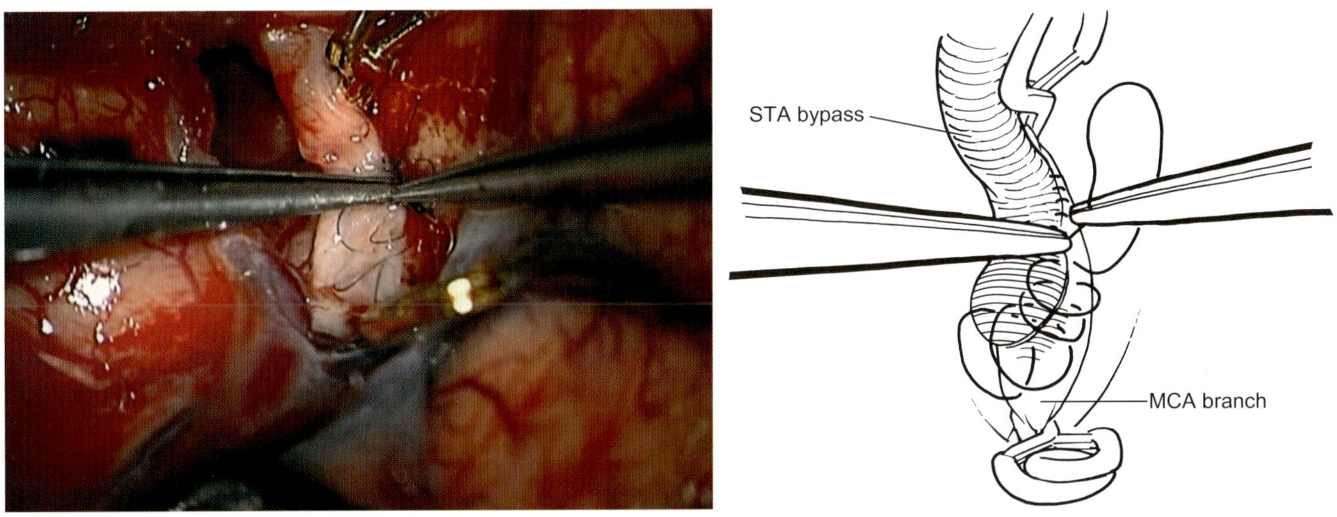

Fig. 2.5l The loops of the running suture are tightened to complete the second anastomosis.

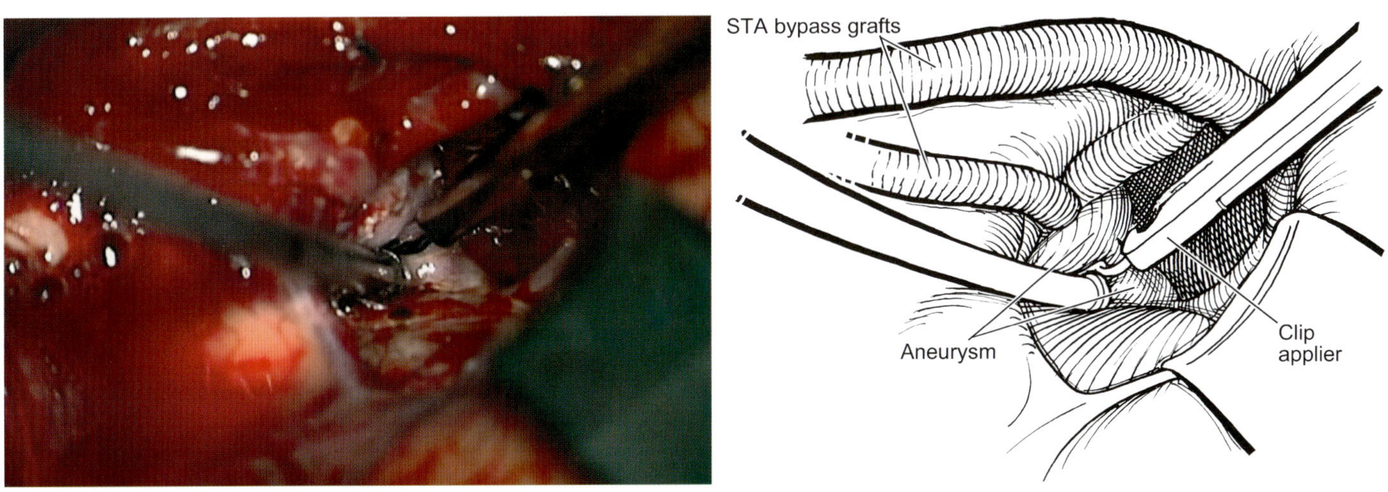

Fig. 2.5m A clip partially occludes the first channel.

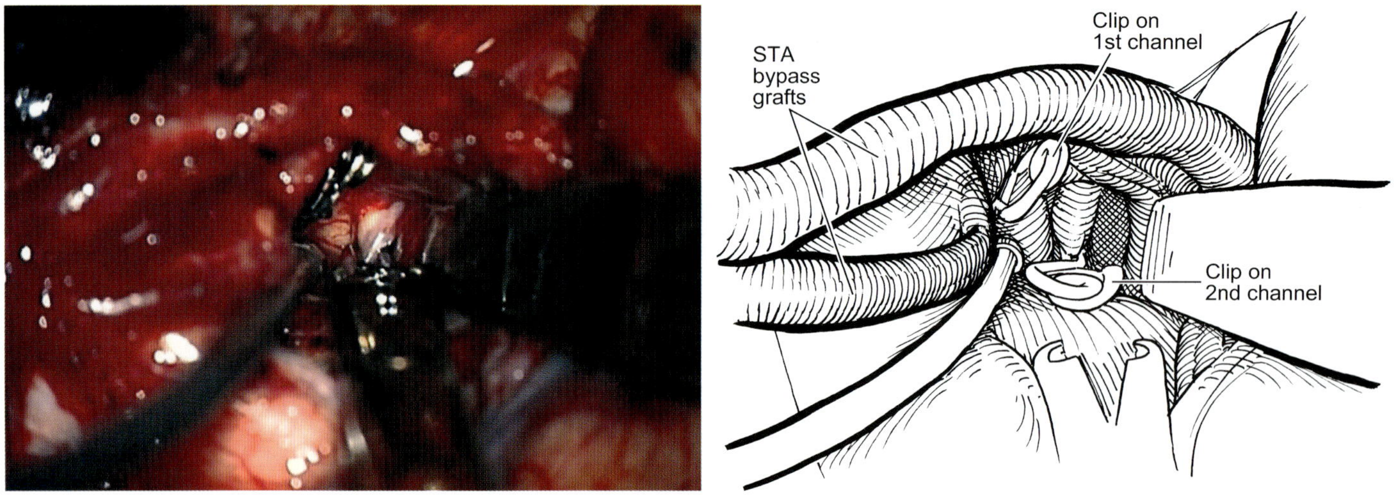

Fig. 2.5n A second clip partially occludes the second channel, reducing flow through the aneurysm by 90% and creating flow demand for the bypass.

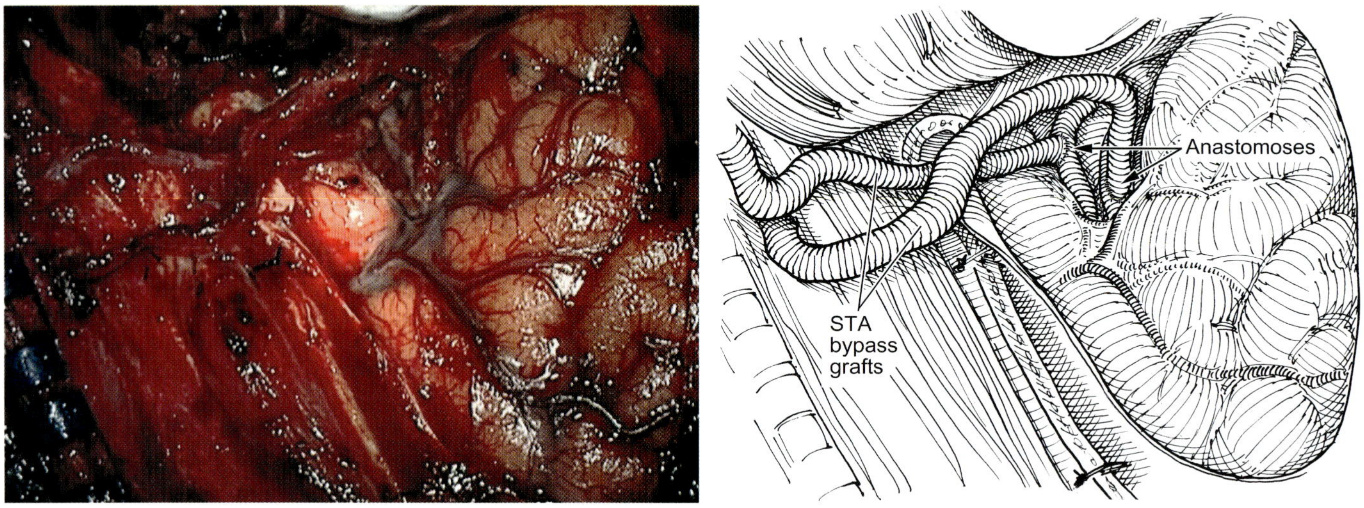

Fig. 2.5o Overview of the two branches of the STA anastomosed to the MCA branches.

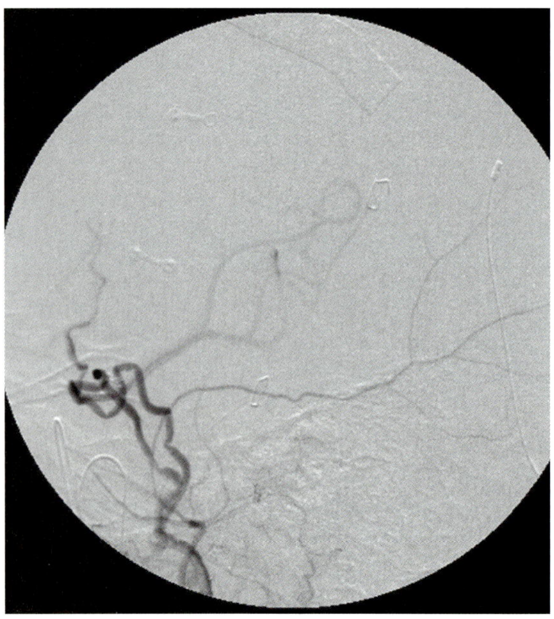

Fig. 2.5p Intraoperative ECA angiogram demonstrates good flow through the two STA branches.

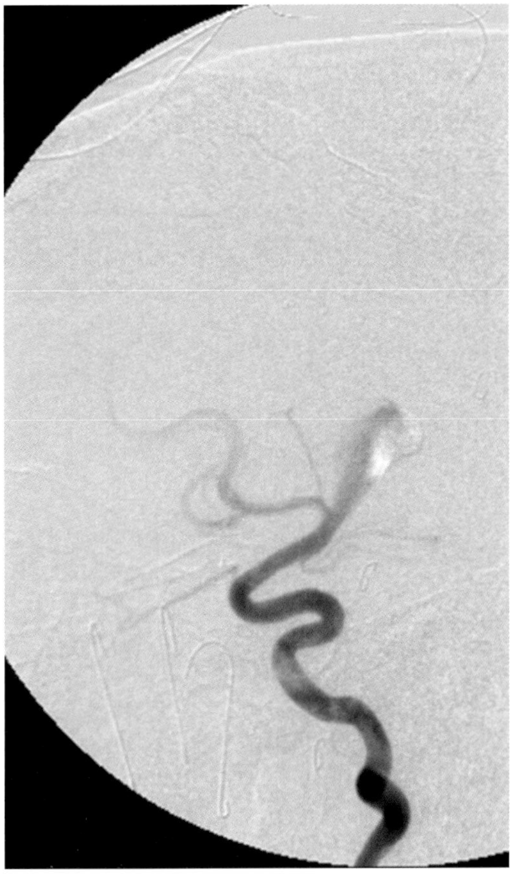

Fig. 2.5q ICA angiogram demonstrates continued flow into the MCA channel.

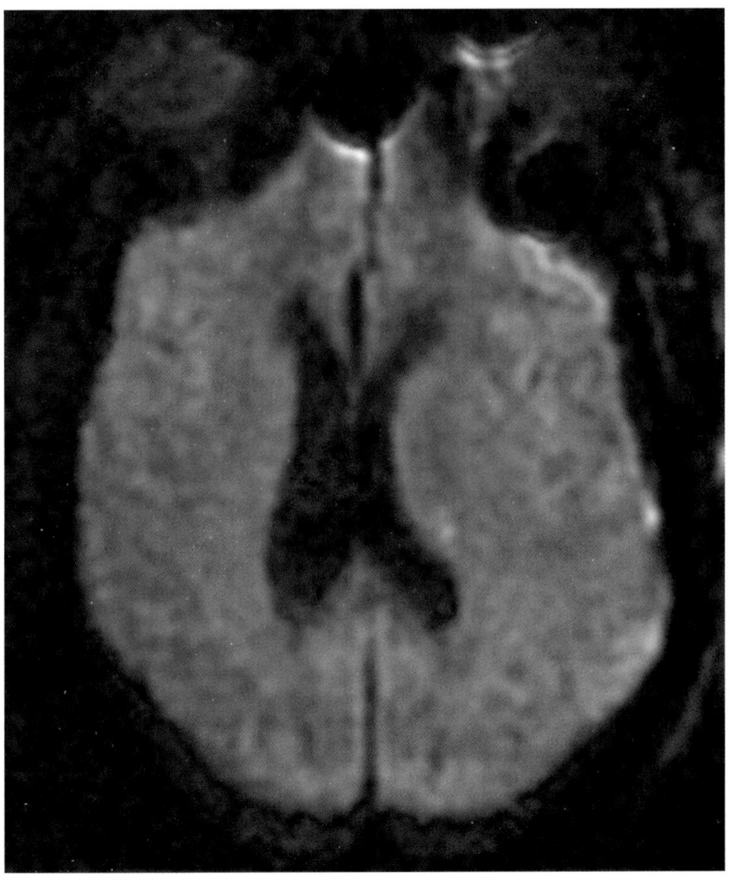

Fig. 2.5r Postoperative MR image demonstrates no ischemic lesions.

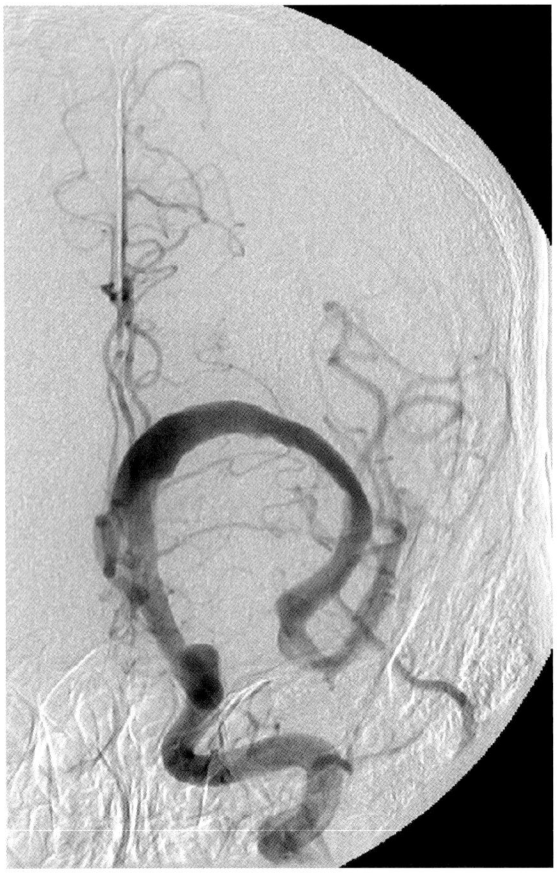

Fig. 2.5s Five days after surgery, an anteroposterior angiogram is obtained in preparation for a balloon occlusion test.

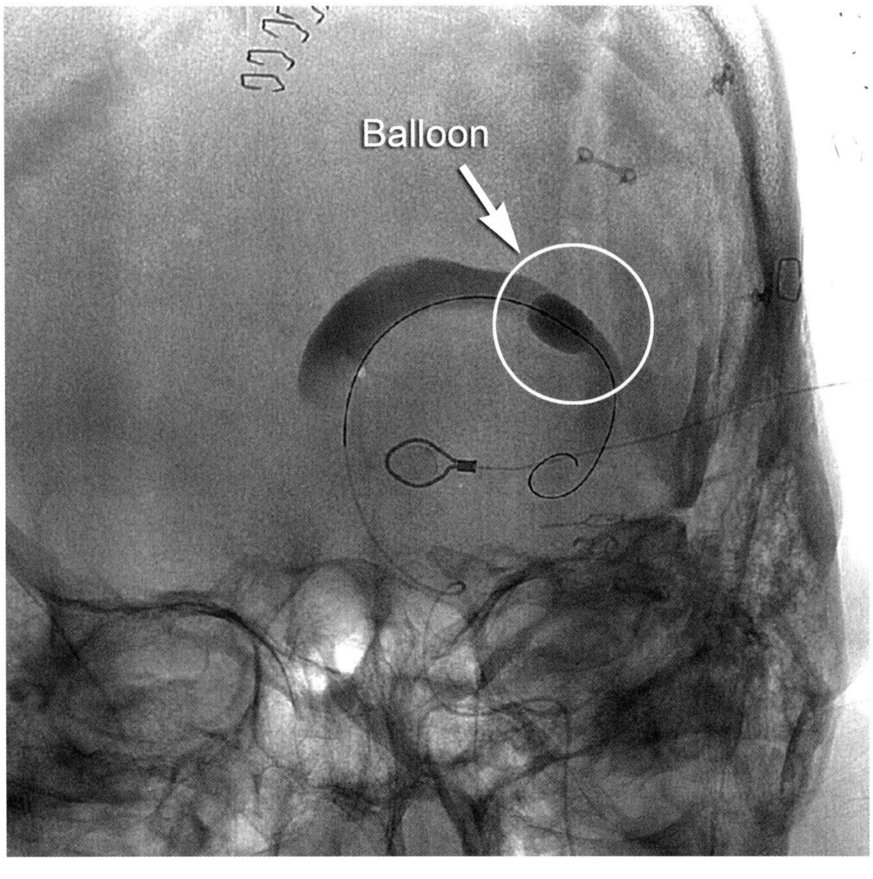

Fig. 2.5t The balloon is inflated in the residual aneurysm lumen to test the bypass.

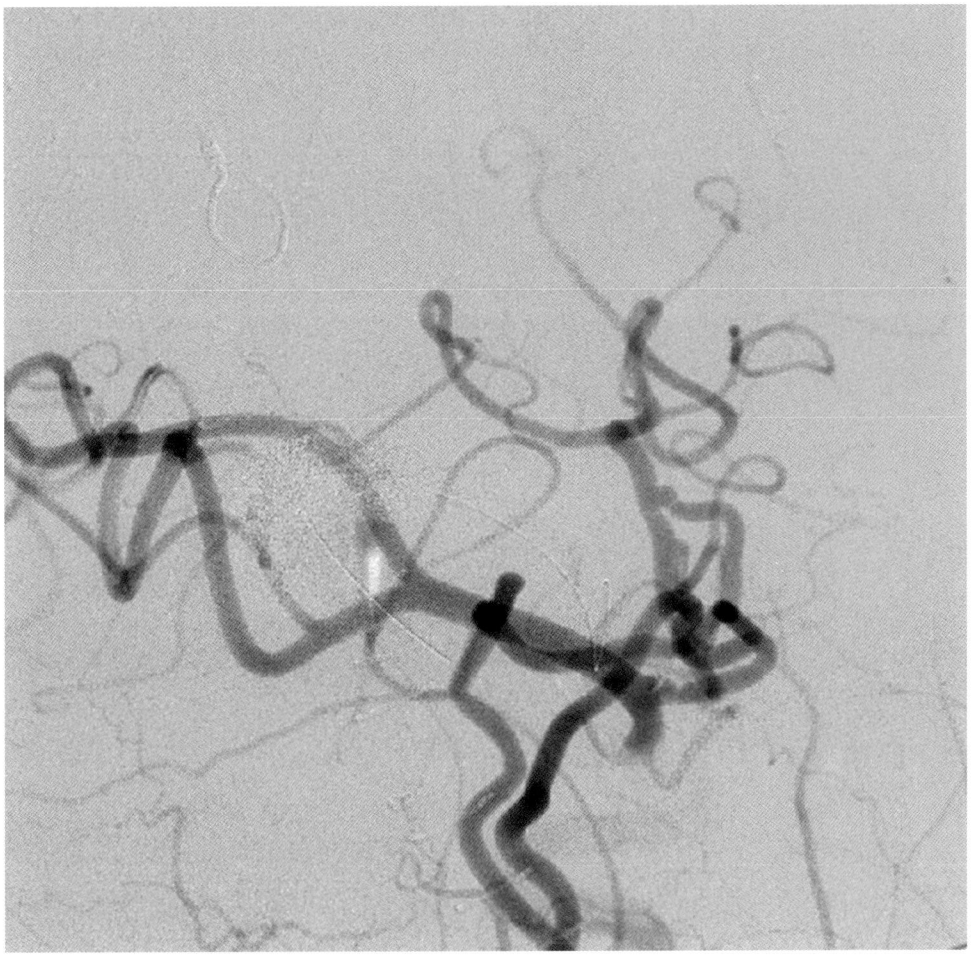

Fig. 2.5u With the balloon inflated, the patency of the bypass is confirmed, as is the significant diameter of the bypass vessels.

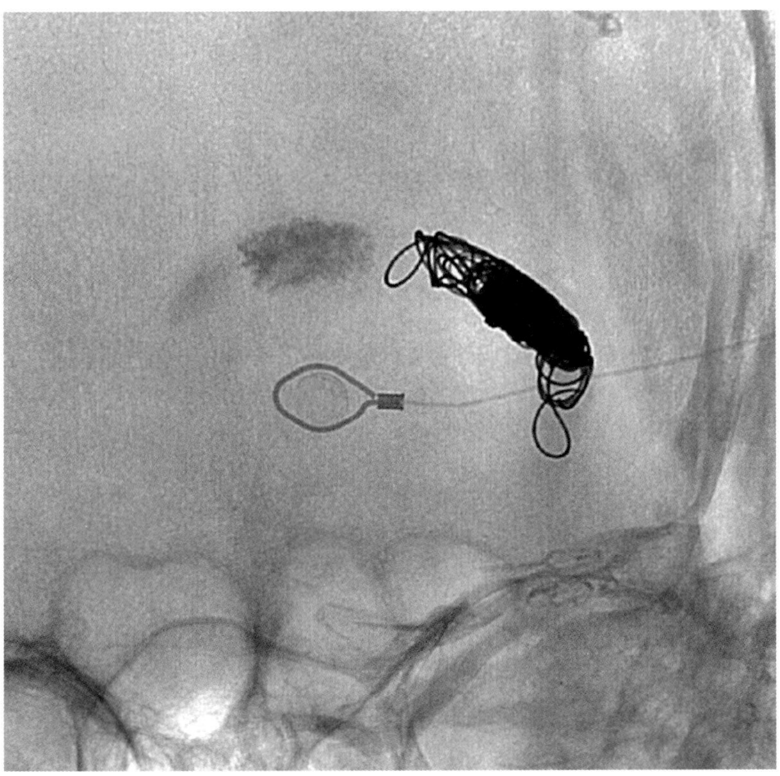

Fig. 2.5v Anteroposterior angiographic projection shows the coils in the channel of the MCA aneurysm occluding the residual lumen of the lesion.

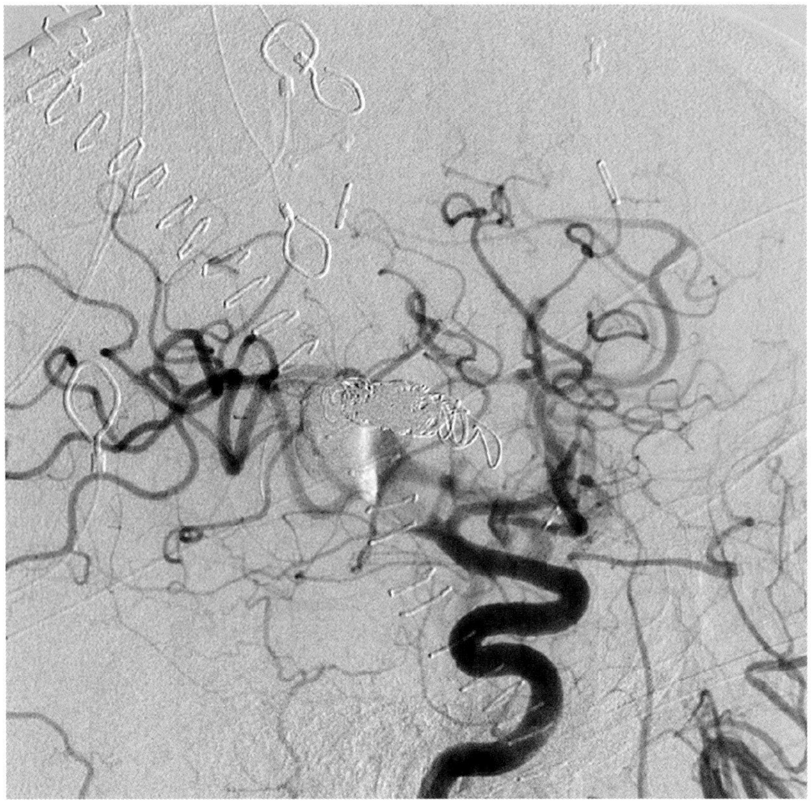

Fig. 2.5w Lateral angiogram confirms absence of flow in the aneurysm and patency of the bypass.

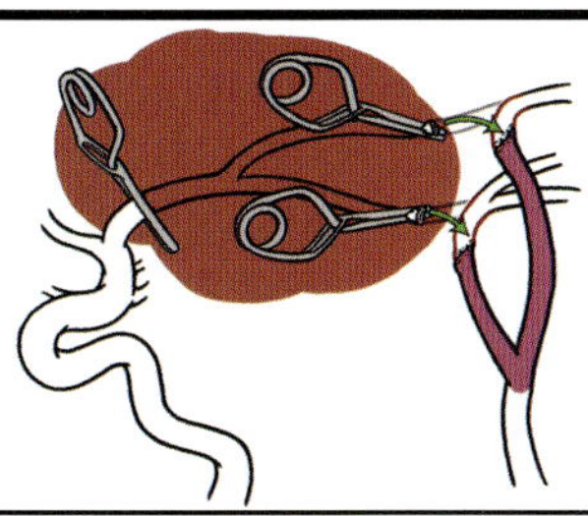

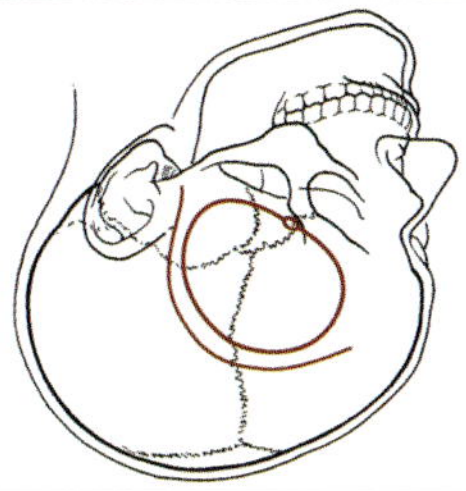

Case 2-6

Diagnosis: Giant left MCA aneurysm

Bypass: Double-barrel STA-to-MCA

Approach: Left pterional

During an evaluation for headache, a giant MCA aneurysm was discovered in a 14-year-old boy.

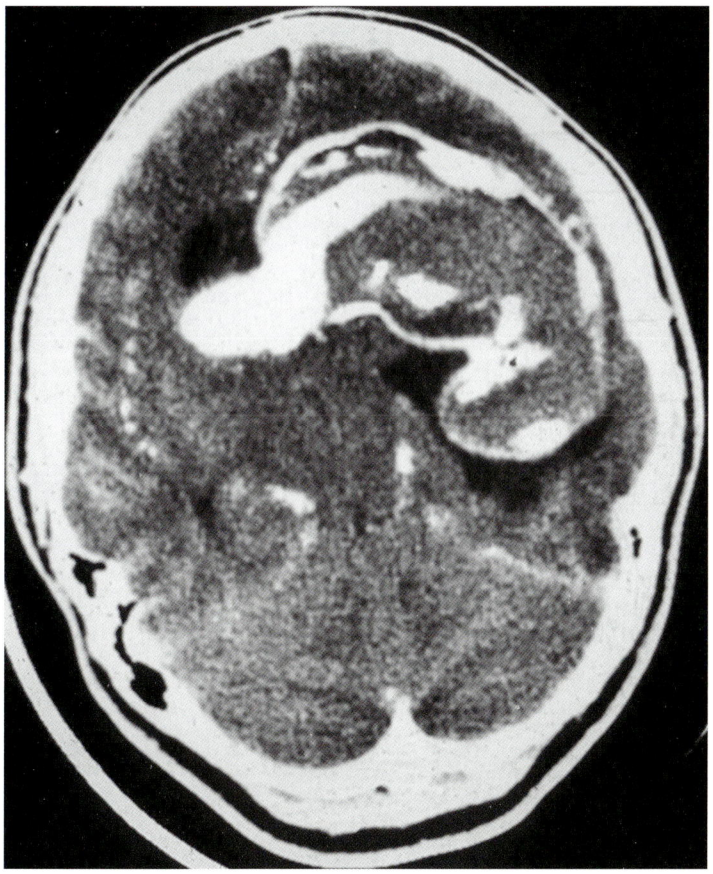

Fig. 2.6a Axial CT scan of the head with contrast shows a giant serpentine MCA aneurysm.

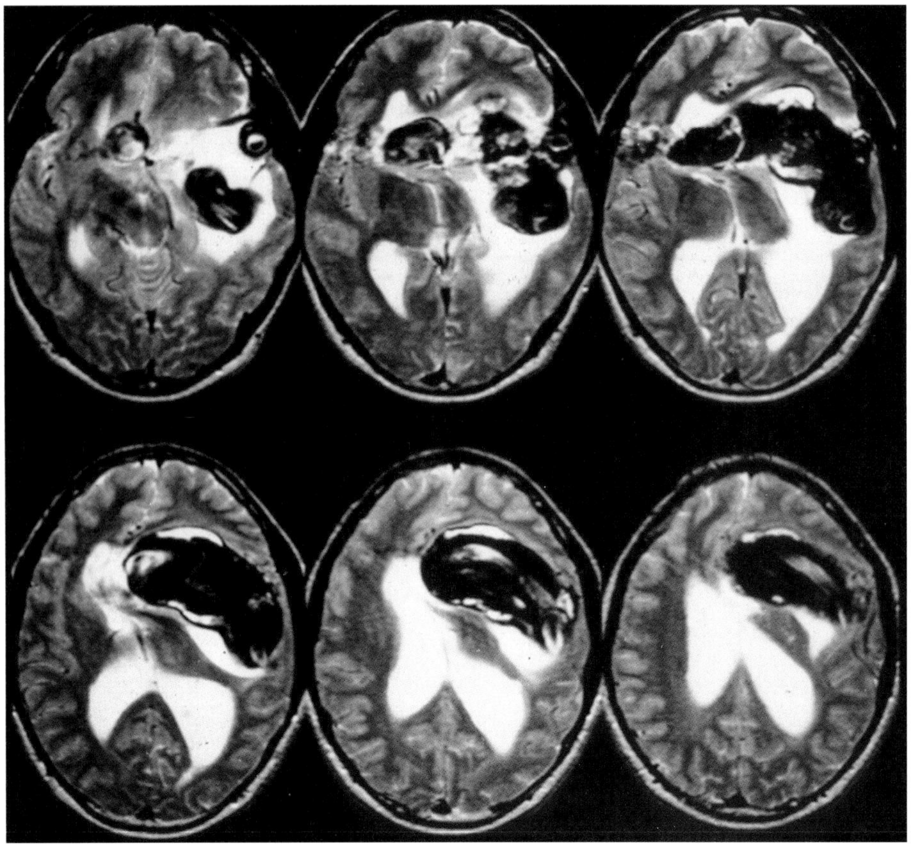

Fig. 2.6b Axial T2-weighted MR images of the brain better define the extremely large area of the mass, which crosses the midline. The variable signal intensity indicates the presence of thrombus in the dome of the aneurysm.

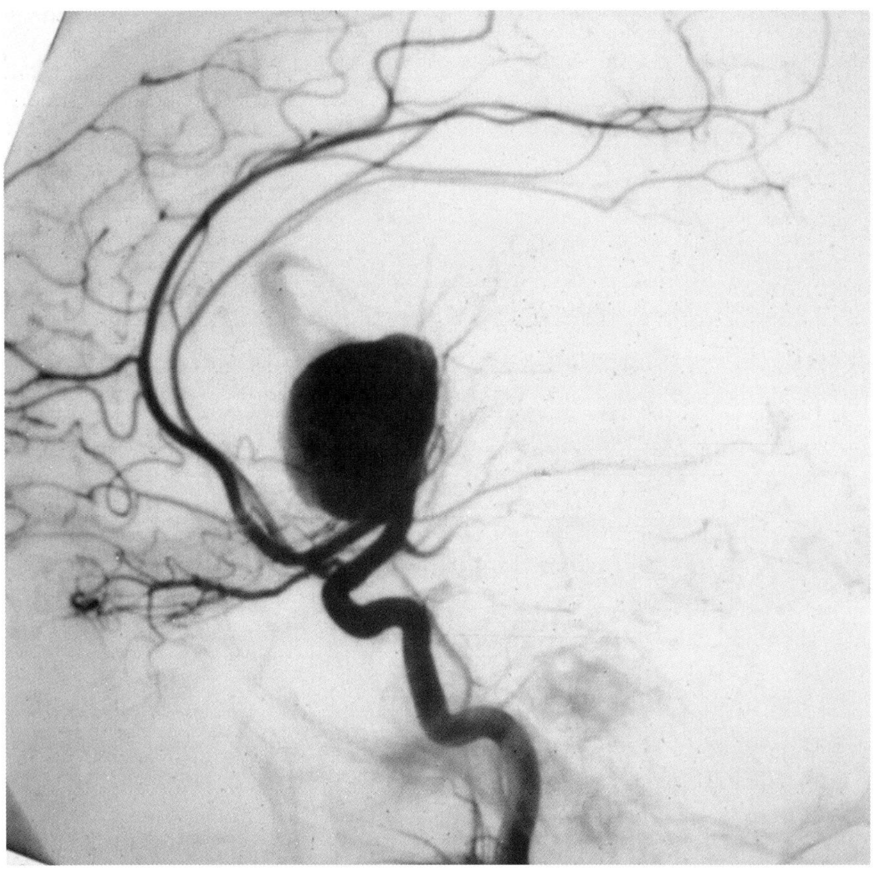

Fig. 2.6c Lateral left ICA angiogram shows that only a small portion of this massive aneurysm fills. Note the bowing of the ACA circulation.

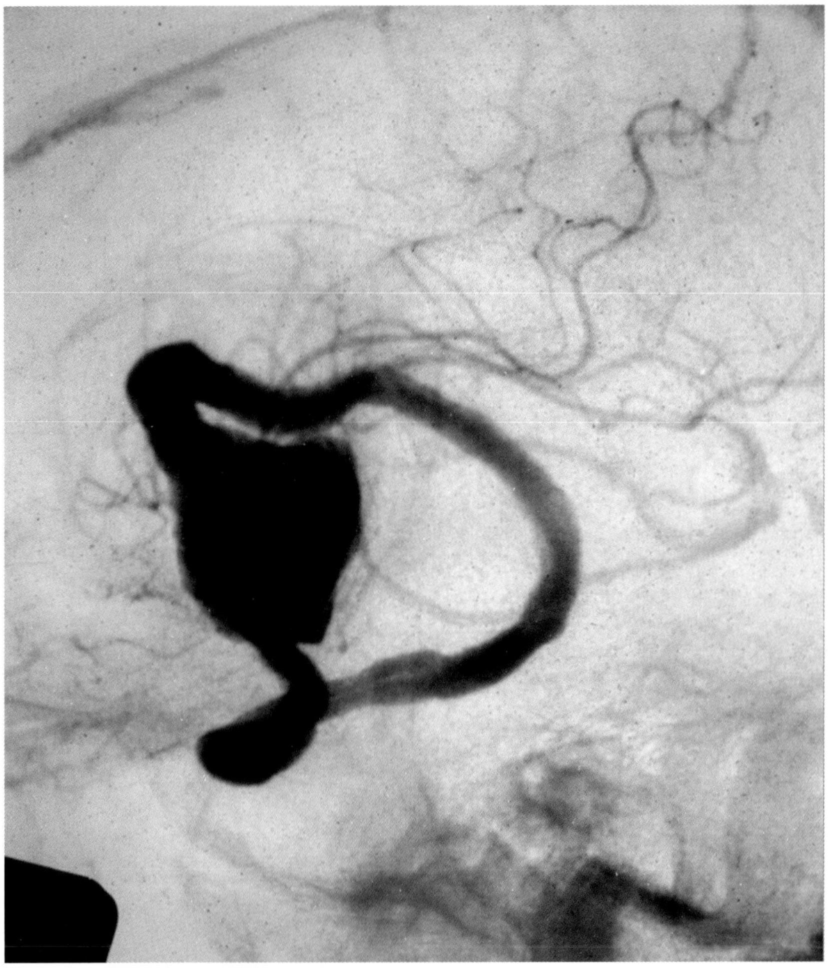

Fig. 2.6d Later phase lateral angiogram shows a large serpiginous channel through the aneurysm.

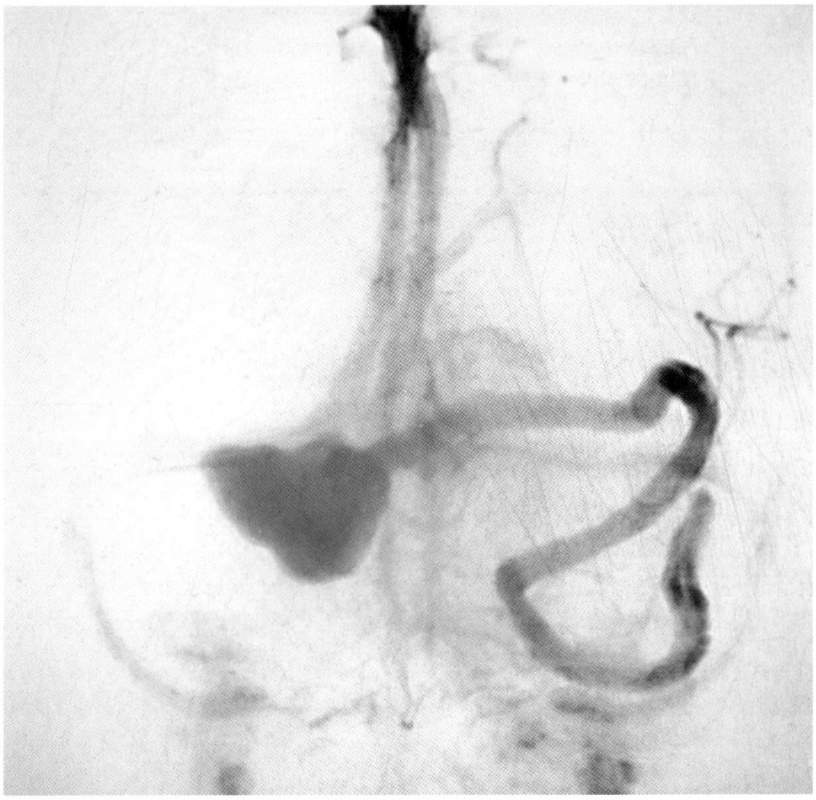

Fig. 2.6e Anteroposterior angiogram shows that the filling portion of this left MCA aneurysm is pushed across the midline to the right. The serpiginous channel crosses to the left side, eventually filling the cortical M4 vessels.

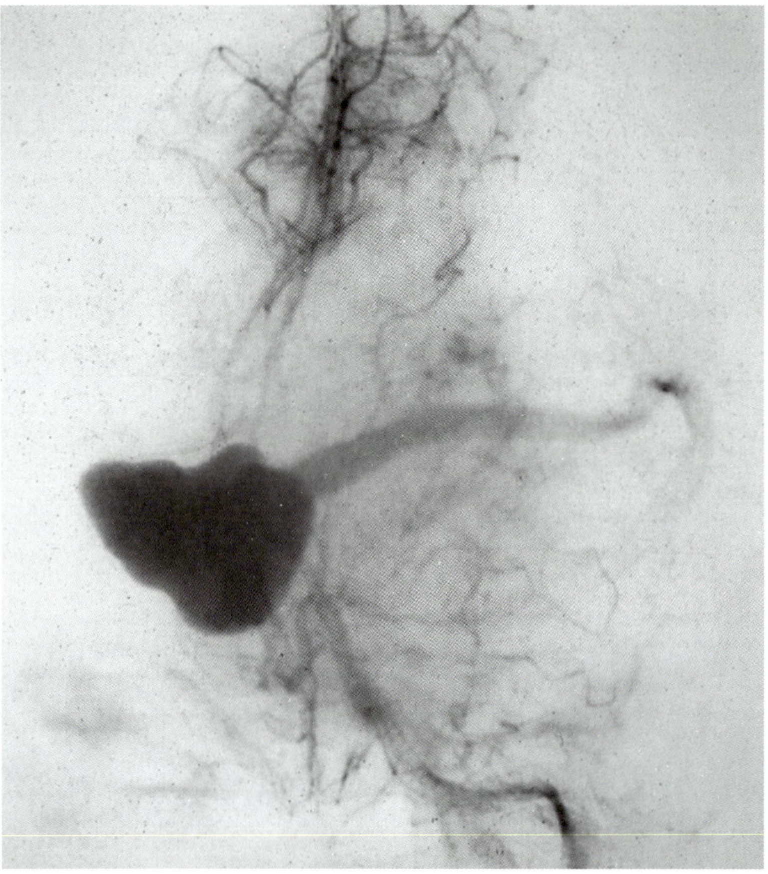

Fig. 2.6f Later phase angiogram shows the blush of cortical vessels, which confirms that the vessels arising from the aneurysm provide significant distal perfusion.

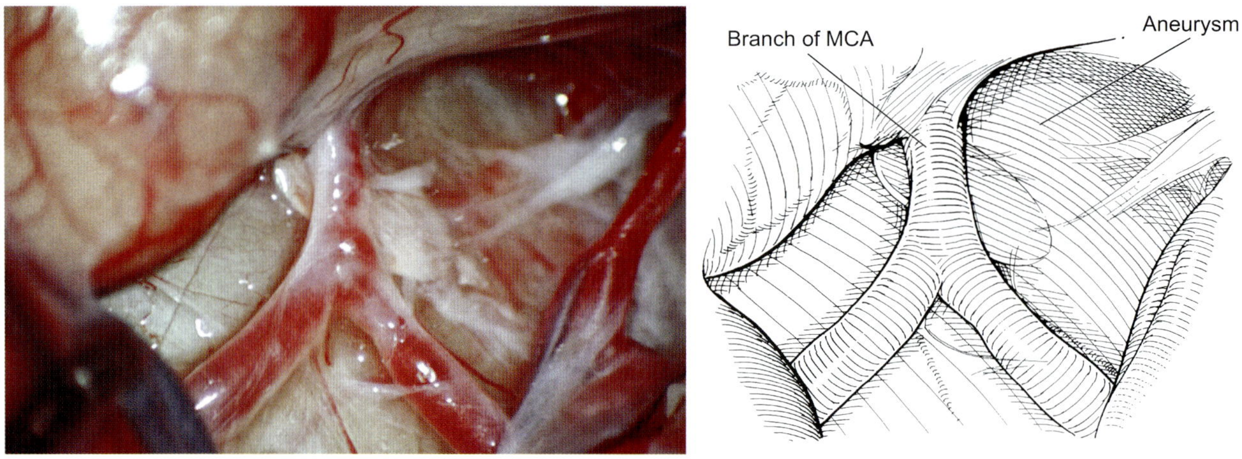

Fig. 2.6g Intraoperative photograph shows the distal MCA vessels arising from the wall of the aneurysm and stretched across its dome.

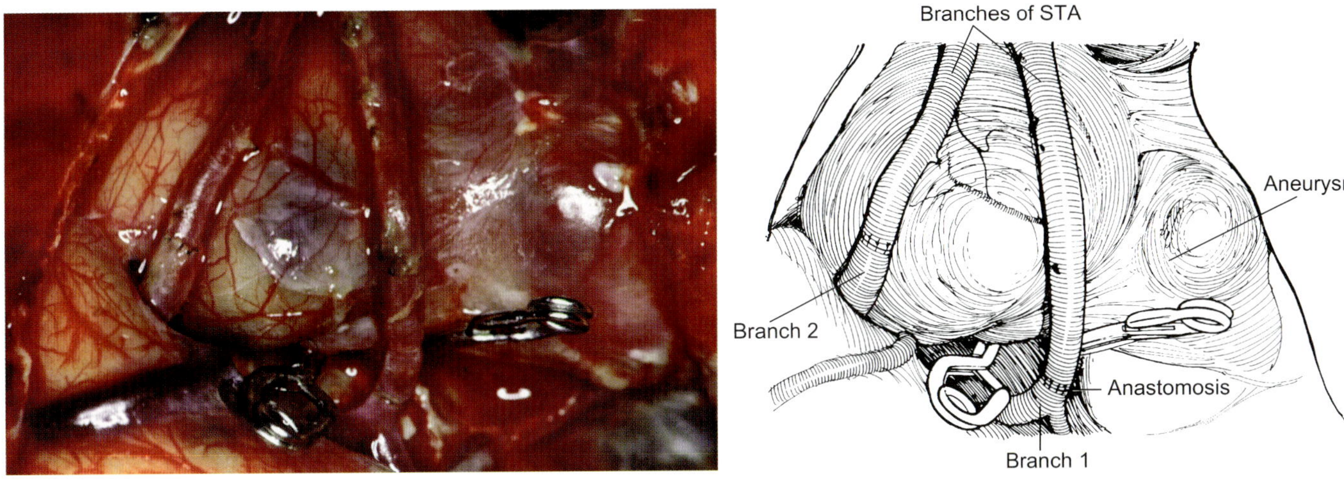

Fig. 2.6h A double-barrel end-to-end STA-to-MCA bypass was performed with the two MCA branches where they exited the aneurysm. Part of the thrombus was removed. A clip placed on the MCA as it entered the aneurysm spared the lenticulostriate arteries. Most of the aneurysm was left in situ.

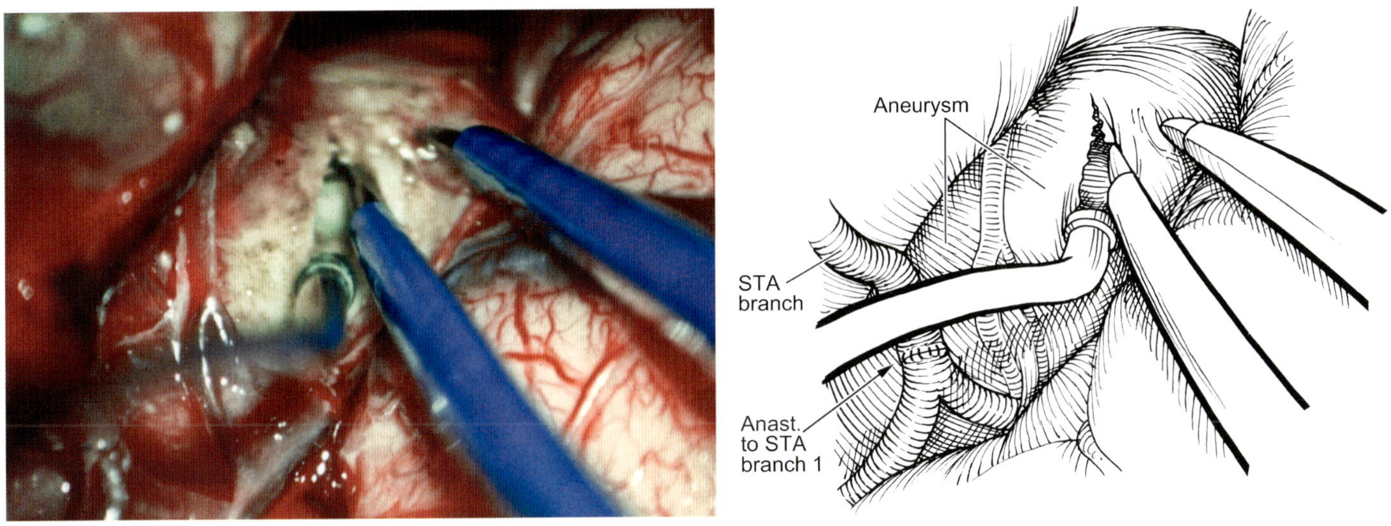

Fig. 2.6i During the second-stage procedure 1 week later, the aneurysm was exposed and incised. The two aneurysm clips placed during the first stage were removed. One of the anastomoses is shown.

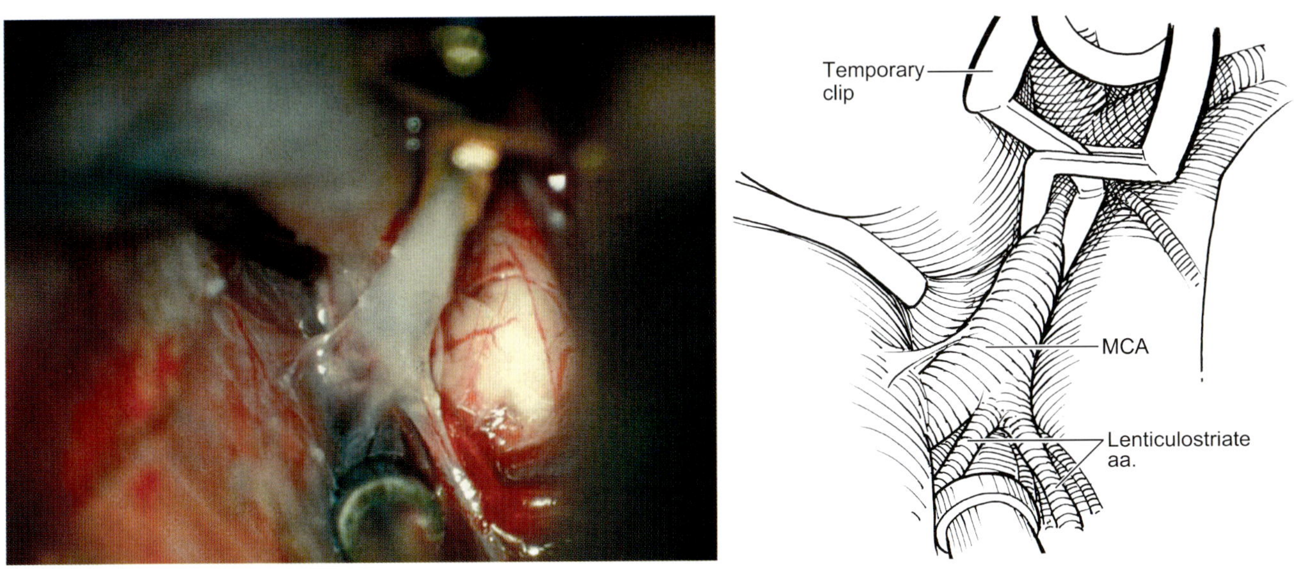

Fig. 2.6j A temporary clip is placed across the MCA. The perforating branches are identified and preserved. A permanent clip will be placed on the MCA distal to the perforating branches at the base of the aneurysm.

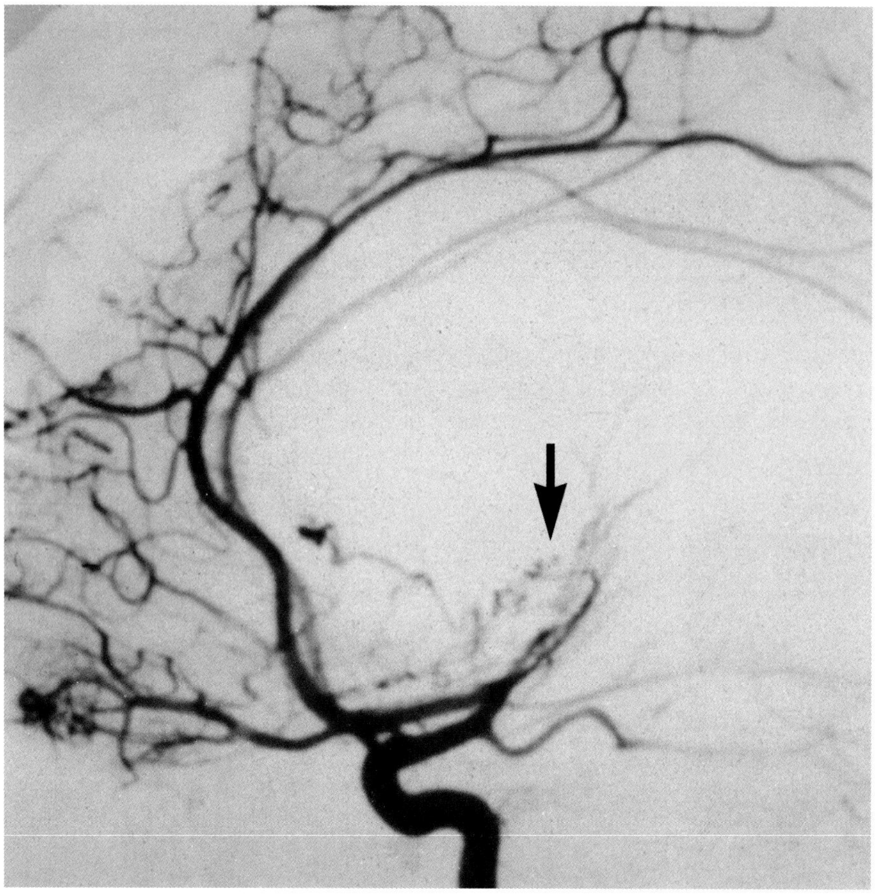

Fig. 2.6k Lateral postoperative angiogram shows no further filling of the aneurysm. The lenticulostriate arteries are visible (*arrow*).

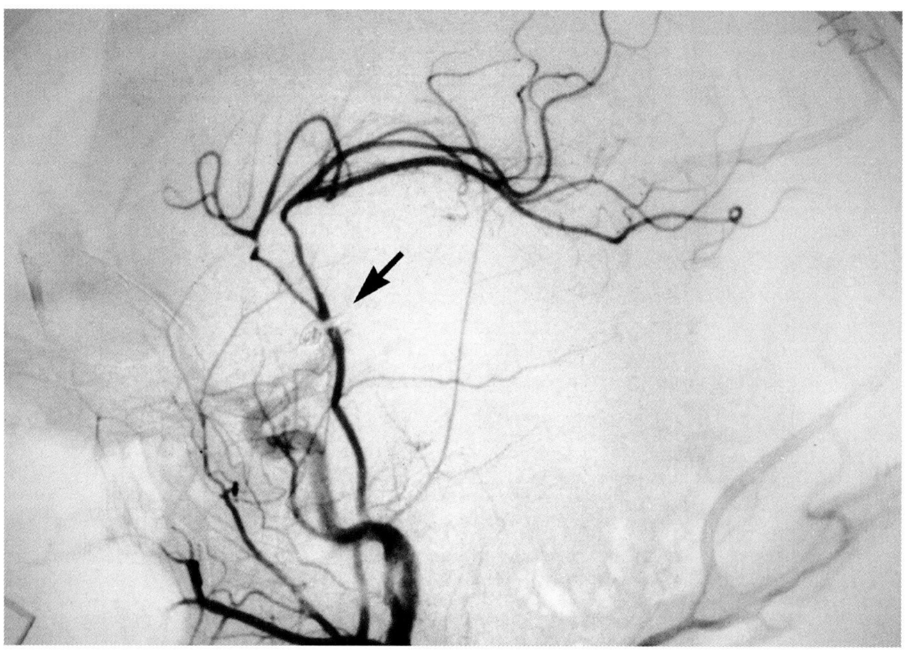

Fig. 2.6l Lateral left ECA angiogram confirms patency of the double-barrel bypass. The discontinuity in the STA is from the shadow of the aneurysm clip (*arrow*). The MCA vessels, which had been stretched by the aneurysm, were elevated and straightened.

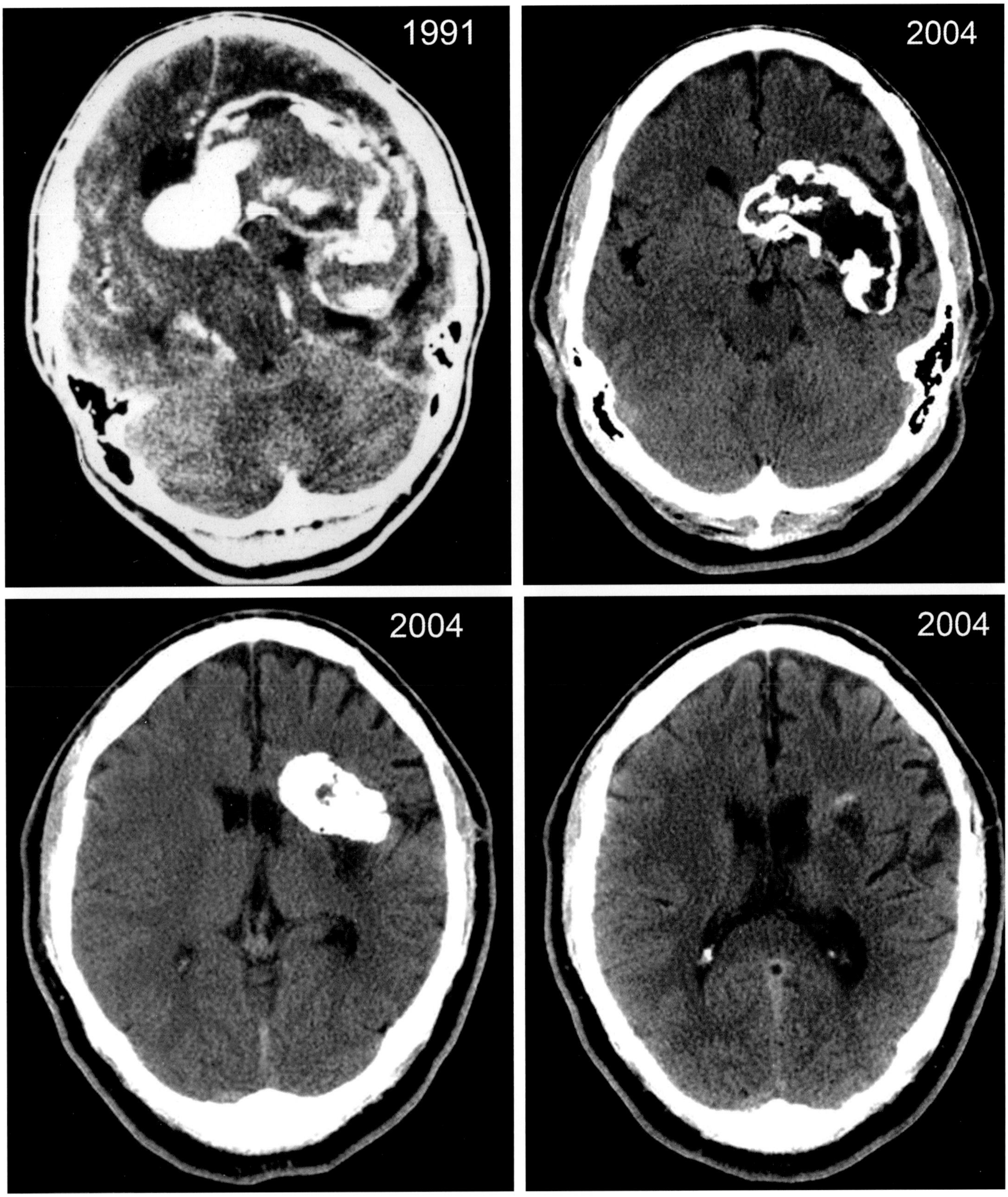

m n o p

Fig. 2.6m–p Preoperative (**m**) and late follow-up (**n, o, p**) CT images show the great reduction in the size of the residual aneurysm. The patient remained completely asymptomatic.

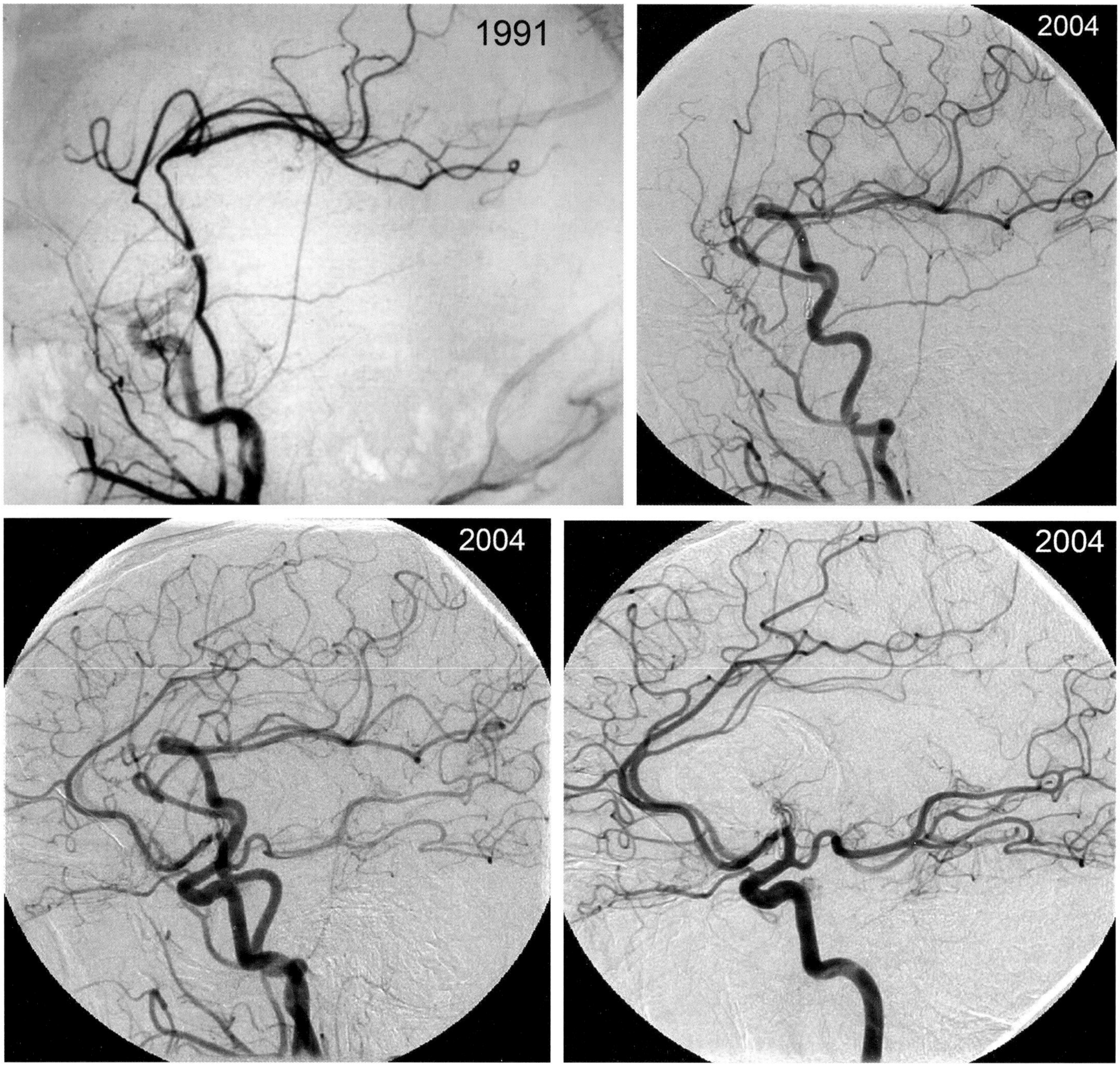

q r s t

Fig. 2.6q–t Postoperative (**q**) and late follow-up (**r, s, t**) angiograms show the robust filling of the MCA territory through the double-barrel bypass and demonstrate the longevity of this artery-to-artery anastomosis. (**Fig. 2.6r and t** used with permission from Springer-Verlag Wien.)

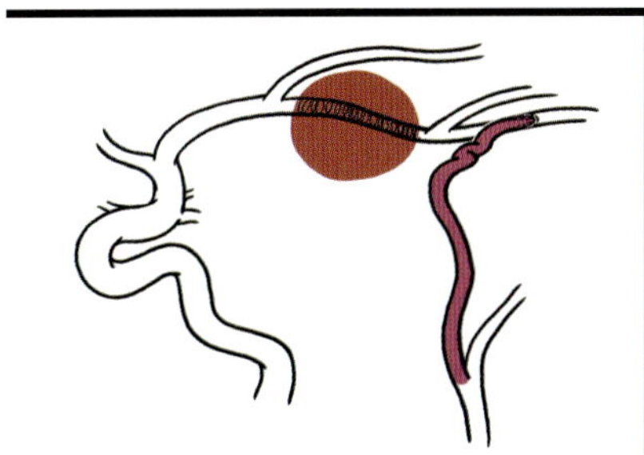

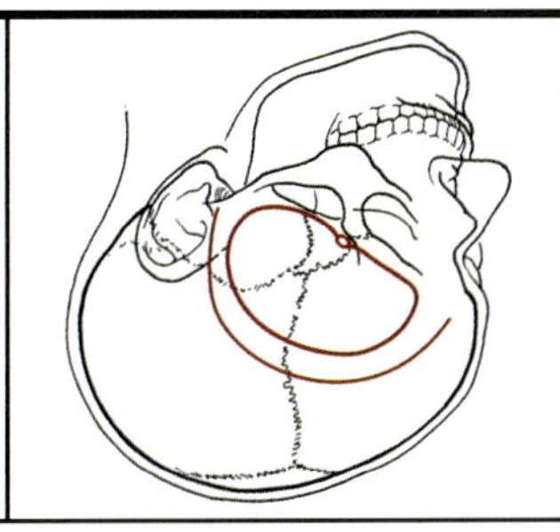

Case 2-7

Diagnosis: Left MCA dissecting fusiform aneurysm

Bypass: STA-to-MCA with endovascular occlusion of aneurysm

Approach: Left frontotemporal

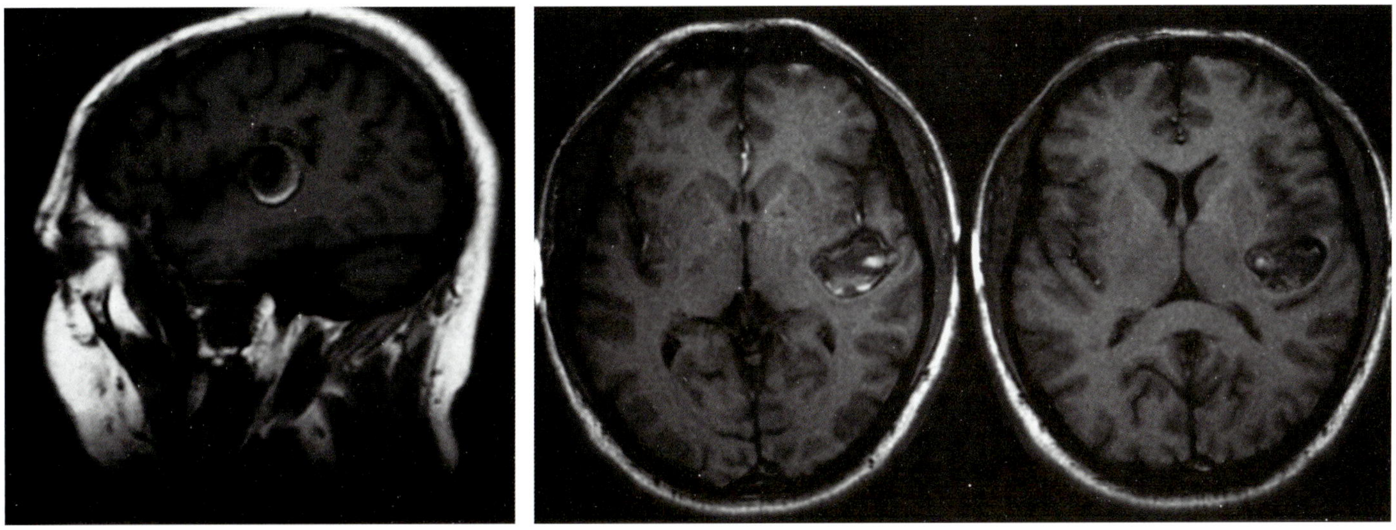

a b

Fig. 2.7a, b Sagittal and axial MR images demonstrate mass effect from a dissecting fusiform aneurysm on the left MCA. This dissecting aneurysm, which had been followed for 7 years, showed growth over a 6-month period. The patient's symptoms included fluctuating periodic aphasia.

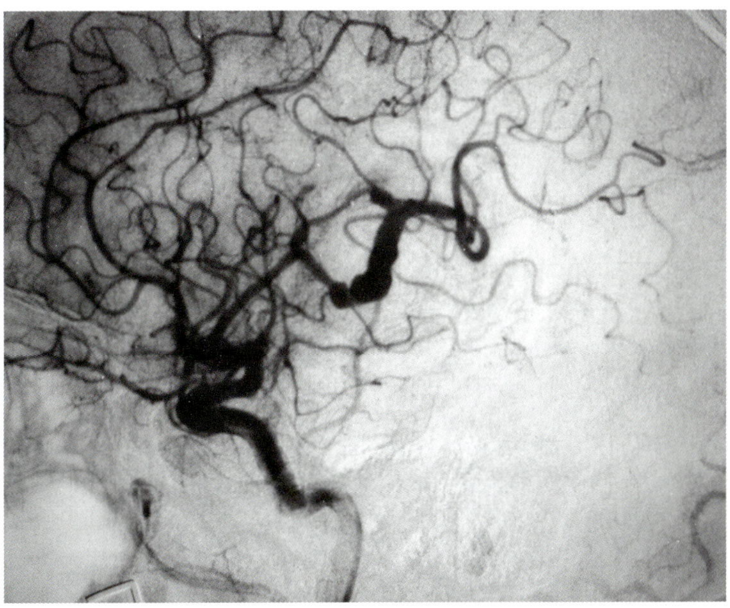

Fig. 2.7c Angiogram demonstrates a fusiform vessel in the distribution of the left MCA.

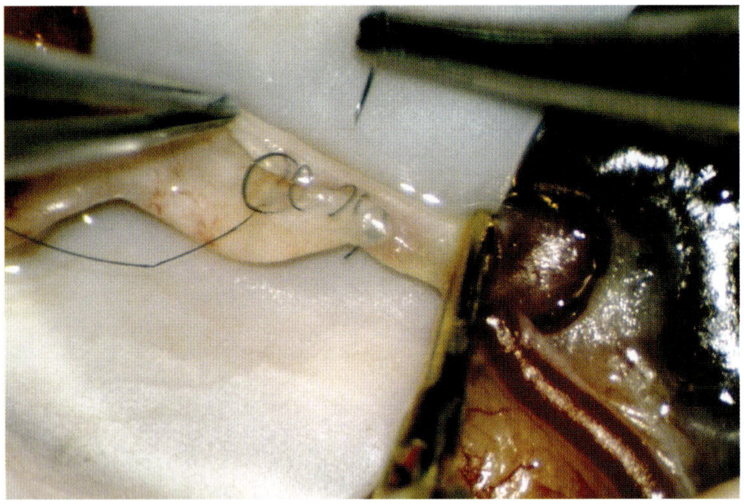

Fig. 2.7d After a frontotemporal craniotomy is performed, the MCA segment distal to the aneurysm is freed from the arachnoid and temporarily clipped. The STA is tacked to the opened MCA with heel and toe stitches and running sutures are loosely placed in one wall.

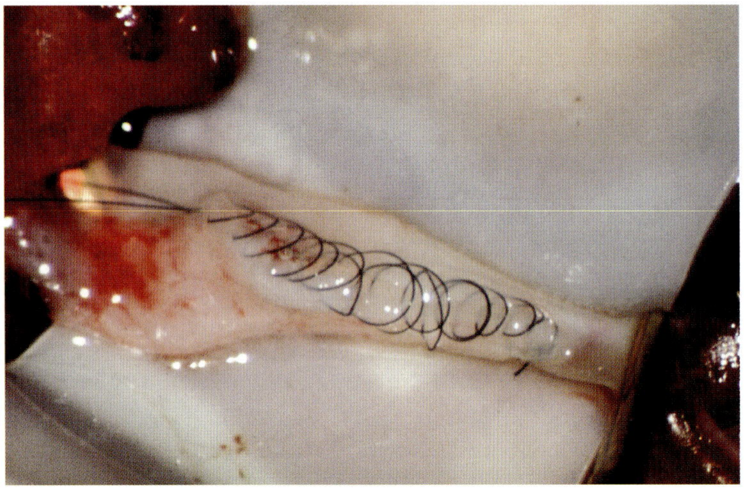

Fig. 2.7e The sutures are tightened and tied to the heel knot.

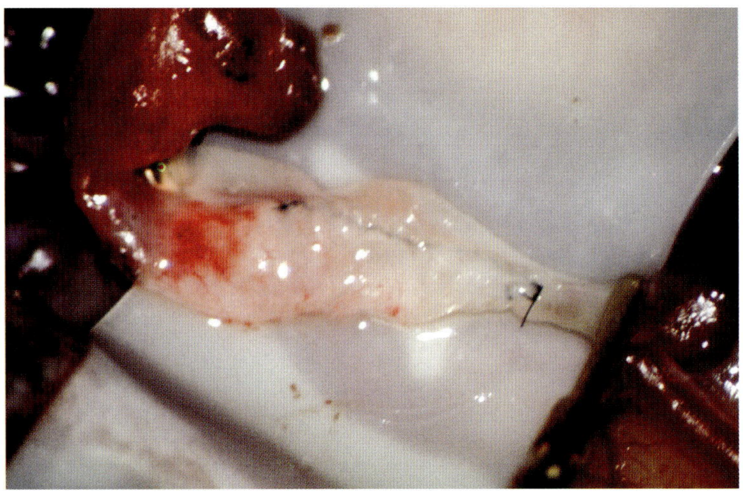

Fig. 2.7f The remainder of the loose running sutures are placed.

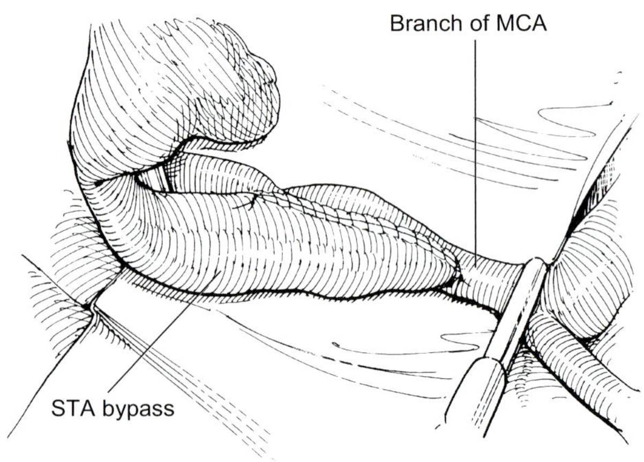

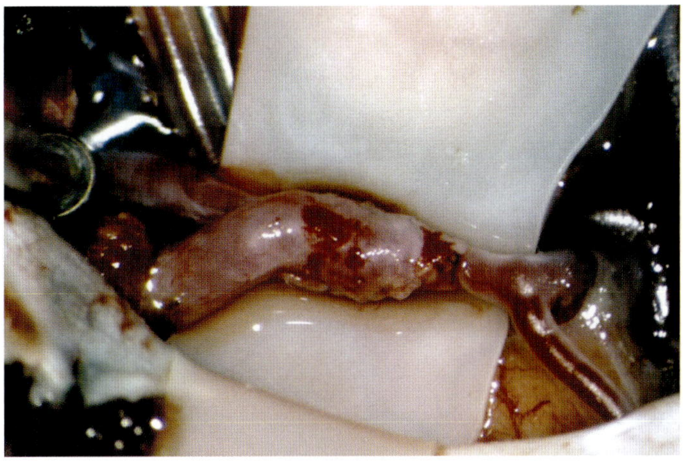

Fig. 2.7g The completed bypass fills robustly.

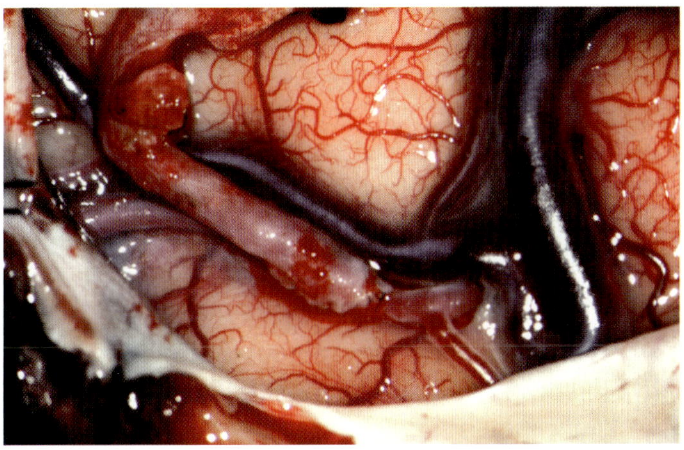

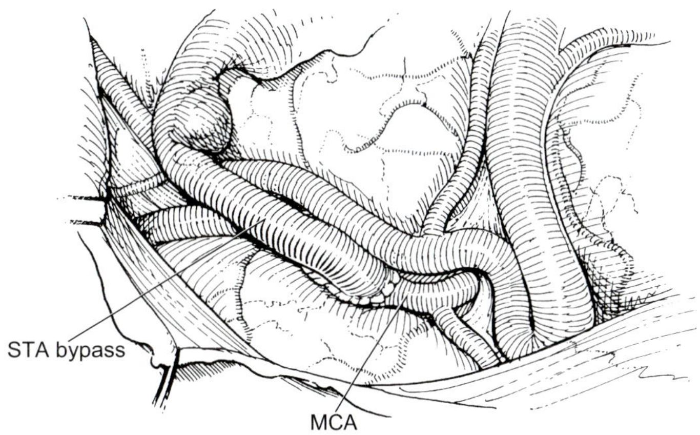

Fig. 2.7h Overview of the completed STA-to-MCA bypass.

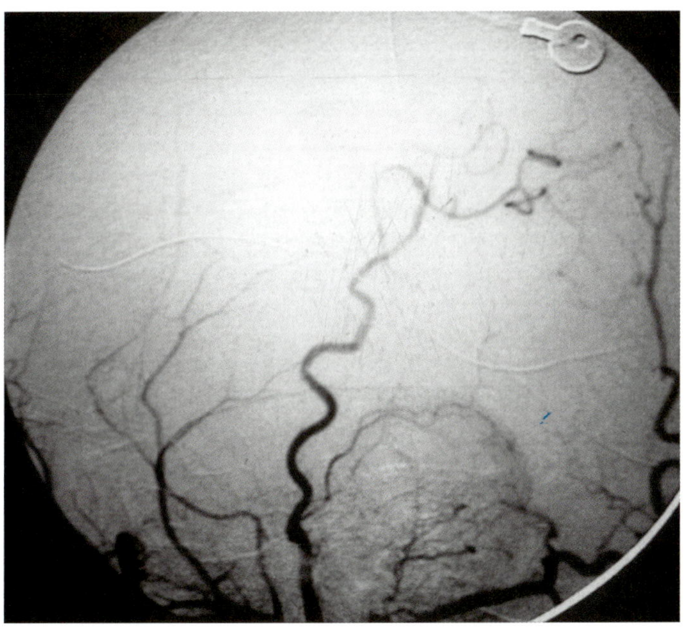

Fig. 2.7i Selective injection of the external vessels on the left demonstrates patency of the bypass.

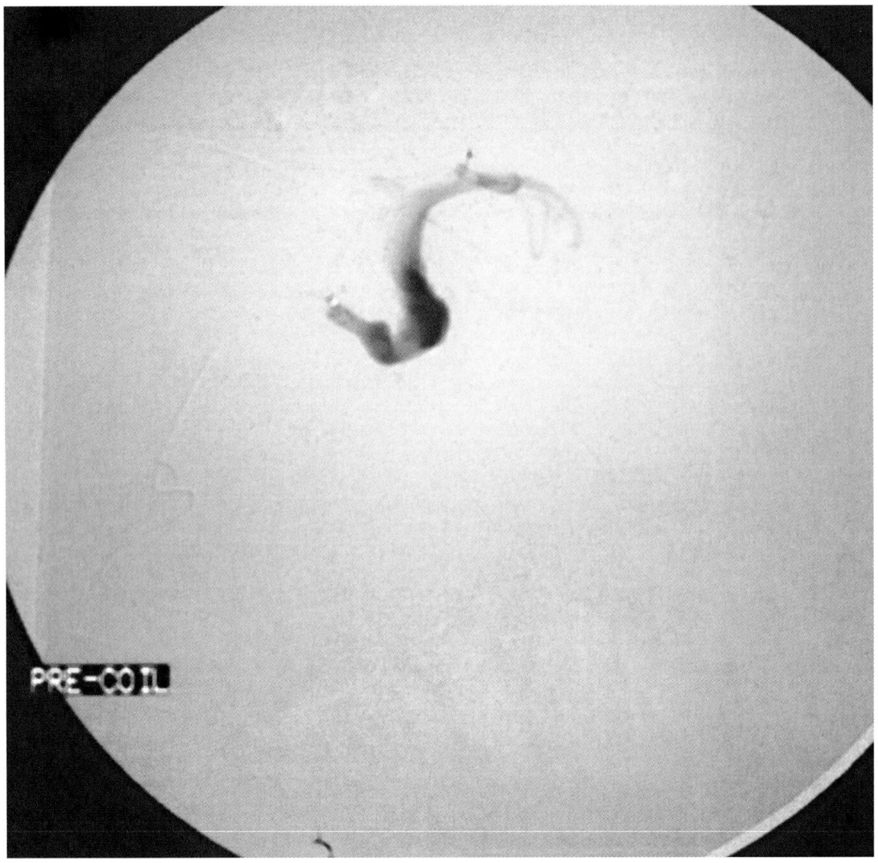

Fig. 2.7j Selective catheterization of the MCA branch involved with the aneurysm is performed. Coils were placed into the vessel until it was obstructed completely.

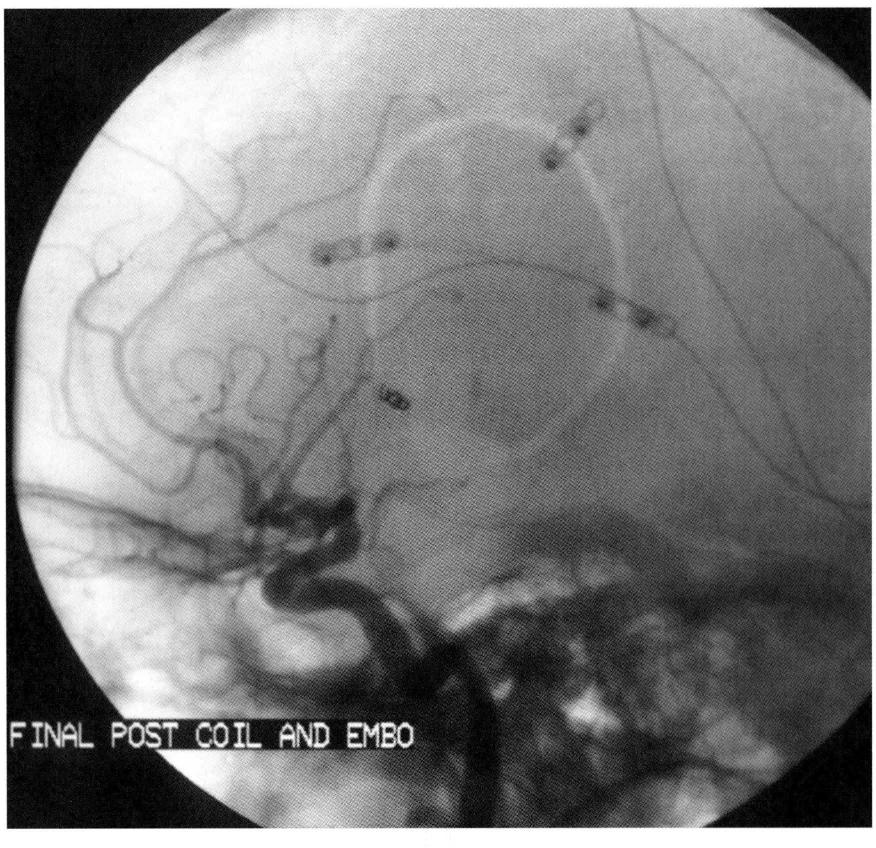

Fig. 2.7k Postoperative ICA angiogram demonstrates the absence of the aneurysm. The patient had no neurologic deficits.

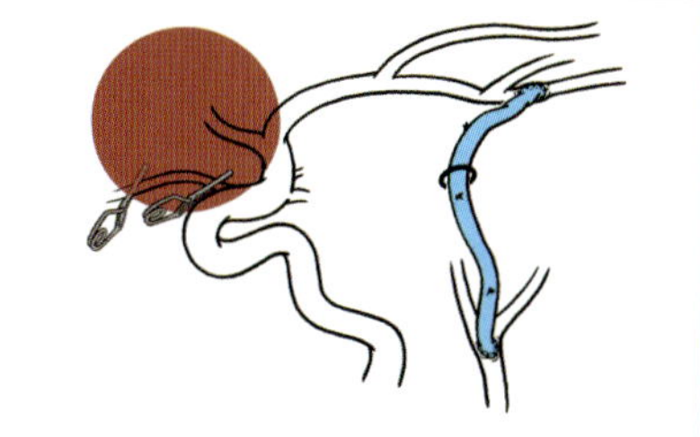

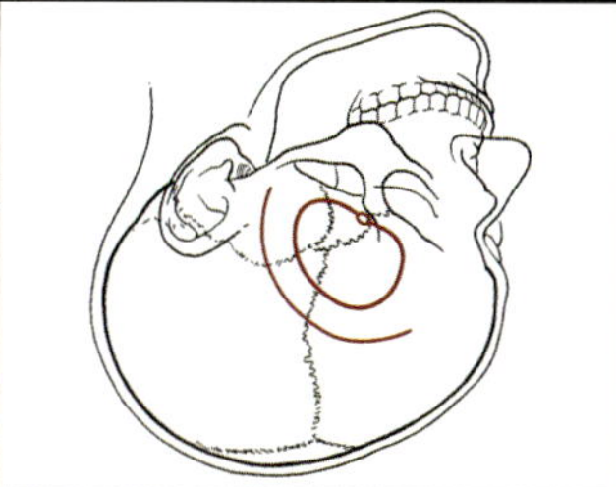

Case 2-8

Diagnosis: Giant left ophthalmic artery aneurysm

Bypass: STA-to-MCA with saphenous vein graft

Approach: Left pterional

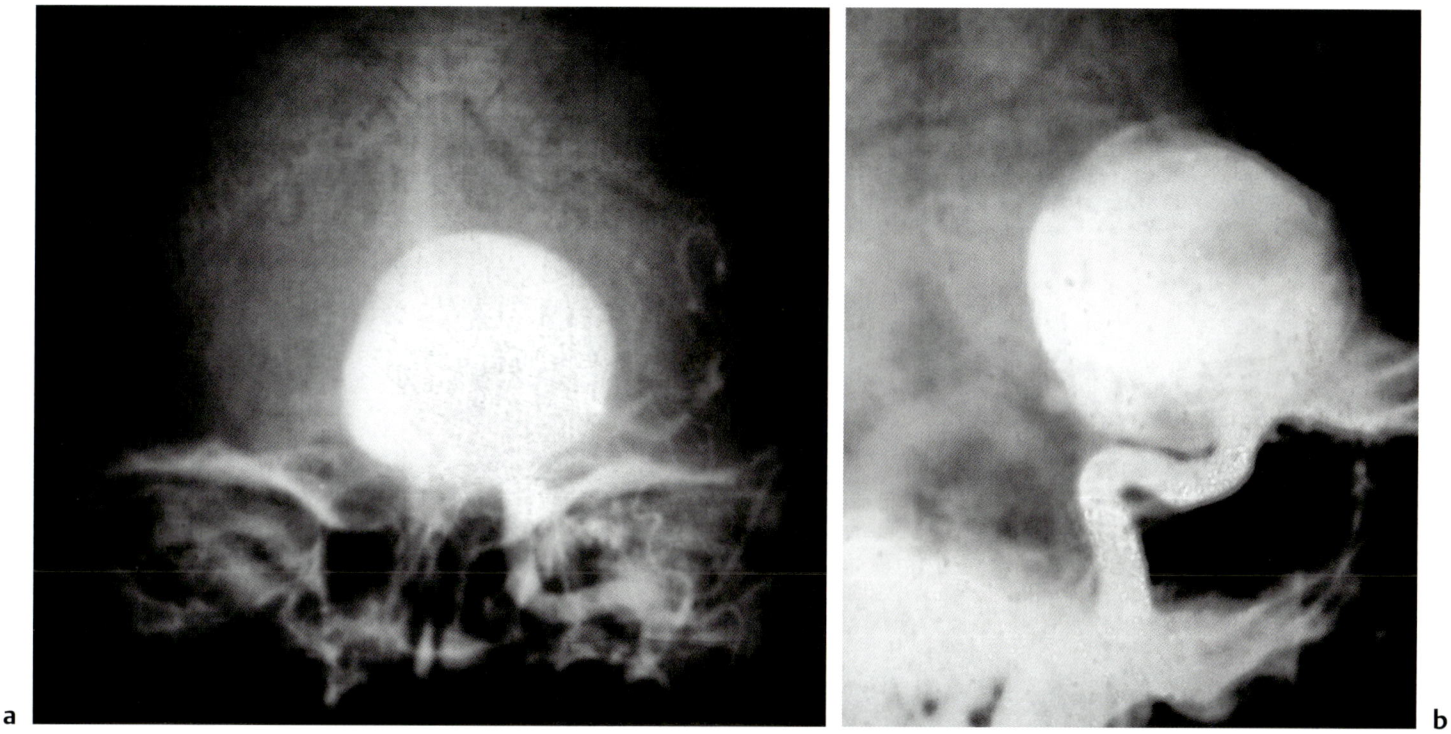

Fig. 2.8a, b Anteroposterior and lateral left ICA angiograms show a giant aneurysm of the left ophthalmic artery in a patient with progressive deterioration of vision and left hemispheric TIAs.

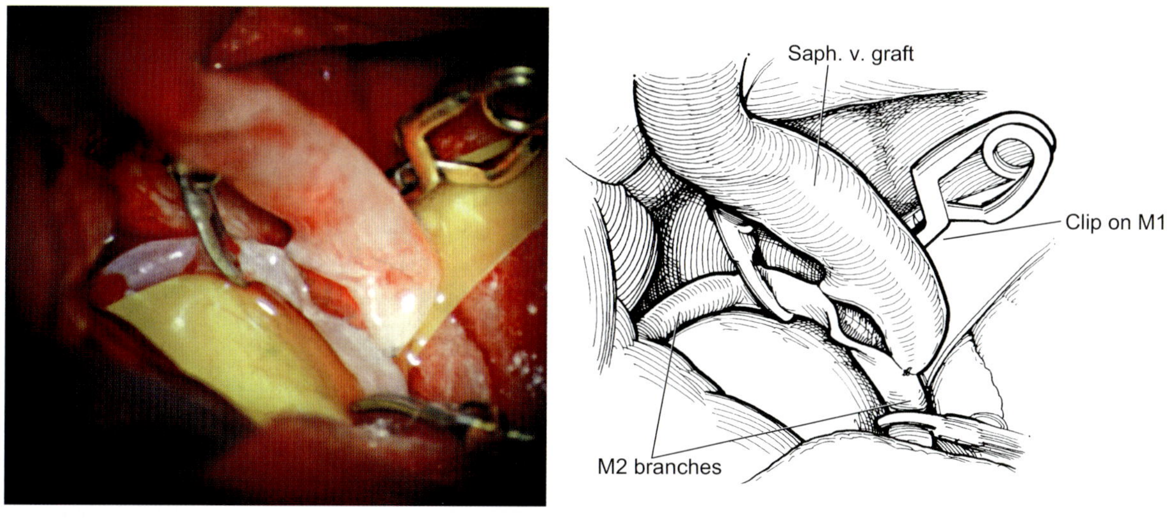

Fig. 2.8c The back wall of a saphenous vein graft–to–MCA anastomosis is completed.

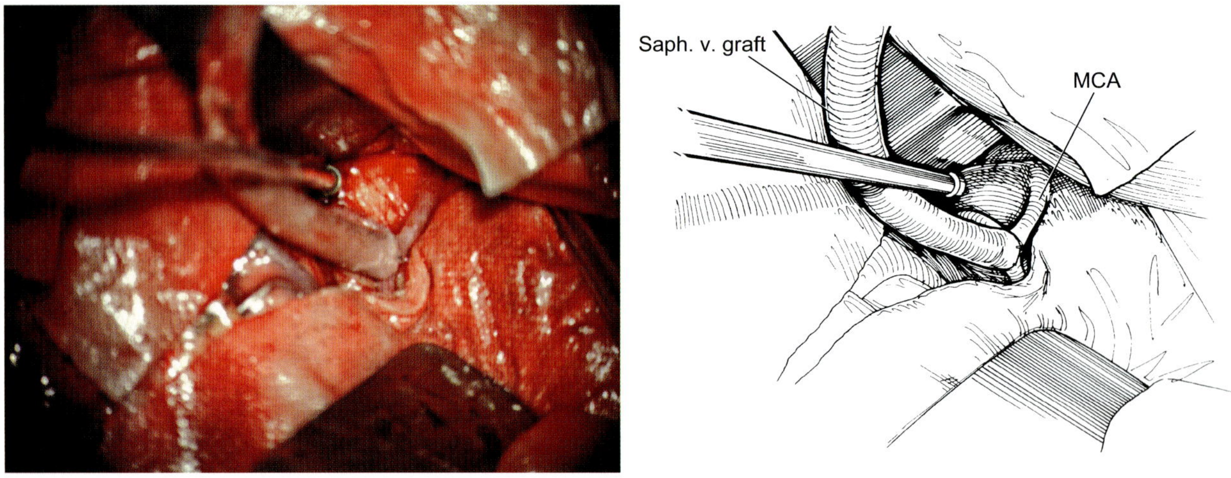

Fig. 2.8d The front wall is completed and the clips are removed, backfilling the graft.

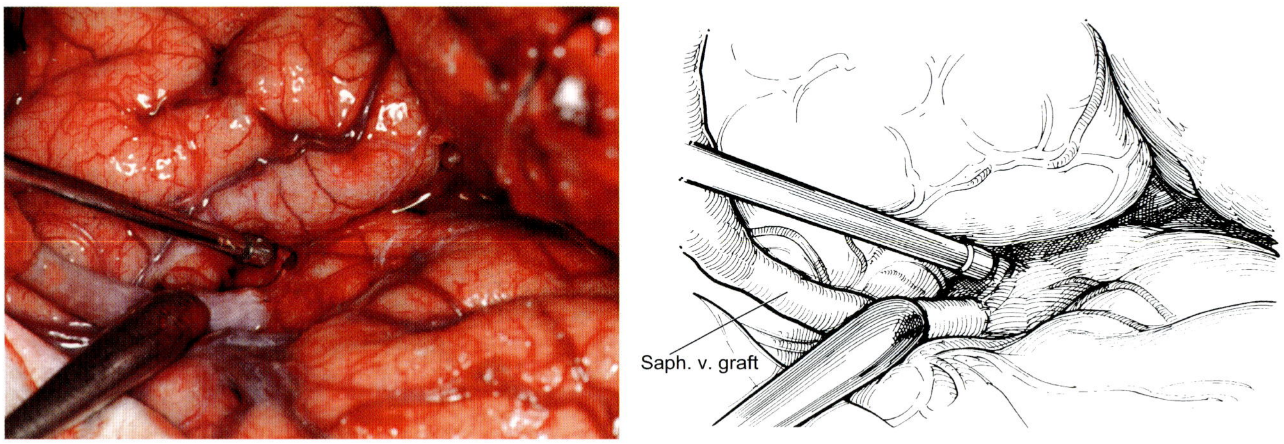

Fig. 2.8e Overview shows the vein graft entering the left sylvian fissure. The aneurysm was then trapped.

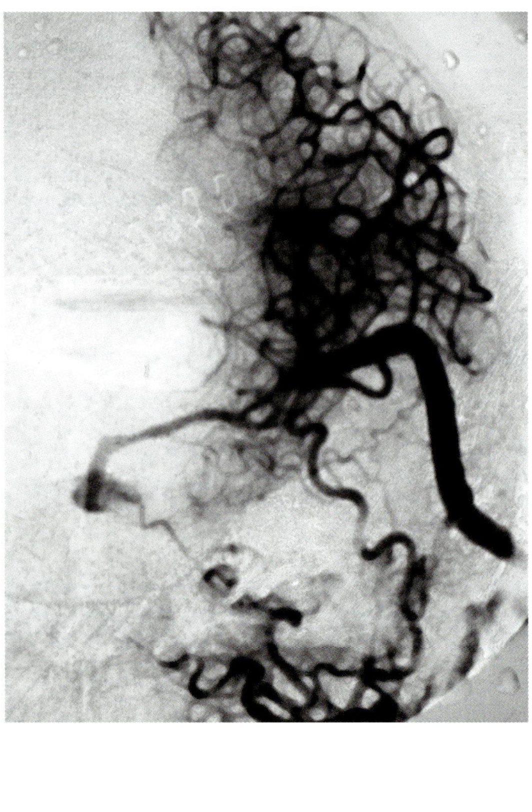

Fig. 2.8f Postoperative left ECA angiographic injection shows excellent filling of the entire distribution of the left MCA. Retrograde filling down to the aneurysm is seen.

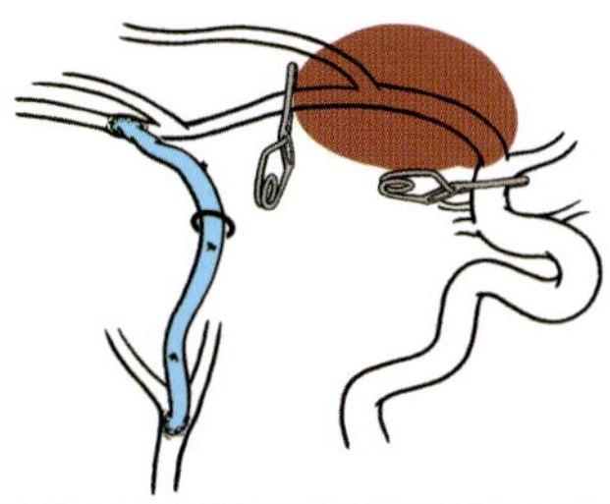

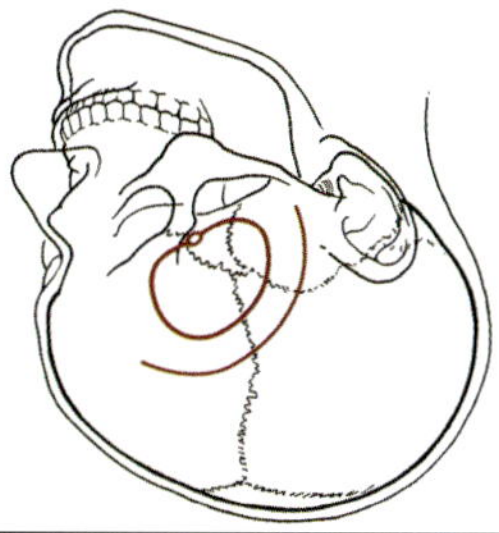

Case 2-9

Diagnosis: Right ICA bifurcation giant fusiform aneurysm

Bypass: STA-to-MCA with saphenous vein graft

Approach: Right pterional

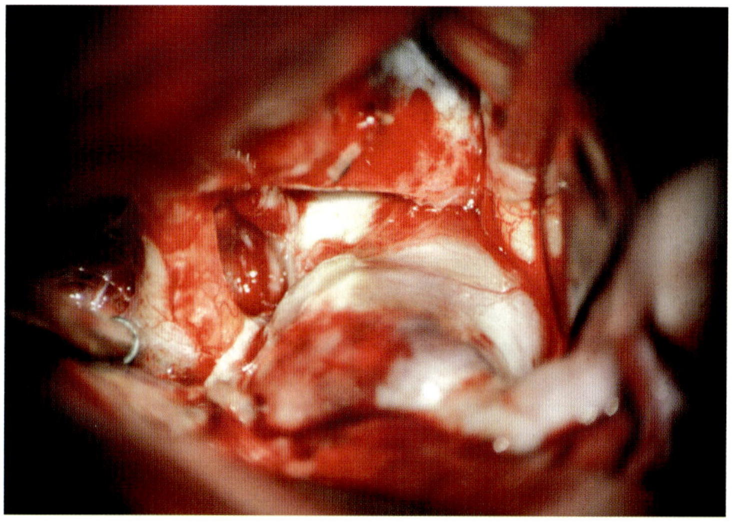

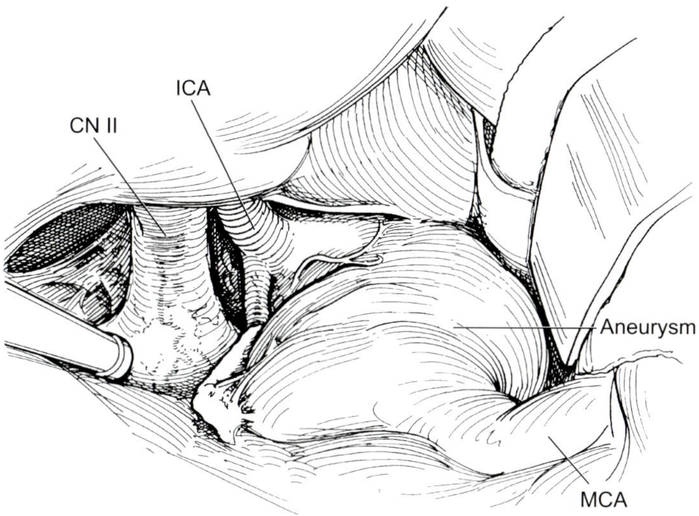

Fig. 2.9a A right pterional craniotomy is performed and the sylvian fissure is split to expose the right MCA and ICA. The PCoA and AChoA were identified.

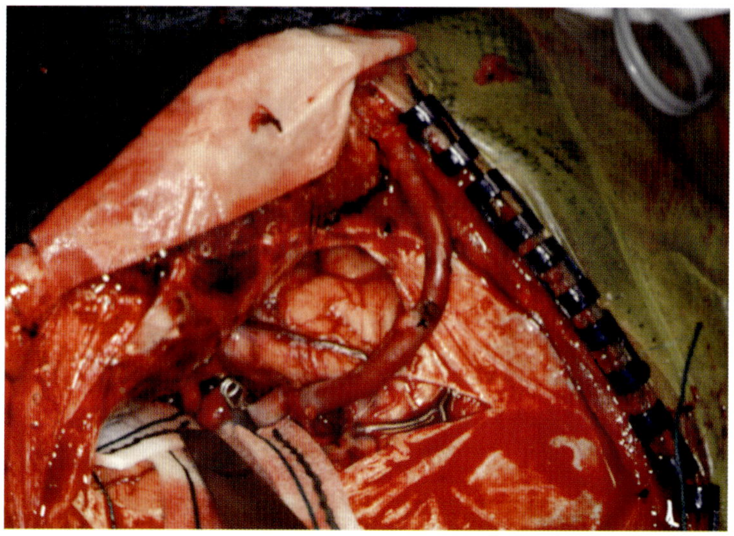

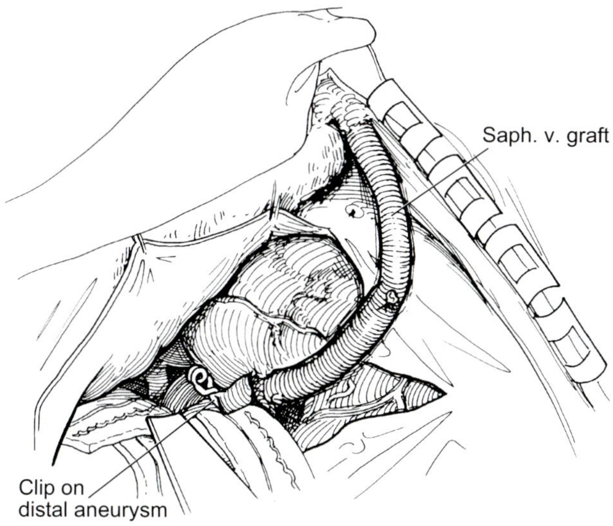

Fig. 2.9b The STA-to-MCA bypass is completed using a saphenous vein graft from the bifurcation of the STA. Clips were placed across the ICA distal to the AChoA and on the MCA distal to the aneurysm to trap the lesion.

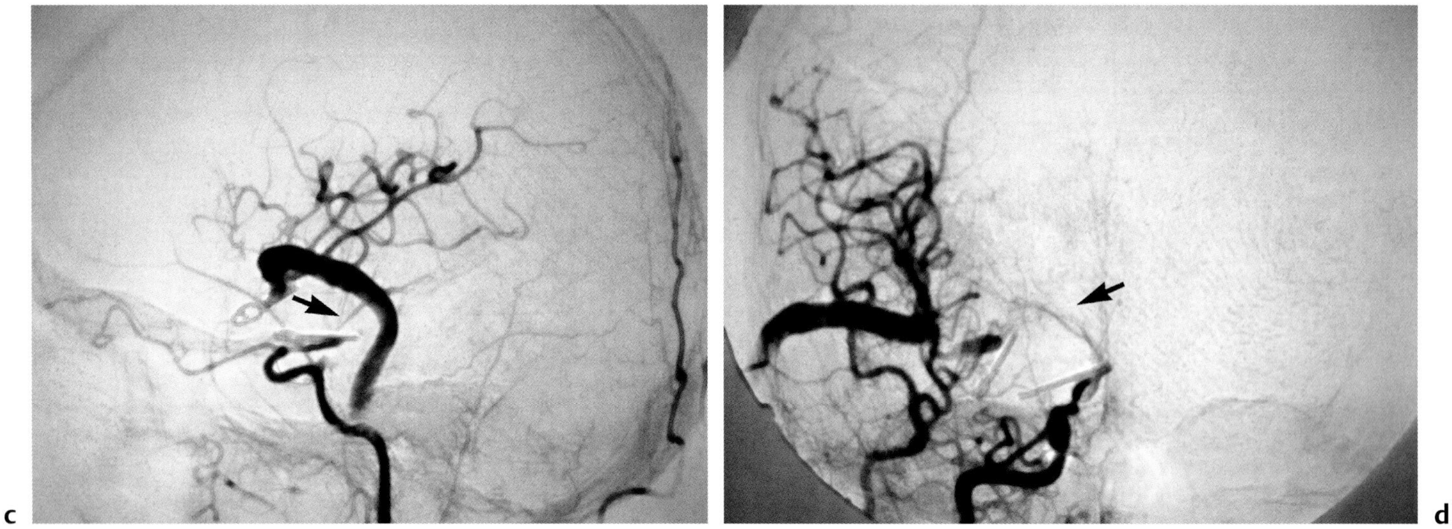

Fig. 2.9c, d Postoperative lateral and anteroposterior angiograms show the clips and the bypass filling the MCA distally. The ICA fills the AChoA (*arrows*).

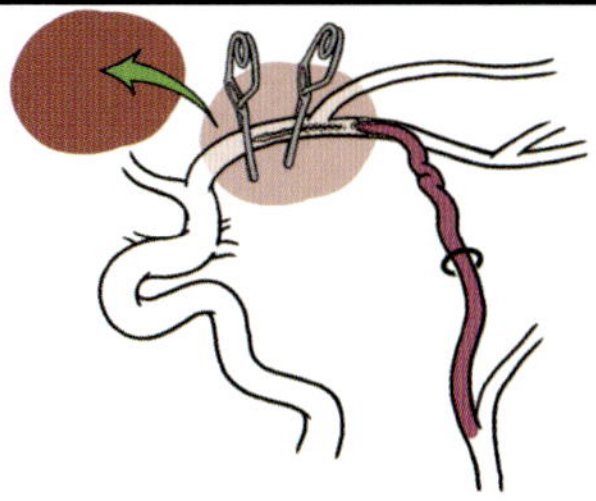

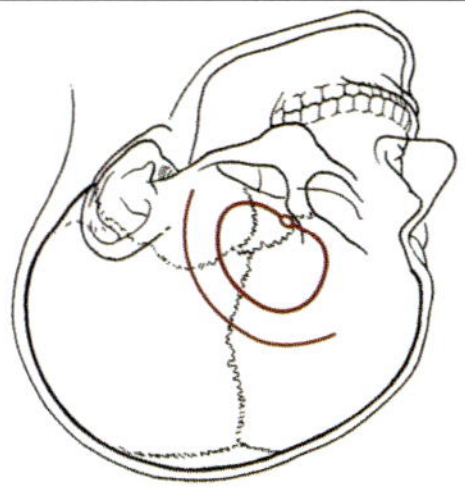

Case 2-10

Diagnosis: Left MCA giant aneurysm

Bypass: STA-to-MCA

Approach: Left pterional

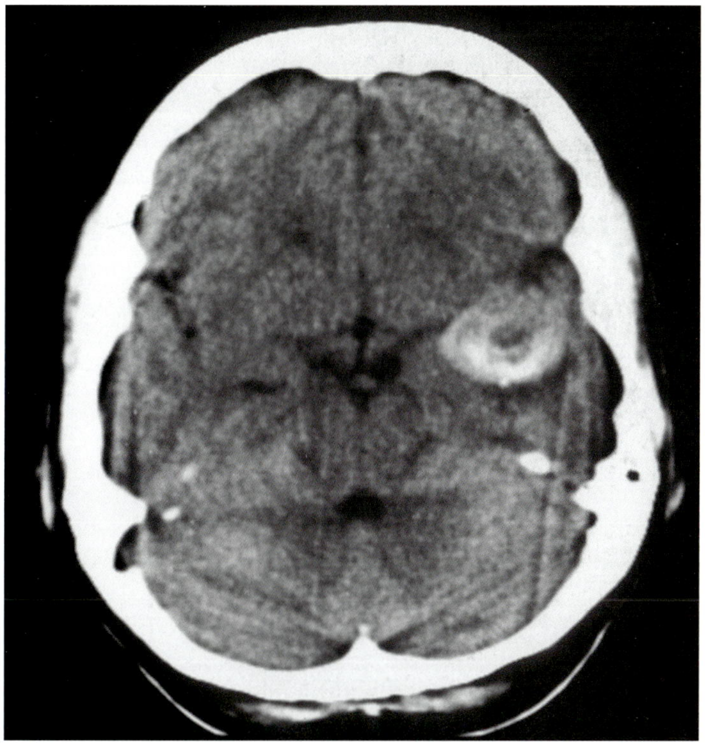

Fig. 2.10a Axial CT scan shows a large, smooth-walled mass in the left sylvian fissure.

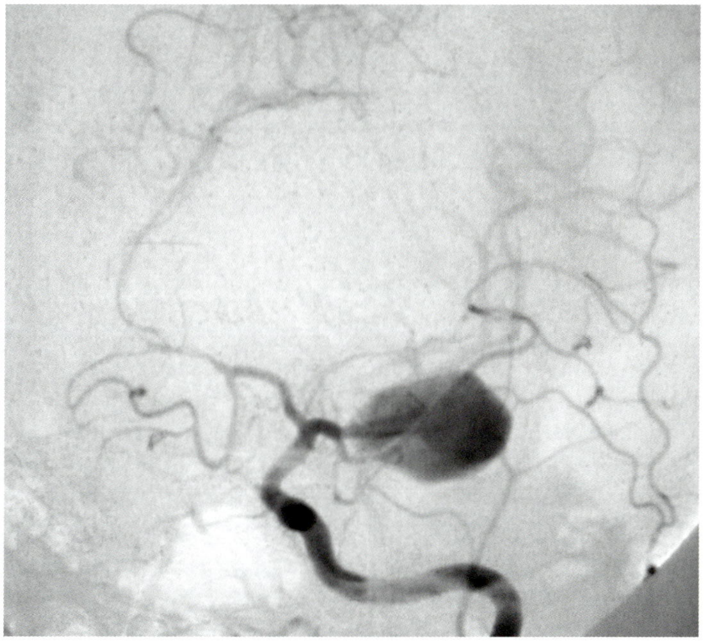

b

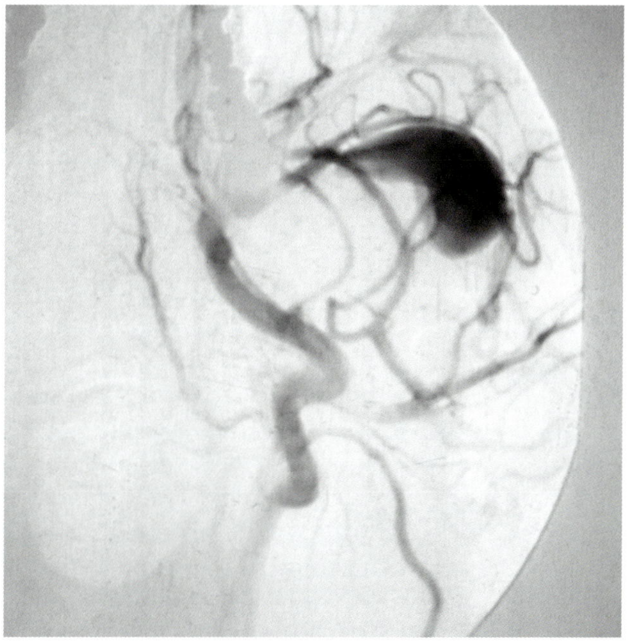

c

Fig. 2.10b, c Anteroposterior and oblique left ICA angiographic injections show a complex aneurysm of the left MCA.

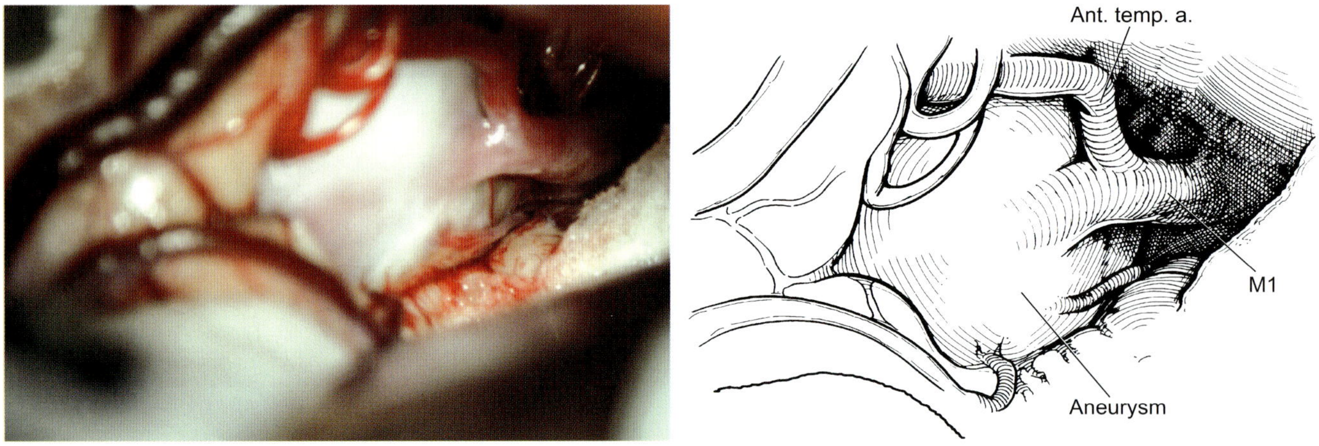

Fig. 2.10d After the sylvian fissure is split, a giant aneurysm of the main trunk of the MCA is visible just distal to the origin of the anterior temporal artery.

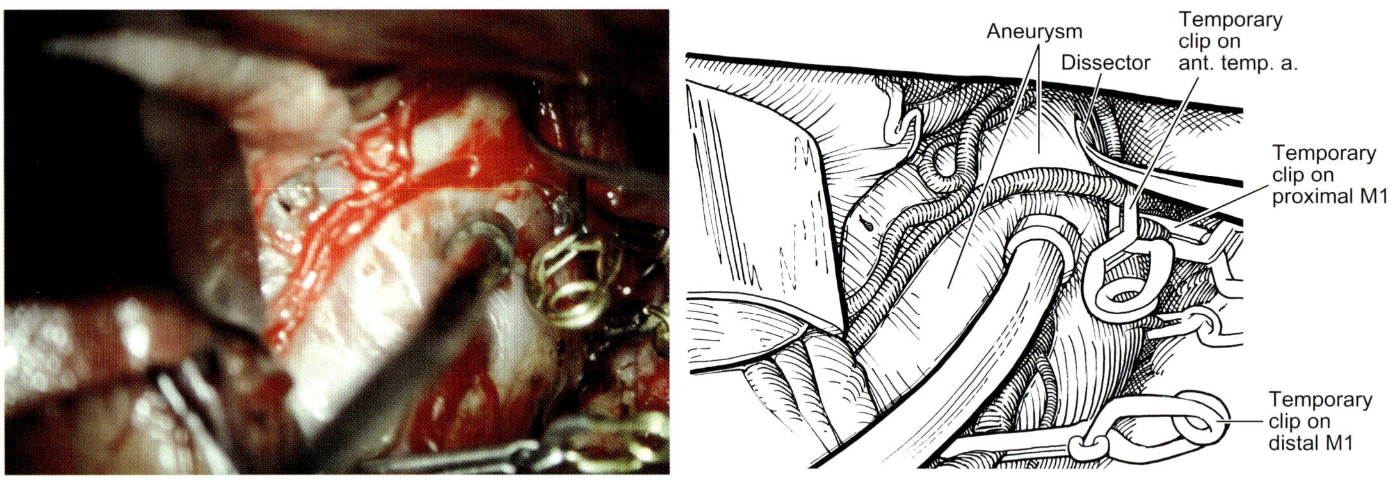

Fig. 2.10e While the MCA branch is temporarily occluded, the aneurysm is exposed further. Abbreviation: ant. temp. a., anterior temporal artery.

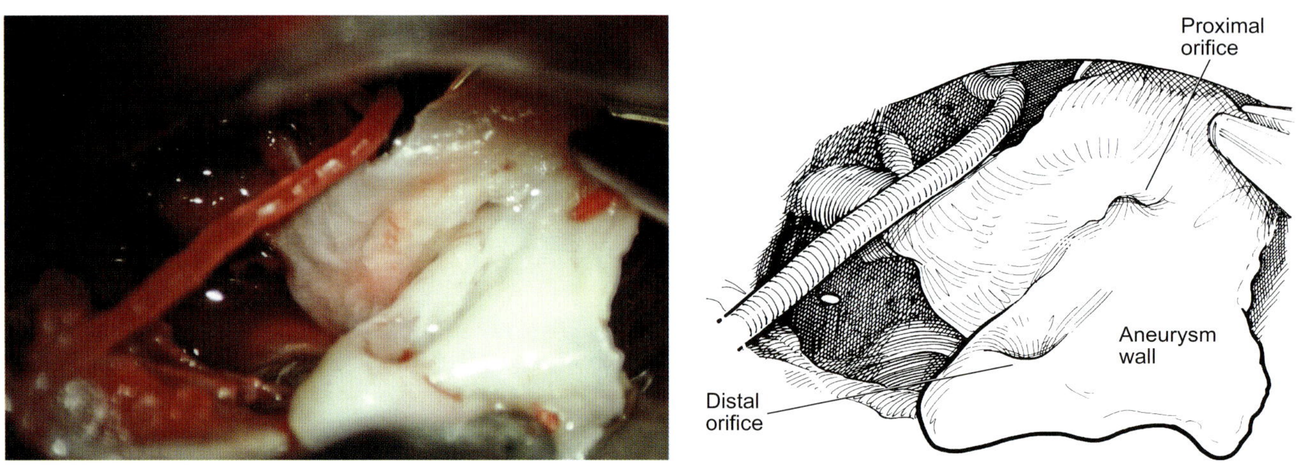

Fig. 2.10f Close-up view after the aneurysm was opened and the thrombus removed. The proximal and distal MCA orifices are visible.

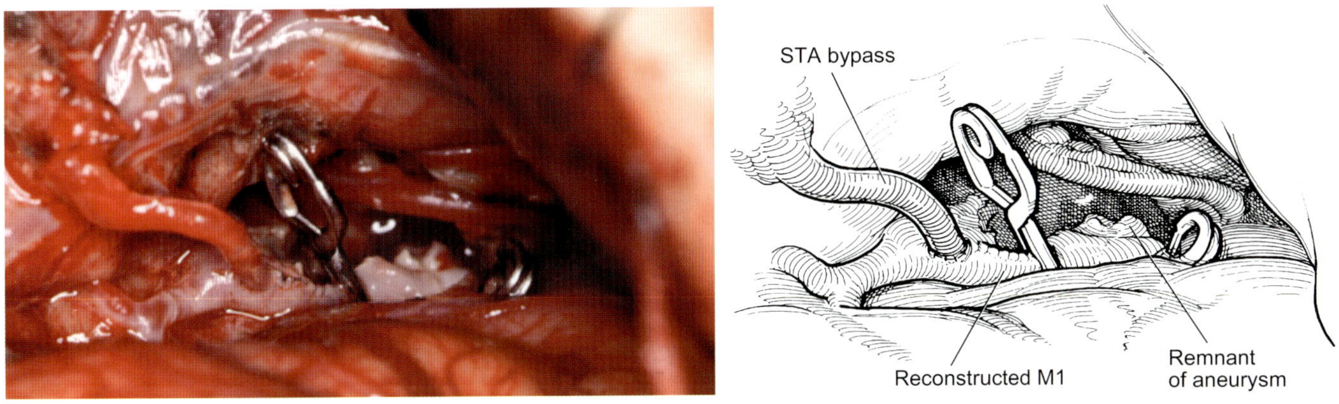

Fig. 2.10g Direct reconstruction of the MCA caused a thrombus to form, occluding the MCA. Therefore, the distal portion of the M1 was reconstructed with 10–0 suture, and the remainder of the aneurysm neck was occluded proximally and distally. An STA-to-distal MCA bypass was used to perfuse the distal MCA.

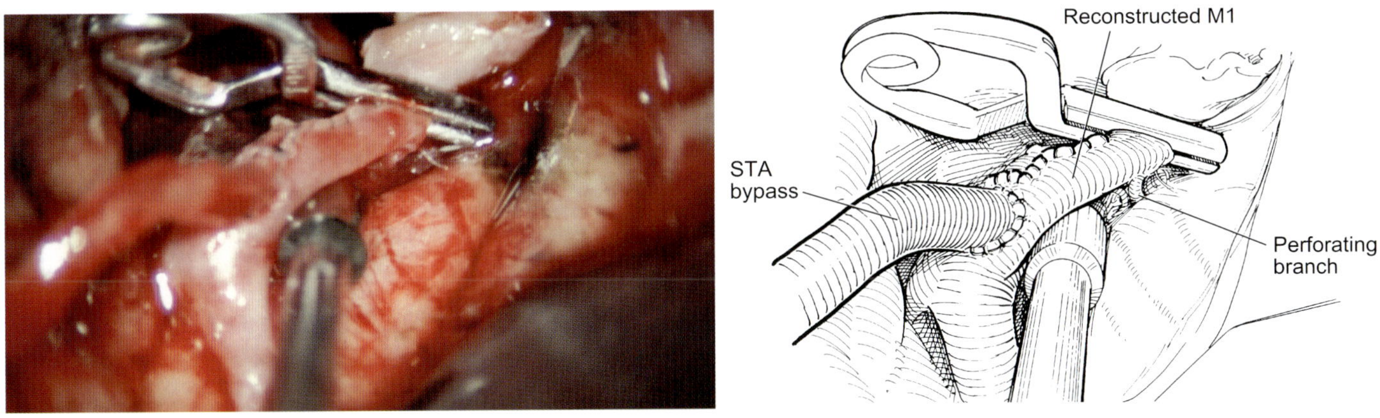

Fig. 2.10h Rotation of the reconstructed distal M1 shows a large perforating branch perfused by retrograde flow through the STA.

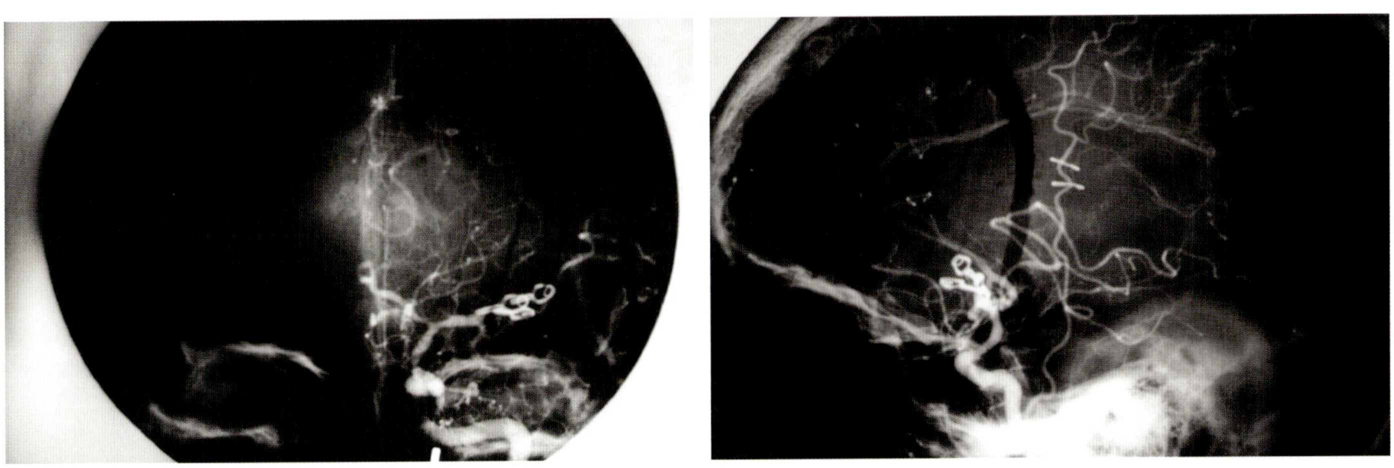

Fig. 2.10i, j Anteroposterior and lateral angiograms demonstrate good filling of the left anterior temporal artery through the ICA. The remaining MCA branches fill through the STA bypass.

3 STA-to-MCA Onlay Bypass

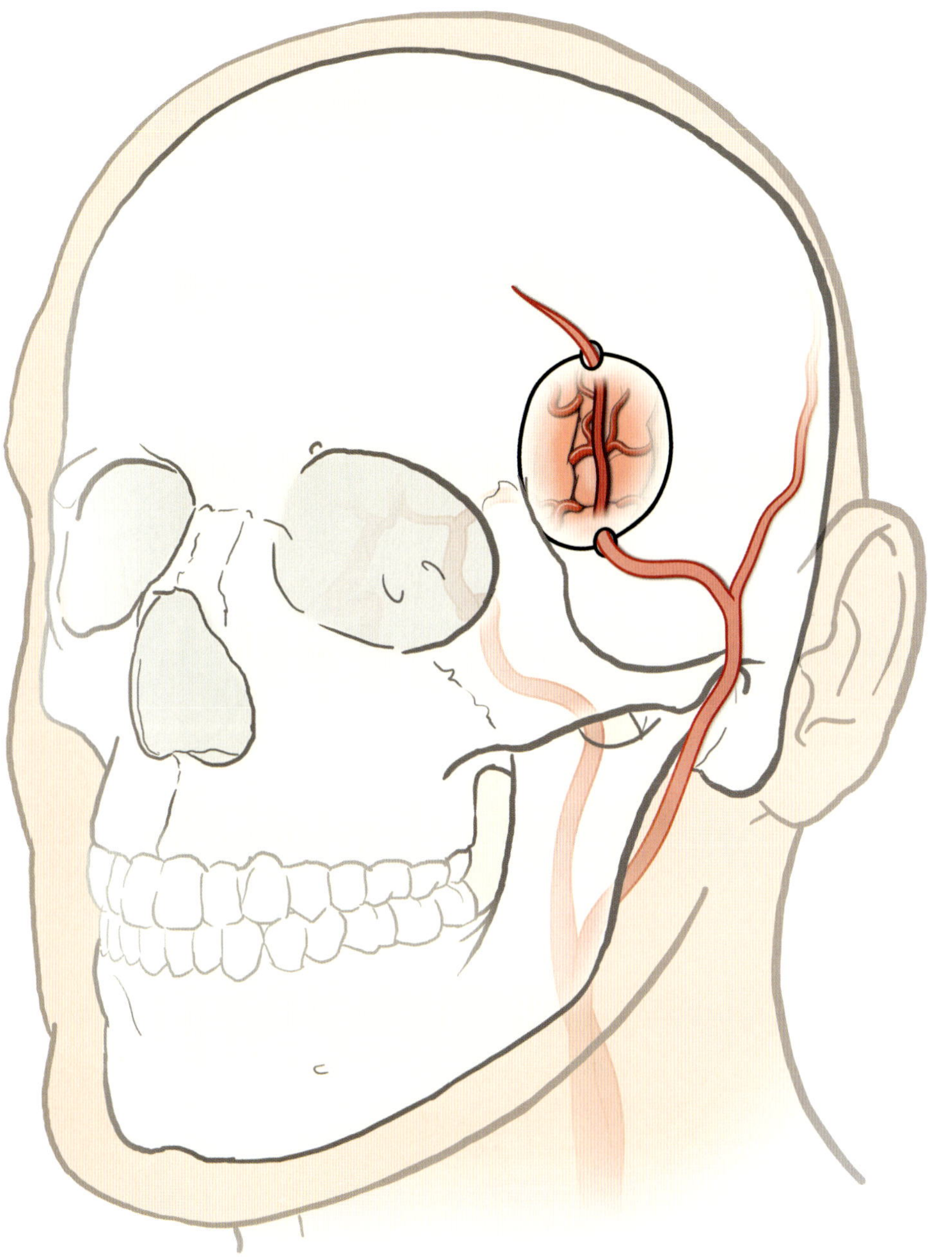

The technique for an onlay STA-to-MCA bypass is almost identical to that for a sutured bypass. However, the continuity of the STA is maintained, and the vessel is placed on the cortex and tacked to the pial edge overlying a dissected surface artery. It is not anastomosed directly. The dural edges are inverted and tucked under the bony edges for further revascularizing potential. In some cases the craniotomy is begun with the intention to perform a direct bypass if possible but is changed to an onlay bypass when no suitable surface vessel is found. In patients with moyamoya disease with fragile vascularity, an onlay bypass is often performed because it minimizes reperfusion risks and is associated with very low rates of morbidity and mortality.

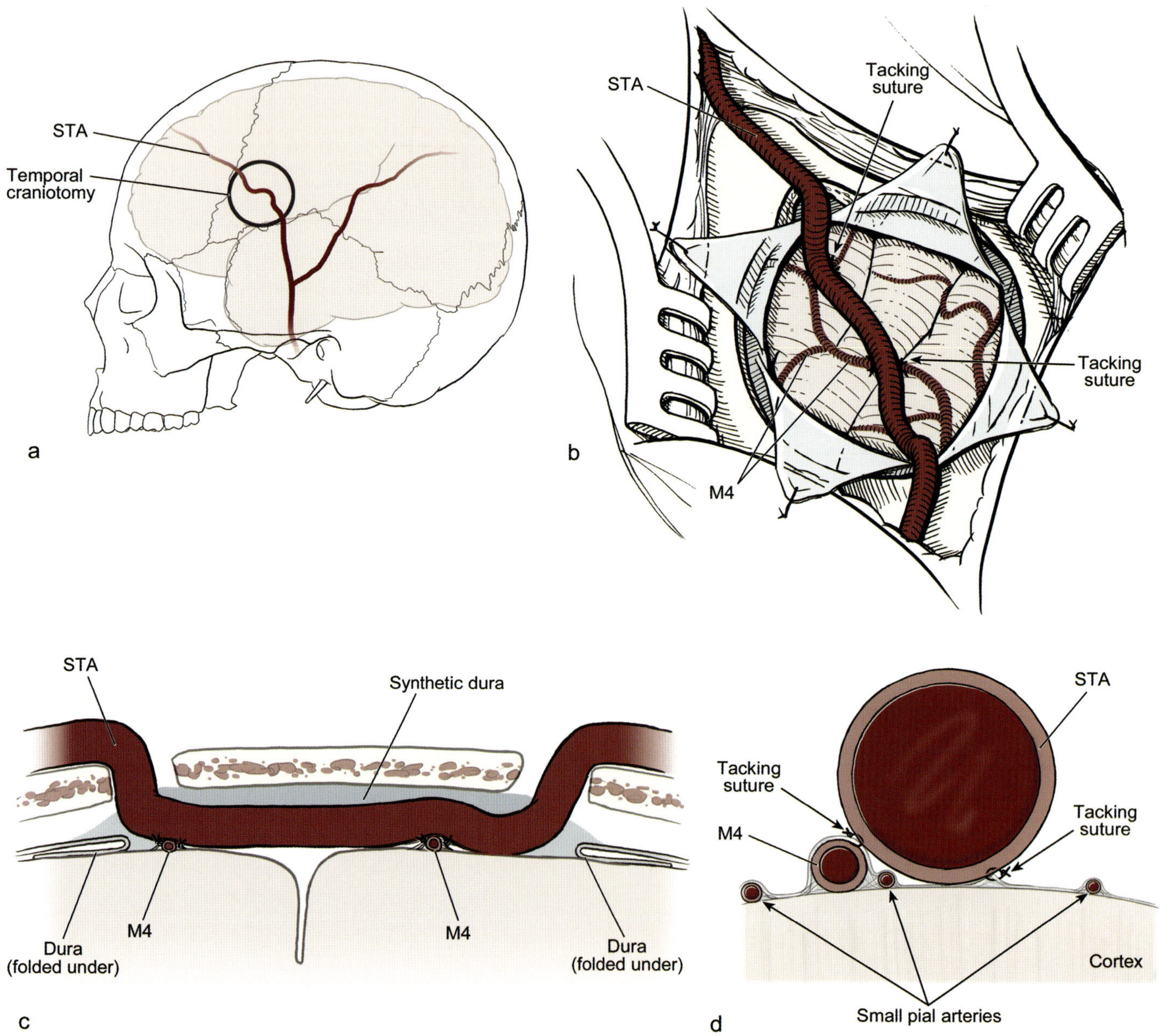

Fig. 3.0a–d Diagram showing the STA-to-MCA onlay bypass. A suitable branch of the STA is identified and a temporal craniotomy is performed over the site of the desired anastomosis (**a**). The dissected STA is placed on the cortex and tacked to the pia near dissected M4 branches (**b**). A cross section shows the en passant placement of the STA on the cortex. The dura is inverted, and a dural substitute is placed over the dural defect. The bone is replaced, leaving generous openings to prevent kinking of the STA (**c**). The pial tacking sutures hold the STA near the surface arteries to facilitate growth of anastomotic vessels (**d**).

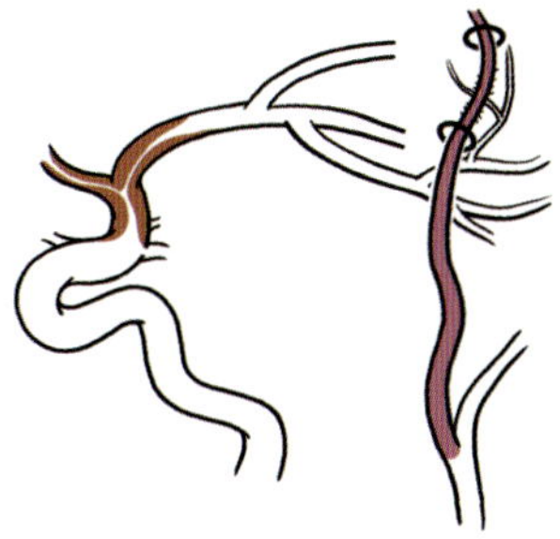

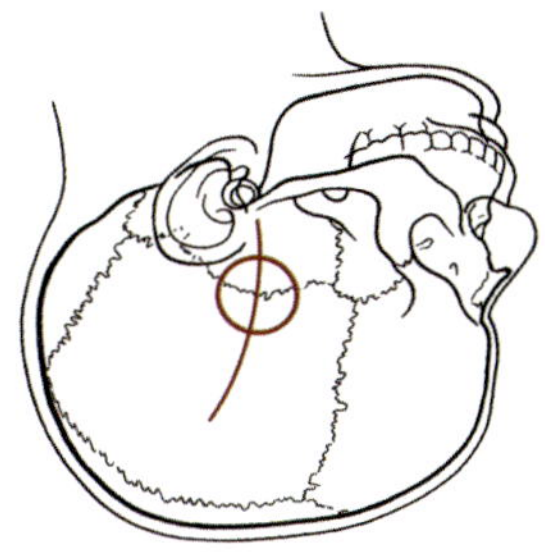

Case 3-1

Diagnosis: Moyamoya disease

Bypass: STA-to-MCA onlay

Approach: Left temporal

Video

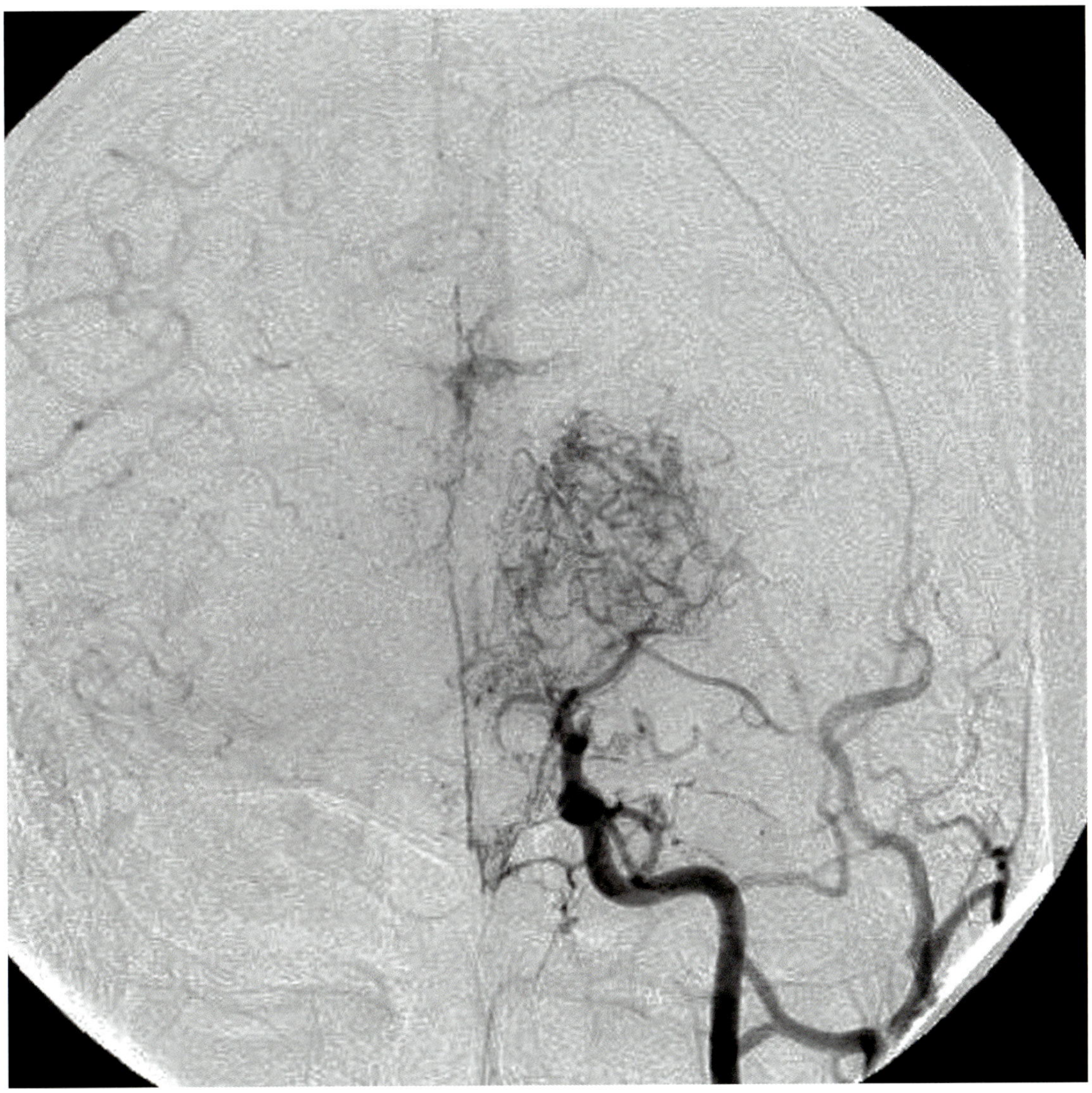

Fig. 3.1a A left ICA anteroposterior angiogram shows a classic moyamoya pattern.

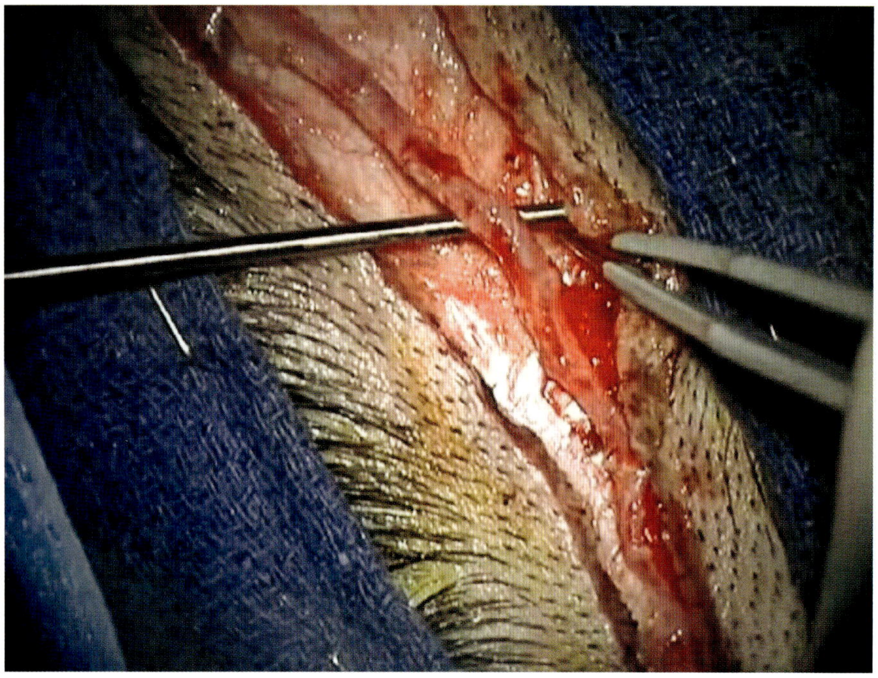

Fig. 3.1b A continuous length of the STA is dissected from the fascia of the temporalis muscle. The top of the head is at the bottom of the frame.

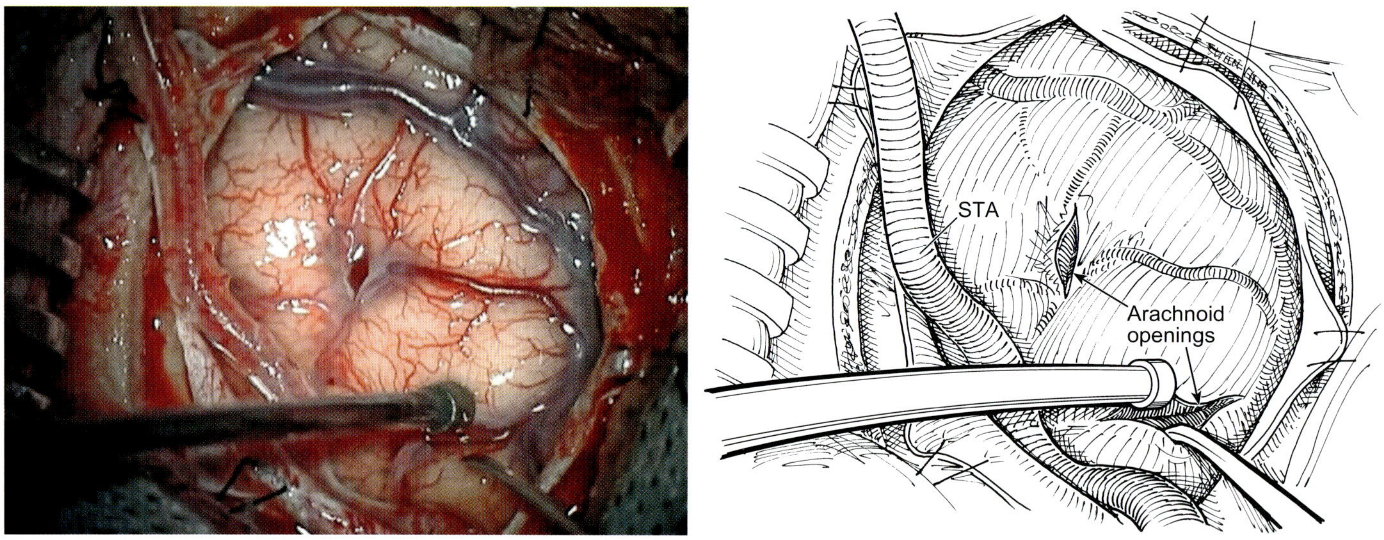

Fig. 3.1c The arachnoid is opened and the surface vessels of the MCA are inspected. No vessel of similar size or larger is found.

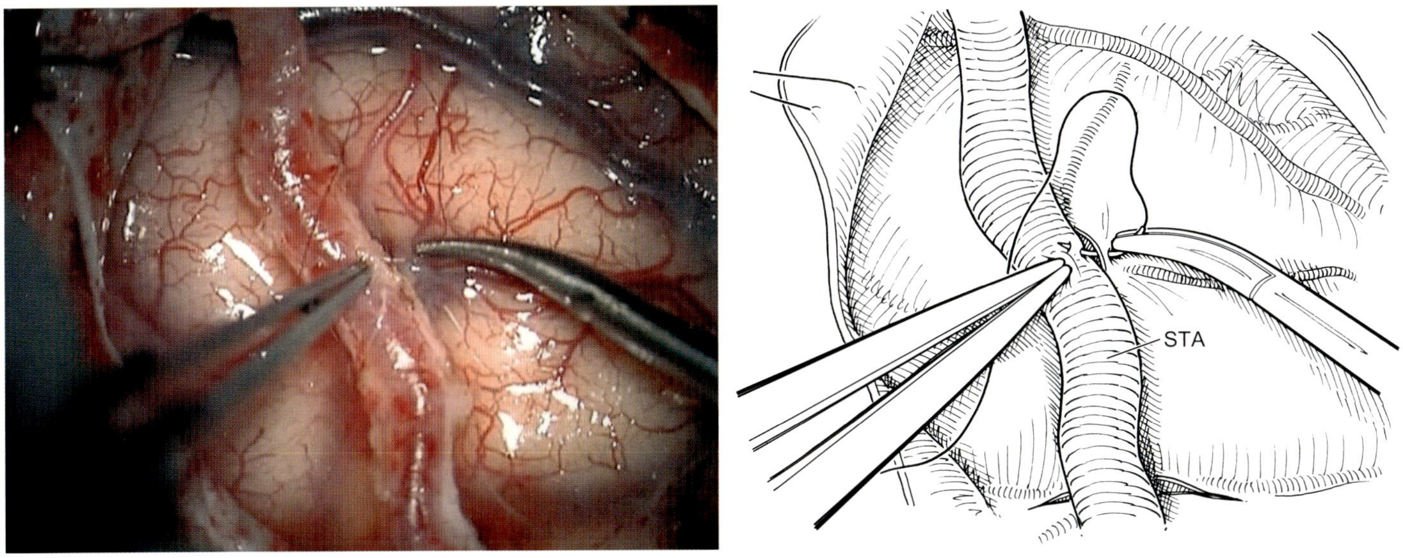

Fig. 3.1d The decision is made to perform an onlay. The STA is sutured to the pia-arachnoid with 10–0 nylon suture.

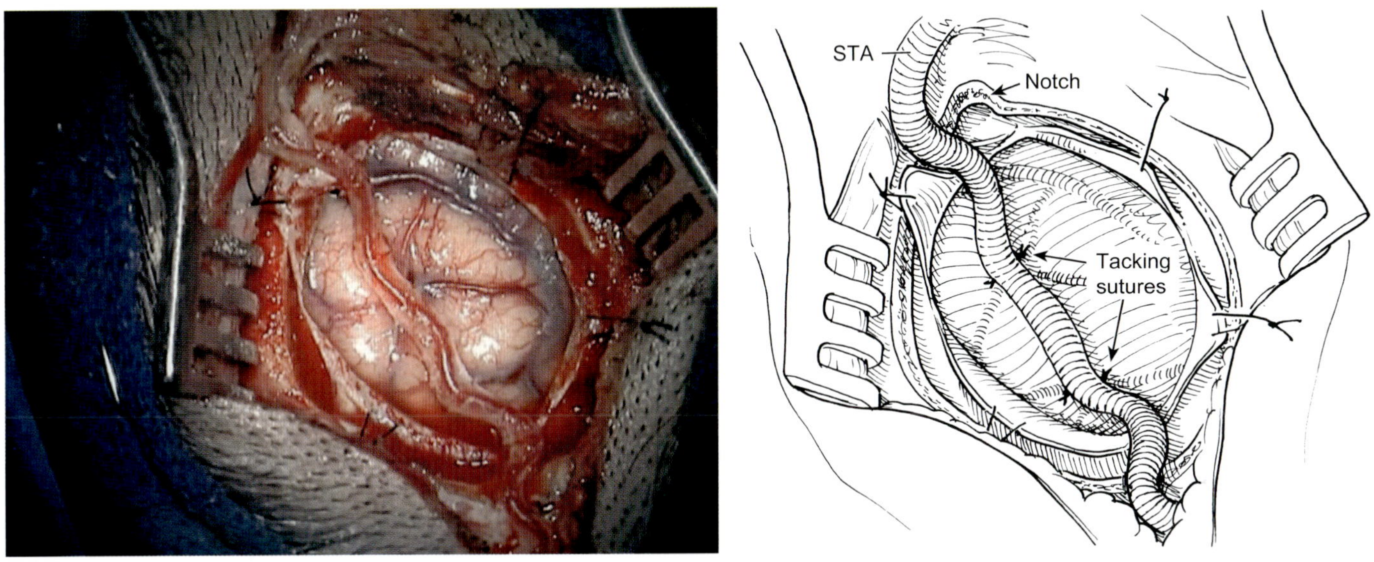

Fig. 3.1e The vessel is left en passant.

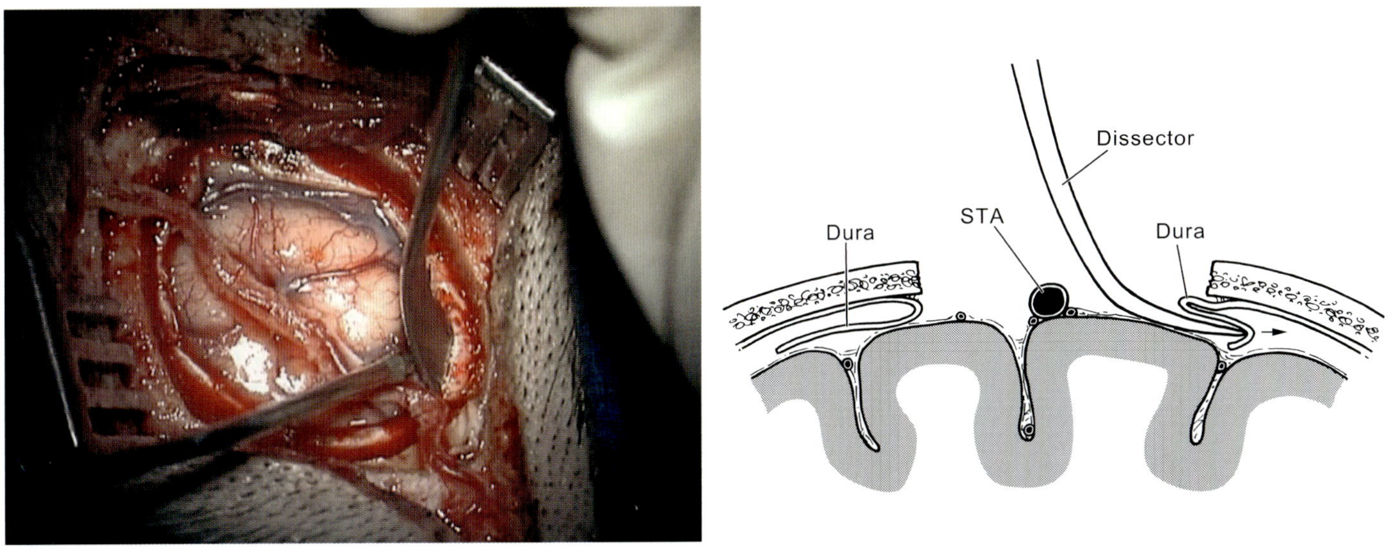

Fig. 3.1f A curved dissector is used to tuck the external surface of the dura under the craniotomy, inverting the dura against the brain. Schematic shows technique in coronal view.

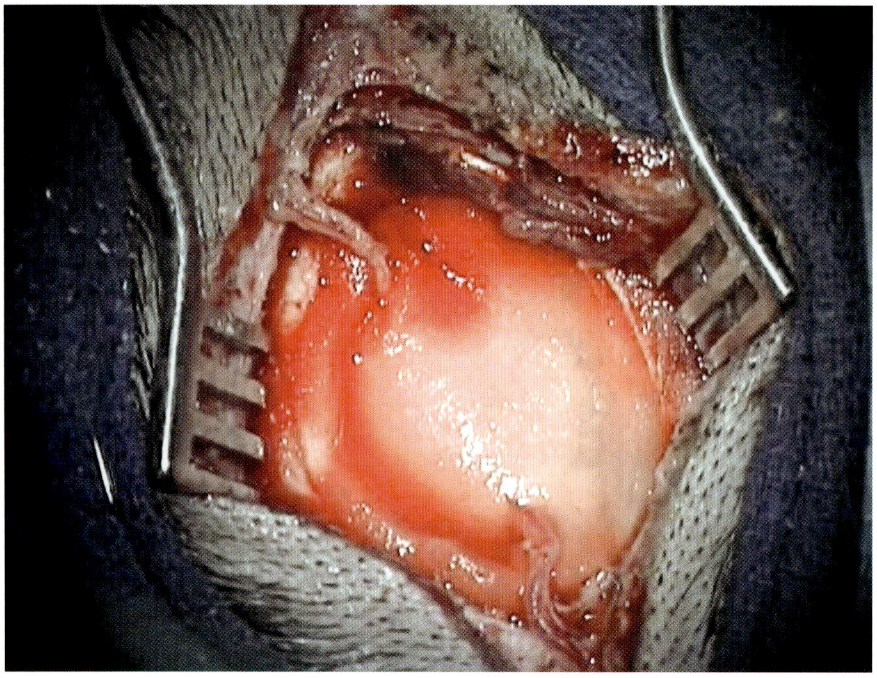

Fig. 3.1g The dural substitute is placed over the dural defect.

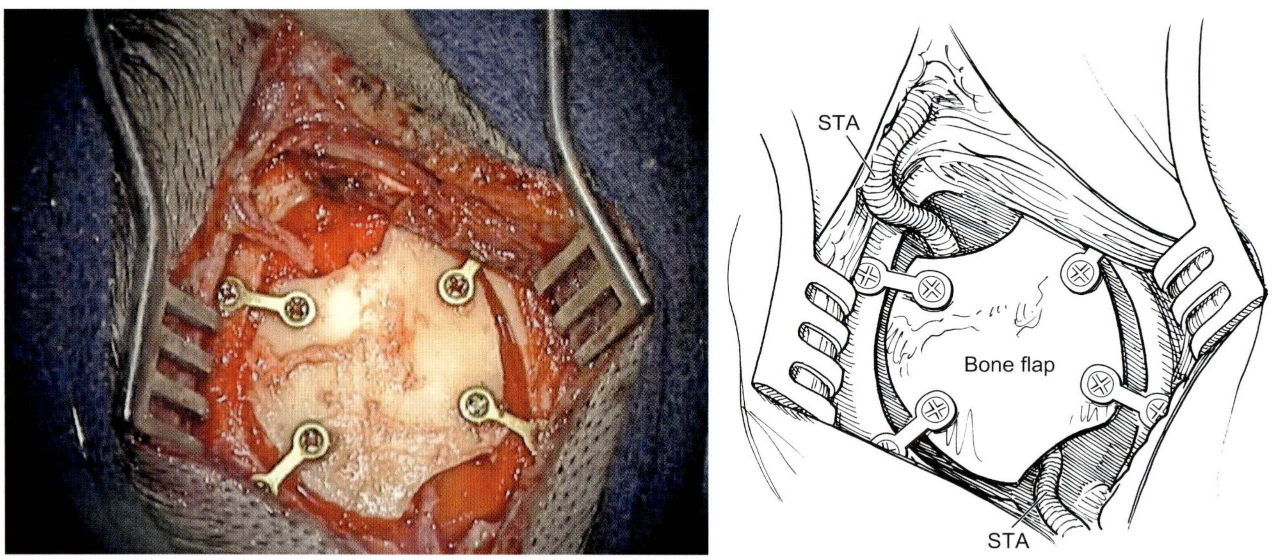

Fig. 3.1h The bone is replaced with generous openings to accommodate the passage of the STA without kinking.

4 MCA-to-MCA Bypass

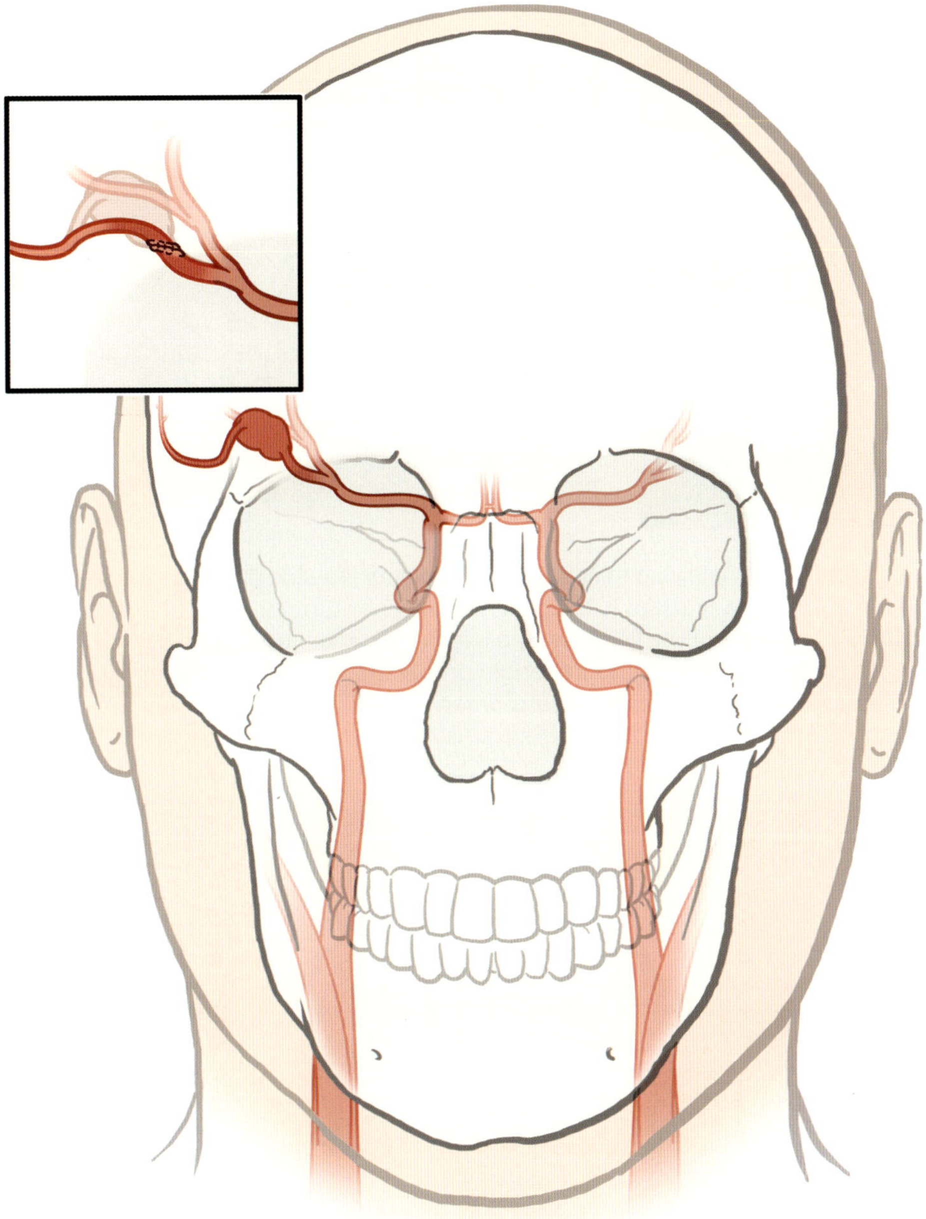

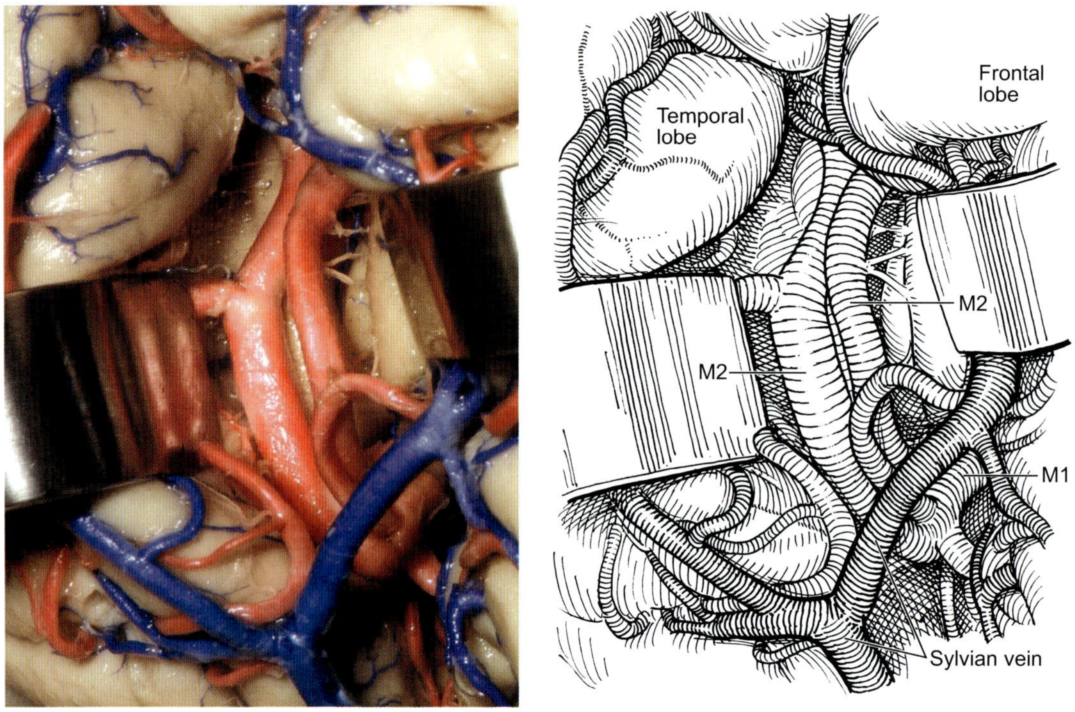

Fig. 4.0a M2 branches distal to an aneurysm may be suitable for side-to-side anastomosis to preserve distal blood flow when the aneurysm is trapped. The anterior temporal artery, which is the first branch off the M1 segment of the MCA, can be used as a donor vessel to bypass an aneurysm that requires M1 occlusion distal to the origin of the anterior temporal artery. (Photograph used with permission from *Journal of Neurosurgery*.)

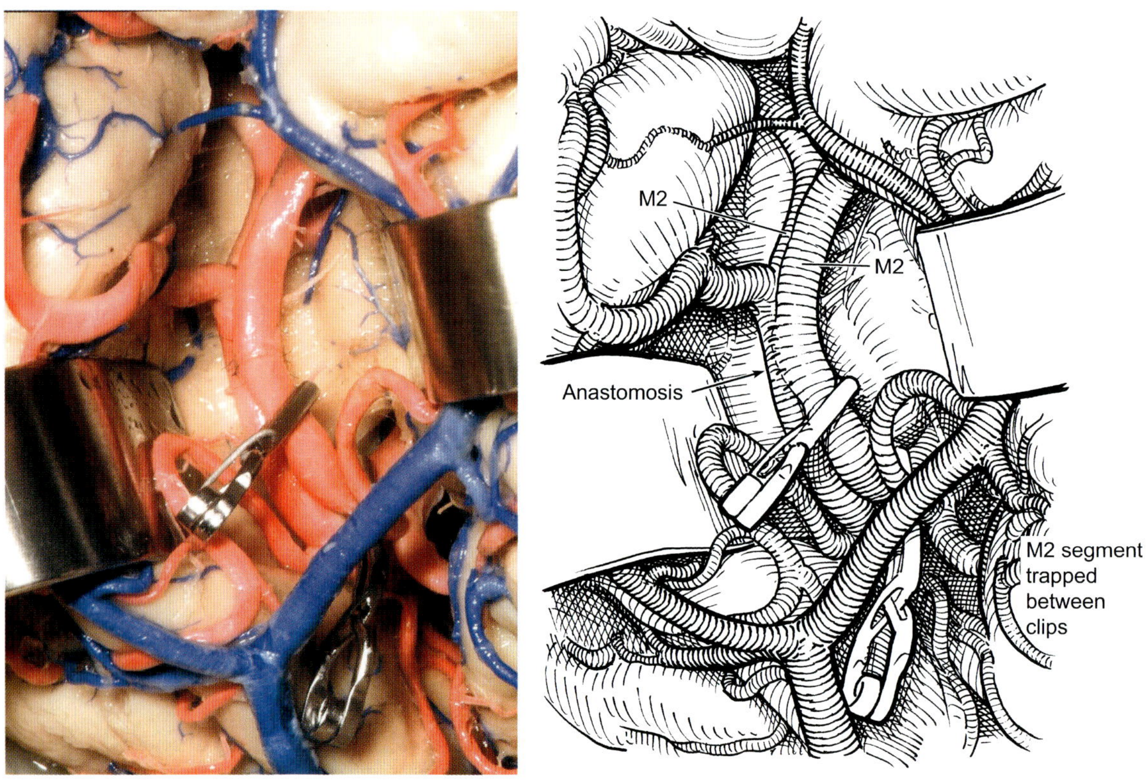

Fig. 4.0b A side-by-side anastomosis has been performed between two adjacent distal M2s. Two clips have been placed to trap a proximal segment of the M2. (Photograph used with permission from *Journal of Neurosurgery*.)

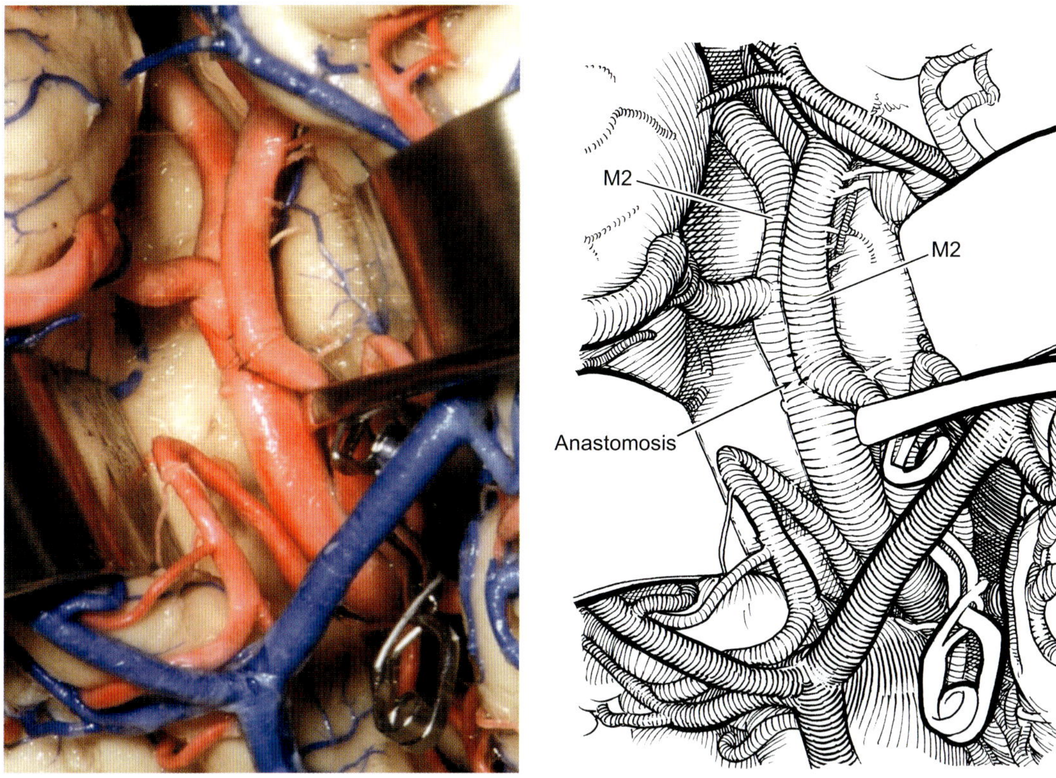

Fig. 4.0c A high-power view of the M2-to-M2 side-to-side anastomosis distal to the trapped segment of one of the M2 branches. (Photograph used with permission from *Journal of Neurosurgery.*)

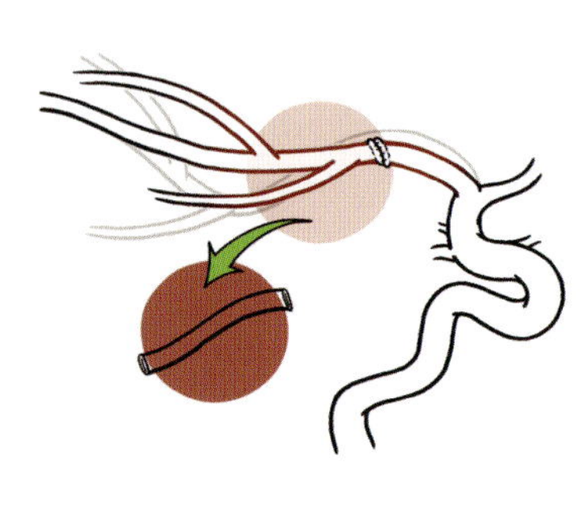

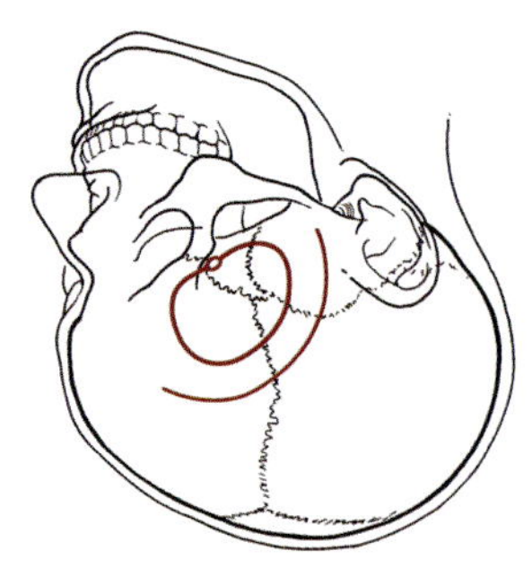

Case 4-1

Diagnosis: Large right MCA aneurysm

Bypass: Primary MCA reanastomosis

Approach: Right pterional

Video

A 74-year-old woman experienced repeated TIAs. Her evaluation showed a large right MCA aneurysm slightly less than 2 cm in diameter. Besides the aneurysm, no other source for the TIAs was identified.

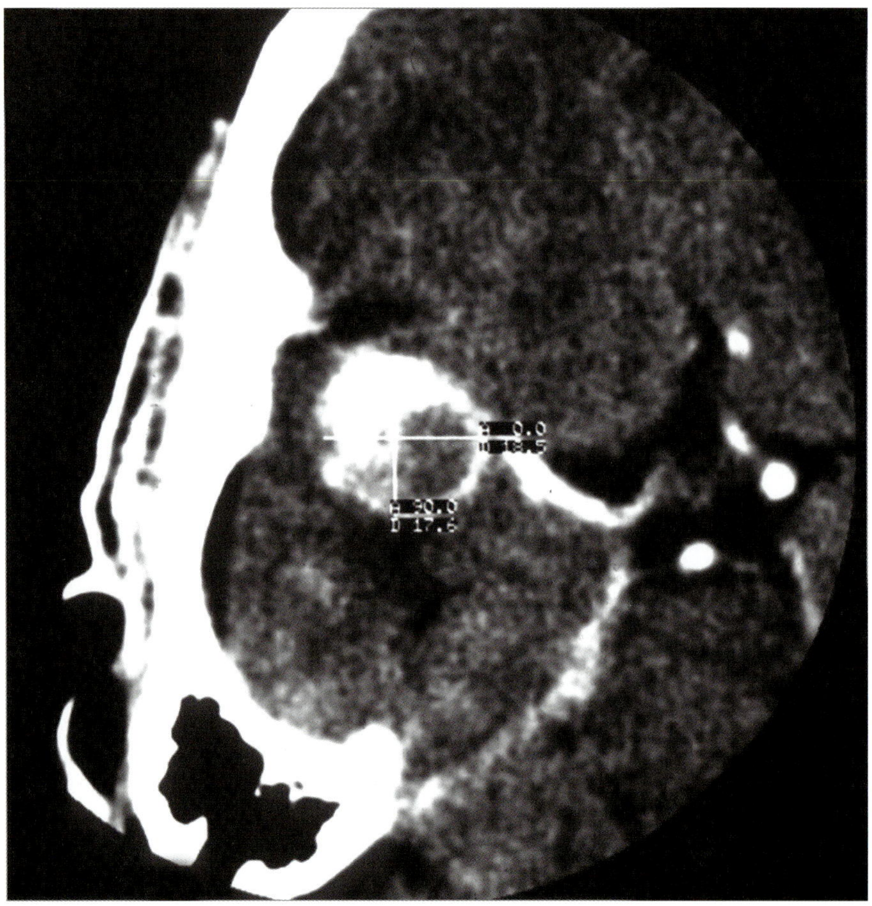

Fig. 4.1a Contrasted axial CT scan of the head shows the well-circumscribed mass in the right sylvian fissure.

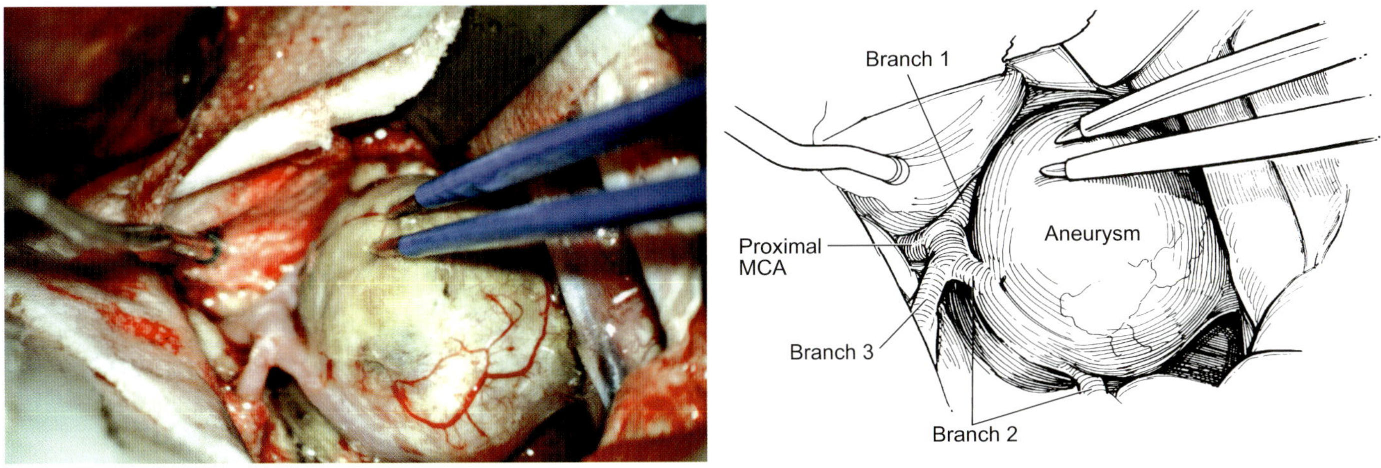

Fig. 4.1b With the sylvian fissure opened, the large aneurysm with its broad neck involving a substantial length of the MCA is visible.

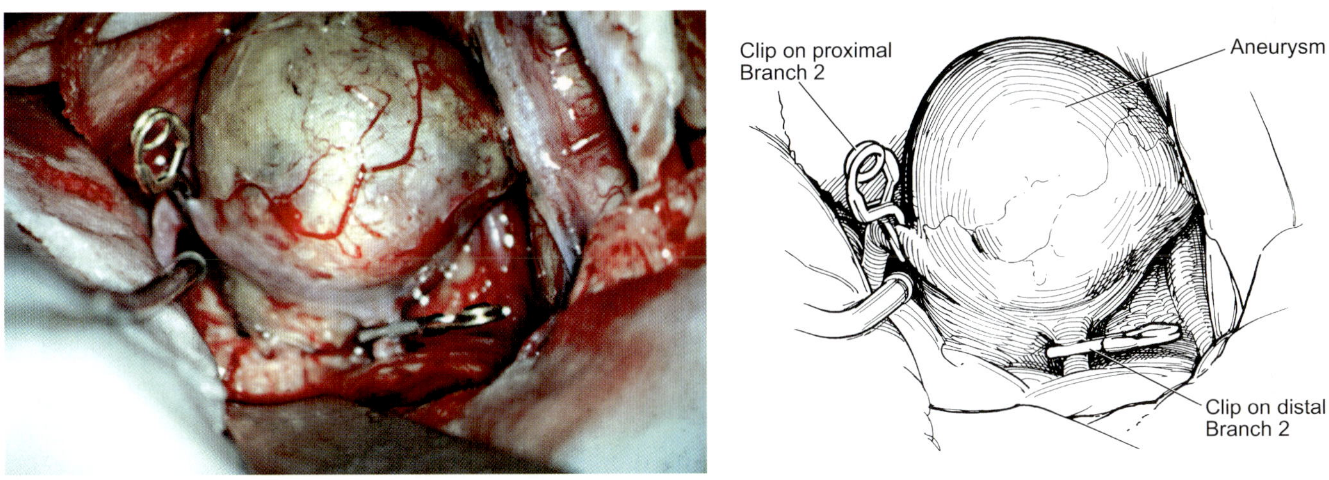

Fig. 4.1c Temporary clips are applied proximal and distal to the neck of the aneurysm.

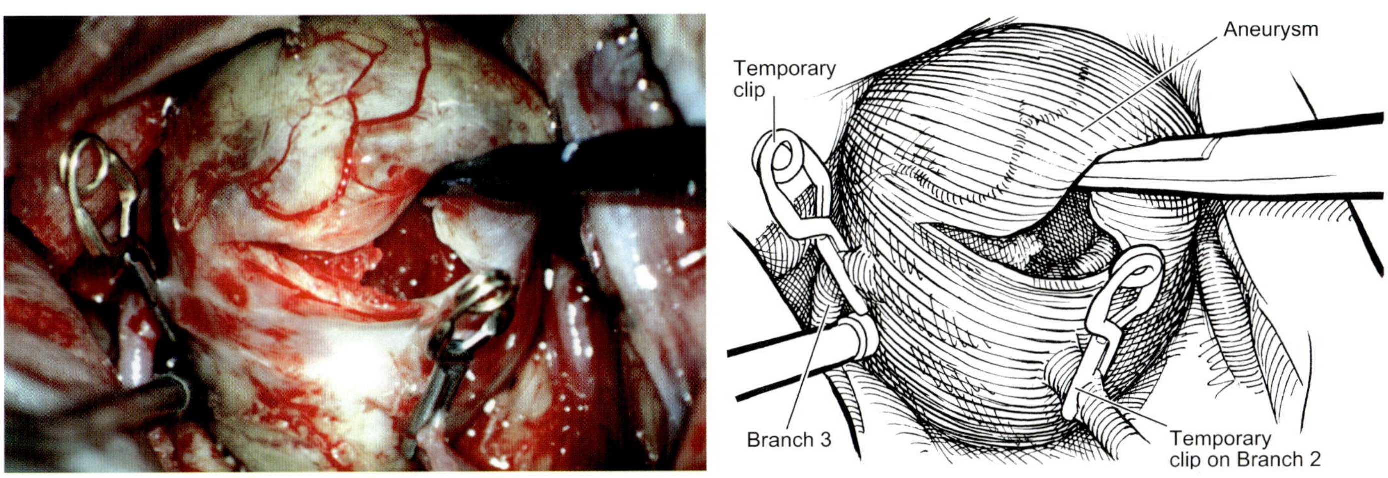

Fig. 4.1d The dome of the trapped aneurysm is opened, exposing a large amount of thrombus.

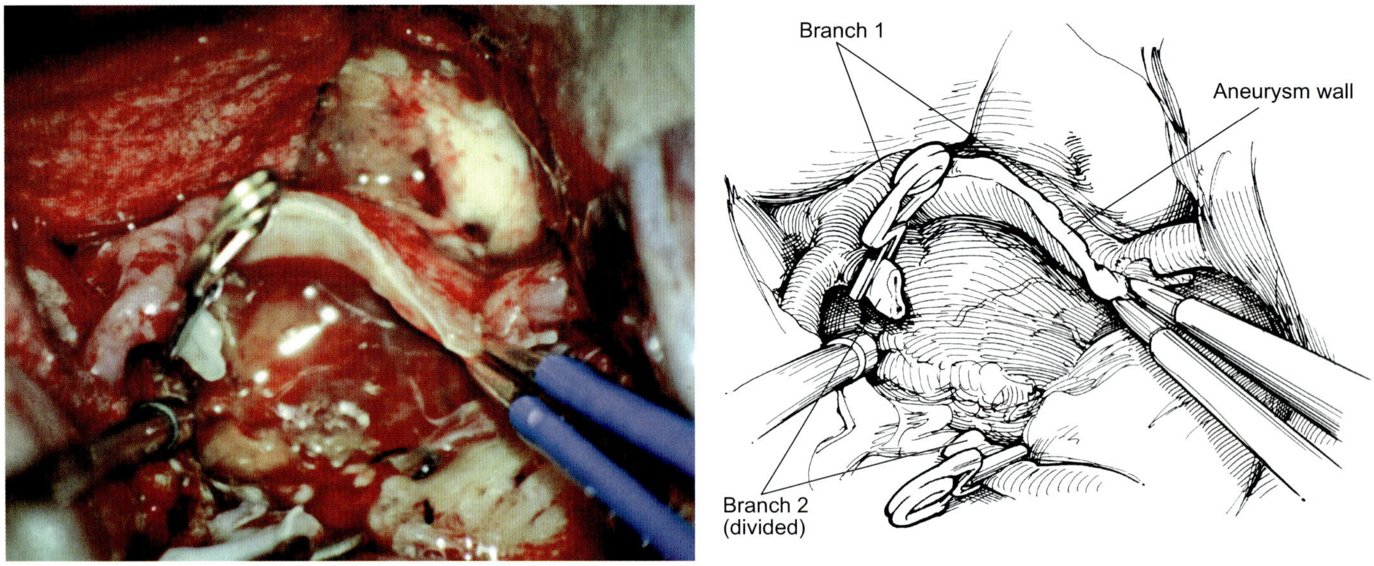

Fig. 4.1e The aneurysm dome and the involved portion of the MCA have been resected except for a portion of the dome firmly adherent to an adjacent branch of the MCA. The cut proximal and distal ends of the MCA are visible.

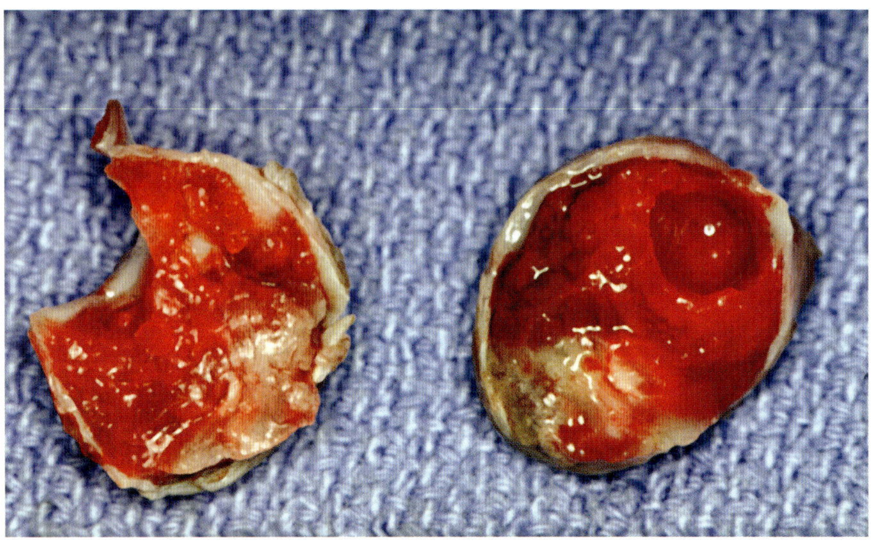

Fig. 4.1f The aneurysmal specimen shows multiple laminations, which are common in large aneurysms. The specimen demonstrates the cause of the patient's embolic events.

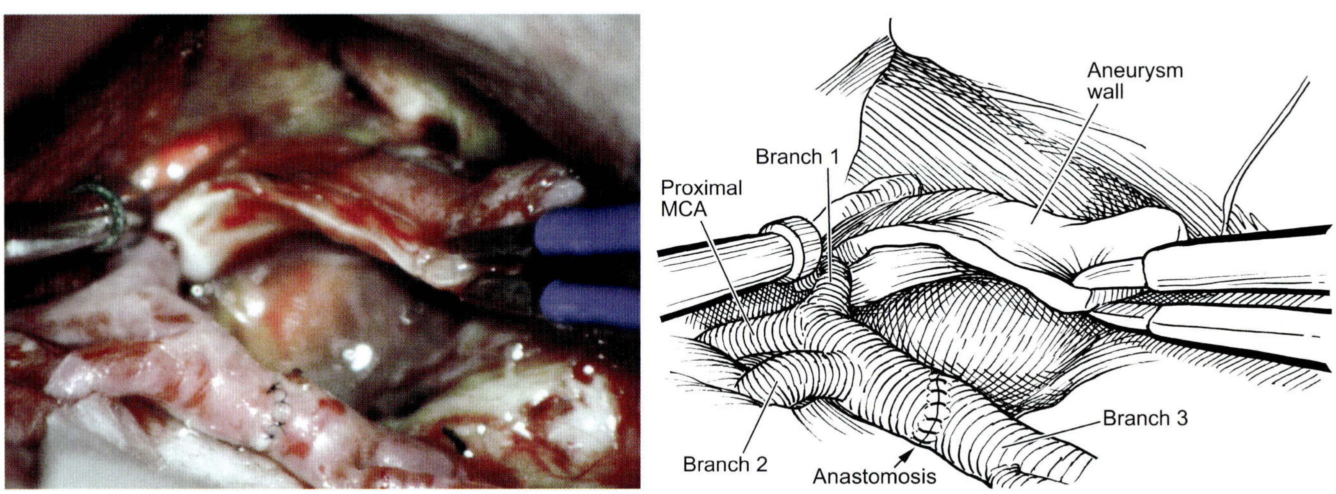

Fig. 4.1g Mobilization and primary reanastomosis of the cut ends of the MCA with 10–0 suture restore normal perfusion.

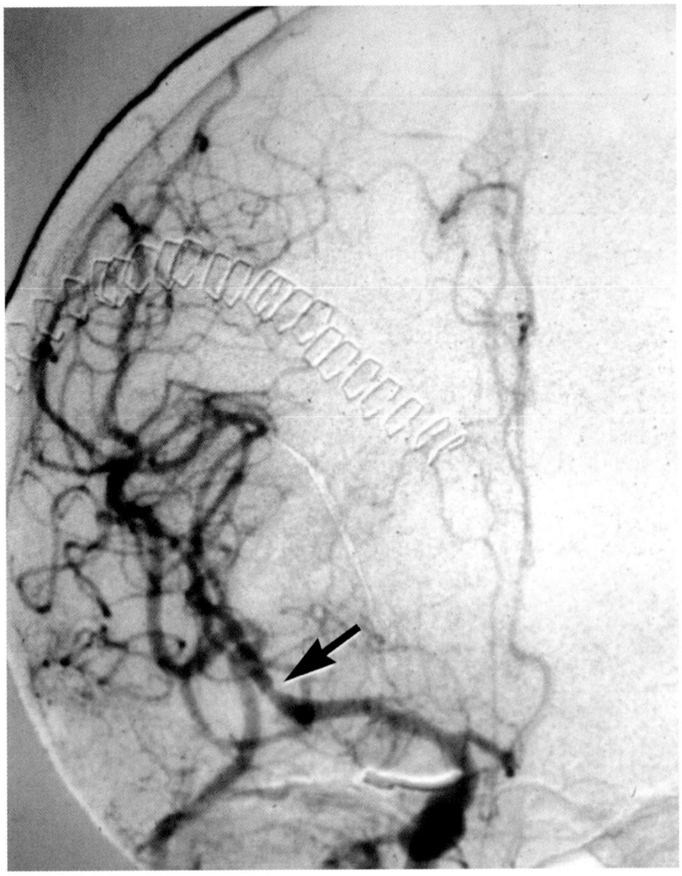

Fig. 4.1h Postoperative anteroposterior angiogram confirms patency of the reanastomosed branch (*arrow*). An incidental ophthalmic artery aneurysm has been obliterated with a clip.

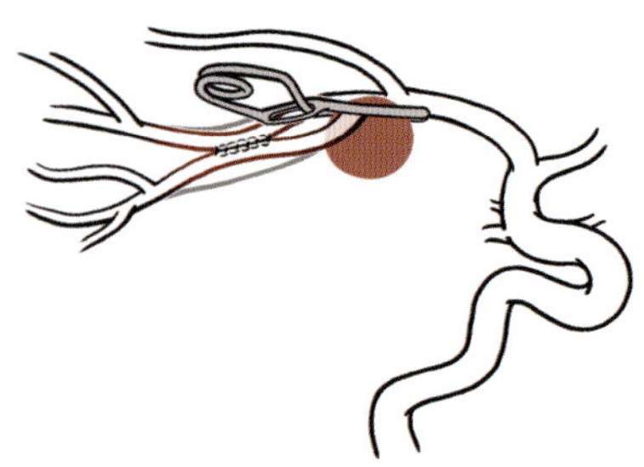

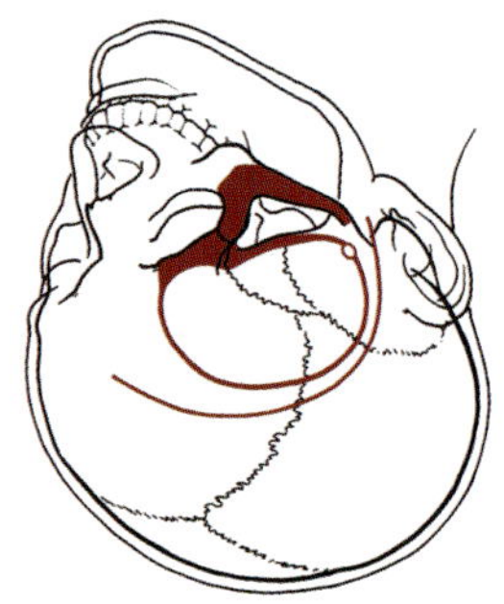

Case 4-2

Diagnosis: Right MCA aneurysm

Bypass: M2-to-M2 side-to-side

Approach: Right orbitozygomatic

Video

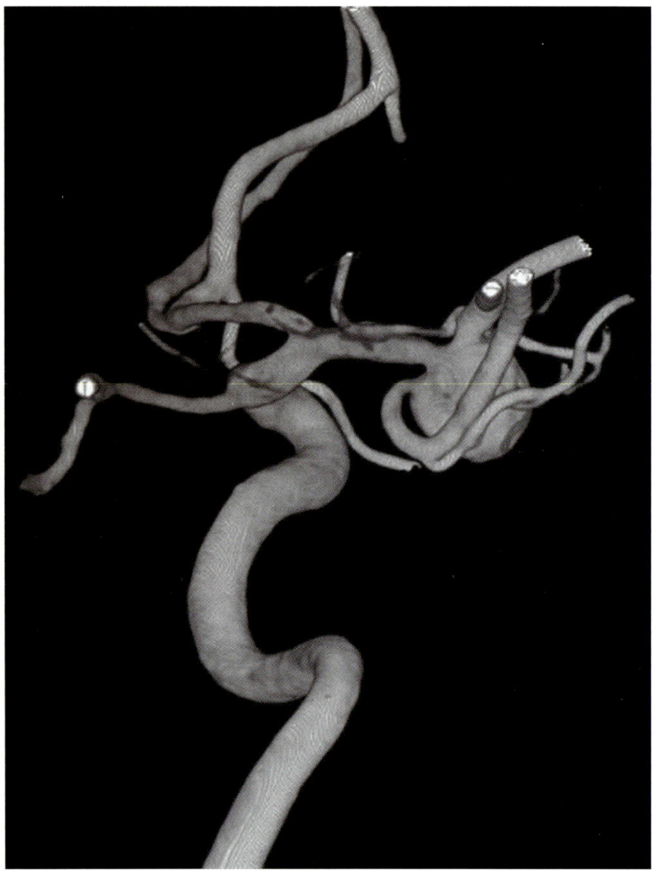

Fig. 4.2a Three-dimensional rotational angiography shows a broad-necked aneurysm of the right MCA.

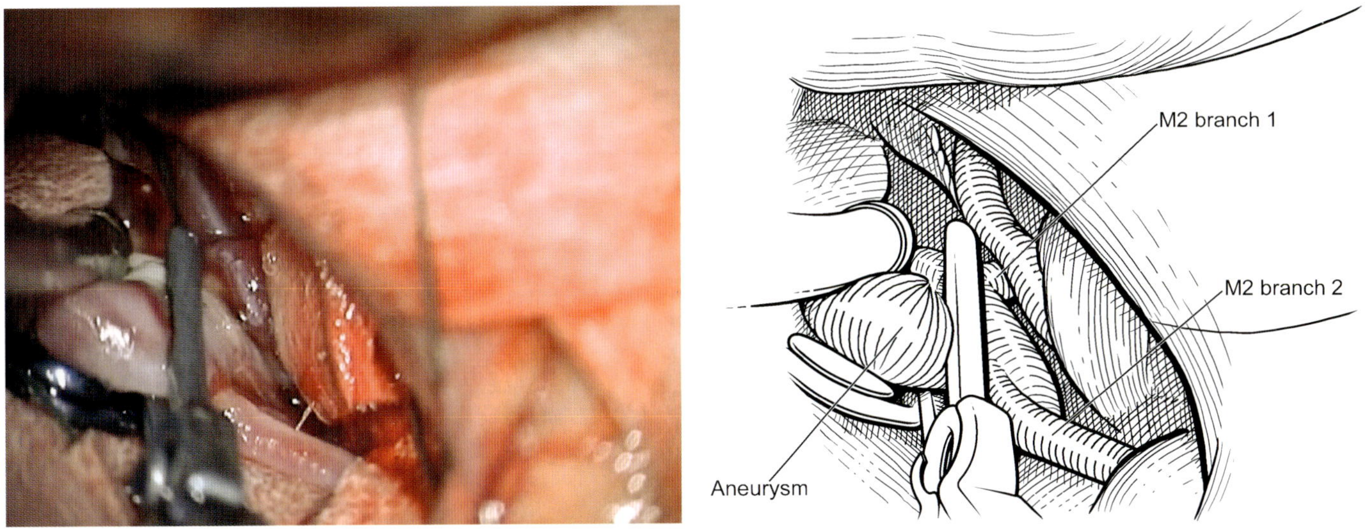

Fig. 4.2b An attempt to apply an aneurysm clip occludes an M2 branch.

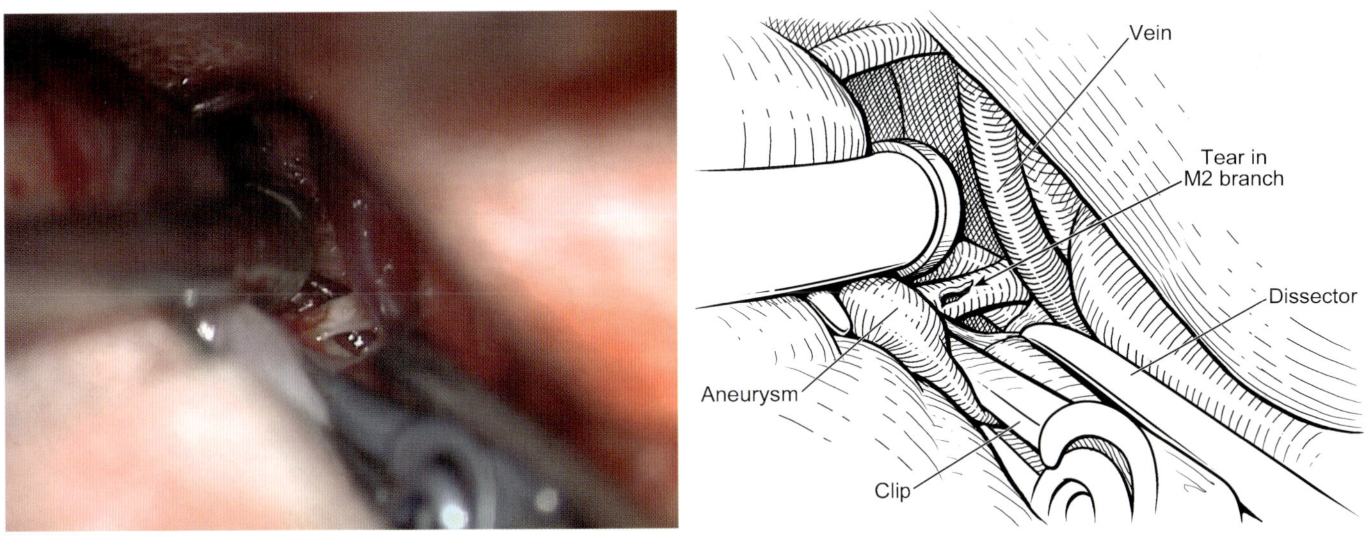

Fig. 4.2c During adjustment, a small tear opens on the shoulder of the M2 branch.

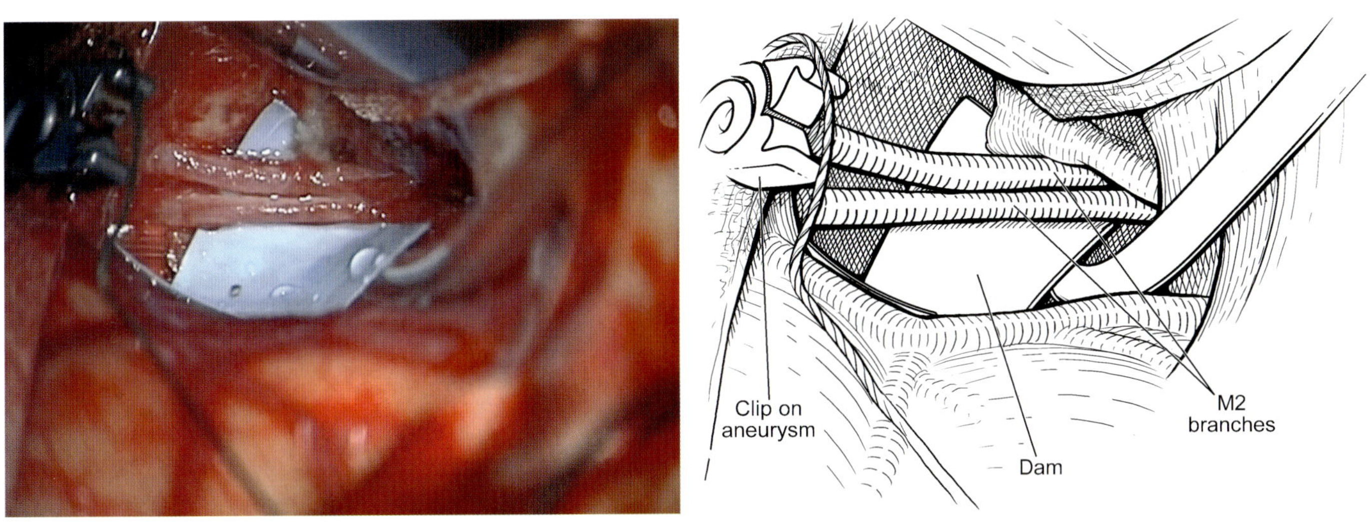

Fig. 4.2d The M2 branches are apposed side to side in the sylvian fissure.

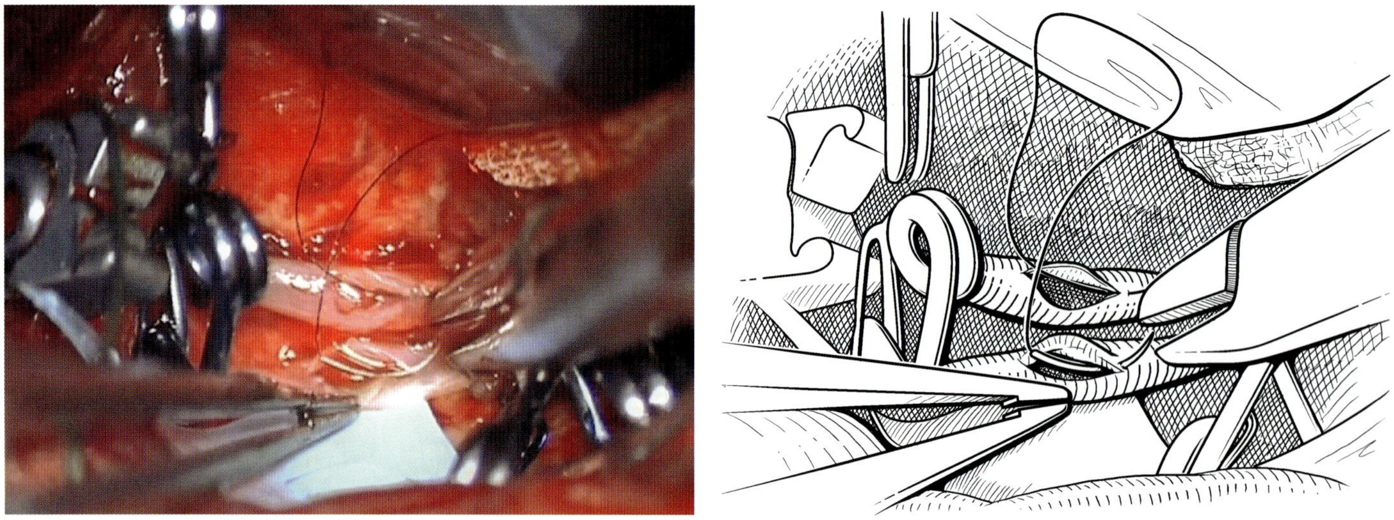

Fig. 4.2e Temporary clips are applied so that the vessels rotate apart slightly. The vessels are opened.

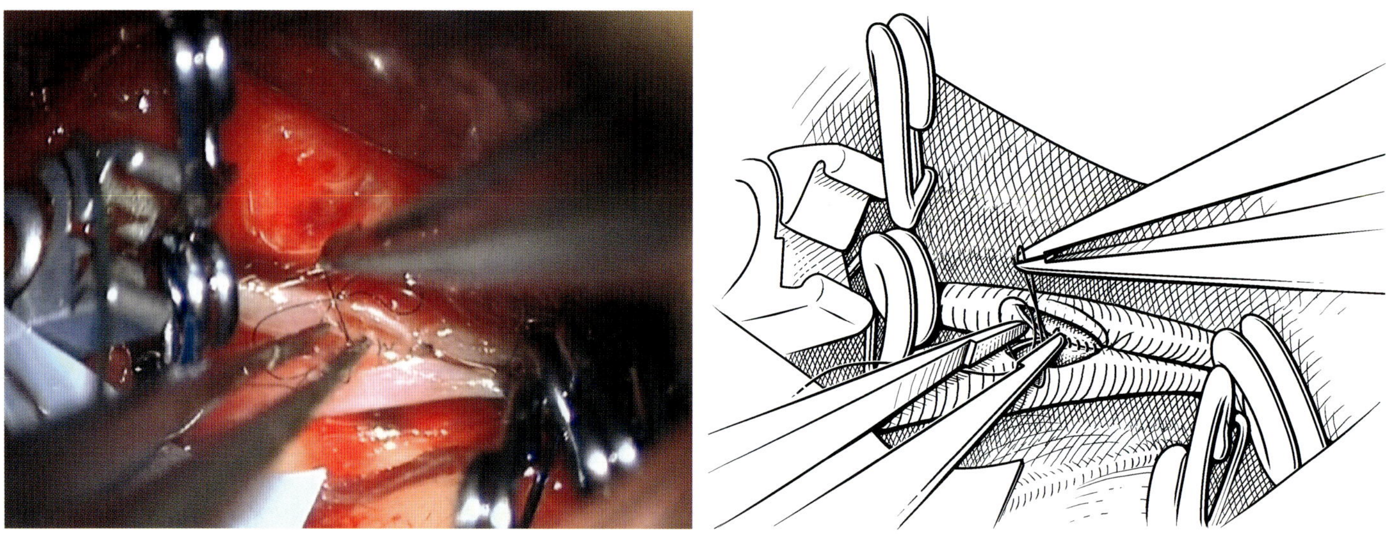

Fig. 4.2f The back wall is sewn with running suture.

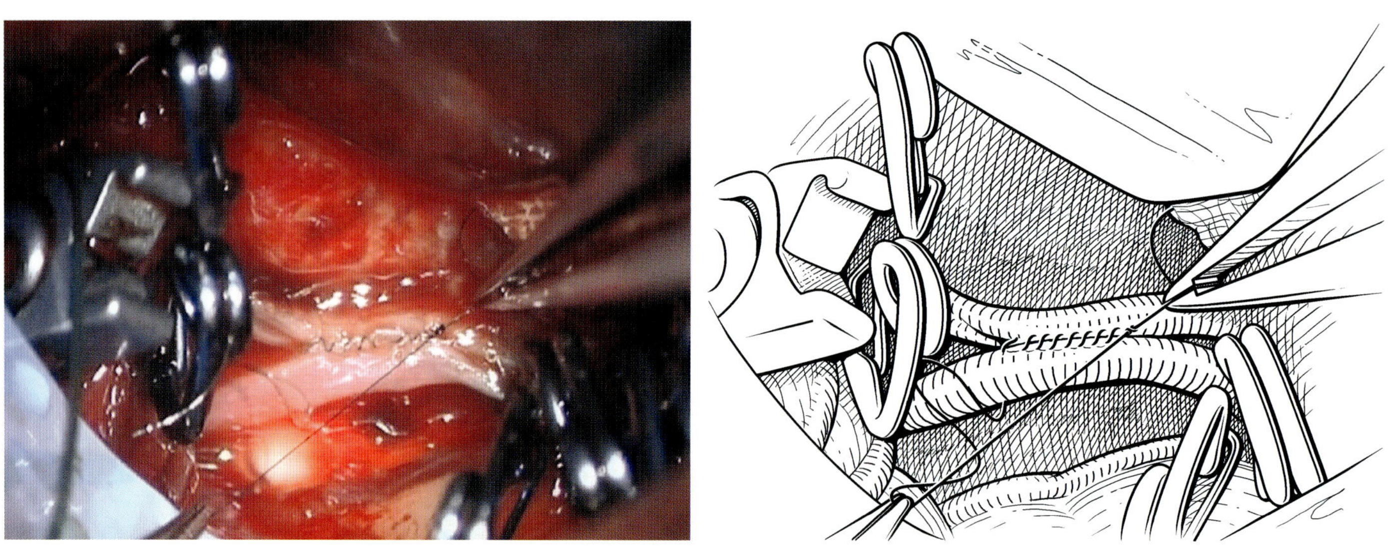

Fig. 4.2g The front wall is sewn with running stitches using the same suture.

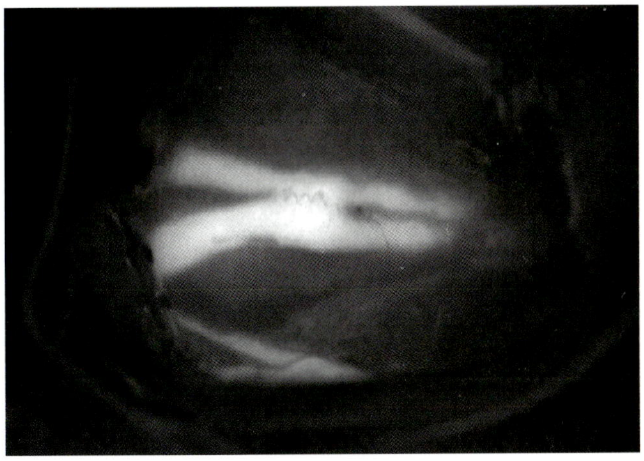

Fig. 4.2h ICG angiography shows brisk filling of all vessels through the bypass.

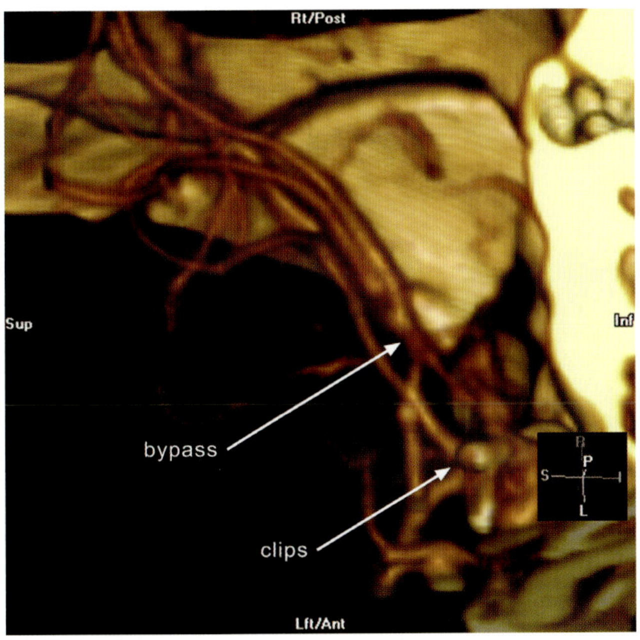

Fig. 4.2i Postoperative three-dimensional reconstructed CT angiogram shows the completed bypass.

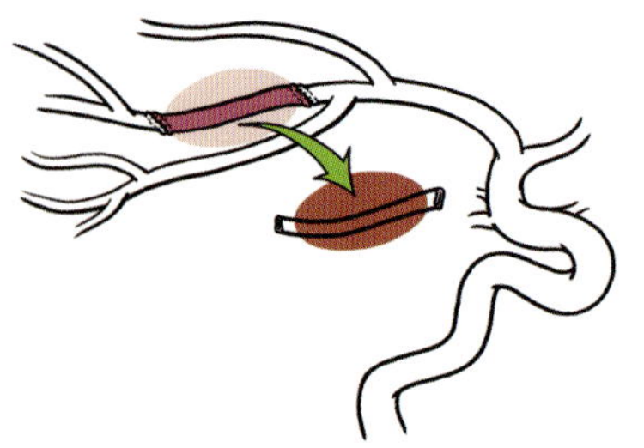

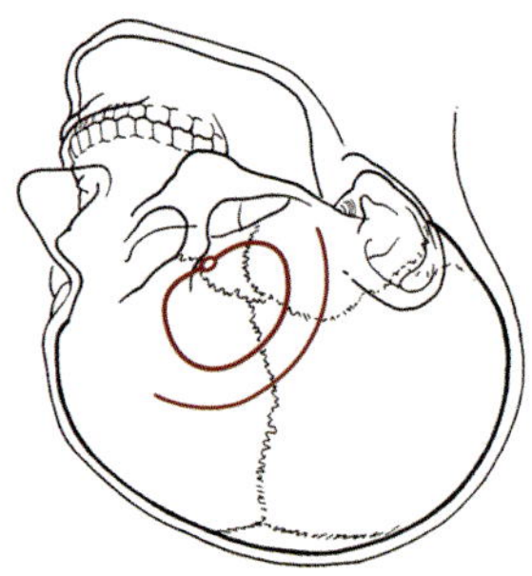

Case 4-3

Diagnosis: Fusiform MCA aneurysm

Bypass: M2-to-M3 interposition radial artery graft

Approach: Right pterional

Video

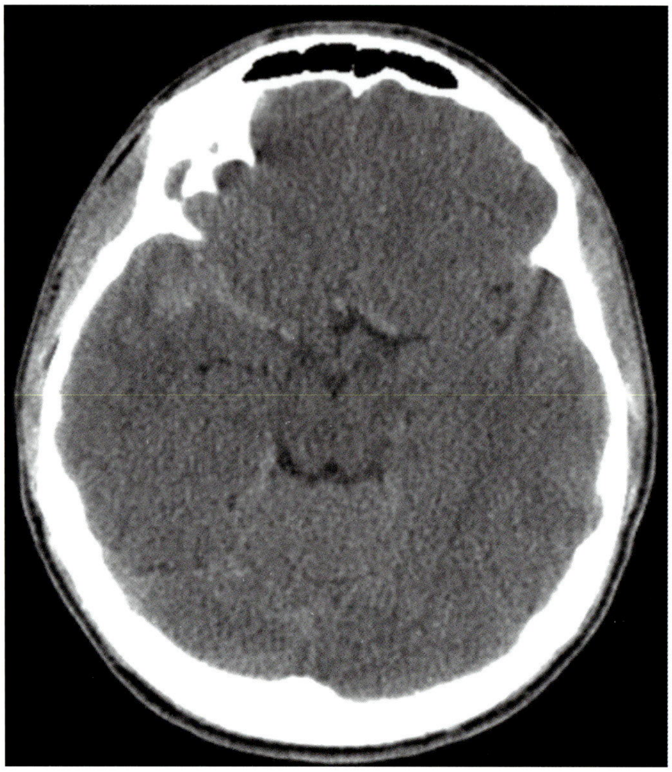

Fig. 4.3a Noncontrast CT scan of the head shows a small amount of blood in the right sylvian fissure.

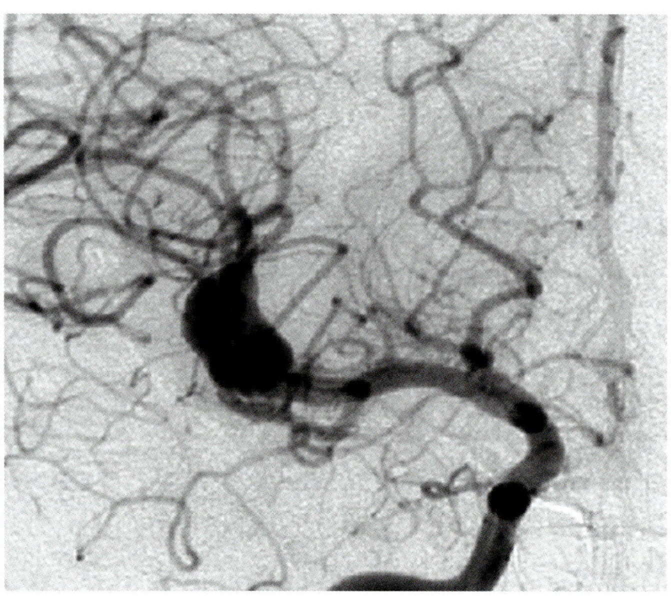

Fig. 4.3b Right ICA angiogram shows a fusiform MCA aneurysm.

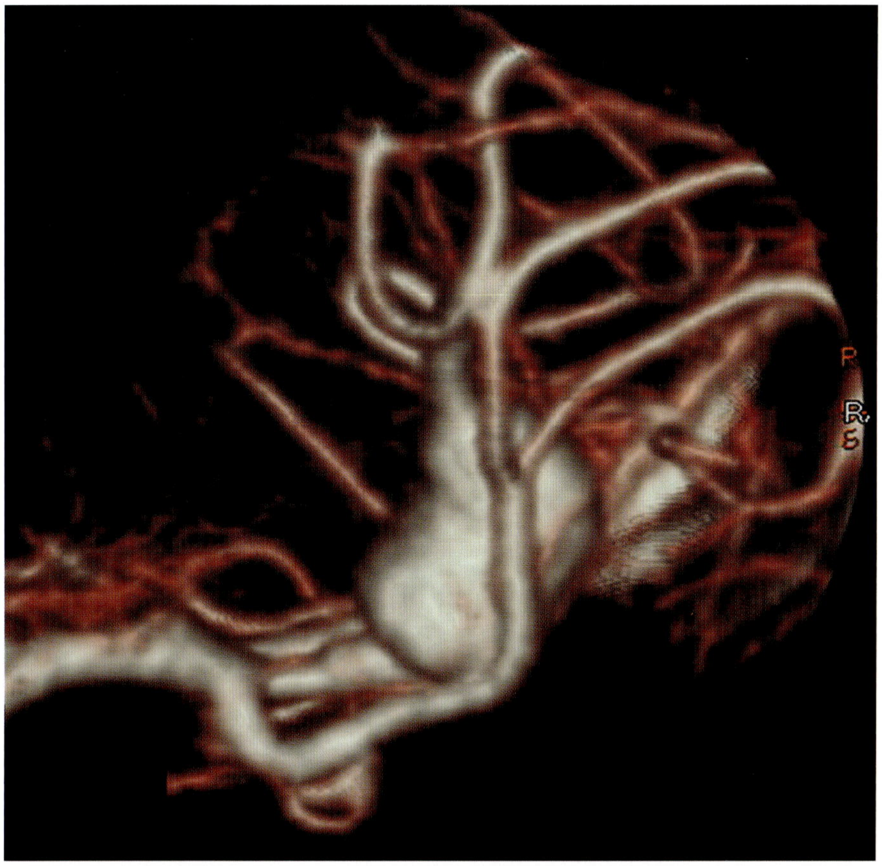

Fig. 4.3c Three-dimensional reconstructed CT shows the involvement of the middle branch of the MCA trifurcation.

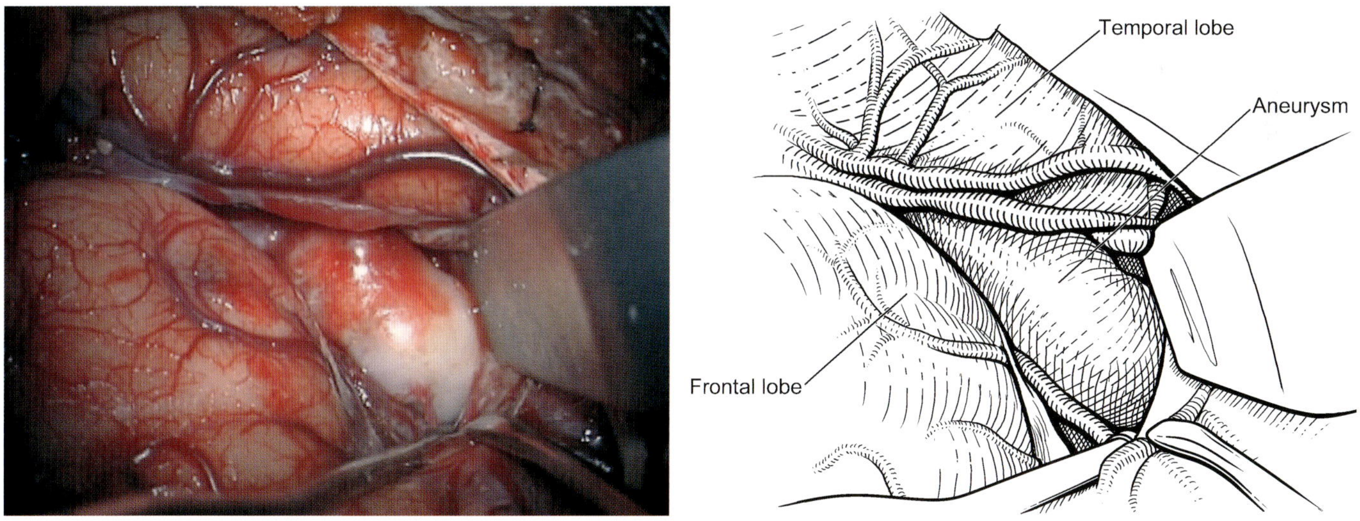

Fig. 4.3d A right pterional craniotomy is performed to expose the aneurysm in the sylvian fissure.

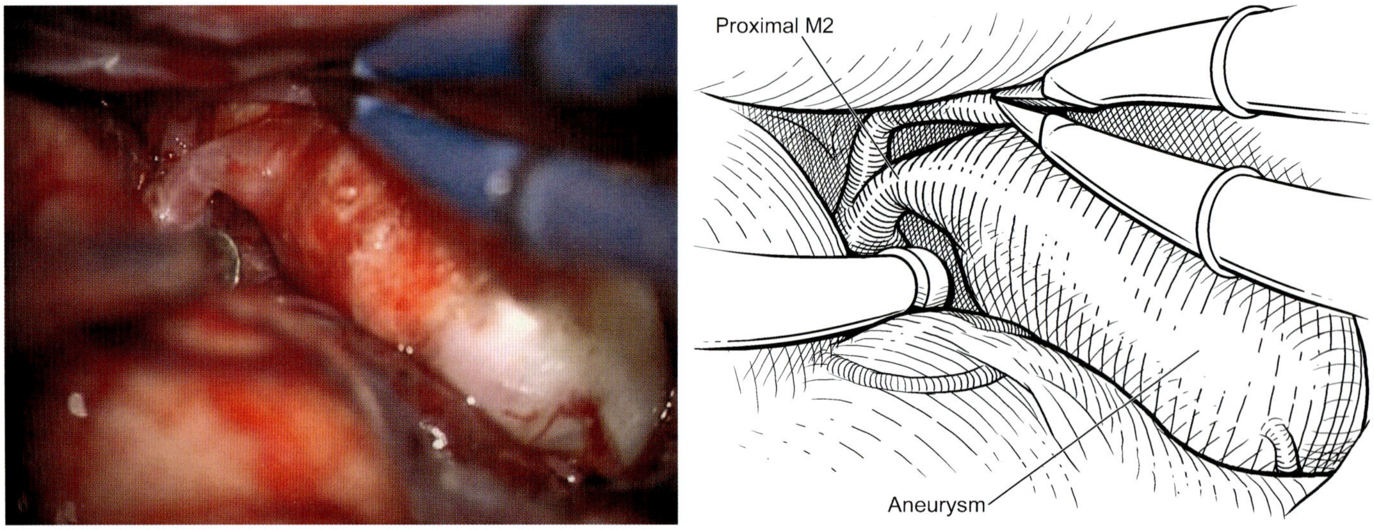

Fig. 4.3e A small segment of the affected branch is found to be normal.

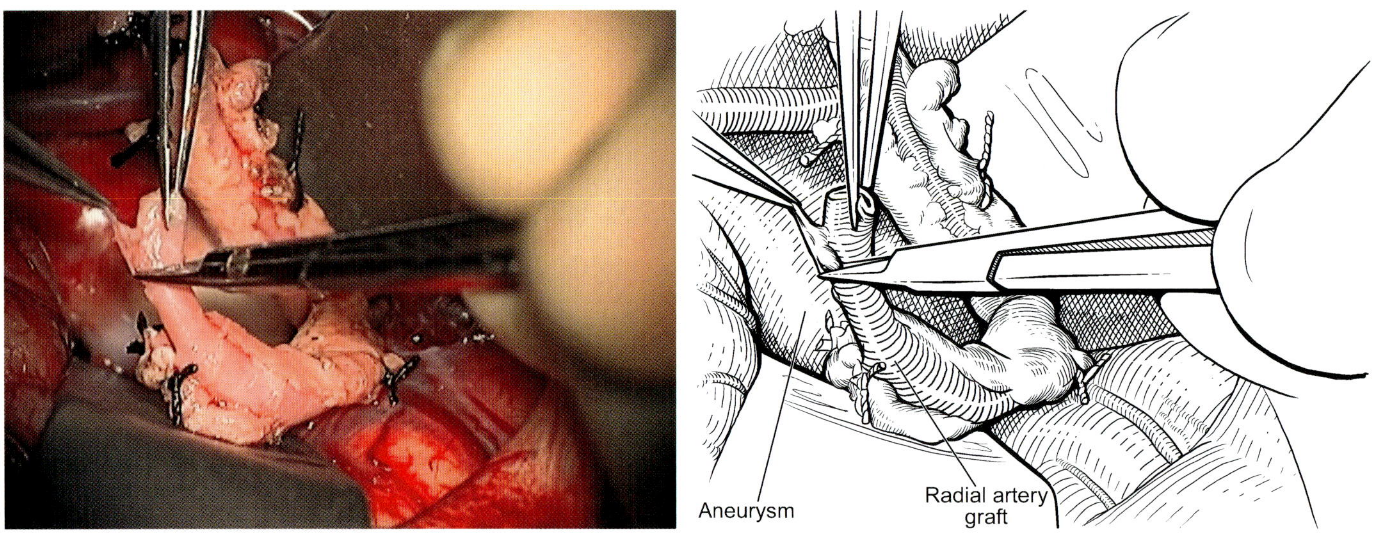

Fig. 4.3f A radial artery graft is prepared.

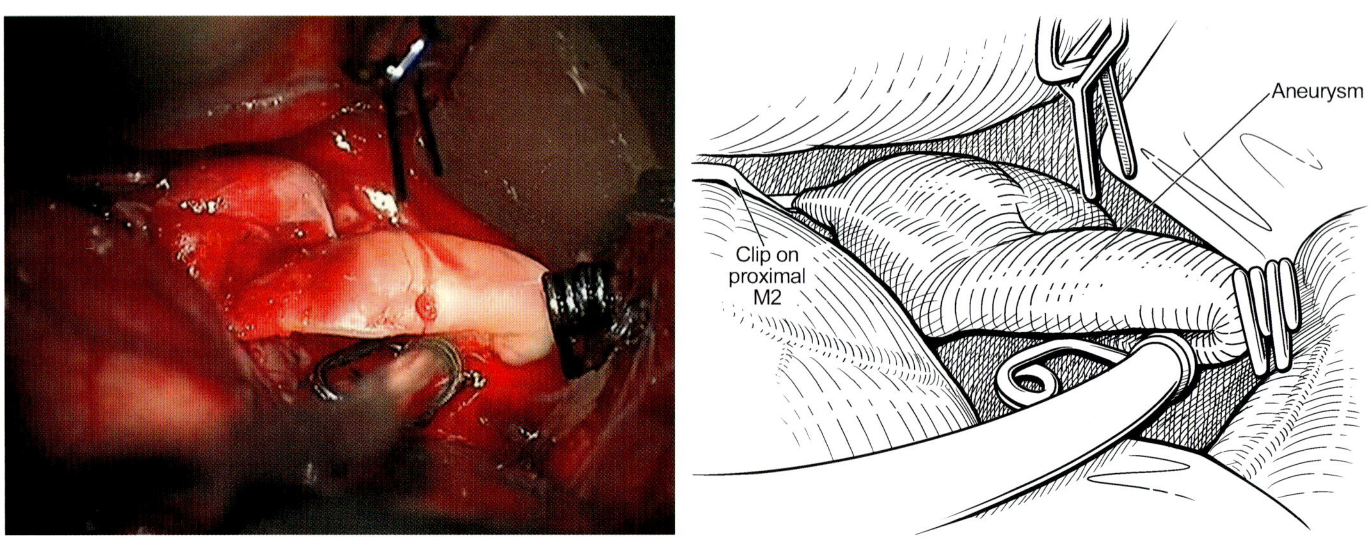

Fig. 4.3g Temporary clips are applied and the aneurysm is collapsed.

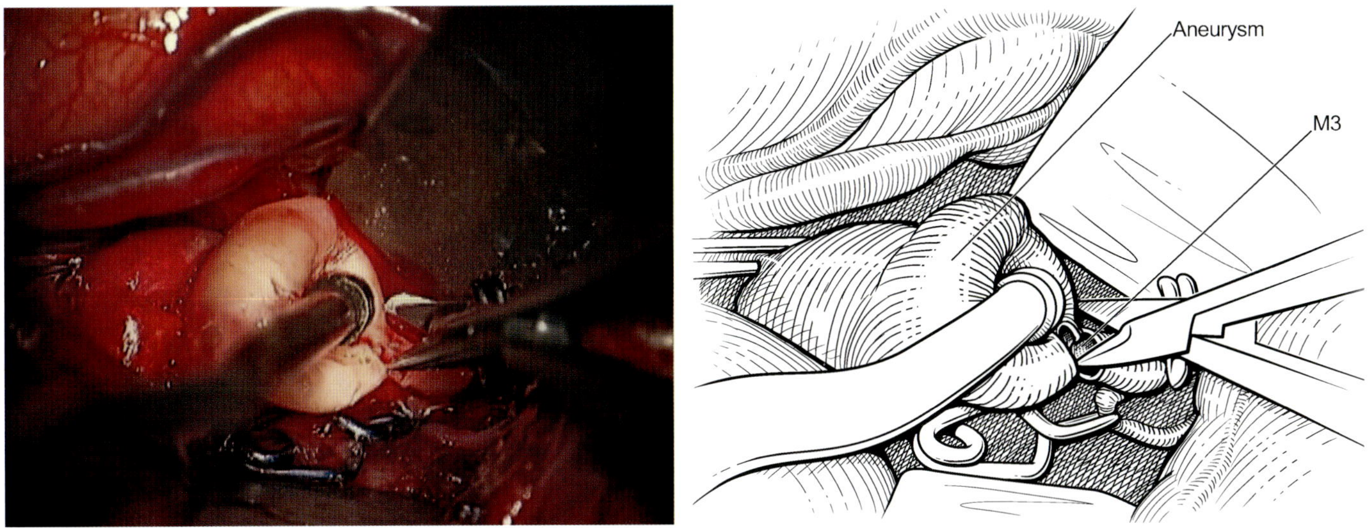

Fig. 4.3h The distal end of the aneurysm, where the M3 is normal, is cut and the aneurysm is excised.

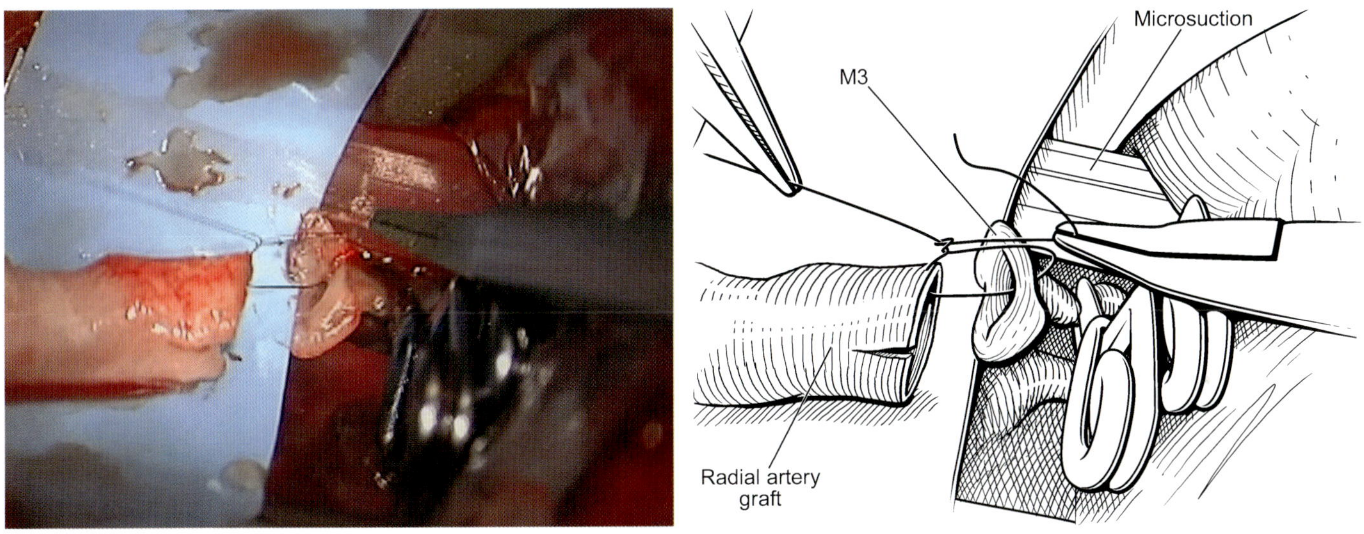

Fig. 4.3i The radial artery graft is sutured to the fishmouthed end of the distal M3 stump.

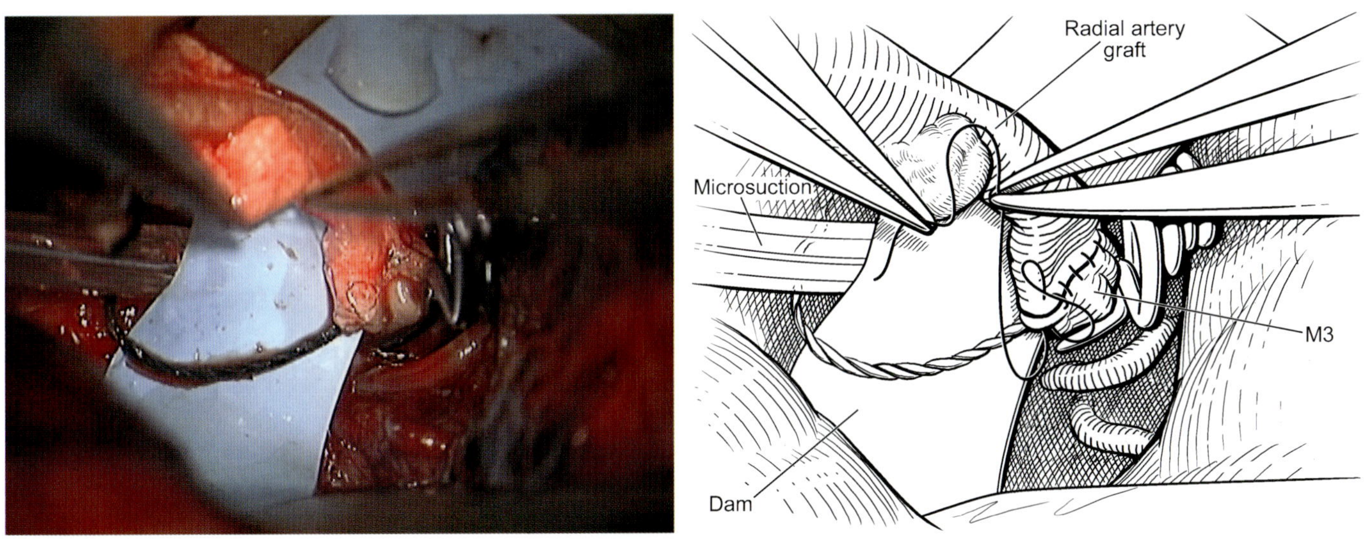

Fig. 4.3j The running suture is cinched tight.

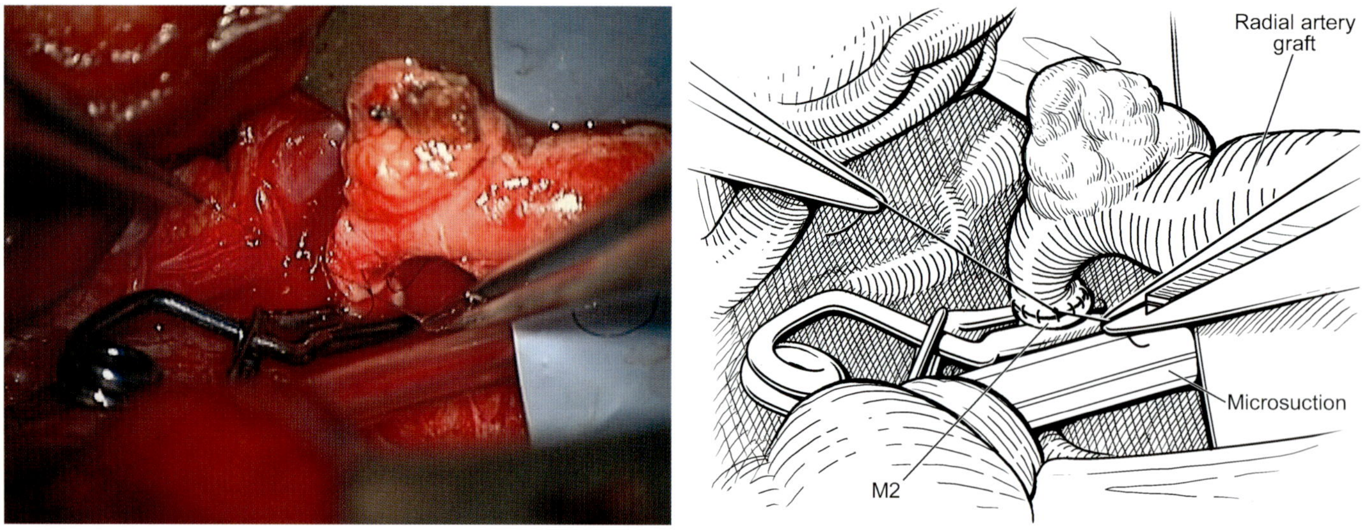

Fig. 4.3k The proximal end of the radial artery graft is anastomosed to the M2 stump with running sutures.

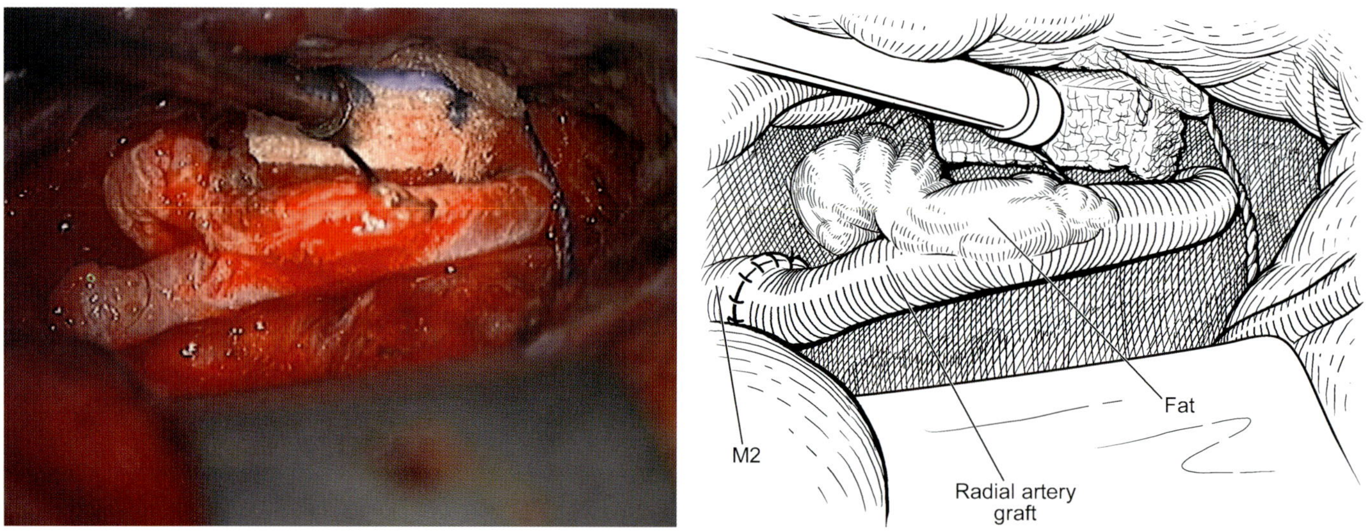

Fig. 4.3l The interposition radial artery graft is seen between the two anastomoses.

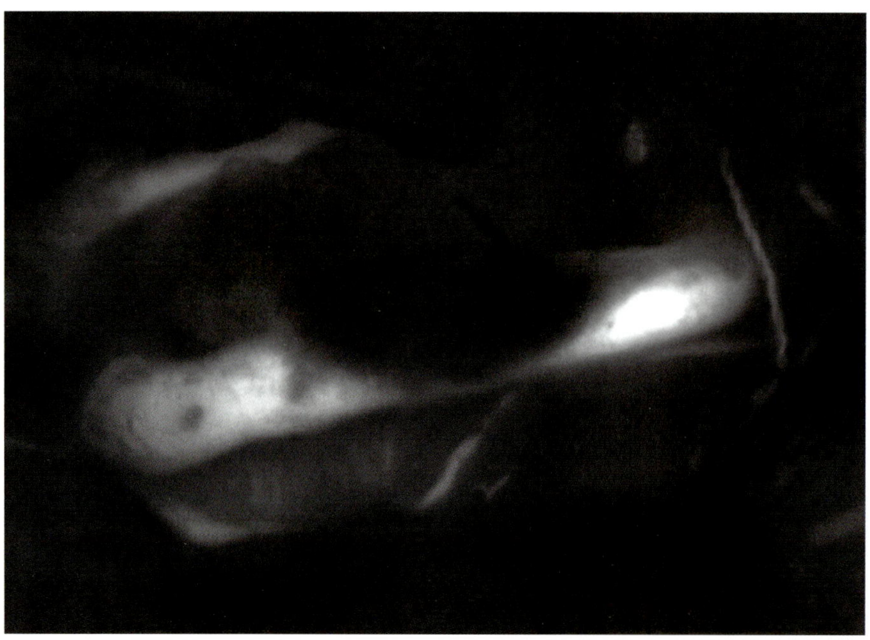

Fig. 4.3m ICG angiogram confirms blood flow through the radial artery graft. The central defect in the image is caused by overlying fat.

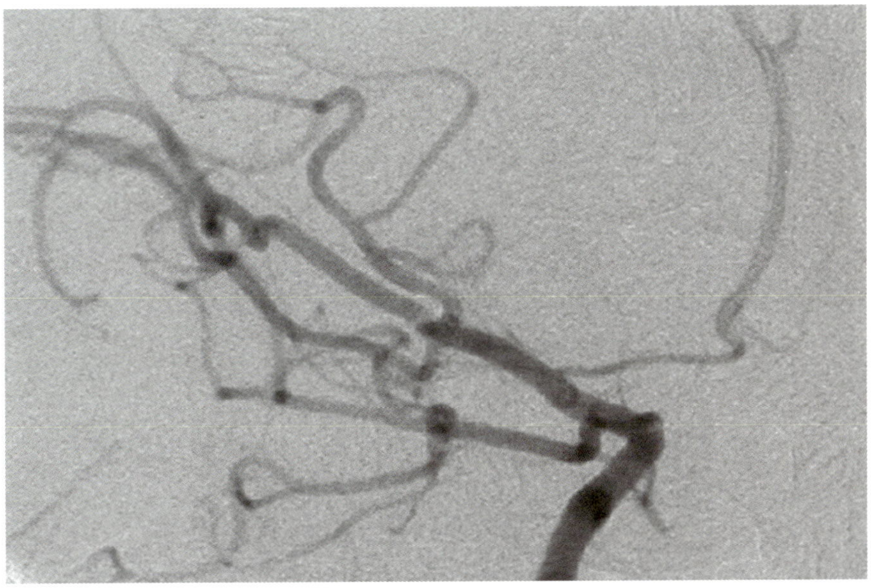

Fig. 4.3n Digital subtraction angiogram confirms patency of the bypass.

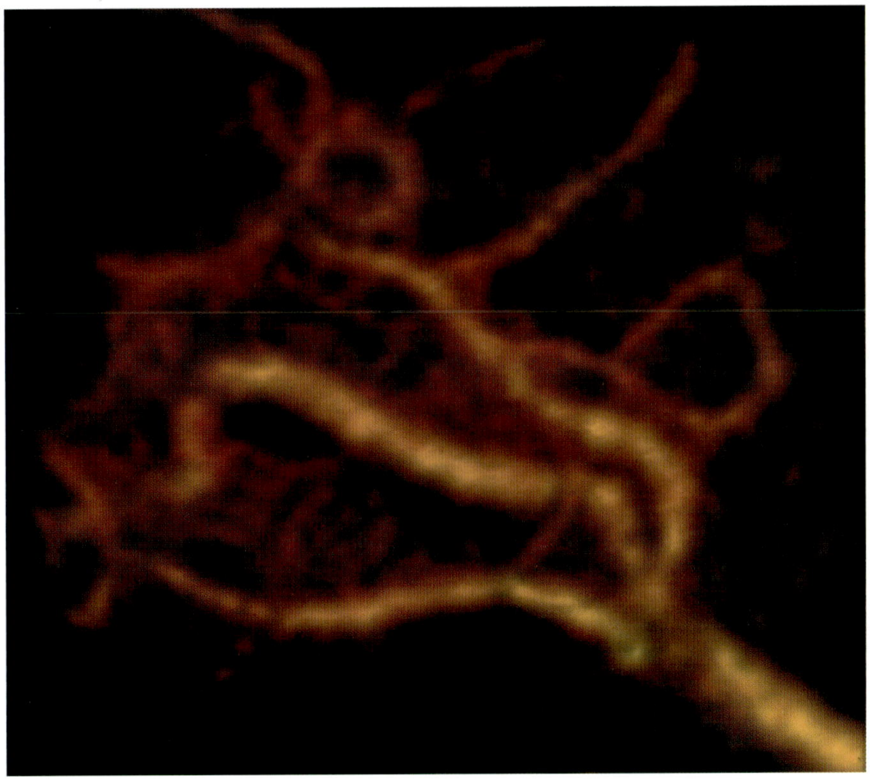

Fig. 4.3o CT angiographic reconstruction shows the interposition radial artery graft in the middle of the MCA trifurcation.

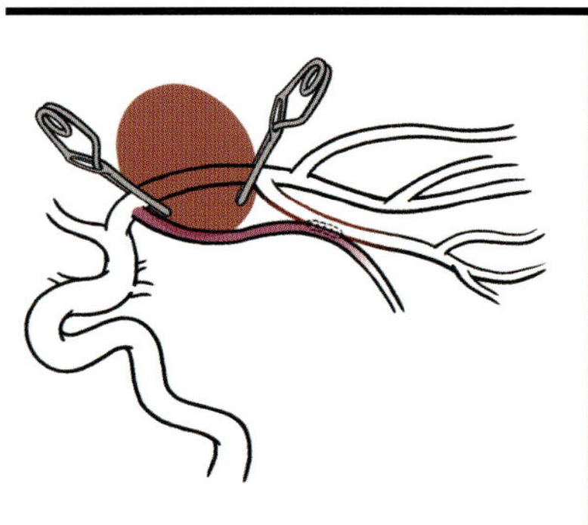

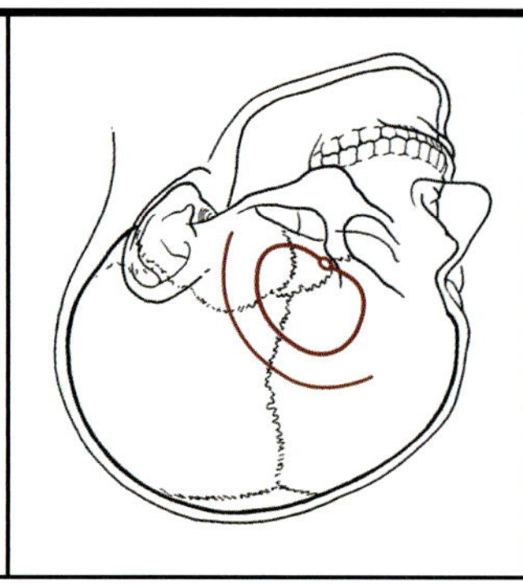

Case 4-4

Diagnosis: Left M1 giant aneurysm

Bypass: Anterior temporal artery–to–MCA

Approach: Left pterional

Video

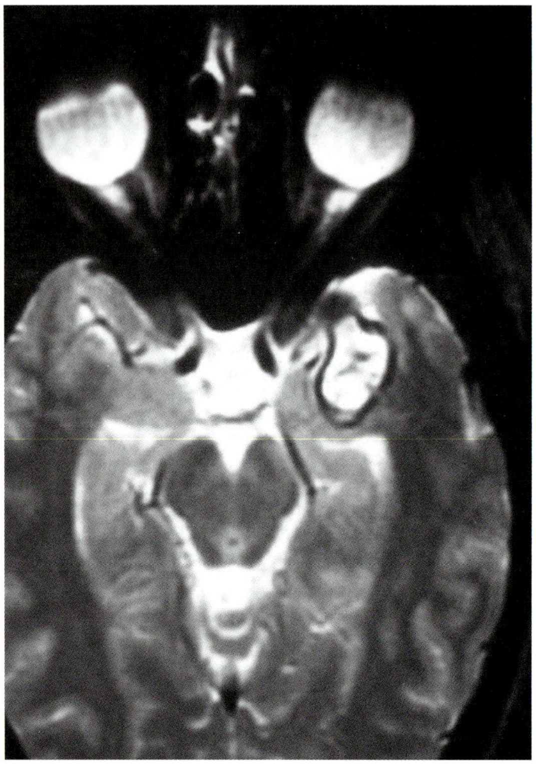

Fig. 4.4a Axial T2-weighted MR image shows a left temporal mass consistent with a thrombosed aneurysm.

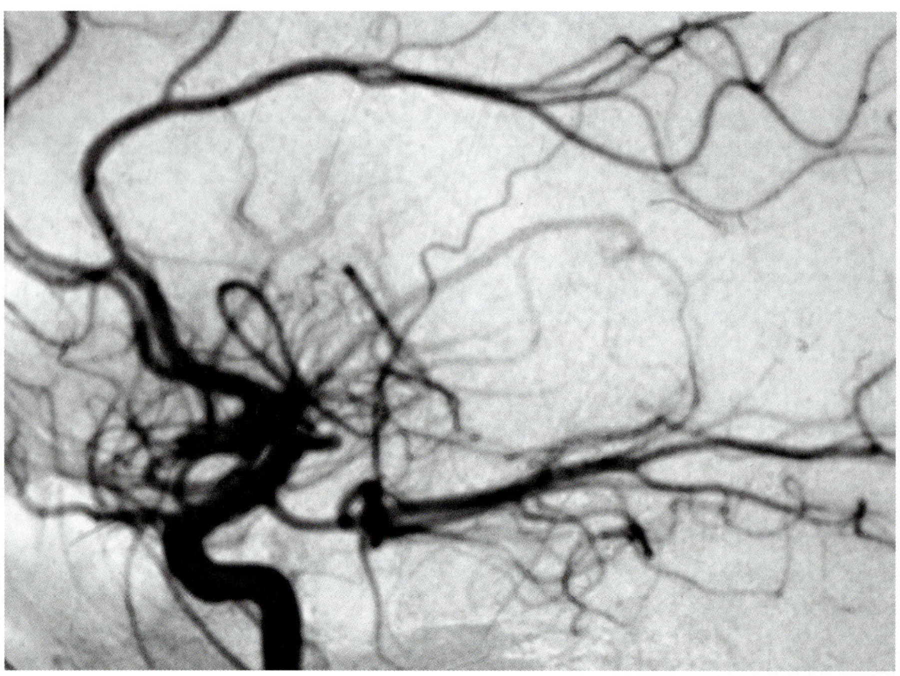

Fig. 4.4b Lateral left ICA angiogram of a 17-year-old girl who presented with thromboembolic symptoms, including left hemispheric TIAs and a small stroke, shows delayed filling of the MCA territory.

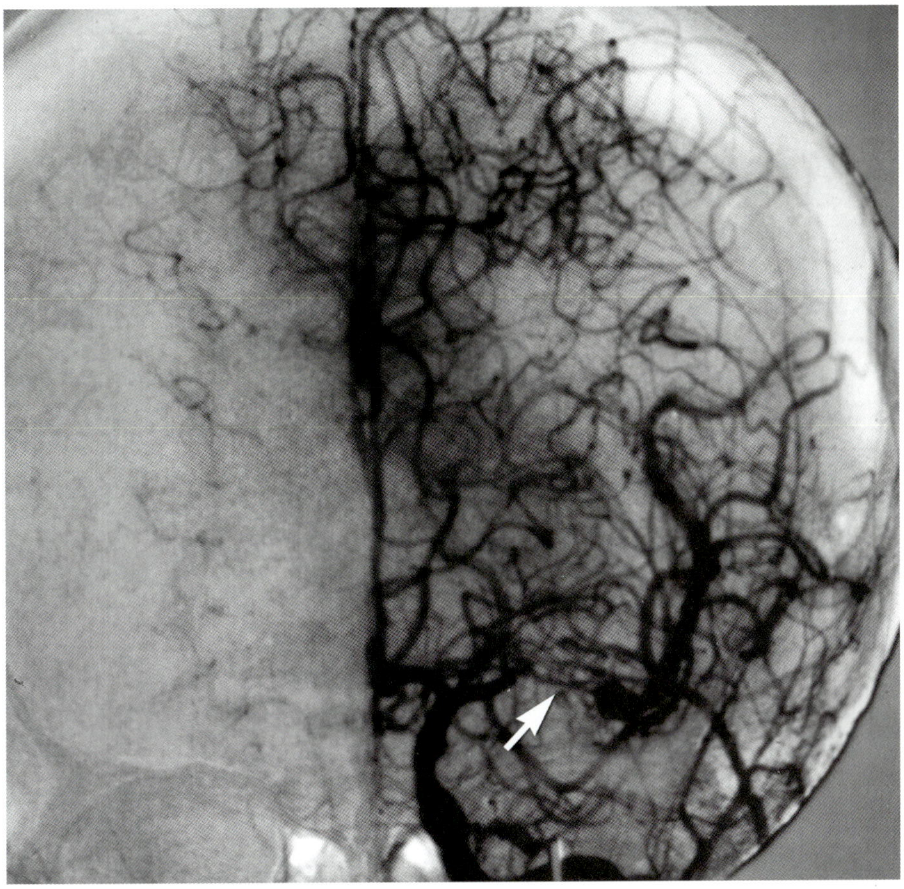

Fig. 4.4c Anteroposterior angiographic view shows severe stenosis of the M1 segment (*arrow*).

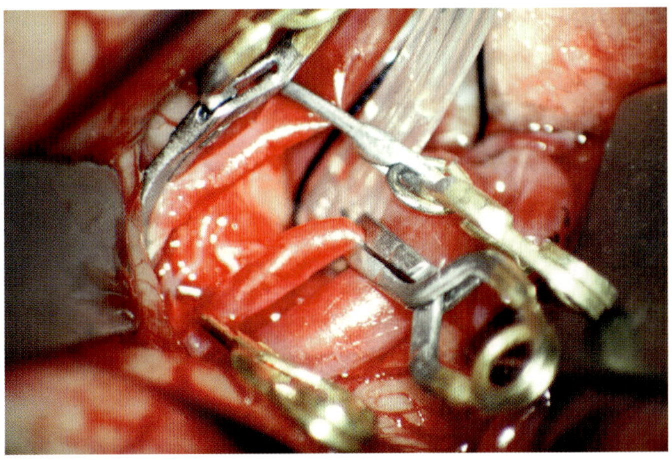

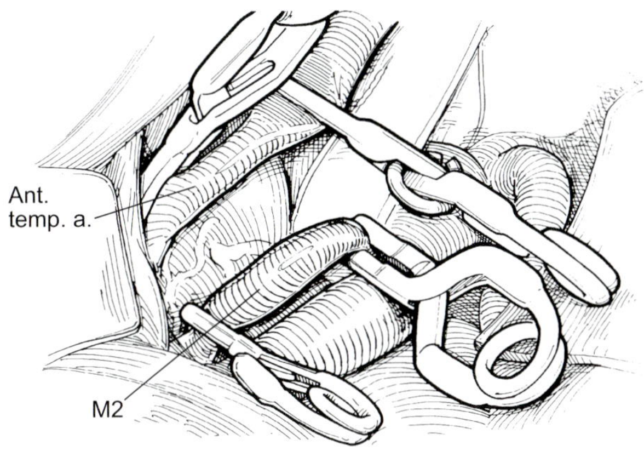

Fig. 4.4d The anterior temporal artery, which originated proximal to the aneurysm, and the M2 branch distal to the aneurysm are prepared for a side-to-side anastomosis. Temporary clips have been placed on both vessels.

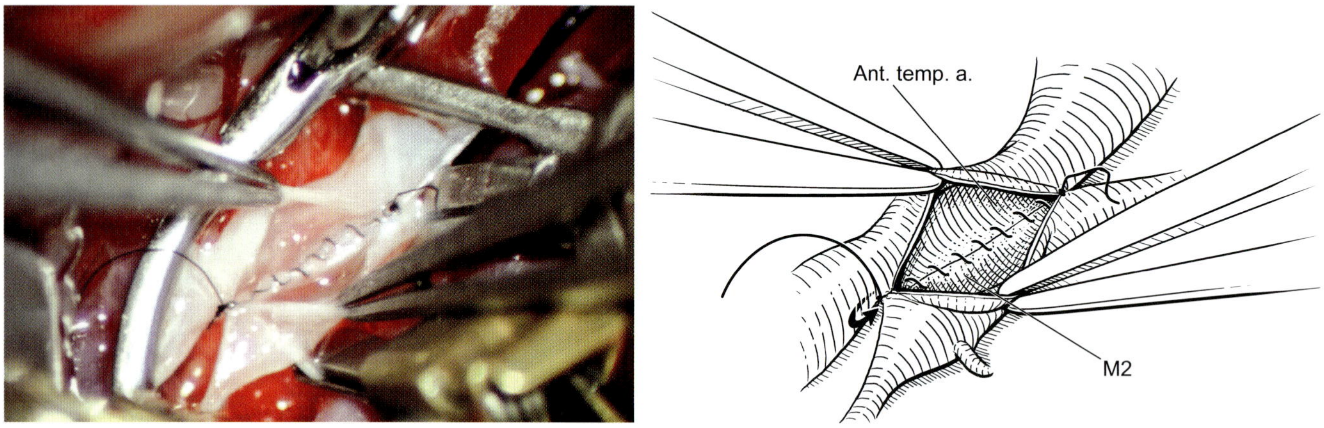

Fig. 4.4e The back wall of the side-to-side anastomosis has been completed. The toe or heel stitch is placed first. The needle is then placed from behind into the lumen, and the bypass is performed on the inside of the vessel walls.

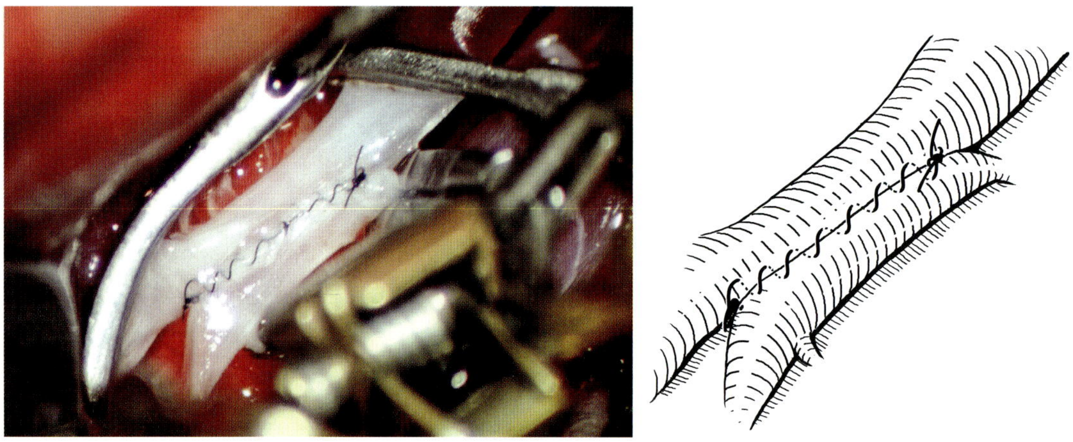

Fig. 4.4f The front wall of the anastomosis has been completed.

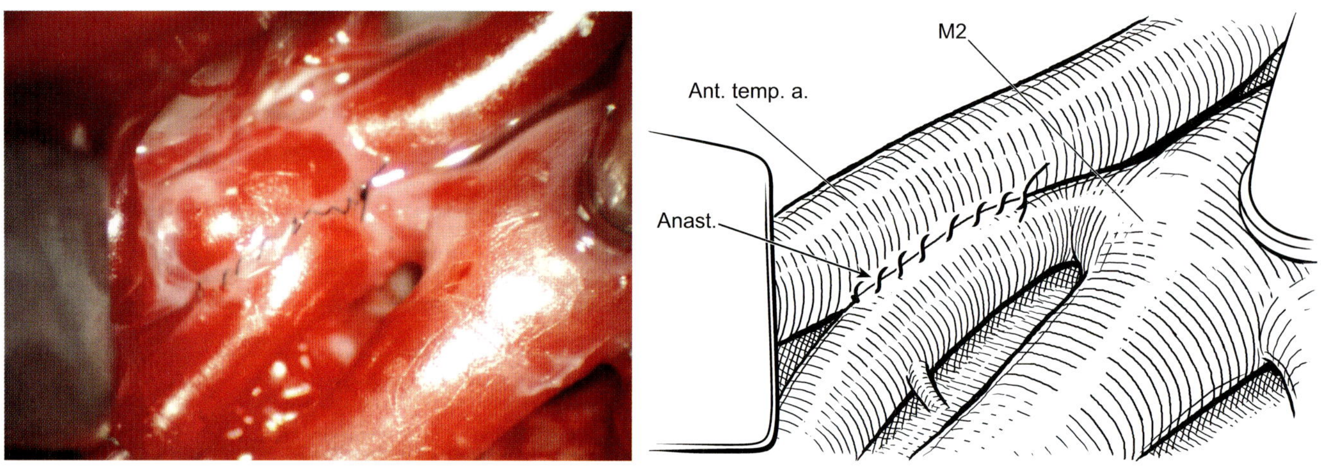

Fig. 4.4g The clips have been removed.

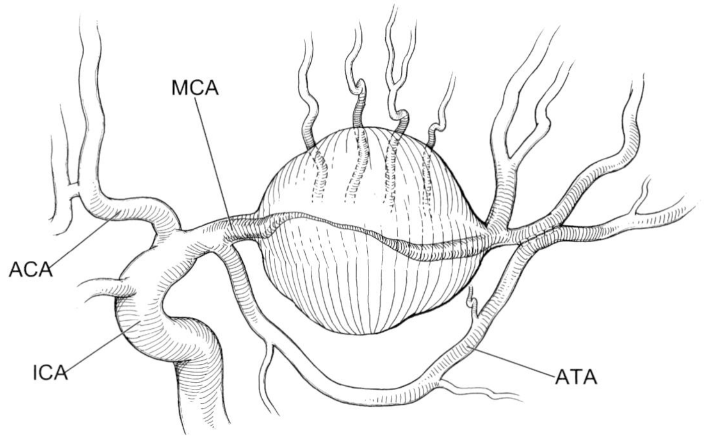

Fig. 4.4h Schematic illustration showing a side-to-side anterior temporal artery-to-M2 bypass to exclude an M1 aneurysm. (Used with permission from *Journal of Neurosurgery*.)

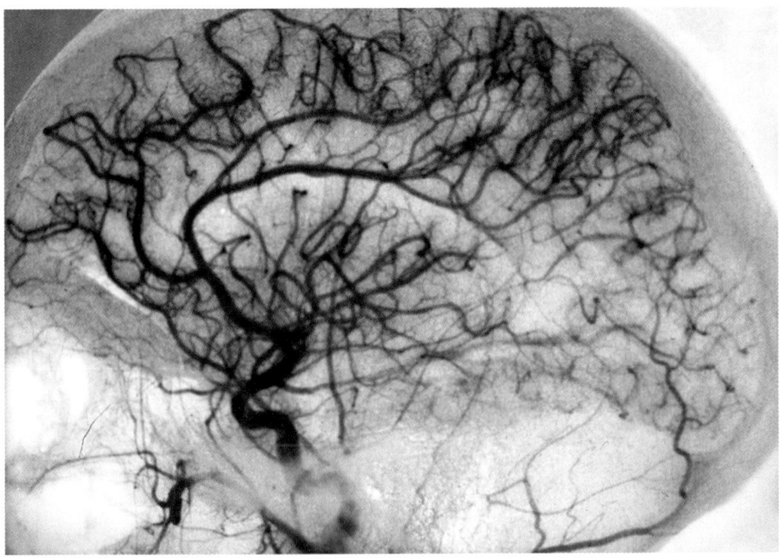

Fig. 4.4i Postoperative lateral left ICA angiogram shows normal filling of the MCA candelabra.

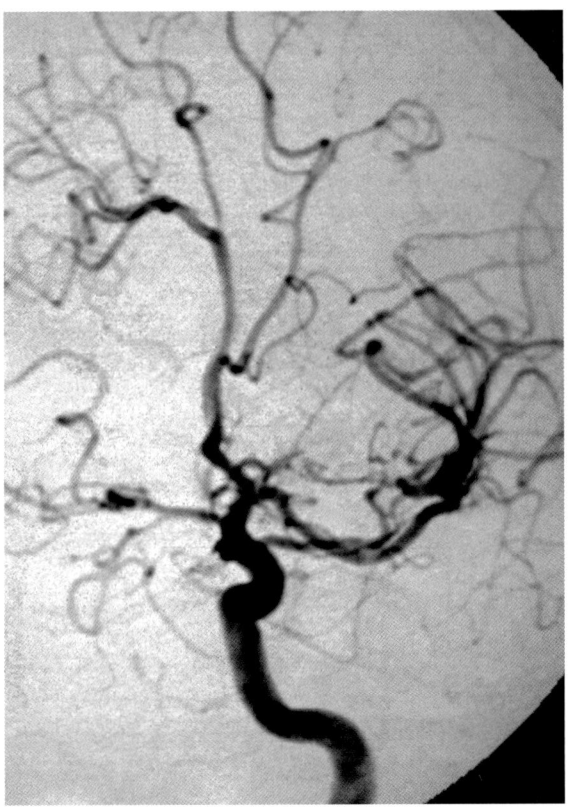

Fig. 4.4j Oblique angiogram shows excellent filling of the MCA via the bypass. Over a follow-up period of more than 8 years, the patient experienced no further symptoms.

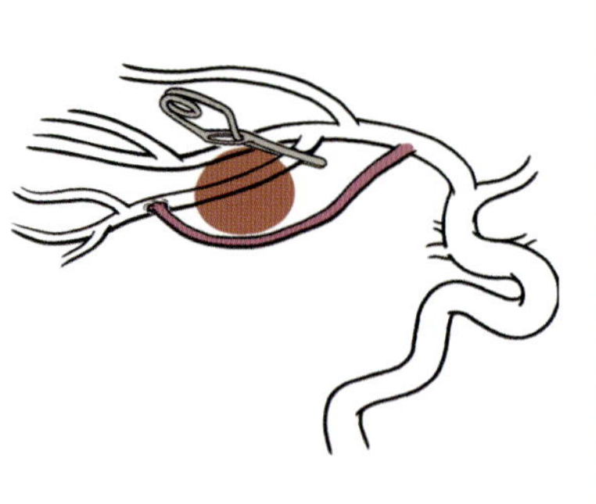

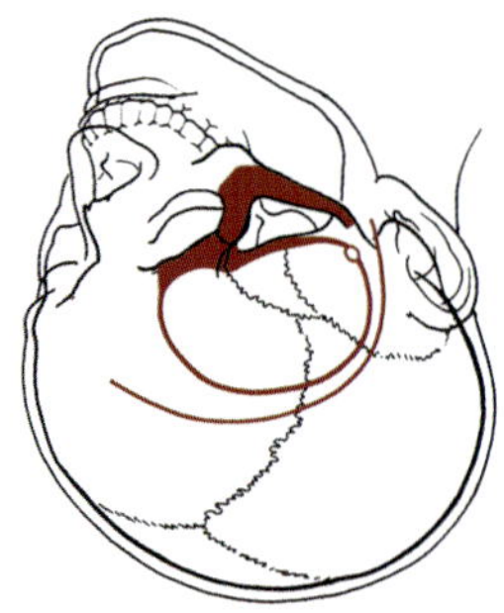

Case 4-5

Diagnosis: Giant recurrent complex right MCA aneurysm

Bypass: Anterior temporal artery–to-distal MCA

Approach: Right orbitozygomatic

Video

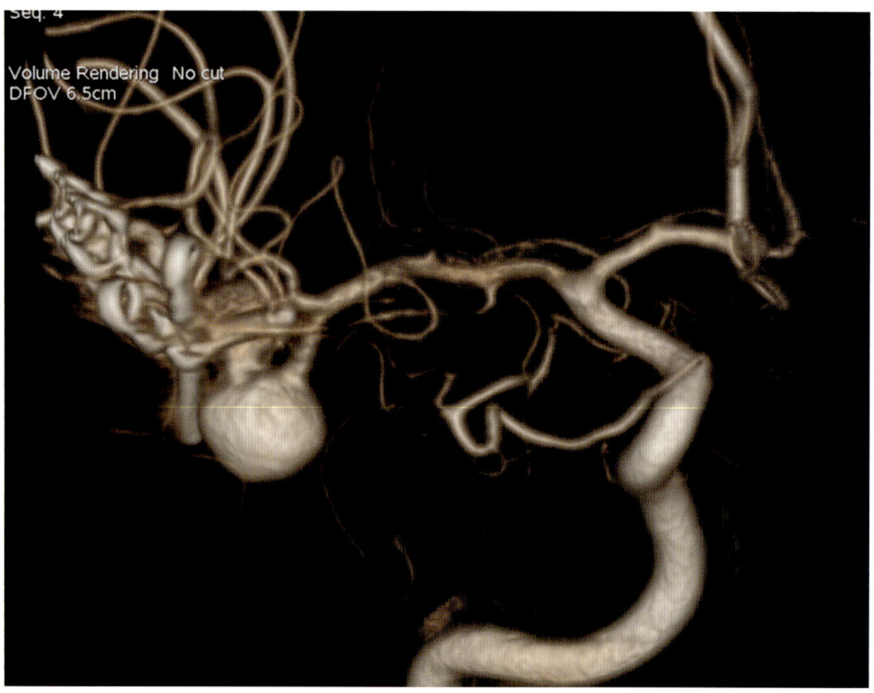

Fig. 4.5a Three-dimensional angiographic reconstruction of the right ICA shows a complex aneurysm of the MCA. In 1991 at the age of 24, the patient had presented with SAH and two clips were applied on the MCA aneurysm. Another clip was applied in 2000, and three more clips were applied in 2001. The patient was referred for this most recent recurrence in 2010.

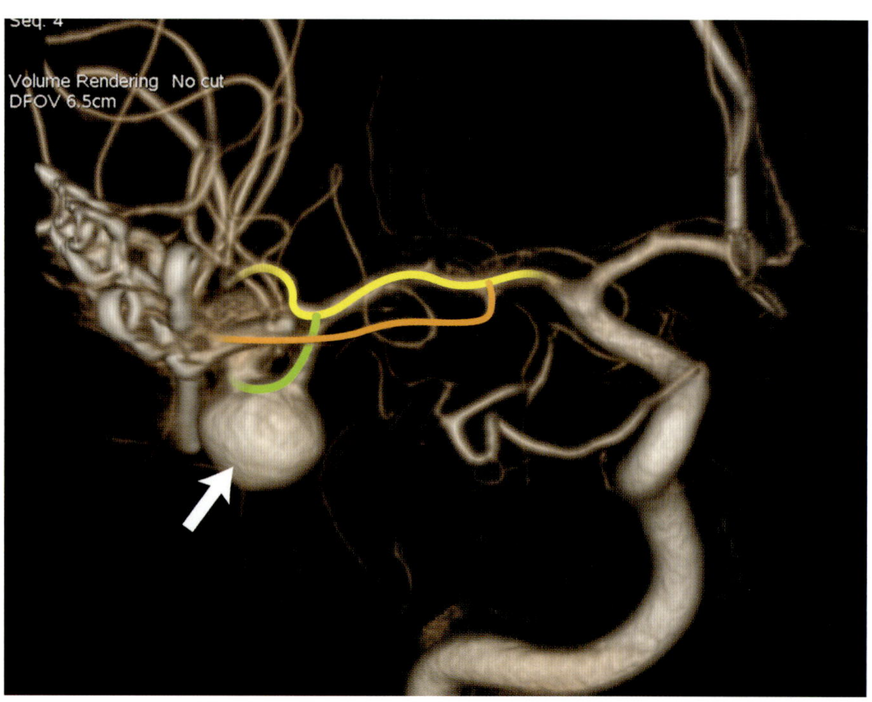

Fig. 4.5b The patient's angiographic study shows several important features. The involved aneurysm (*arrow*) is located relatively distally. This configuration would allow the normal proximal MCA branches (*yellow*) to be preserved if it were possible to place a clip at the base of the aneurysm. Such clipping would occlude the distal outflow of the M2 branch. The anterior temporal artery (*orange*) is clearly visible as it courses along the aneurysm in the sylvian fissure. This configuration allows surgical planning to incorporate the anterior temporal artery as an anastomotic vessel to supply distal outflow of the vessel involving the aneurysm. *Green*, M2 branch into aneurysm.

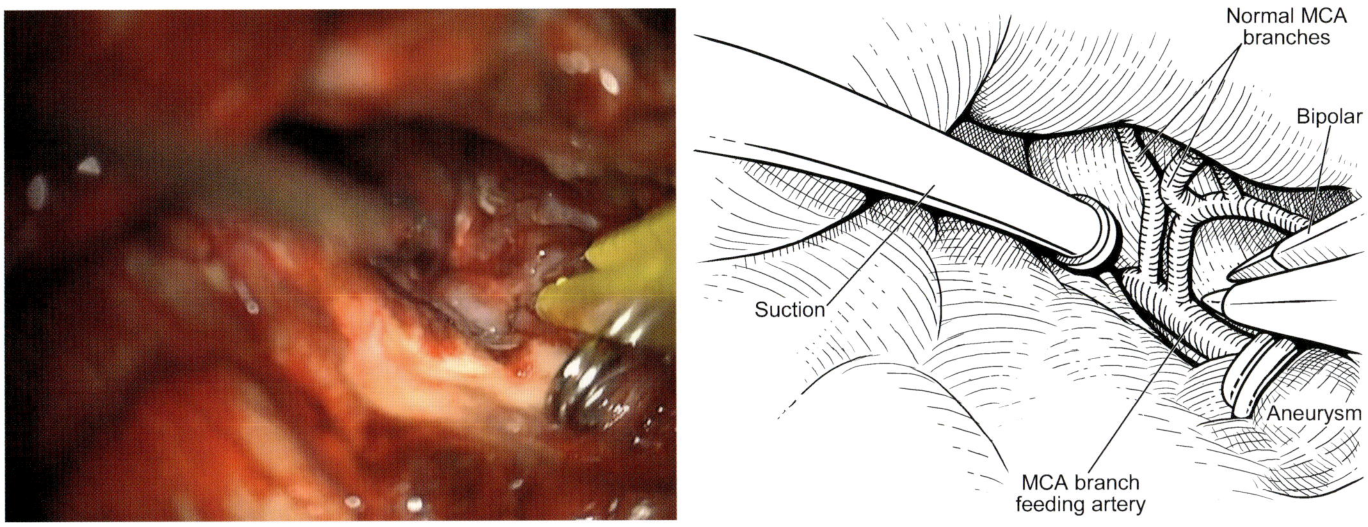

Fig. 4.5c The sylvian fissure is opened and the MCA branch feeding the aneurysm and its normal branches are identified.

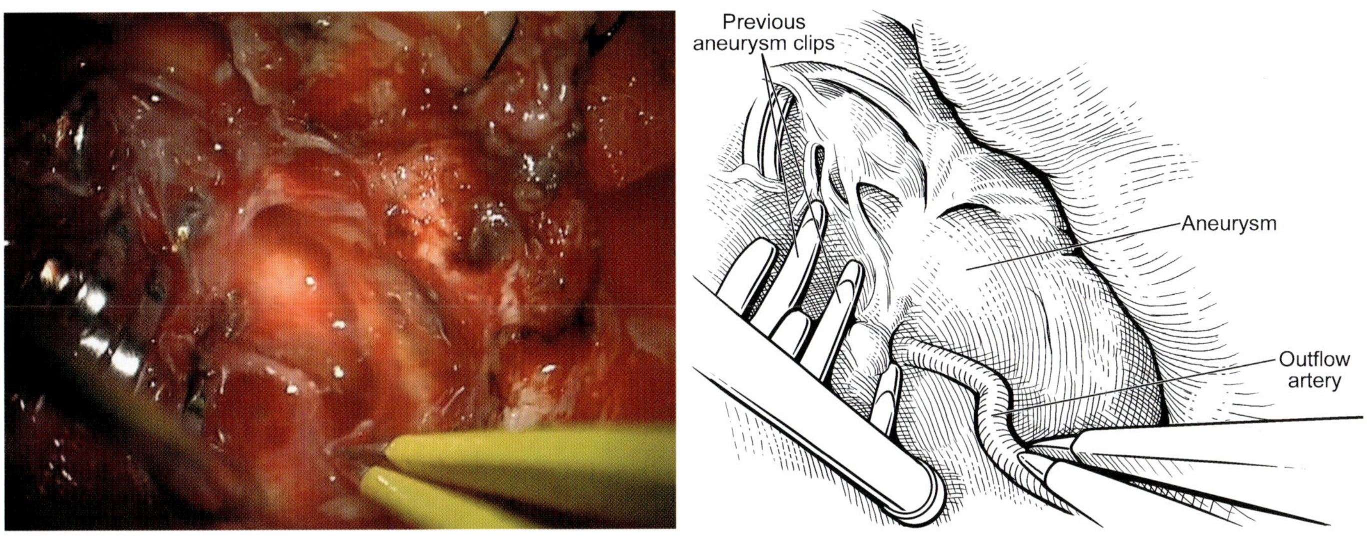

Fig. 4.5d The outflow vessel distal to the aneurysm clips is exposed.

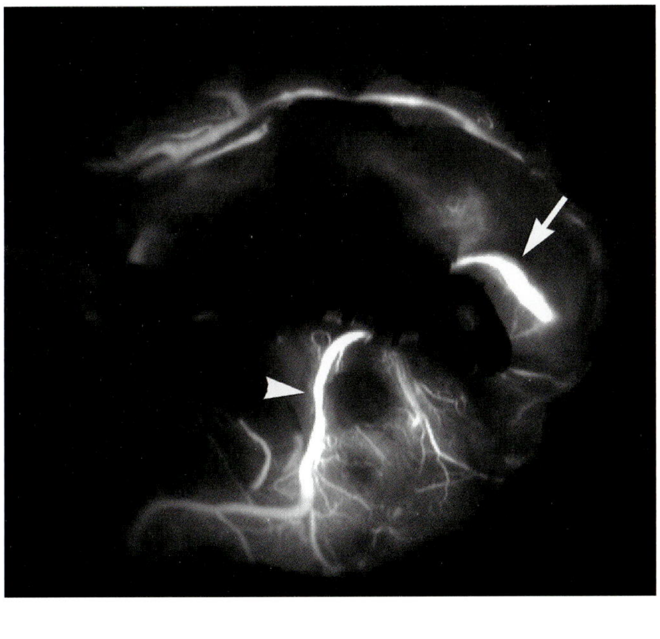

Fig. 4.5e An ICG angiogram demonstrates continued filling of the proximal MCA branch (*arrowhead*) and the more distal branch, which is part of the aneurysm (*arrow*).

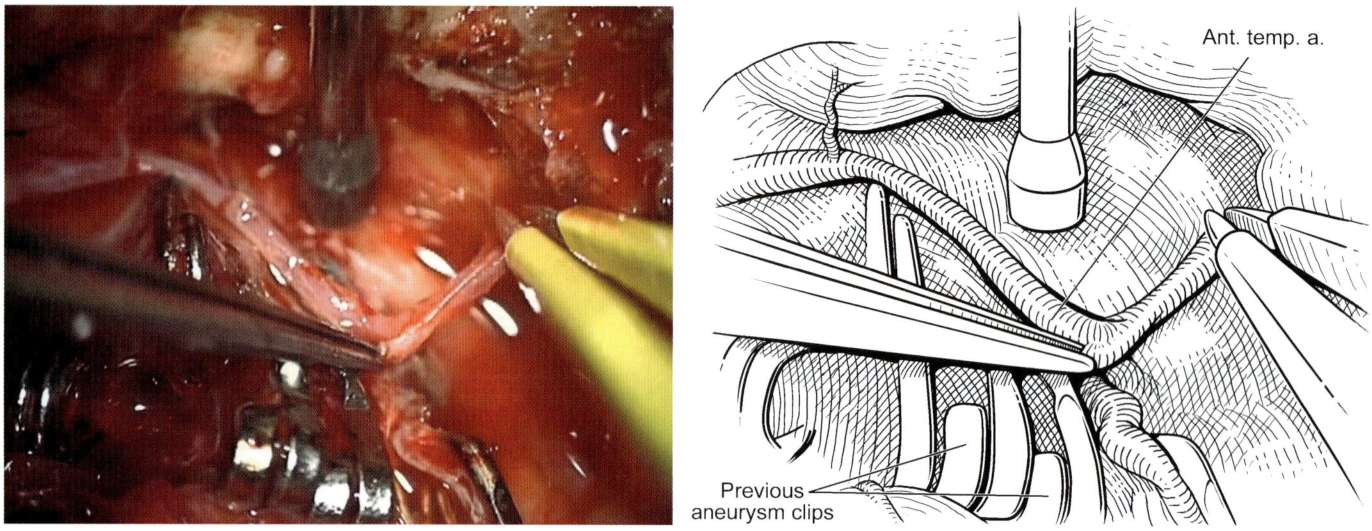

Fig. 4.5f The anterior temporal artery is dissected free.

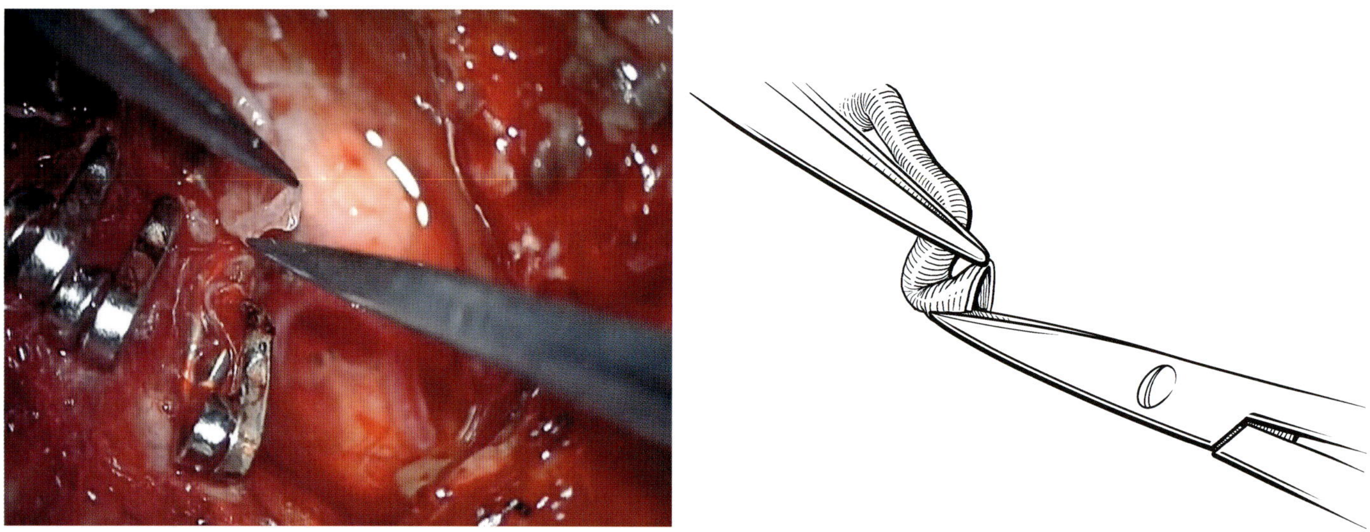

Fig. 4.5g The anterior temporal artery is cut.

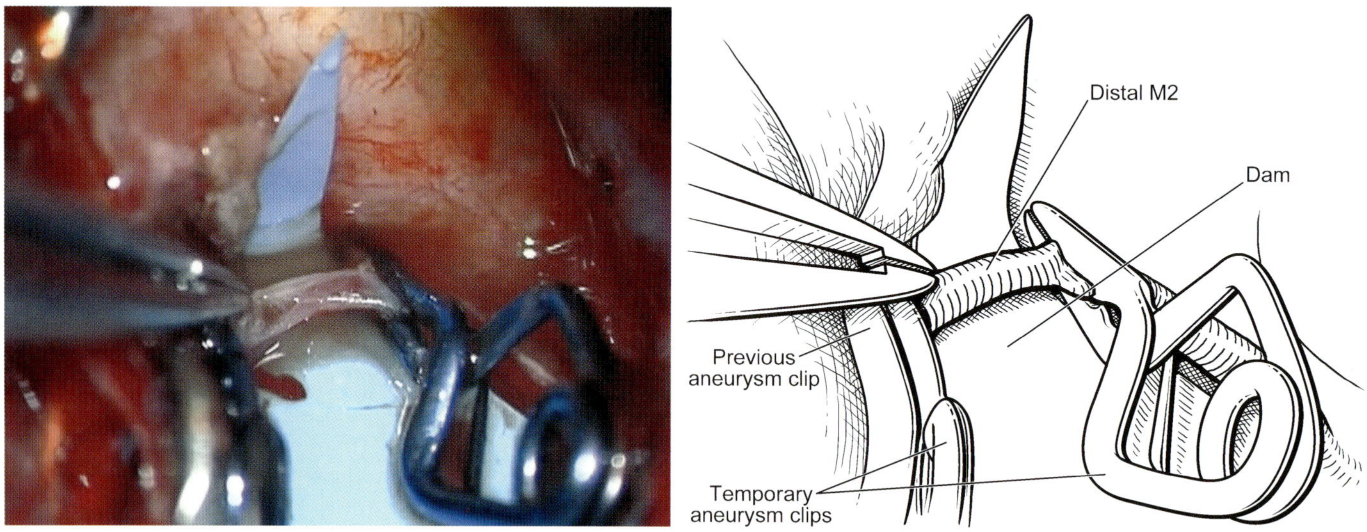

Fig. 4.5h The MCA branch distal to the aneurysm is exposed.

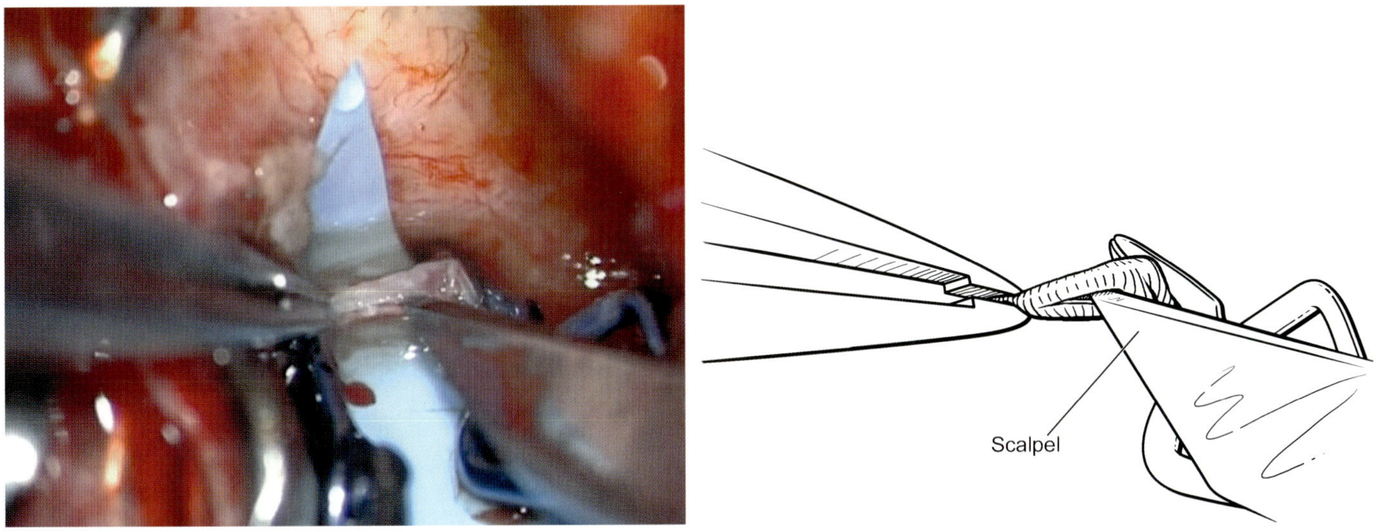

Fig. 4.5i The arteriotomy of the MCA branch is performed.

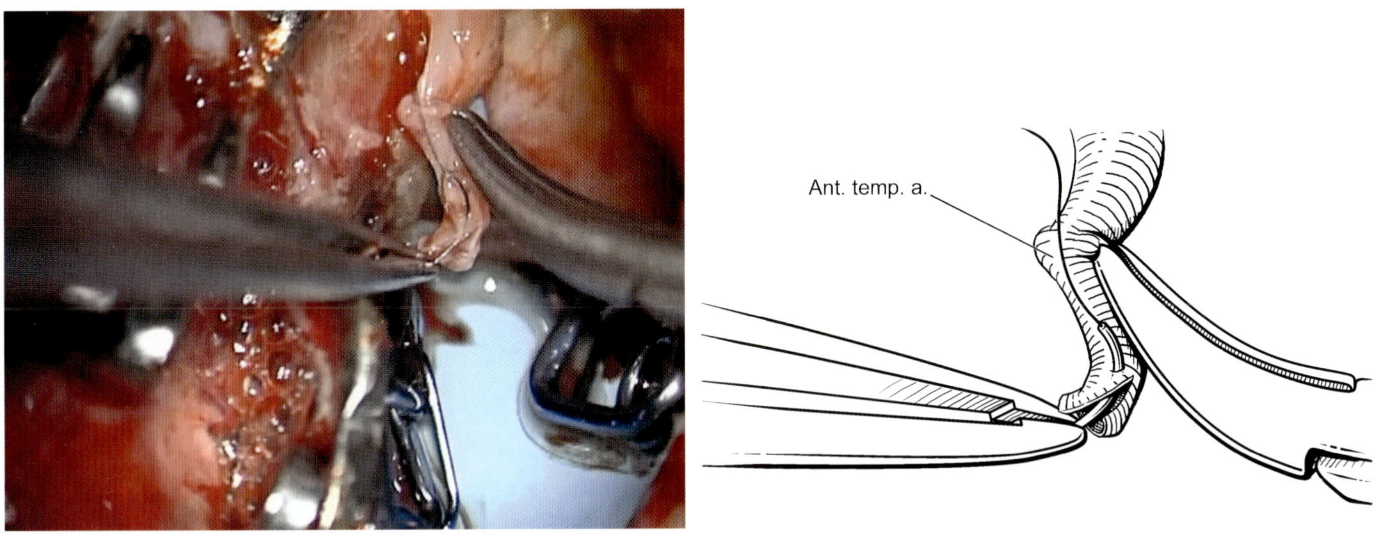

Fig. 4.5j The heel stitch is placed in the anterior temporal artery.

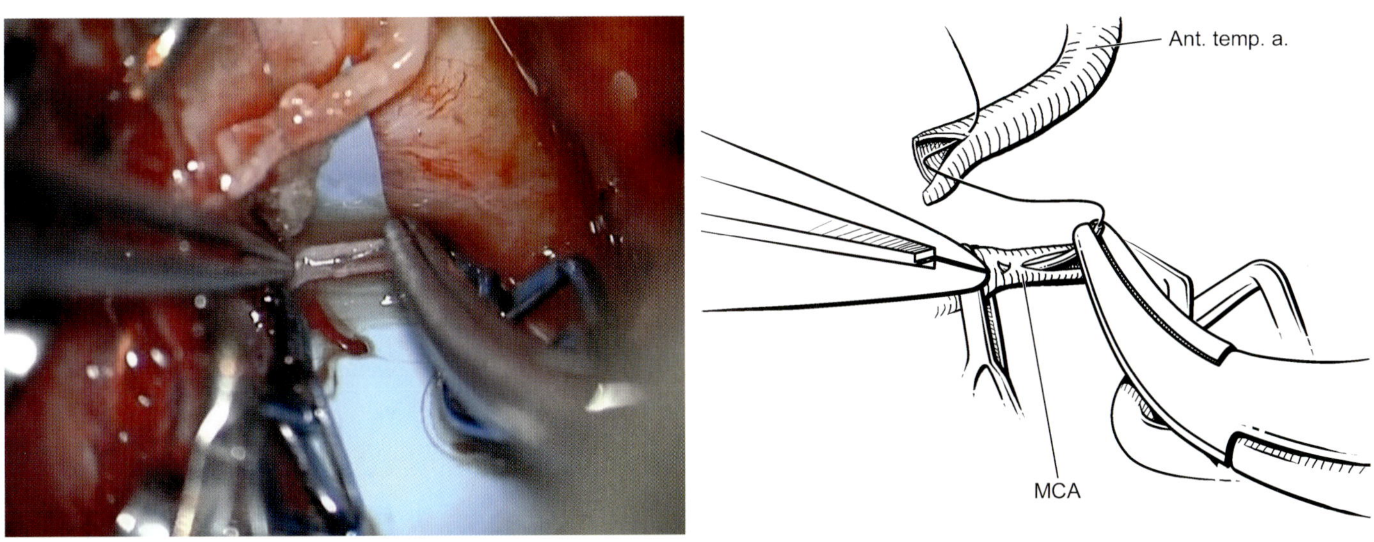

Fig. 4.5k The suture is passed through one end of the MCA arteriotomy.

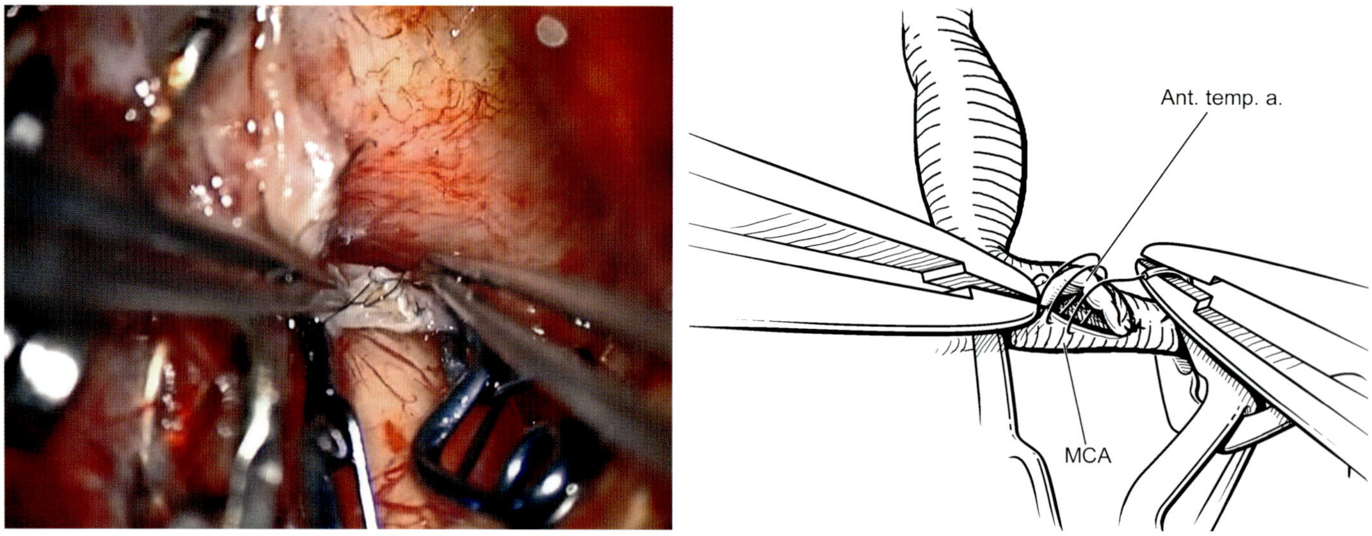

Fig. 4.5l The loose 11–0 running sutures are placed.

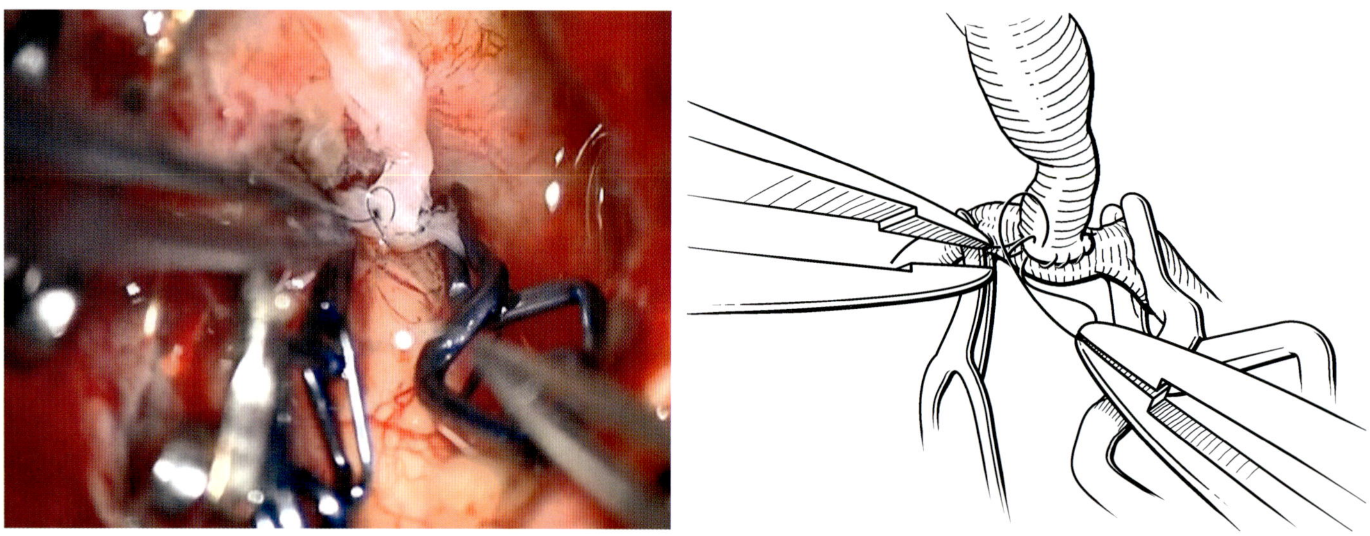

Fig. 4.5m The sutures are tightened.

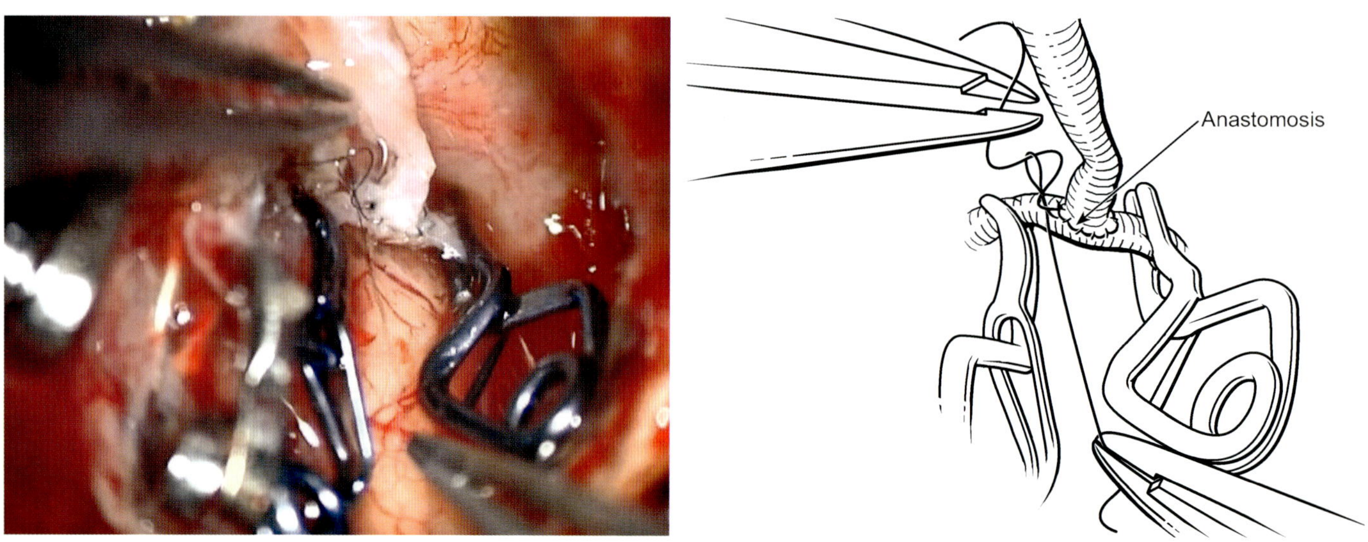

Fig. 4.5n The anastomosis is completed.

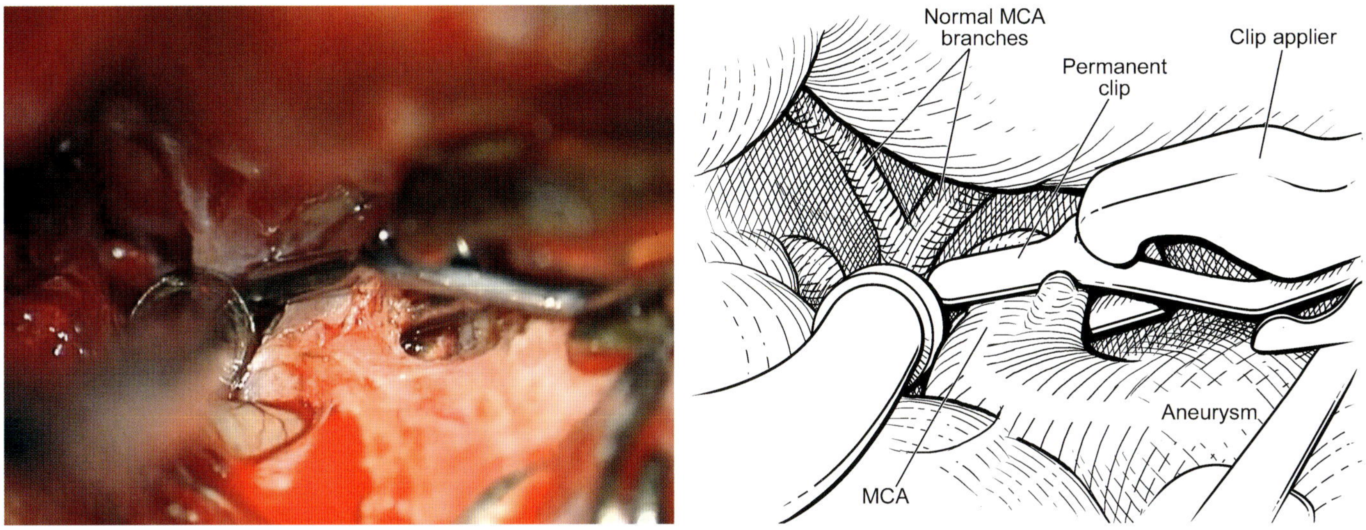

Fig. 4.5o A permanent clip is placed on the MCA distal to the exit of the normal MCA branch and proximal to the MCA aneurysm.

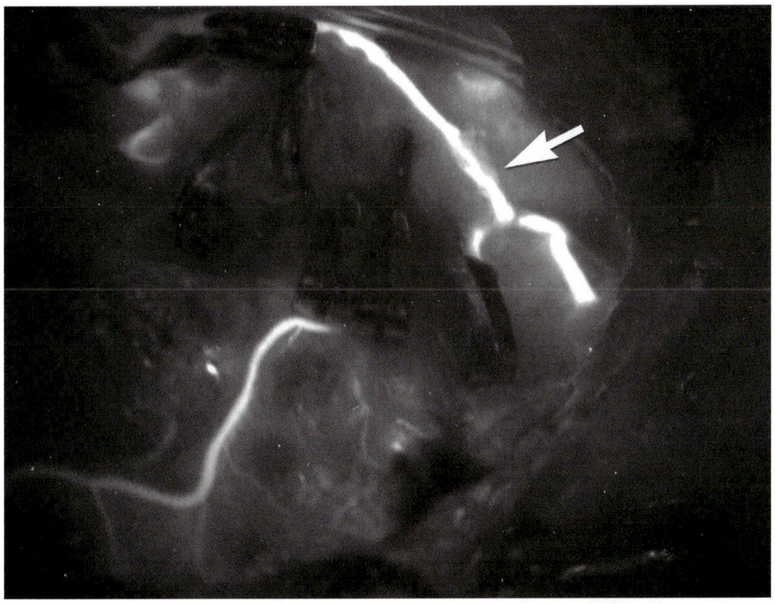

Fig. 4.5p ICG angiogram confirms patency of the bypass (*arrow*).

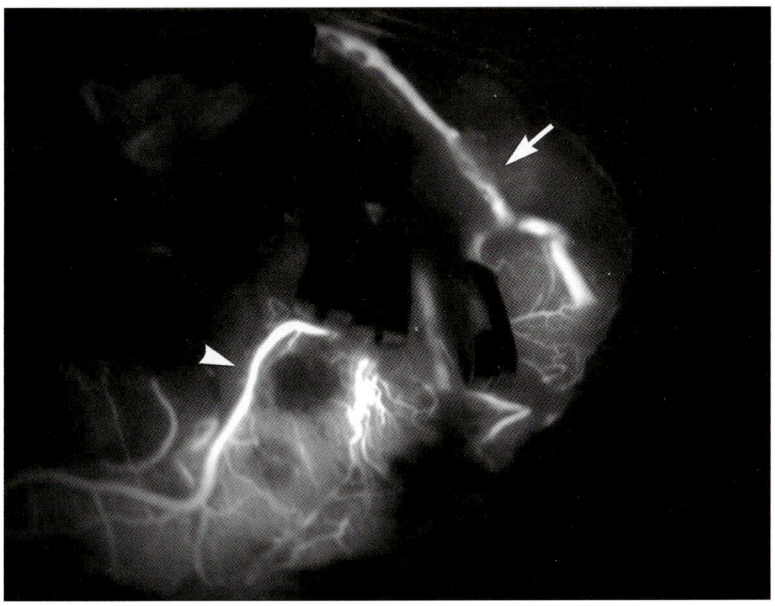

Fig. 4.5q A later view of the ICG angiogram shows good filling of the hemisphere through the bypass (*arrow*) and proximal branch of the MCA (*arrowhead*).

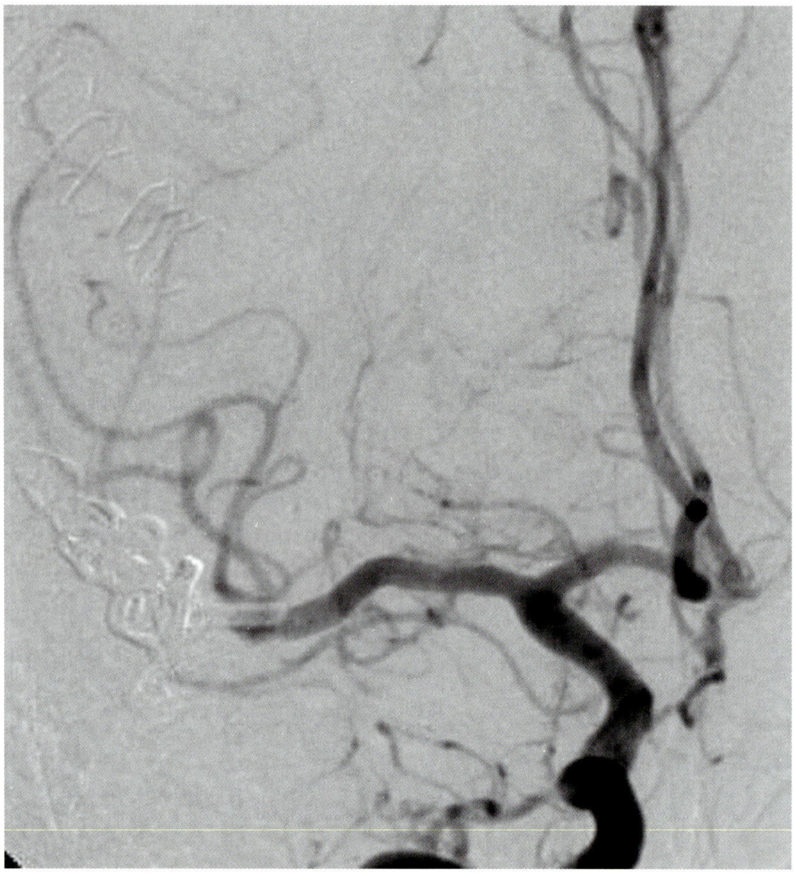

Fig. 4.5r Anteroposterior angiogram demonstrates absence of the aneurysm and patency of the anterior temporal artery.

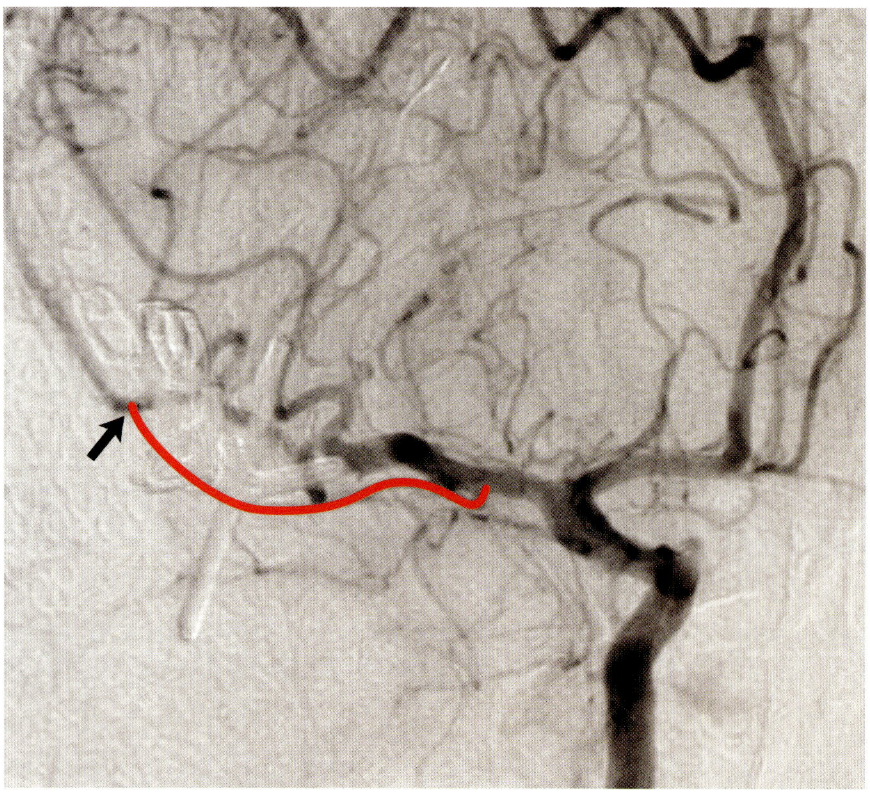

Fig. 4.5s An *orange line* has been placed over the anterior temporal artery demonstrating the anastomosis (*arrow*). The patient had no postoperative deficits.

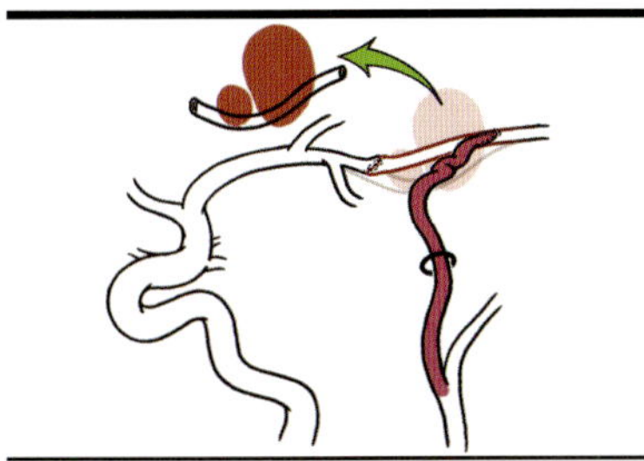

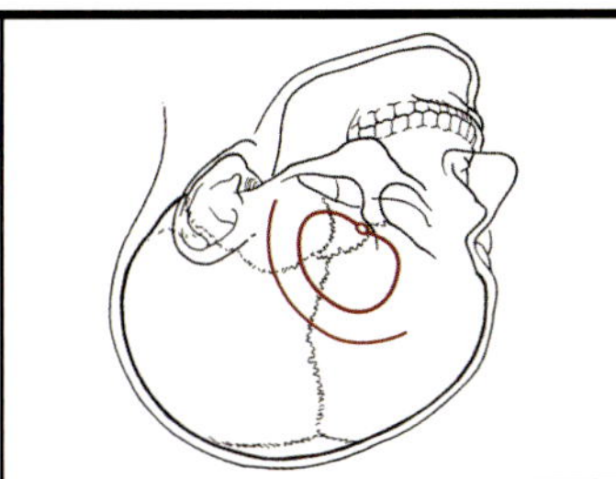

Case 4-6

Diagnosis: Giant left MCA aneurysm

Bypass: Direct MCA-to-MCA and STA-to-MCA

Approach: Left pterional

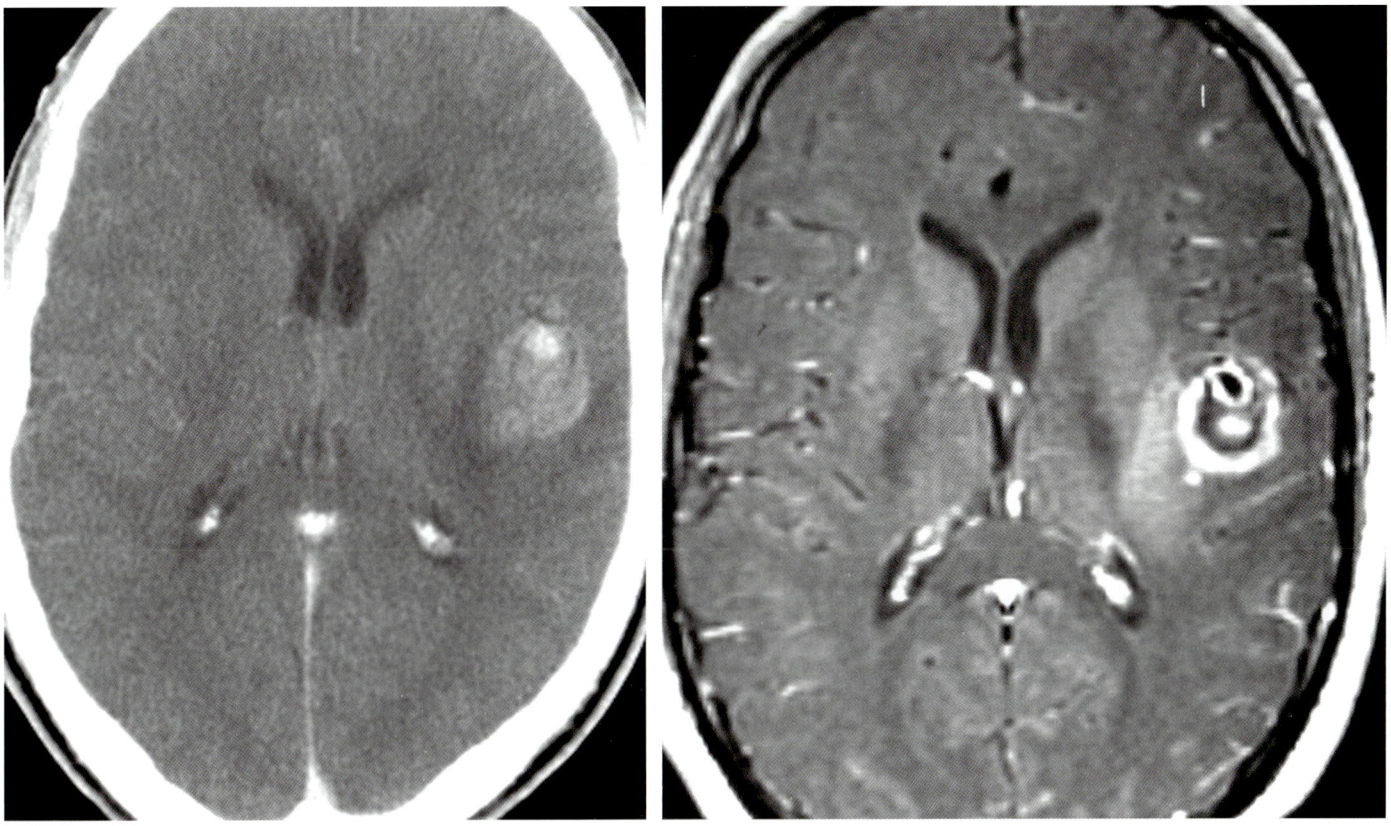

a b

Fig. 4.6a, b Axial CT and MR images demonstrate a complex MCA aneurysm in a 22-year-old man who experienced the sudden onset of headache, aphasia, and weakness, which all improved over several weeks.

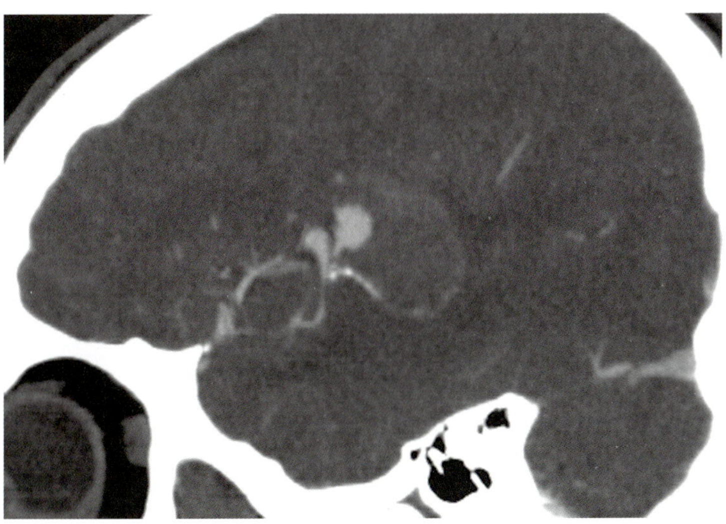

Fig. 4.6c CT angiogram shows two complex MCA aneurysms.

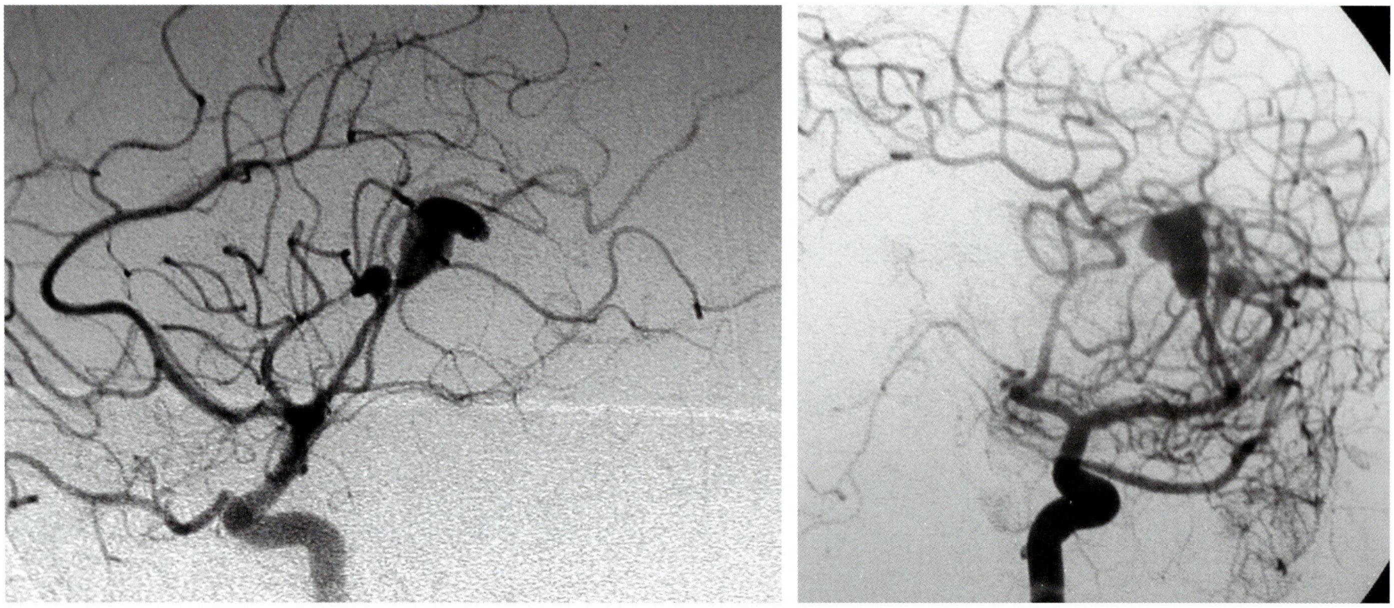

d e

Fig. 4.6d, e Lateral and oblique angiograms show two complex MCA aneurysms on the angular branch of the left MCA.

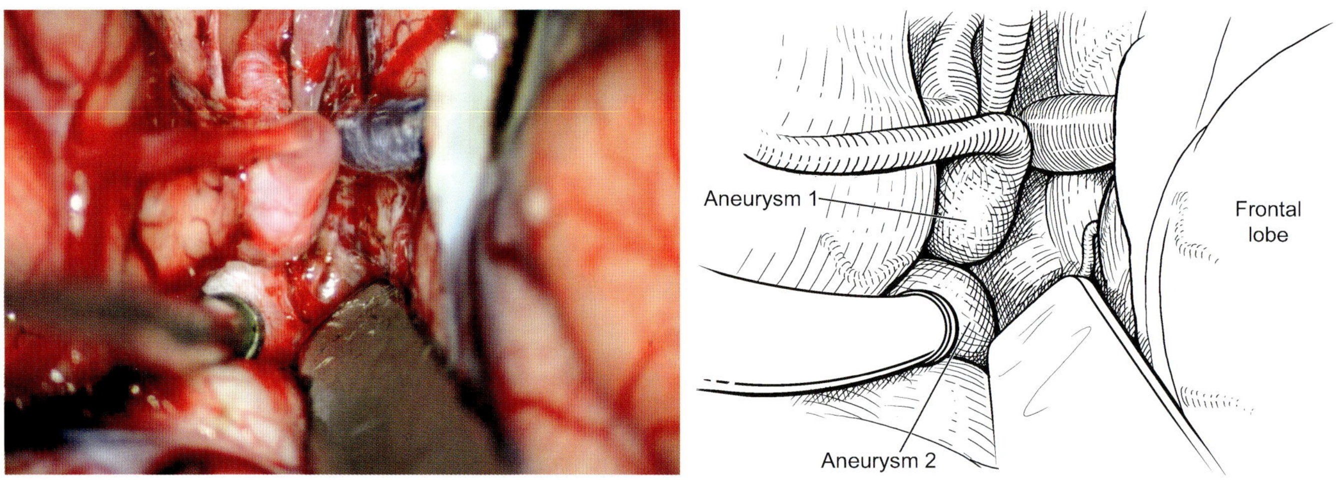

Fig. 4.6f The distal sylvian fissure is opened and the aneurysms are exposed.

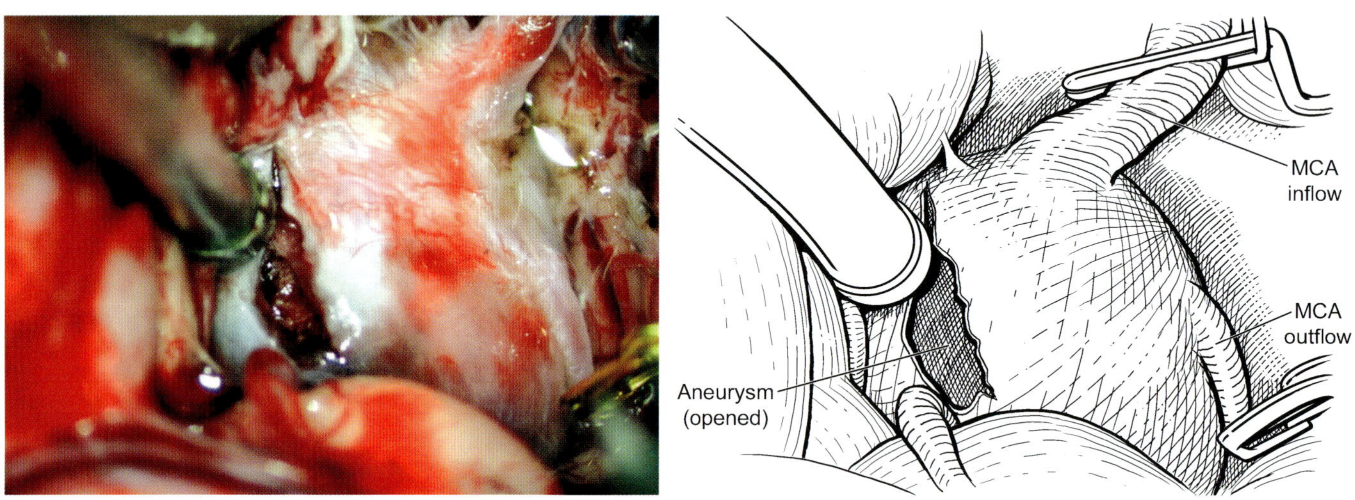

Fig. 4.6g The large MCA aneurysm has been incised to assess the feasibility of clip reconstruction, which is impossible.

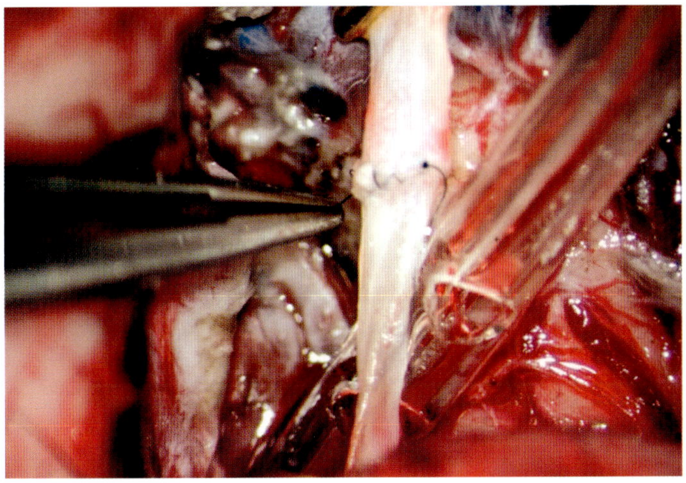

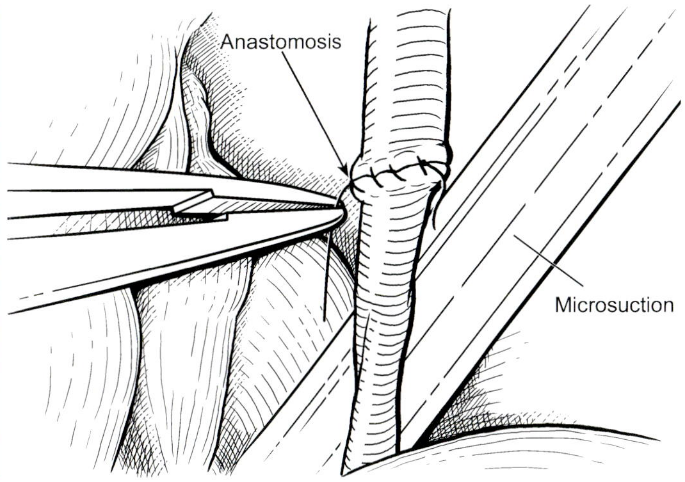

Fig. 4.6h The inflow and outflow branches of the giant MCA aneurysm have been cut and anastomosed end to end.

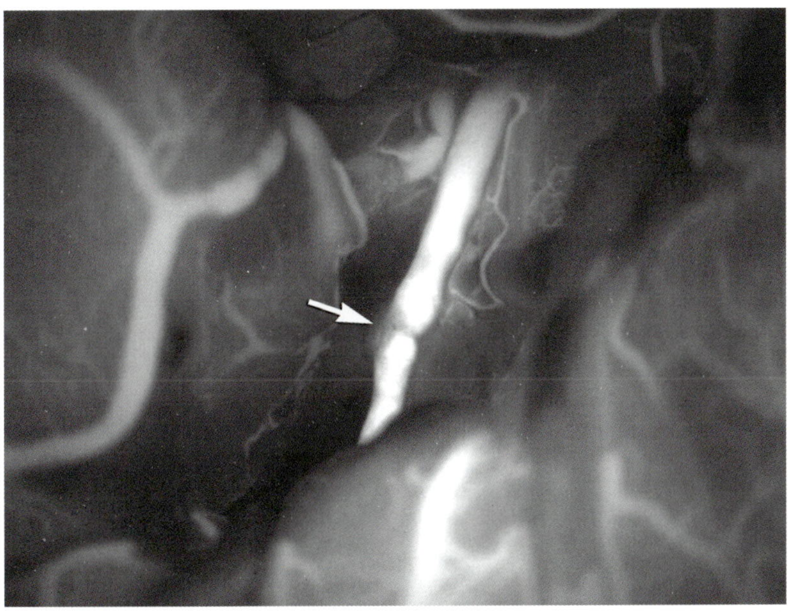

Fig. 4.6i ICG angiogram confirms patency of the direct anastomosis although a clump of platelets appears at the anastomotic site (*arrow*).

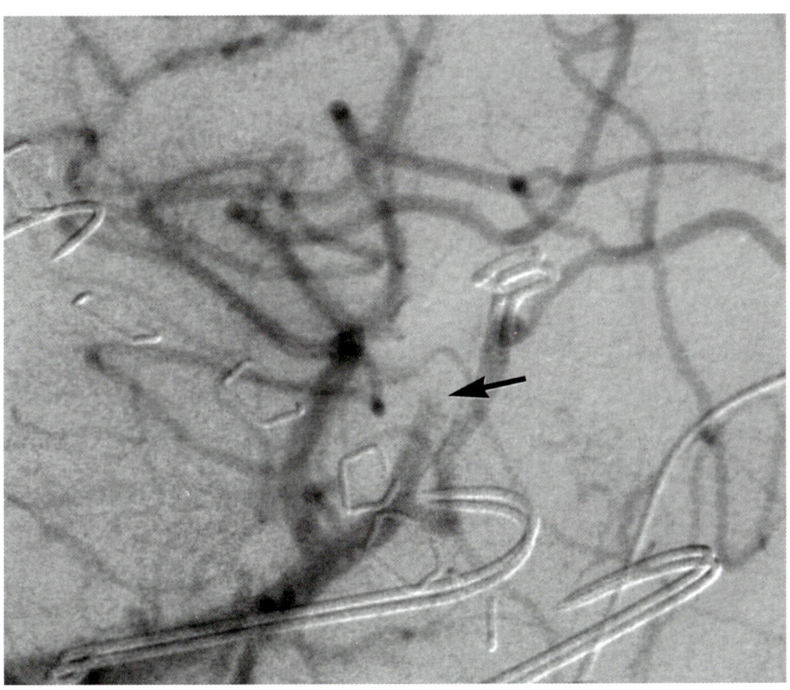

Fig. 4.6j Intraoperative angiogram demonstrated occlusion (*arrow*) of the direct anastomosis of the MCA-to-MCA branches. The anastomosis was reexamined and patency was reestablished.

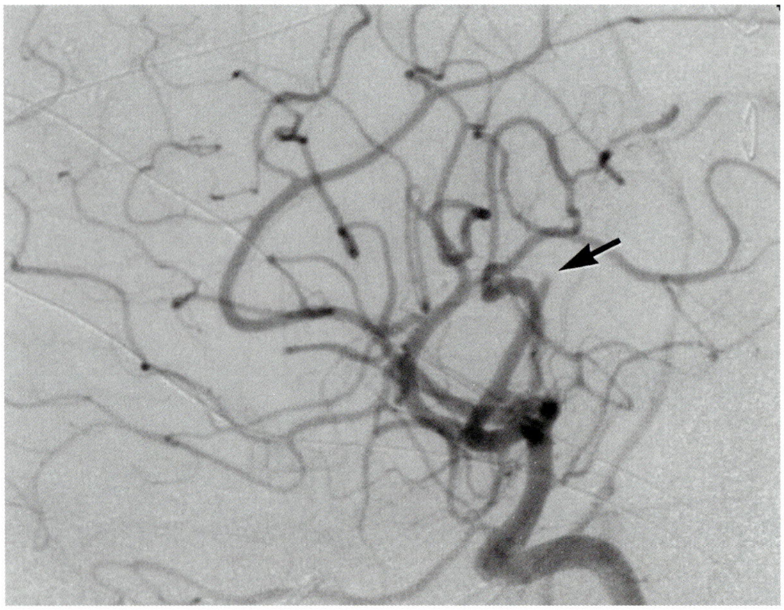

Fig. 4.6k After the anastomosis was reopened, a repeat intraoperative angiogram again demonstrates occlusion (*arrow*) of the direct anastomosis.

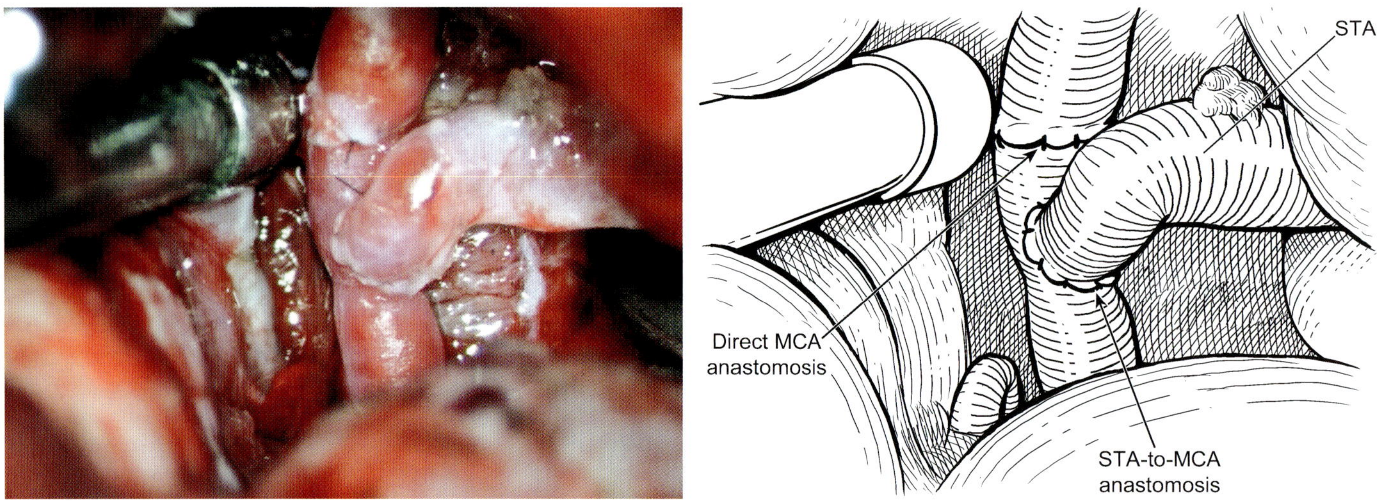

Fig. 4.6l Because the direct MCA anastomosis twice failed to maintain patency, an STA bypass was anastomosed to the angular MCA branch distal to the direct anastomosis. The direct anastomosis was also reopened.

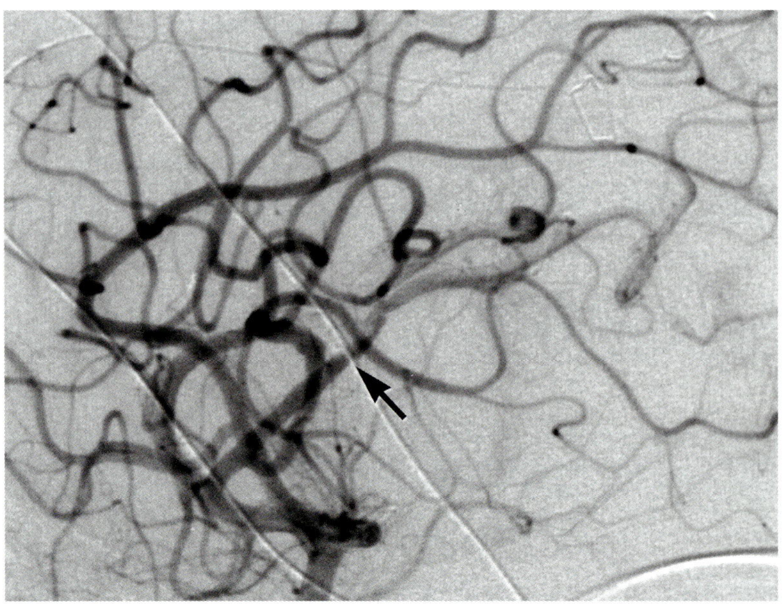

Fig. 4.6m Postoperative angiogram demonstrates that the previously occluded direct anastomosis (*arrow*) is now patent.

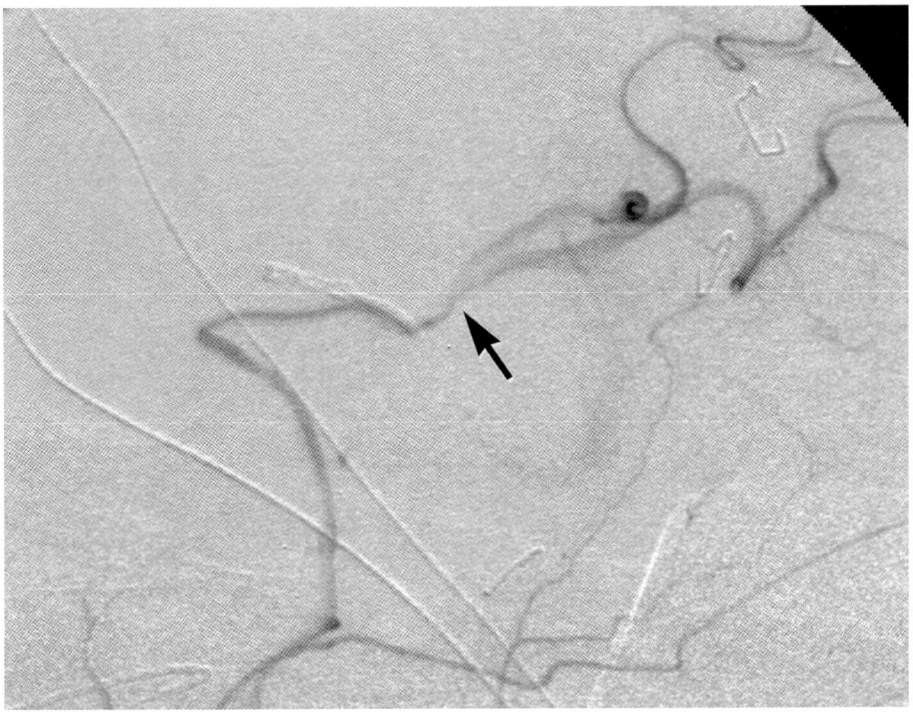

Fig. 4.6n ECA angiogram also confirms patency of the STA-to-MCA bypass (*arrow*).

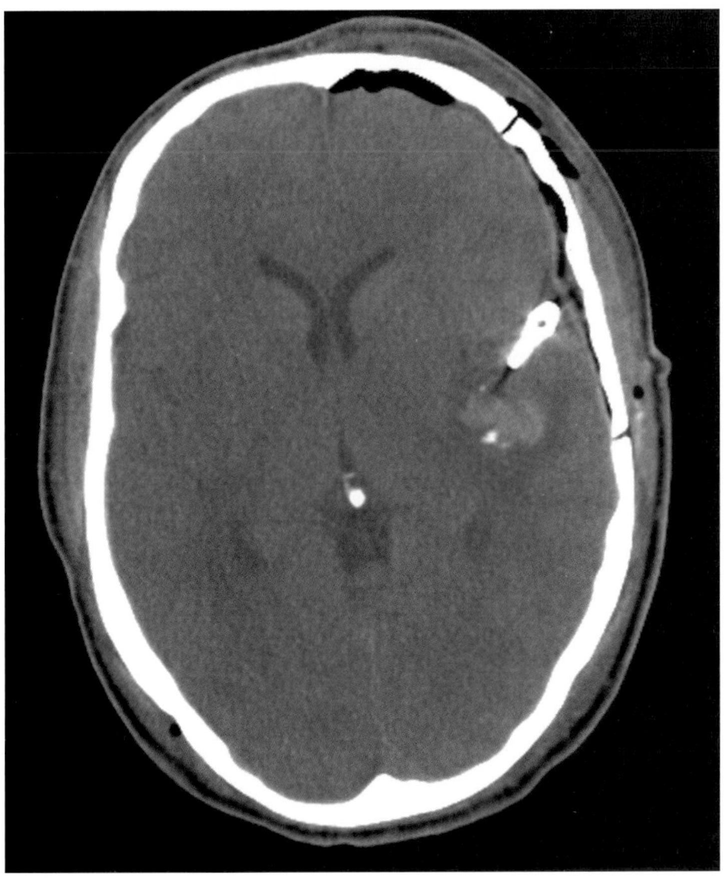

Fig. 4.6o Postoperative CT shows the residual portion of the thrombosed aneurysm and absence of any infarction. The patient's postoperative course was uncomplicated.

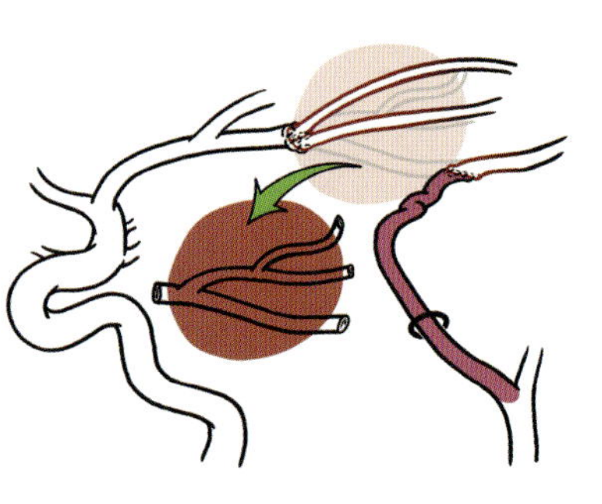

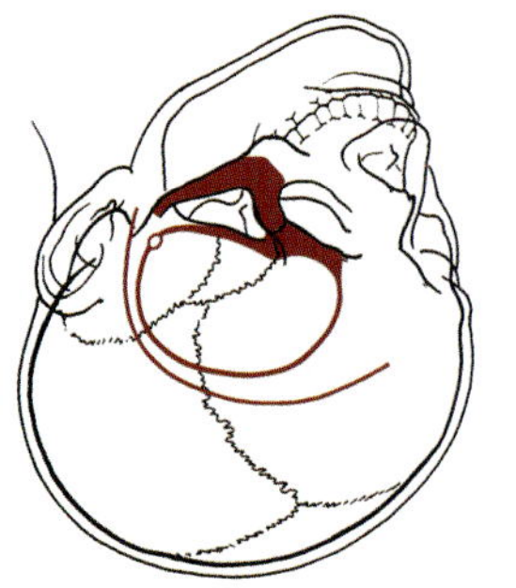

Case 4-7

Diagnosis: Large complex left MCA aneurysm

Bypass: Excision of aneurysm, direct MCA-to-MCA and STA–to–distal MCA

Approach: Left orbitozygomatic

Video

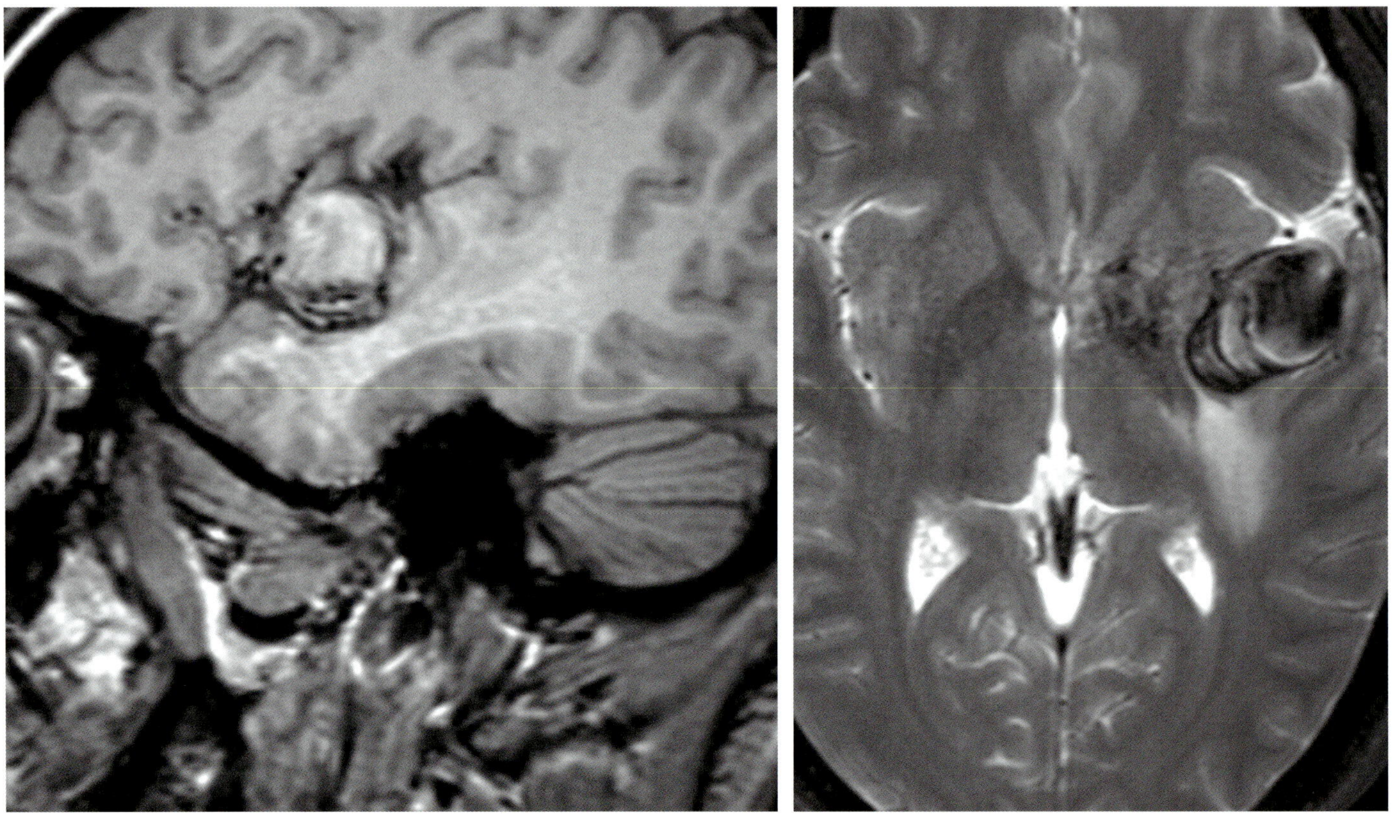

Fig. 4.7a, b Parasagittal and axial MR images of a 39-year-old man with memory loss and fluctuating aphasia show a large complex left MCA aneurysm.

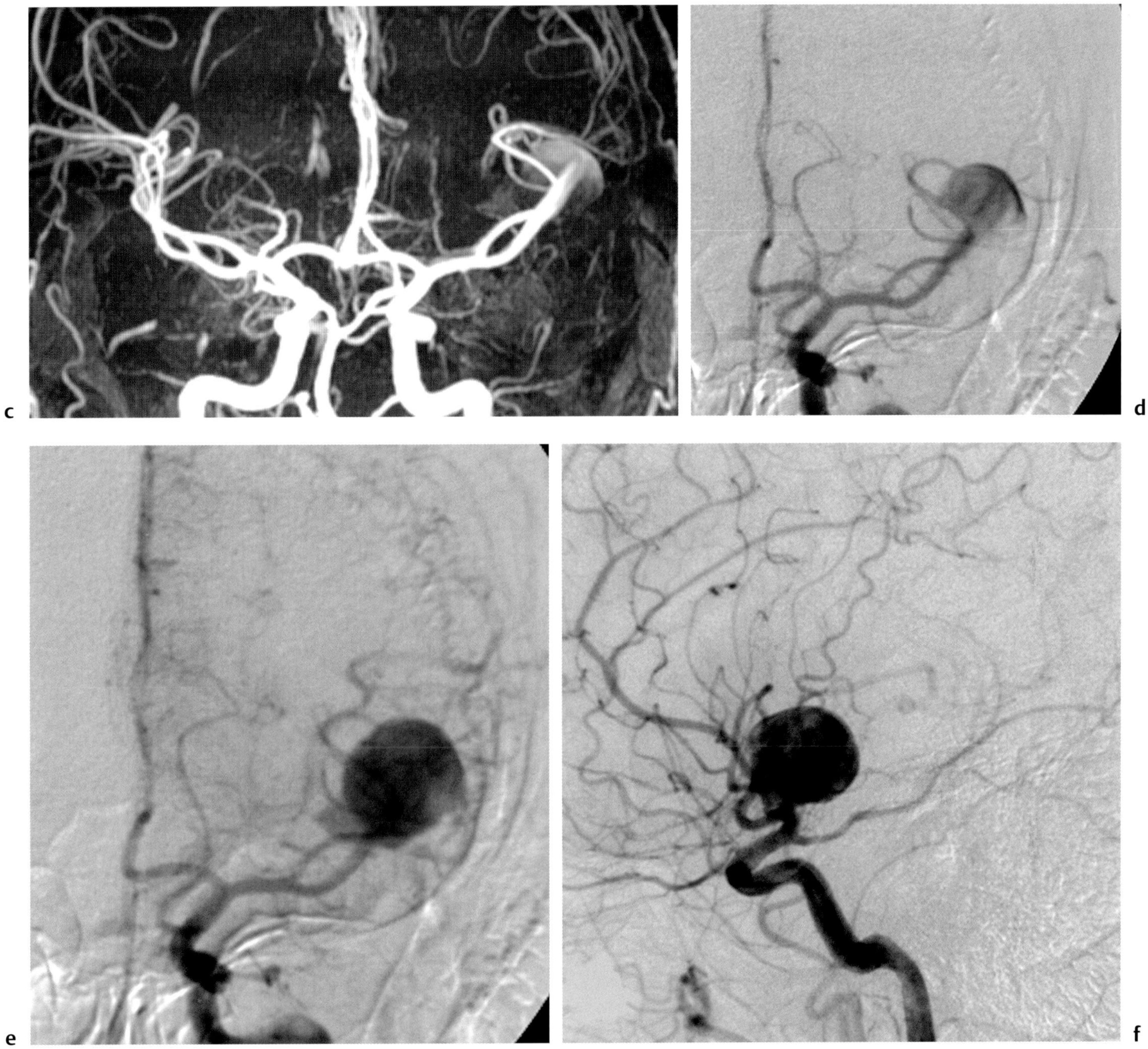

Fig. 4.7c–f Anteroposterior (**c, d, e**) and lateral (**f**) views of a large left M2 aneurysm.

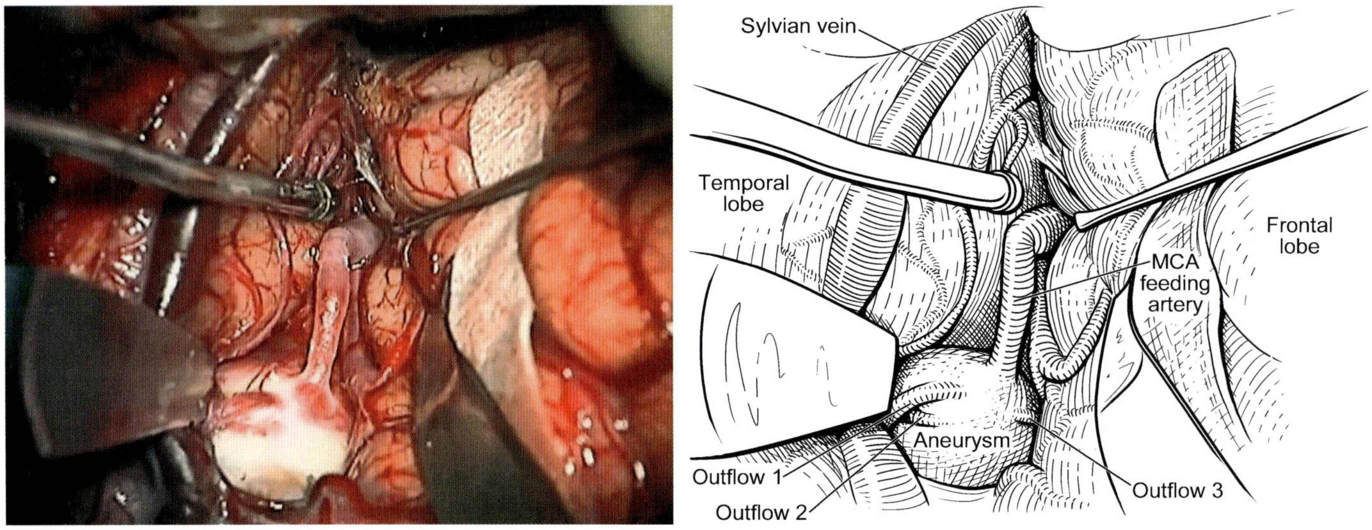

Fig. 4.7g Through a left orbitozygomatic approach, the sylvian fissure is opened, exposing the large aneurysm, feeding vessel, and three outflow vessels.

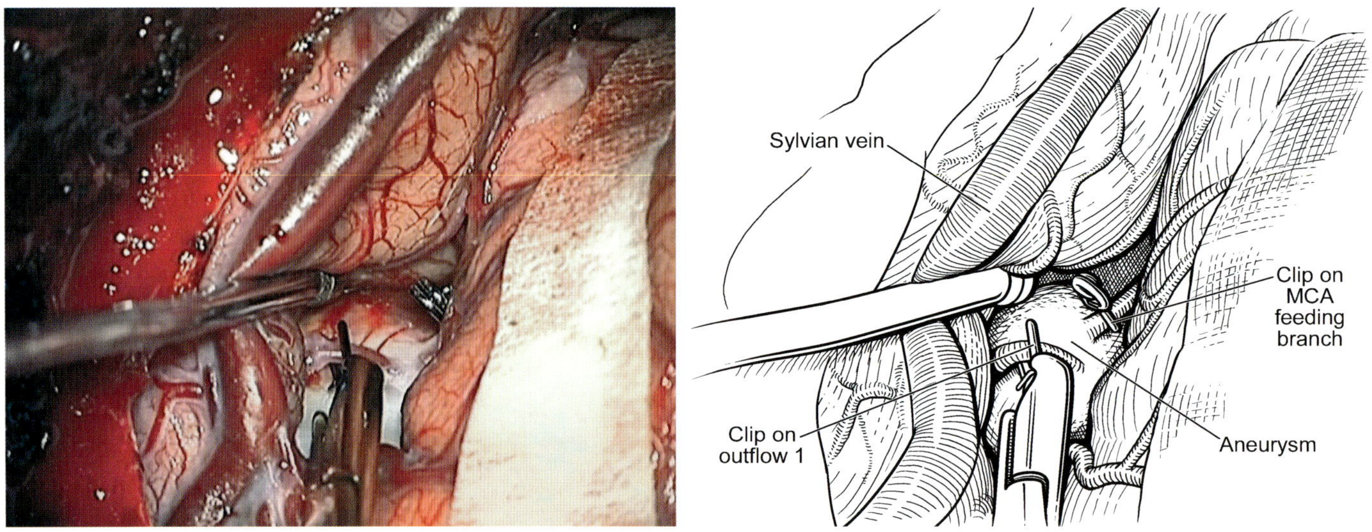

Fig. 4.7h The MCA feeding branch and the distal MCA outflow branches are clipped.

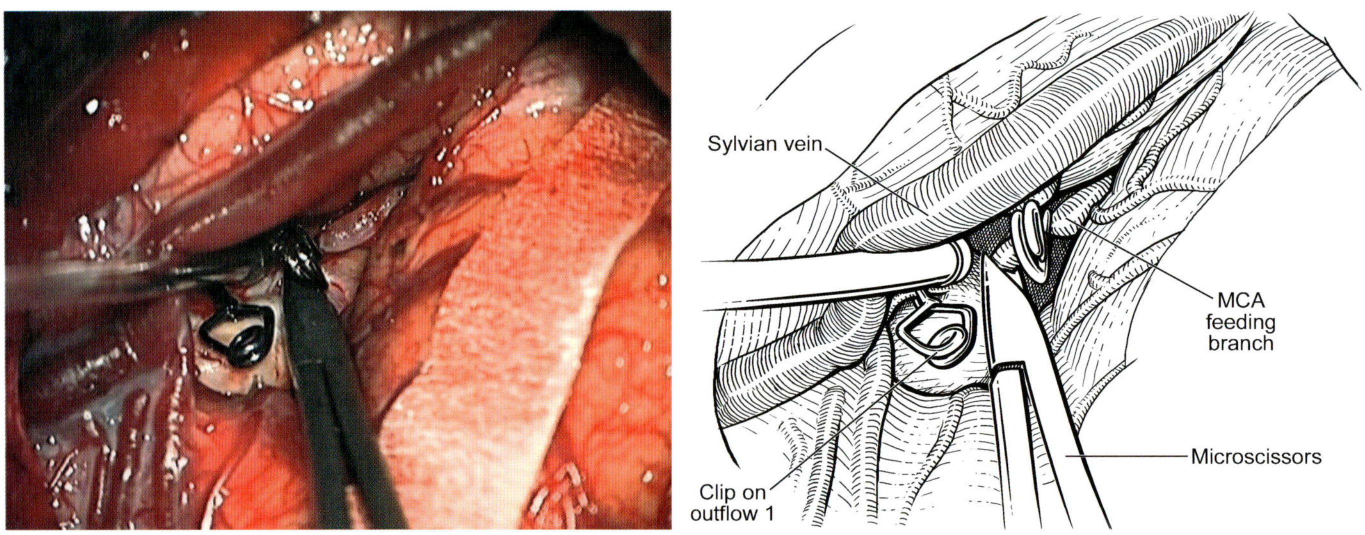

Fig. 4.7i The MCA feeding branch and the distal MCA outflow branches are cut.

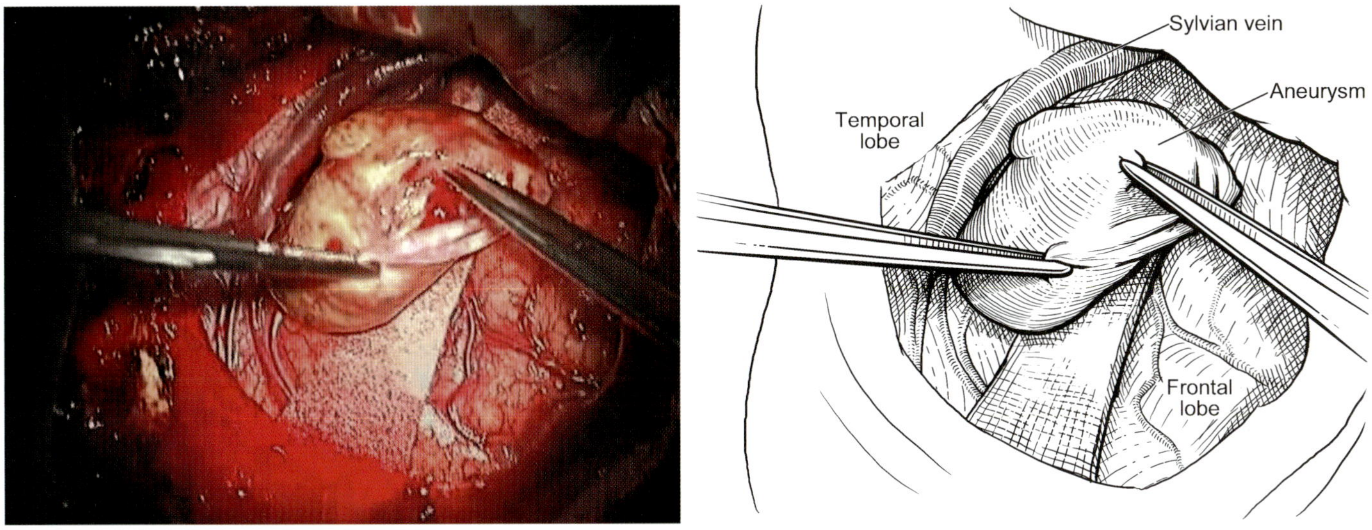

Fig. 4.7j After the clipped branches have been cut, the aneurysm is excised.

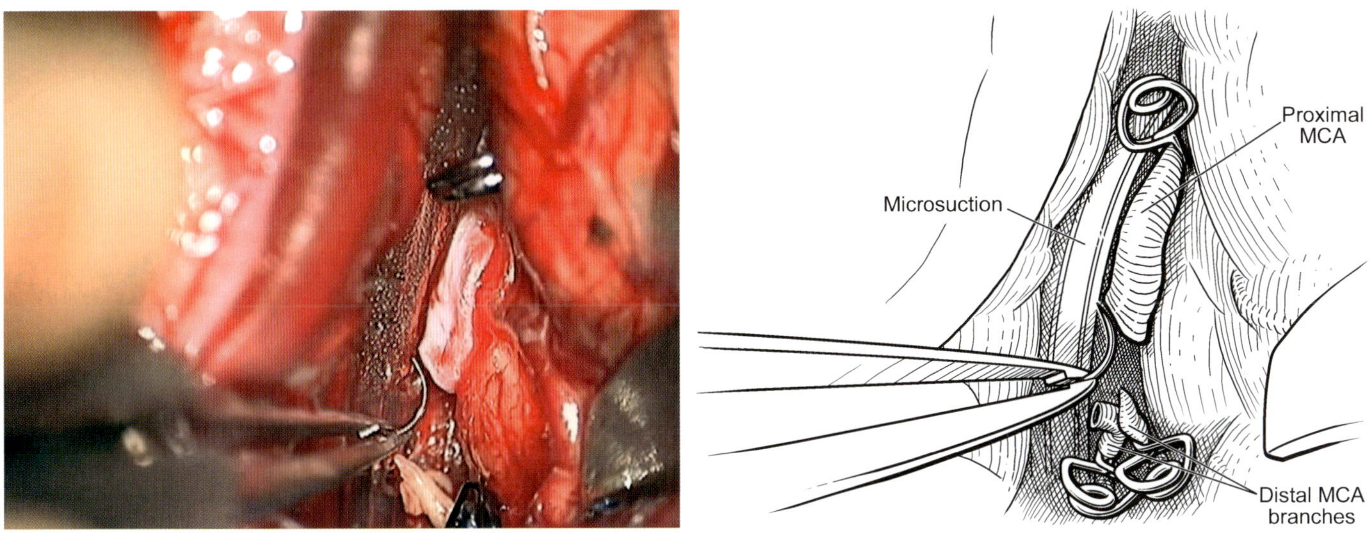

Fig. 4.7k The cut ends of the proximal MCA and two distal MCA branches are prepared for a Figure 8 anastomosis.

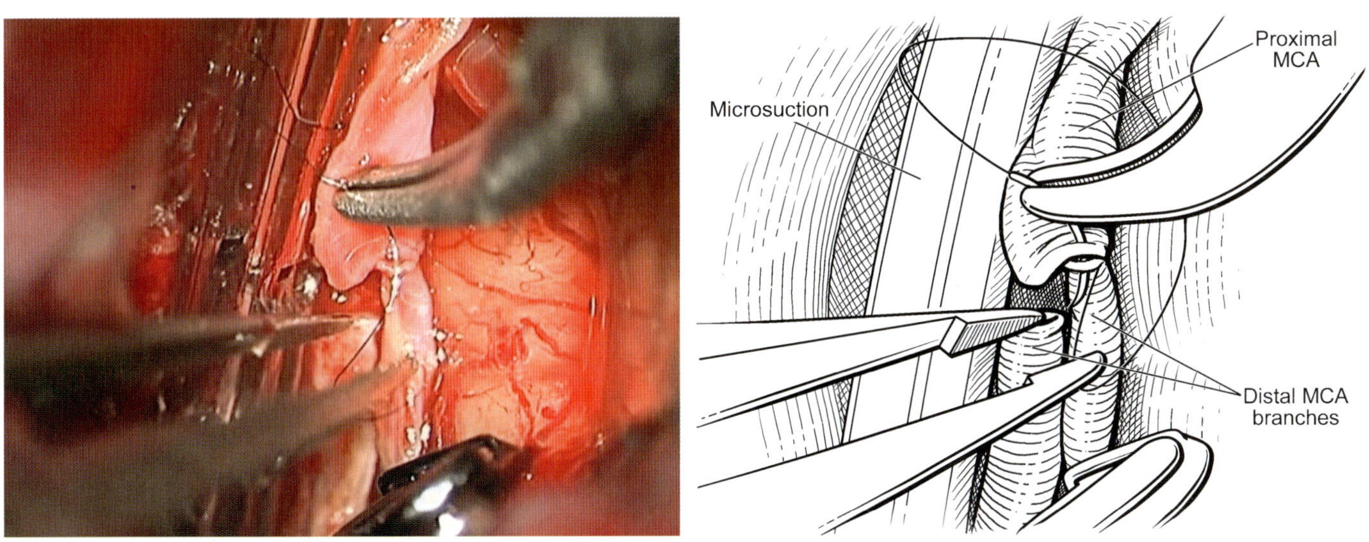

Fig. 4.7l The first distal MCA branch is anastomosed to the proximal MCA with a running suture.

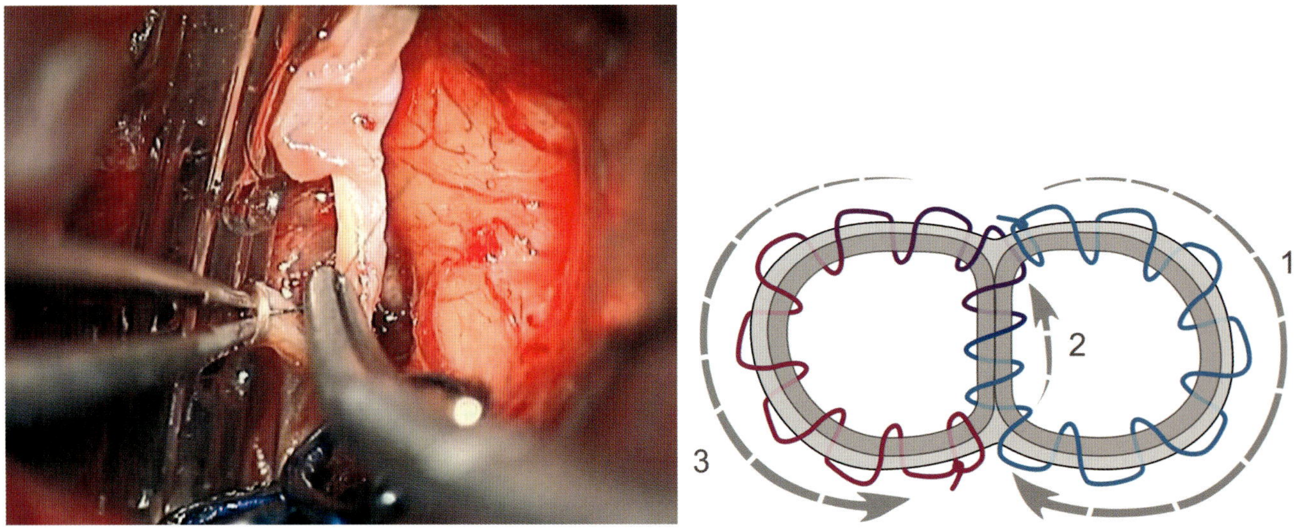

Fig. 4.7m The anastomosis of the first distal MCA branch to the proximal MCA is three-quarters complete. A running suture is started in the second distal branch to join the two medial walls. Diagram of continuous Figure 8 shows suturing sequence.

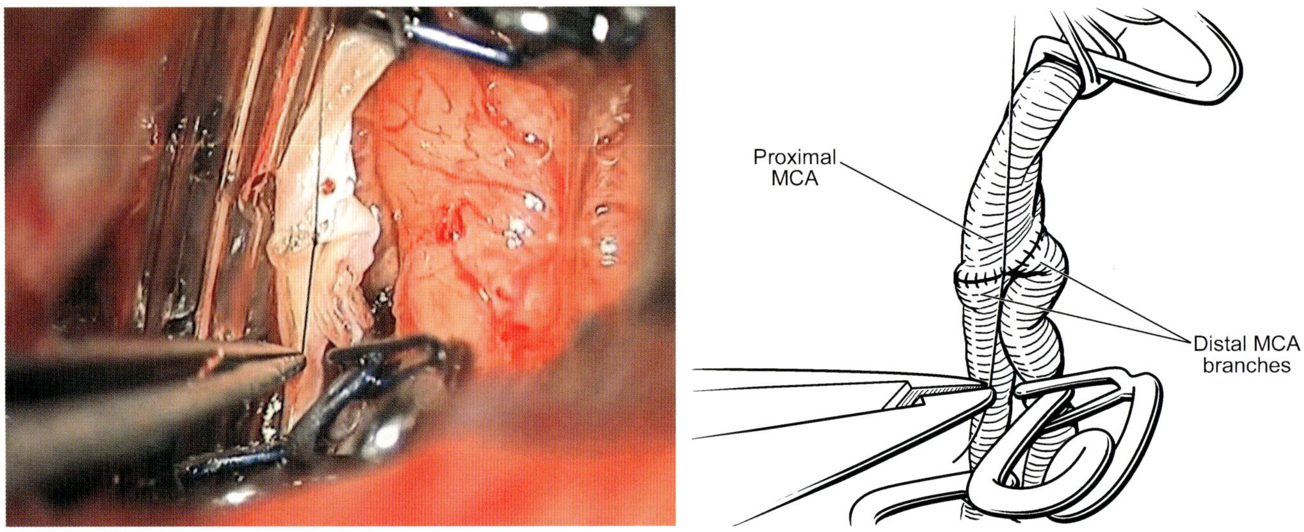

Fig. 4.7n The running suture continues around the second distal branch to complete the Figure 8 anastomosis.

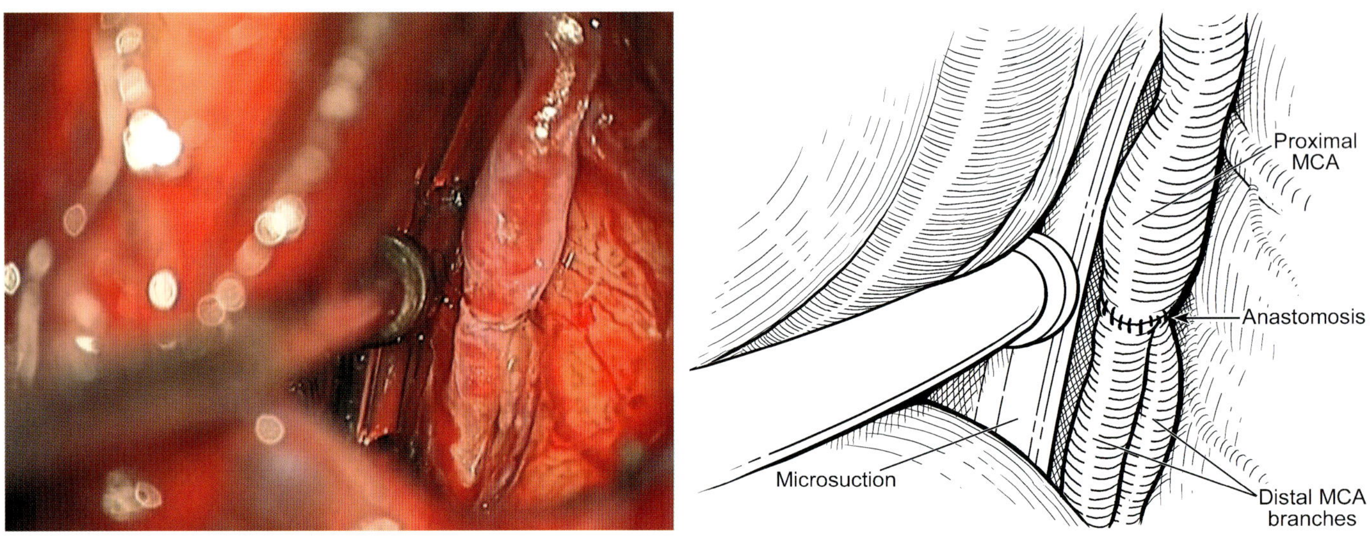

Fig. 4.7o The Figure 8 anastomosis from the proximal MCA to the two distal branches is completed. The temporary clips are removed to check the patency of the bypass.

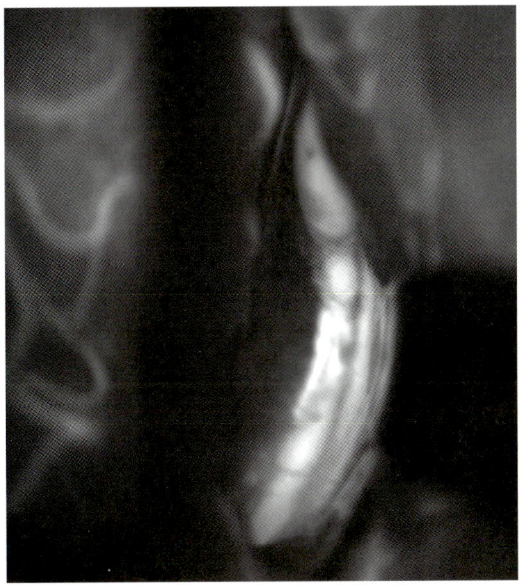

Fig. 4.7p Intraoperative ICG angiogram confirms patency of both channels.

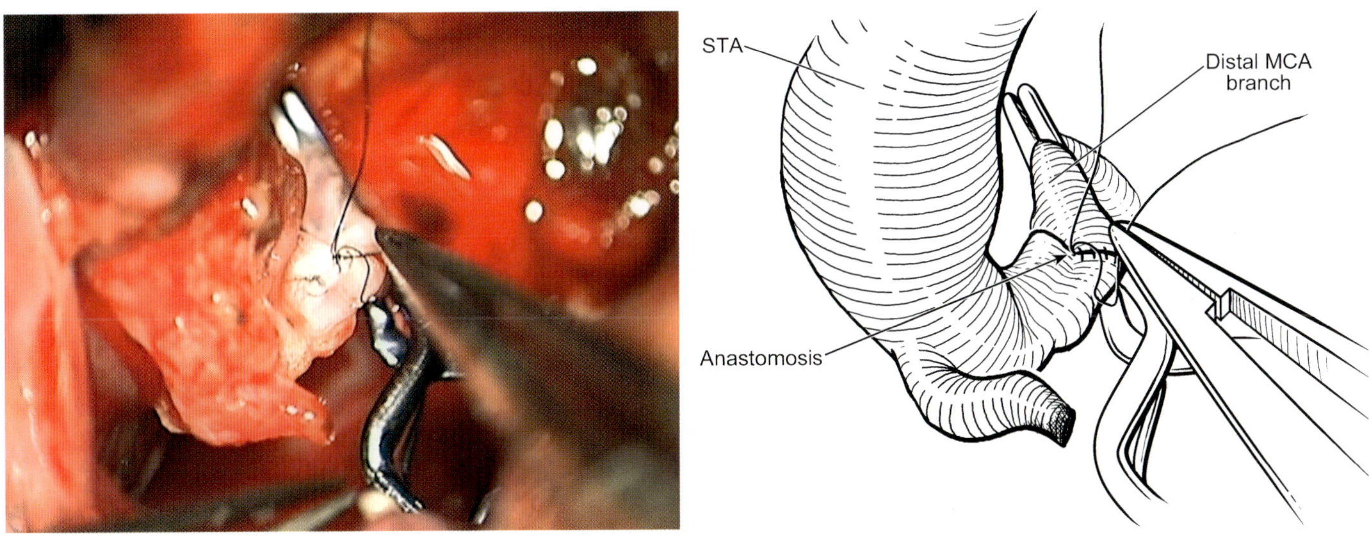

Fig. 4.7q An STA-to-distal MCA anastomosis is performed to vascularize the remaining distal branch of the MCA aneurysm.

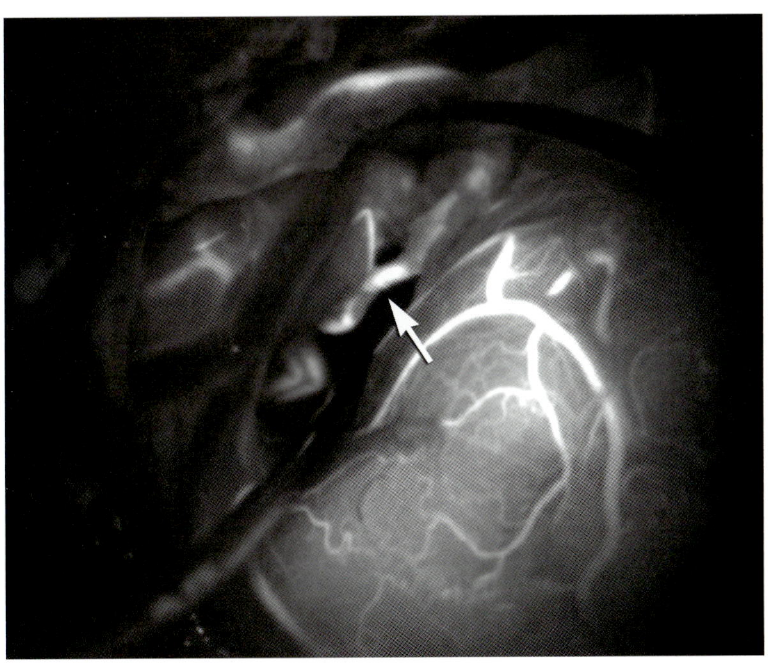

Fig. 4.7r Intraoperative ICG angiogram demonstrates patency of the STA-to-MCA bypass (*arrow*).

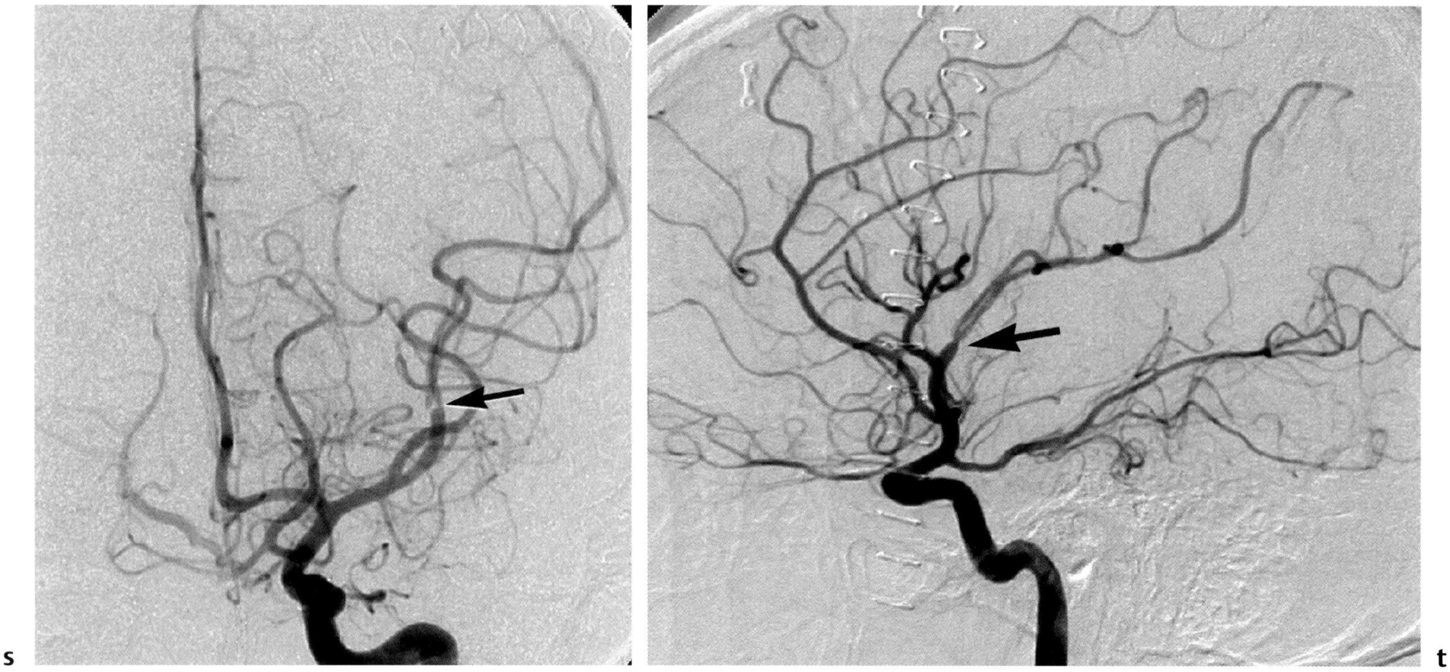

Fig. 4.7s, t Anteroposterior and lateral ICA angiograms confirm patency of the bypass (*arrows*) of the proximal MCA branch to the two distal MCA branches.

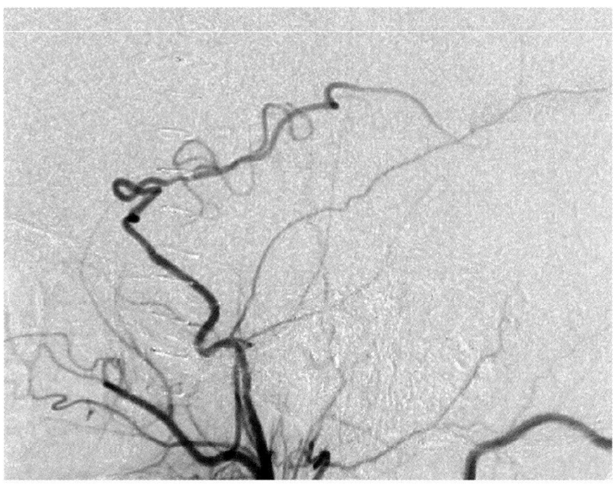

Fig. 4.7u Lateral ECA angiogram demonstrates patency of the STA to the remaining MCA branch.

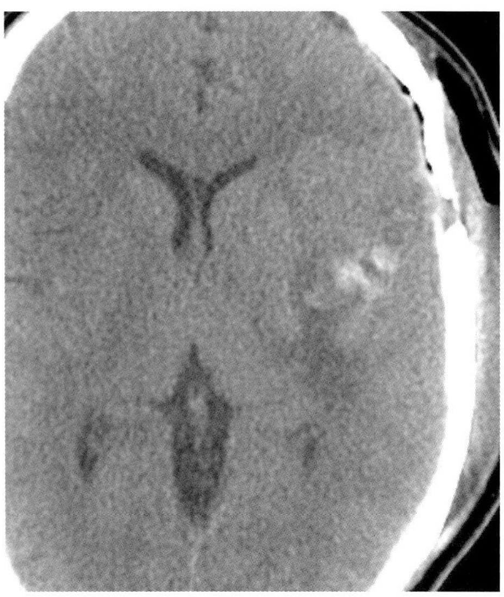

Fig. 4.7v Postoperative CT shows no ischemic regions. The patient made an excellent recovery.

5 MMA-to-MCA Bypass

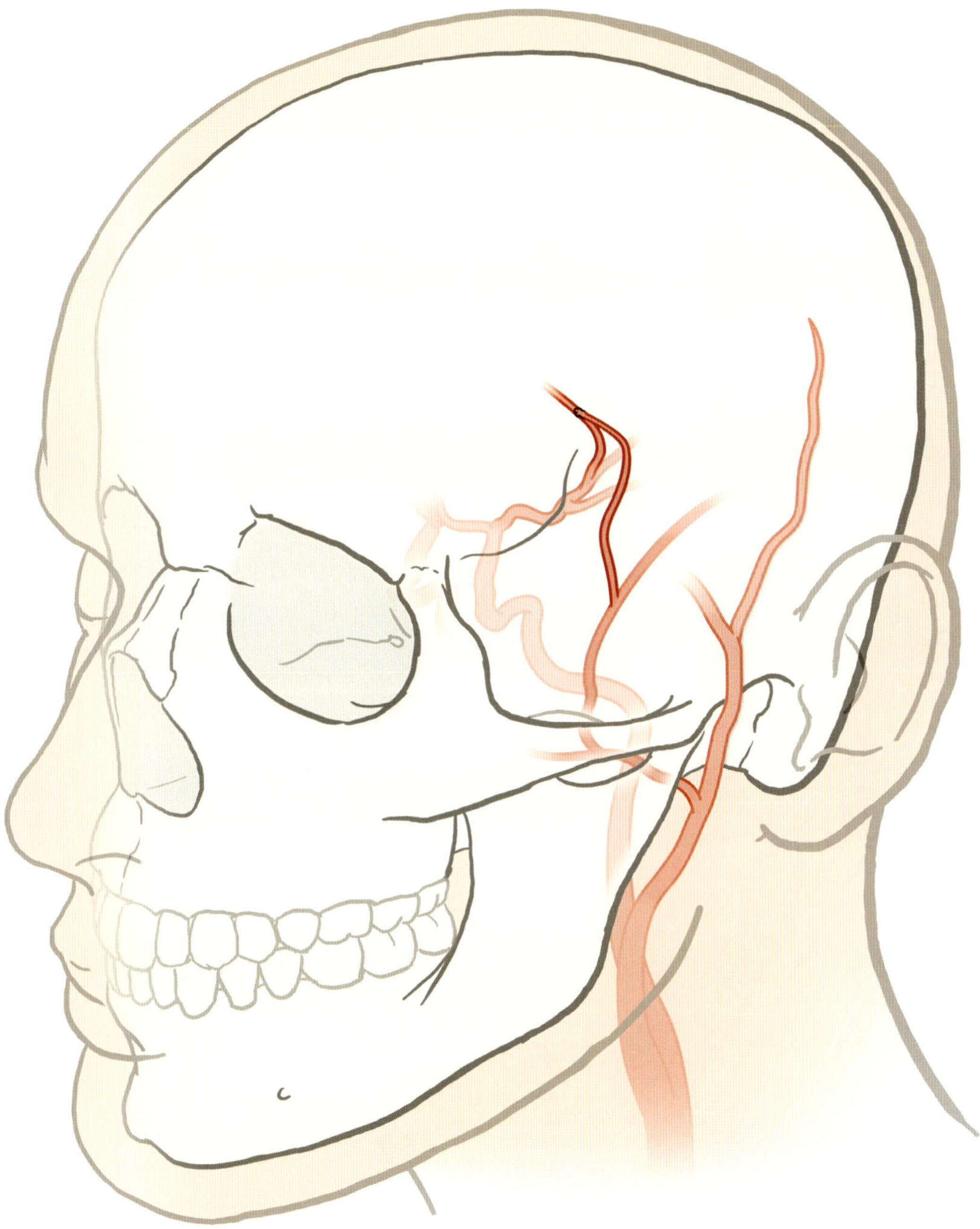

The MMA is a small vessel with fairly robust flow under normal conditions. If the STA is unsuitable or if a second vessel is needed for bypass to the territory of the MCA, the MMA may be considered as a donor vessel. In certain pathological conditions, such as in the presence of some tumors, the MMA substantially enlarges, making it more suitable for use in a bypass.

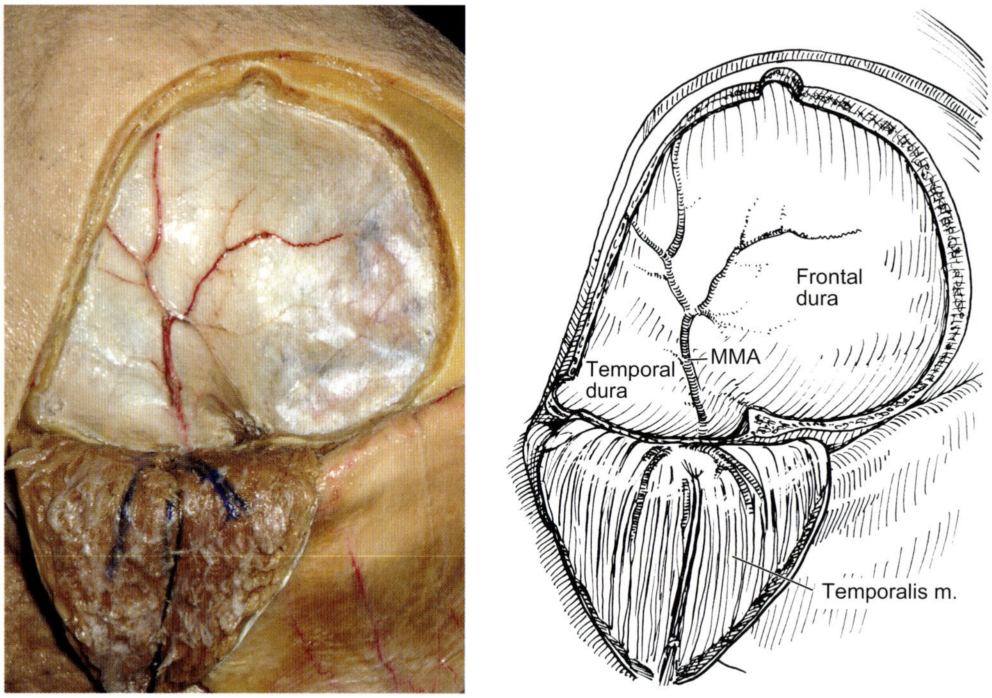

Fig. 5.0a In this anatomical specimen, the MMA is visible through a frontotemporal craniotomy. (Photograph used with permission from *Journal of Neurosurgery*.)

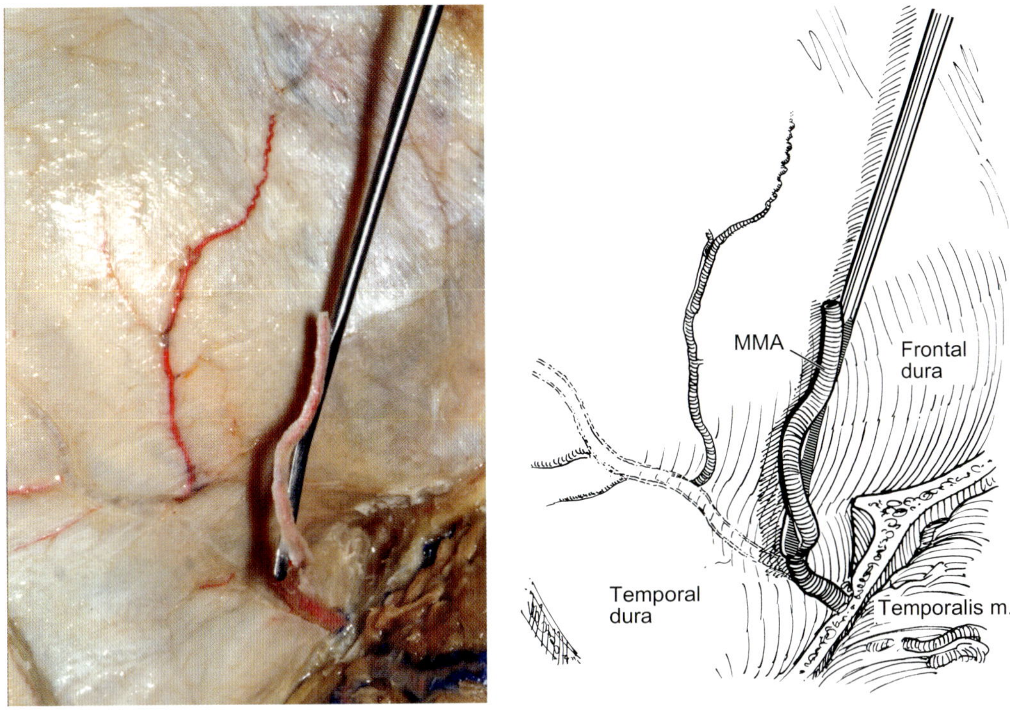

Fig. 5.0b The major trunk of the MMA has been dissected free. (Photograph used with permission from *Journal of Neurosurgery*.)

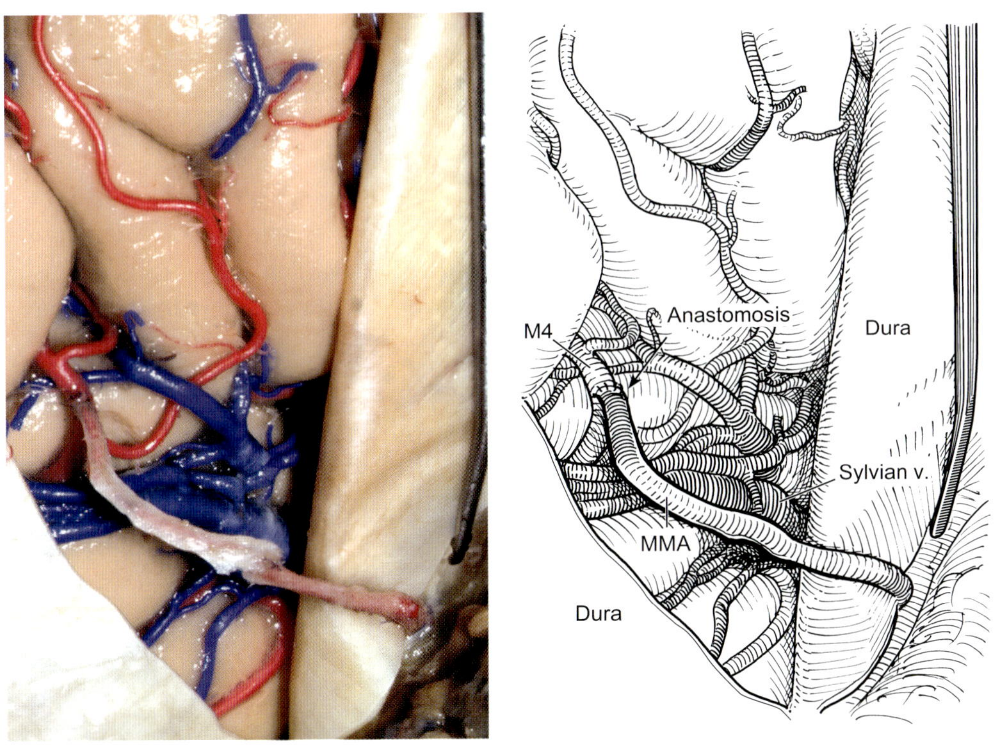

Fig. 5.0c The MMA has been anastomosed to a cortical branch of the MCA. (Photograph used with permission from *Journal of Neurosurgery*.)

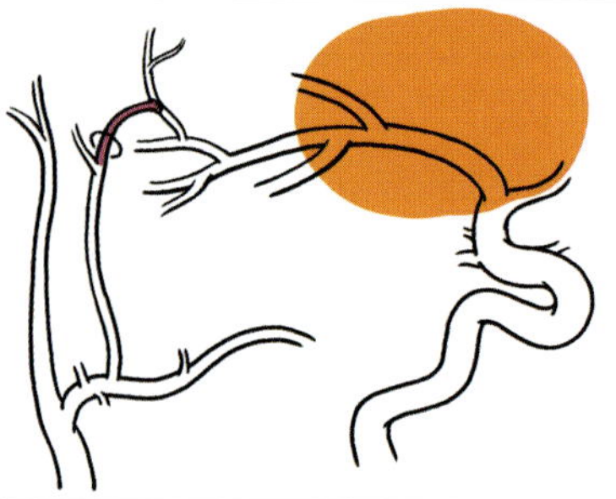

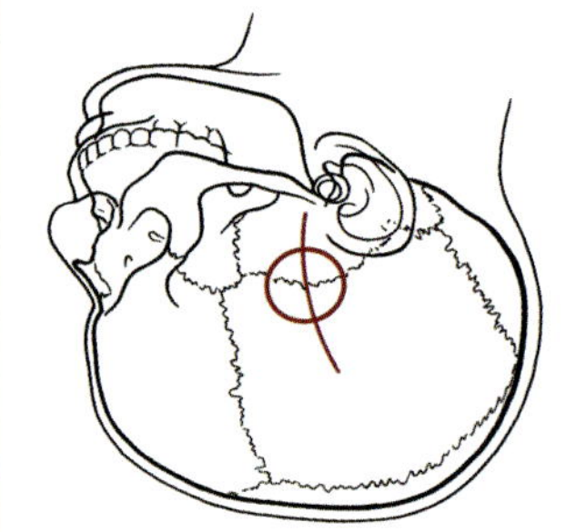

Case 5-1

Diagnosis: Left parafalcine meningioma with MCA occlusion and ACA-to-MCA collateralization

Bypass: MMA-to-MCA

Approach: Right temporal

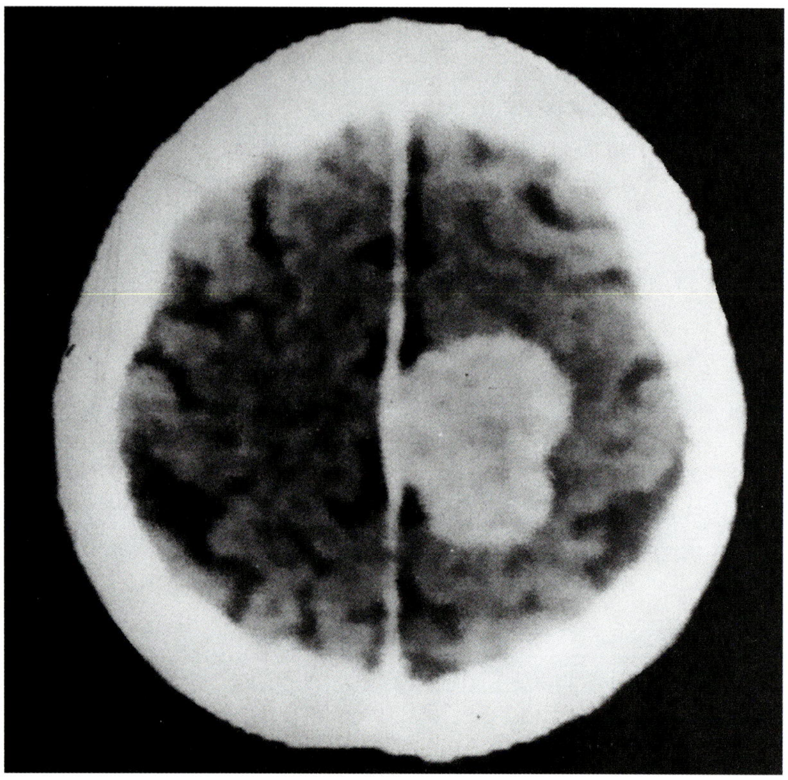

Fig. 5.1a Axial CT shows a high-density lesion consistent with a right falcine meningioma. (Used with permission from *Journal of Neurosurgery*.)

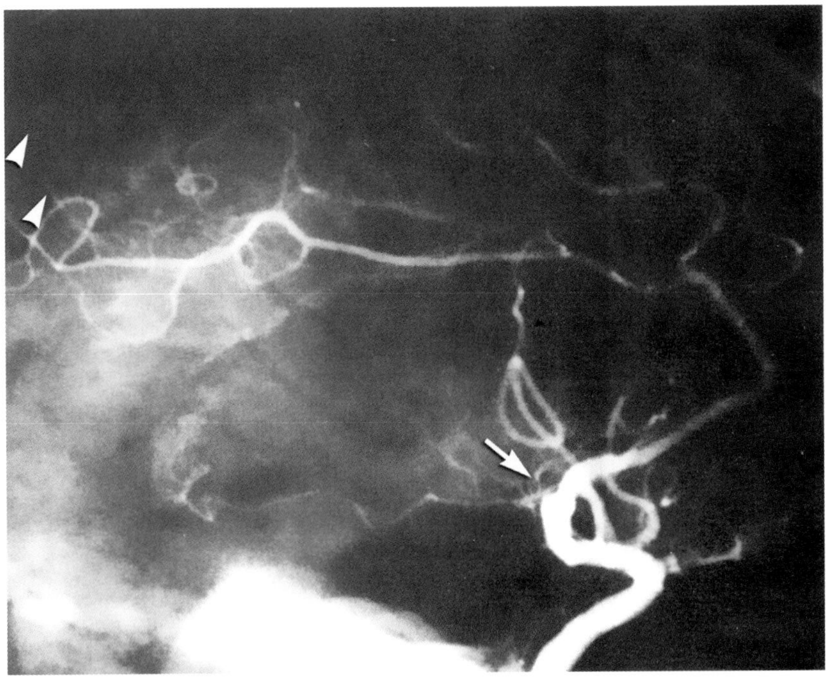

Fig. 5.1b Right ICA angiogram shows draped vessels (*arrowheads*) and an unrelated occlusion (*arrow*) of the MCA. (Used with permission from *Journal of Neurosurgery*.)

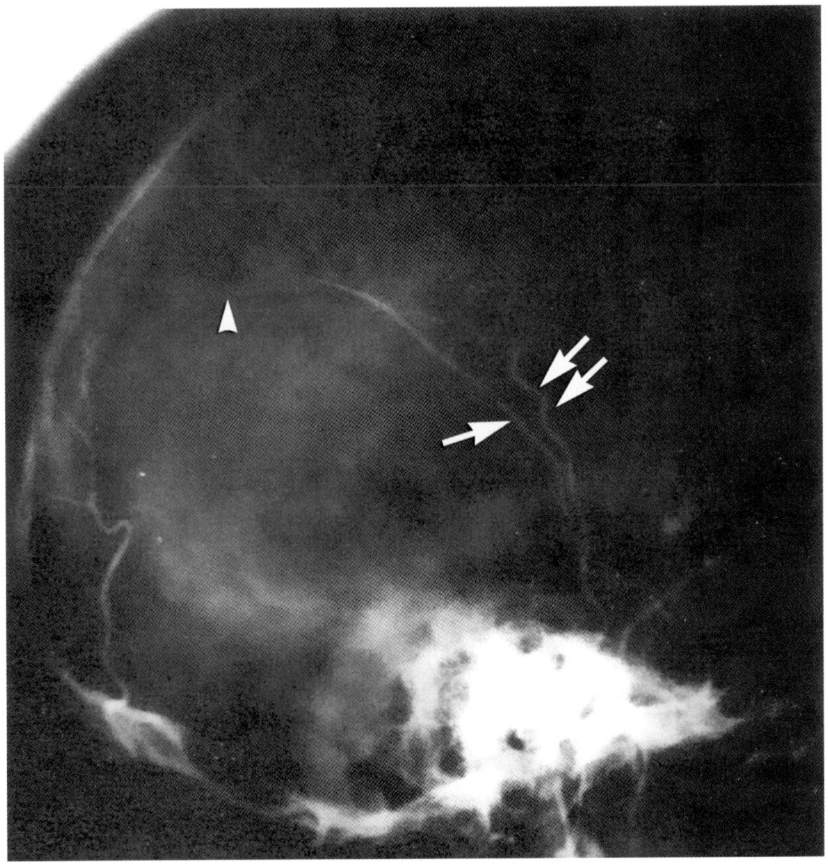

Fig. 5.1c Right ECA angiogram shows the STA (*double arrows*) and large-caliber MMA (*arrow*). Distal branches of the MMA (*arrowhead*) feed the tumor. (Used with permission from *Journal of Neurosurgery*.)

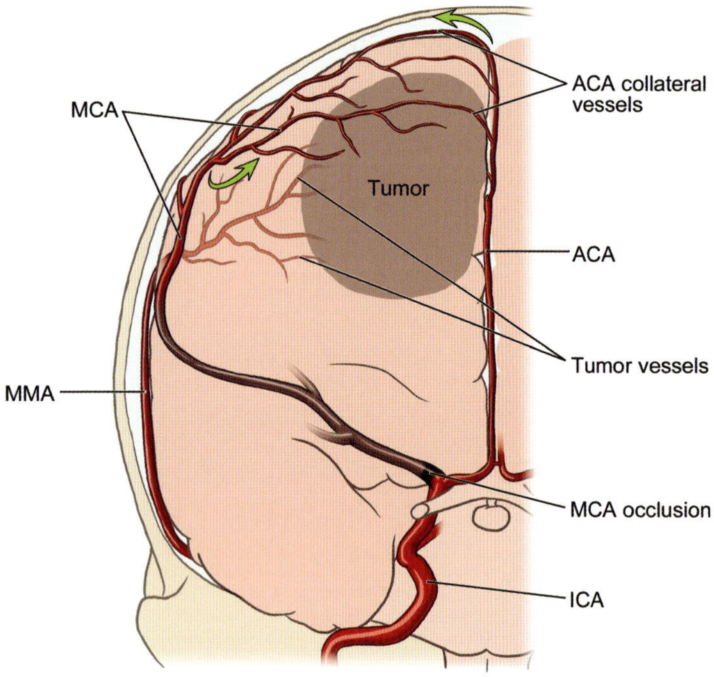

Fig. 5.1d Overview shows the blood supply of the tumor, which is fed by the enlarged MMA and its branches as well as by the distal vessels of the MCA. In response to the occlusion at the origin of the MCA, the distal MCA is supplied by retrograde flow (*arrows*) through collateral vessels of the ACA.

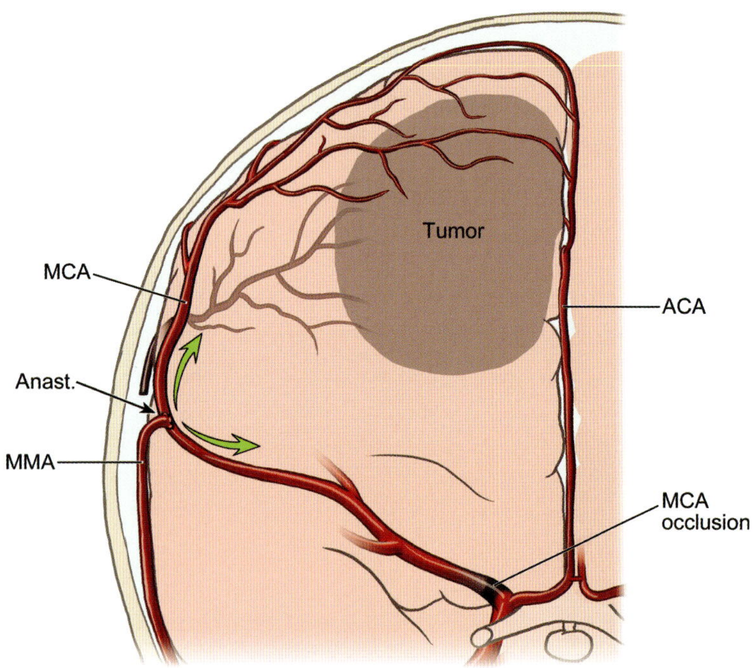

Fig. 5.1e The MMA-to-MCA bypass diverts MMA blood flow away from the tumor and supplies the proximal and distal distribution (*arrows*) of the MCA.

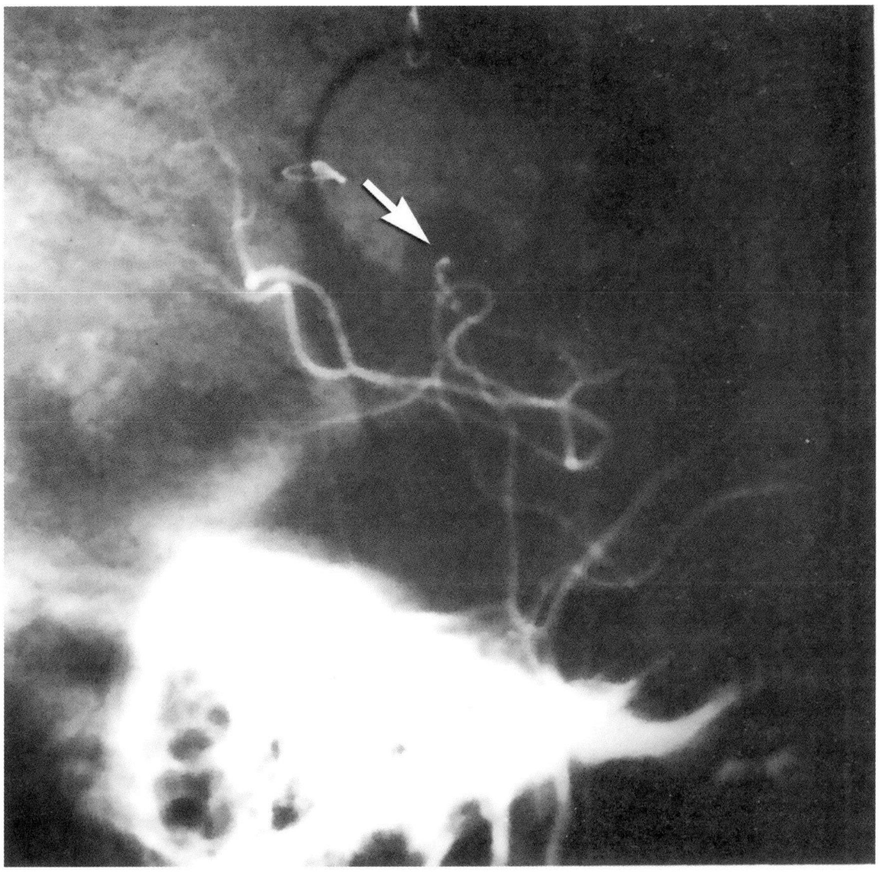

Fig. 5.1f Right ECA angiogram obtained 2 weeks after surgery shows the patent anastomosis (*arrow*) between the MMA and MCA. (Used with permission from *Journal of Neurosurgery*.)

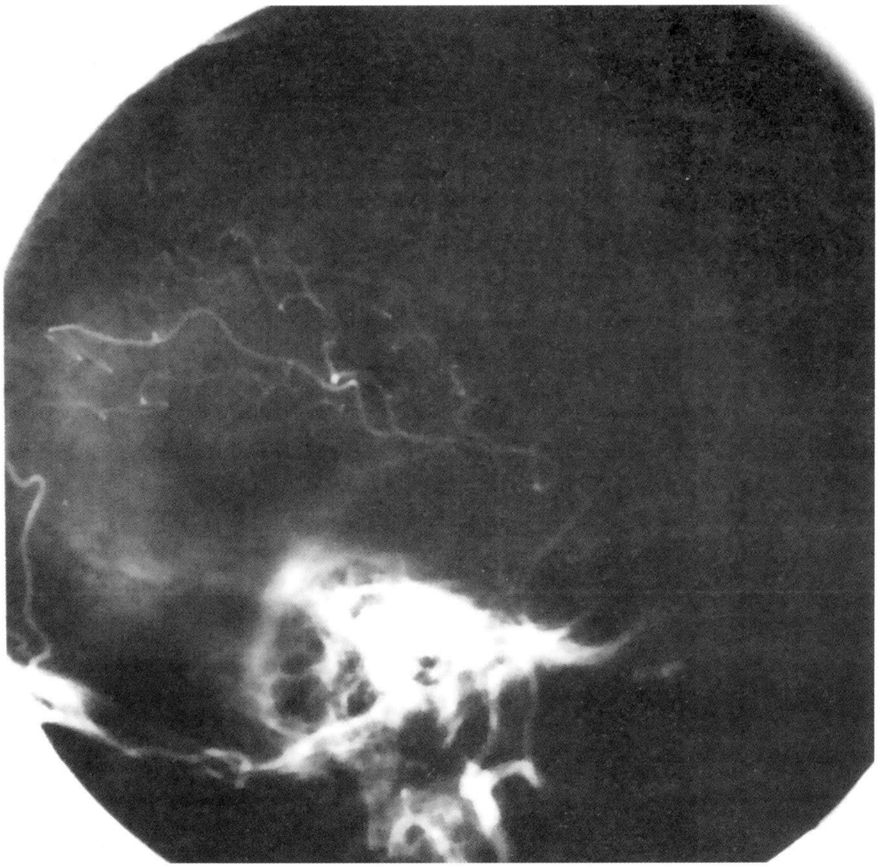

Fig. 5.1g A later phase angiogram demonstrates significant perfusion of the MCA territory through the anastomosis. The MMA-to-MCA bypass facilitated later resection of the tumor. (Used with permission from *Journal of Neurosurgery*.)

6 Bonnet Bypass

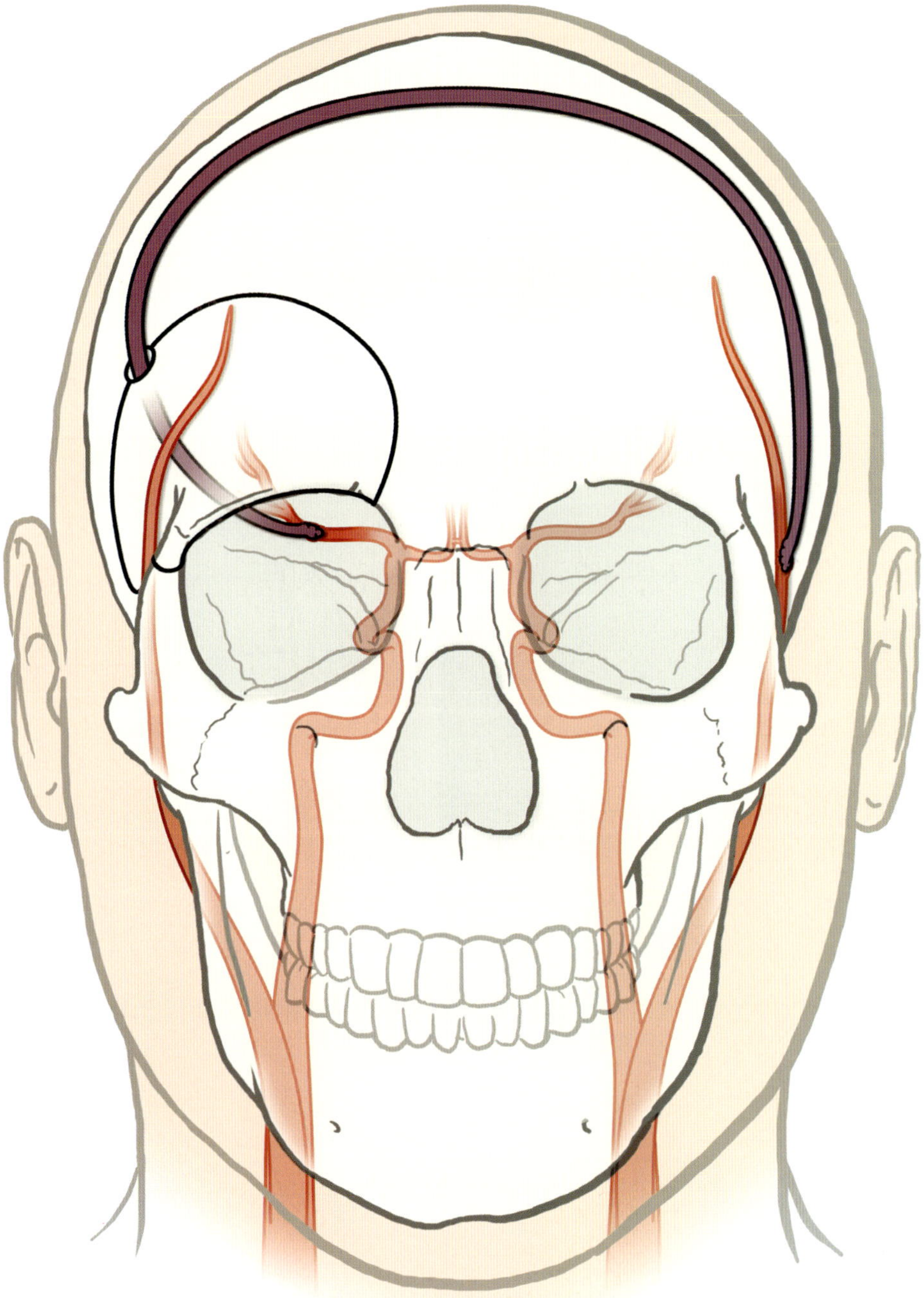

The bonnet bypass is a long interposition graft bypass that crosses the dome of the calvarium to reach the MCA on the contralateral side. The bonnet bypass was developed to allow an EC-to-IC bypass to be created in patients lacking an ipsilateral donor vessel. The typical indications are pathology in the ipsilateral neck that requires resection of the ECA and ICA.

The vessel of origin for a bonnet bypass is usually the bifurcation of the STA or, on rare occasions, the ECA in the neck. The interposition graft is obtained by harvesting the radial artery or saphenous vein. The technique for the bonnet bypass differs from that for an STA-to-MCA bypass or for an ICA-to-MCA bypass only in that the graft itself crosses over the top of the head to reach the MCA.

The patient should be positioned supine with the head in a neutral position and firmly secured to the table. The head is placed into a headholder with the pins low and posterior so that a bicoronal incision can be made and the patient can be rolled side to side to bring both sides into position for easy access.

A frontotemporal craniotomy is made on the recipient side to allow access to the sylvian fissure and MCA. A groove the width of the graft is drilled in the frontal bone from the donor vessel side to the recipient side to protect the graft from external compression. The MCA anastomosis is performed first. The graft is placed into the bony groove, and then the proximal graft is anastomosed to the STA bifurcation, allowing an incision that perfectly matches the diameter of the graft.

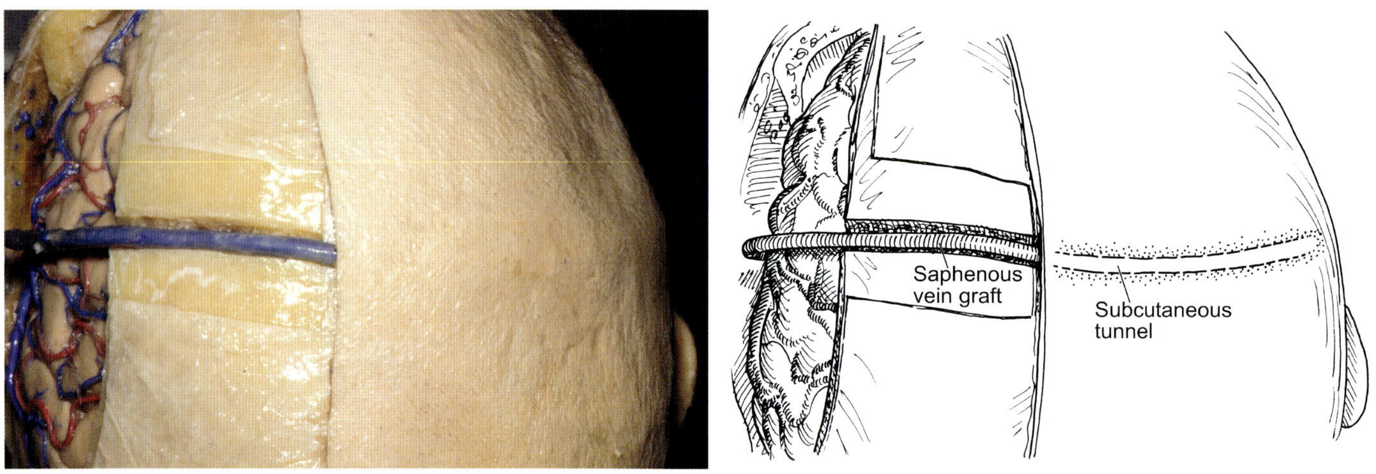

Fig. 6.0a This specimen shows the course of the graft, which is lying in a bony groove (*dashed lines*), from one side to the other side. (Photograph used with permission from *Journal of Neurosurgery*.)

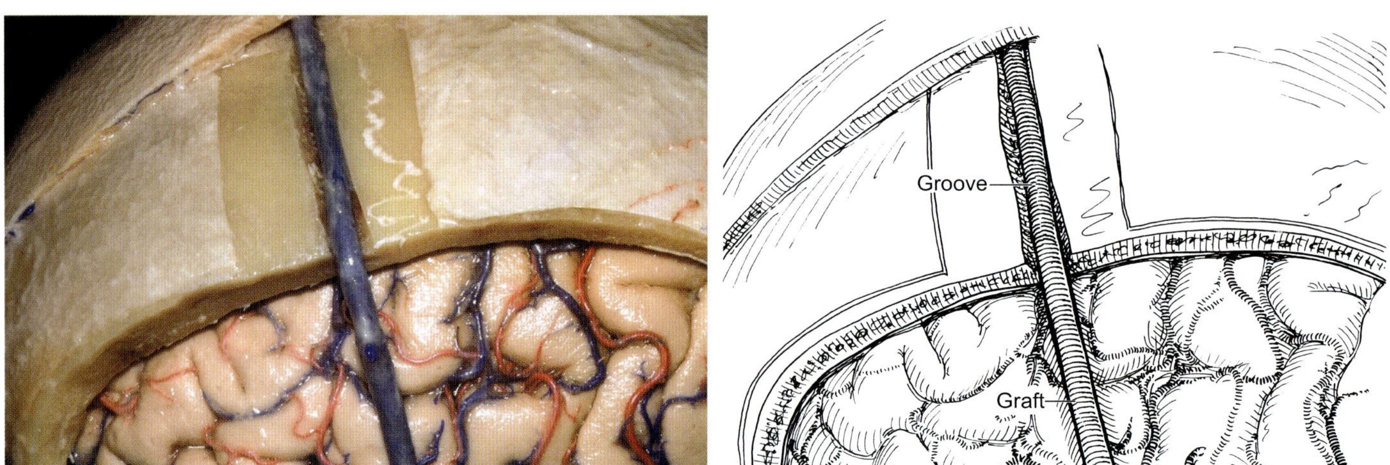

Fig. 6.0b Side view shows the graft in the groove. (Photograph used with permission from *Journal of Neurosurgery*.)

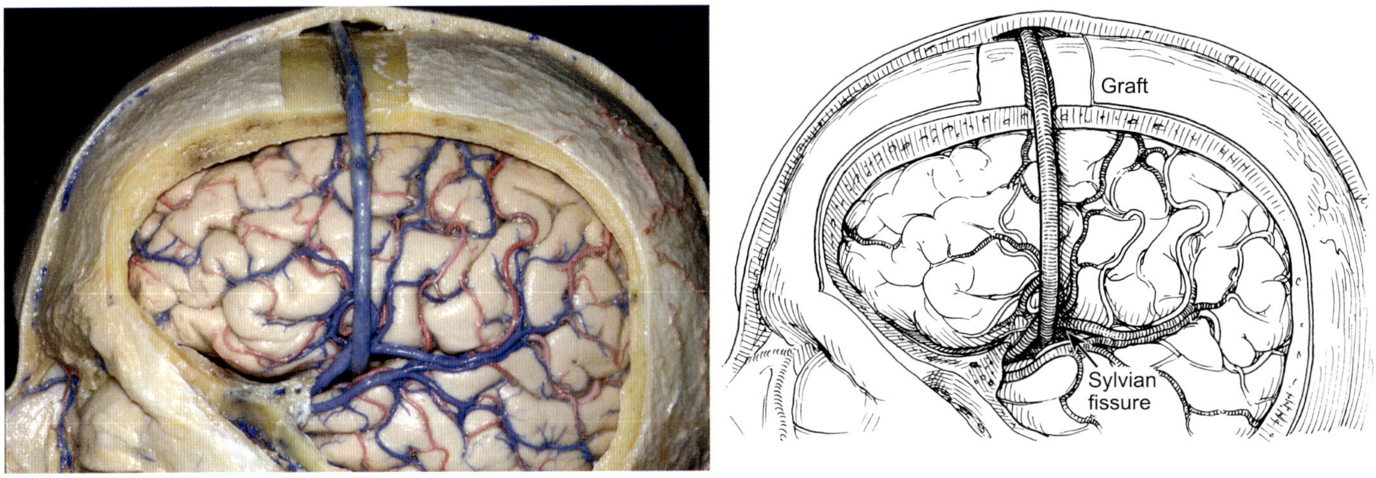

Fig. 6.0c Overview shows the graft as it enters the sylvian fissure. (Photograph used with permission from *Journal of Neurosurgery*.)

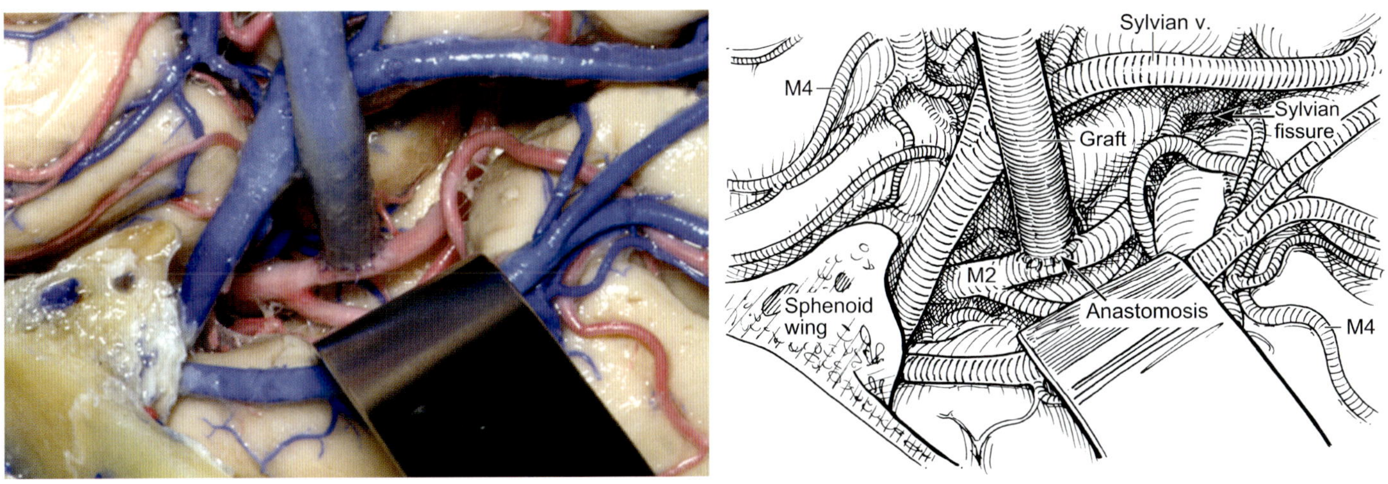

Fig. 6.0d High-power view shows the graft anastomosed to M2. (Photograph used with permission from *Journal of Neurosurgery*.)

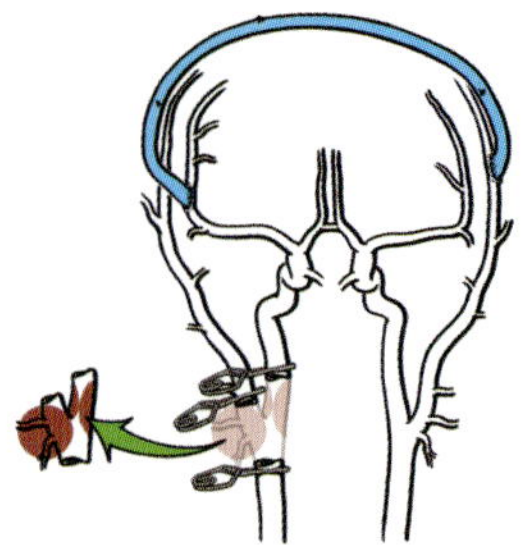

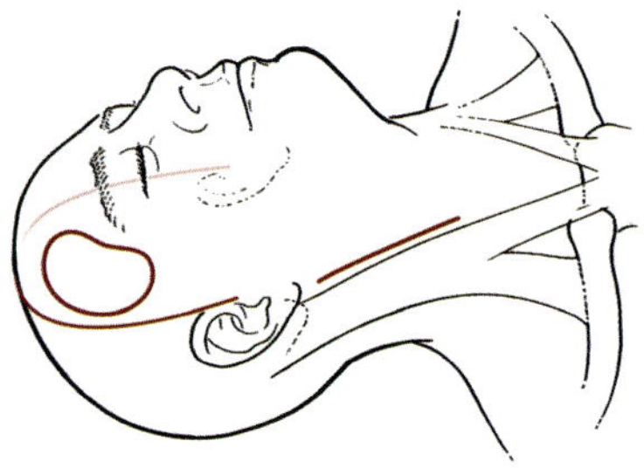

Case 6-1

Diagnosis: Complex mycotic pseudoaneurysm of right carotid bifurcation

Bypass: Bonnet

Approach: Right anterior cervical and right pterional

Video

This patient had a history of oral pharyngeal carcinoma and had undergone a radical neck dissection. He had recurrent infections and a chronic draining orocutaneous fistula. He reached neurosurgical attention after he experienced recurrent TIAs involving the right hemisphere.

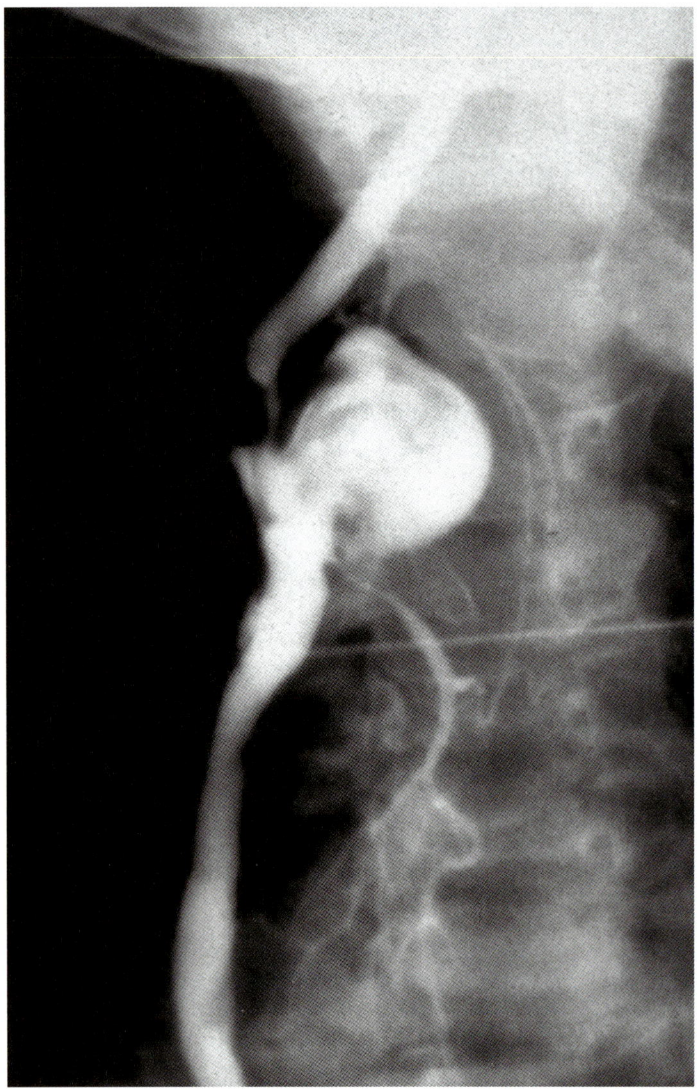

Fig. 6.1a Unsubtracted right CCA angiogram shows a complex mycotic pseudoaneurysm at the carotid bifurcation and marked stenosis of the ICA.

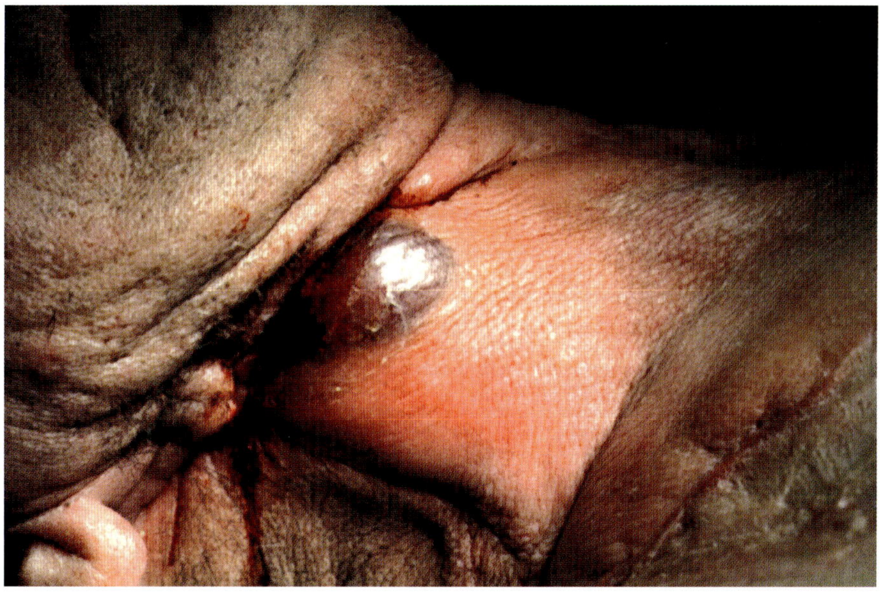

Fig. 6.1b Extensive postoperative scarring and radiation-induced changes on the right side of the patient's neck have made this tissue unsuitable for a bypass.

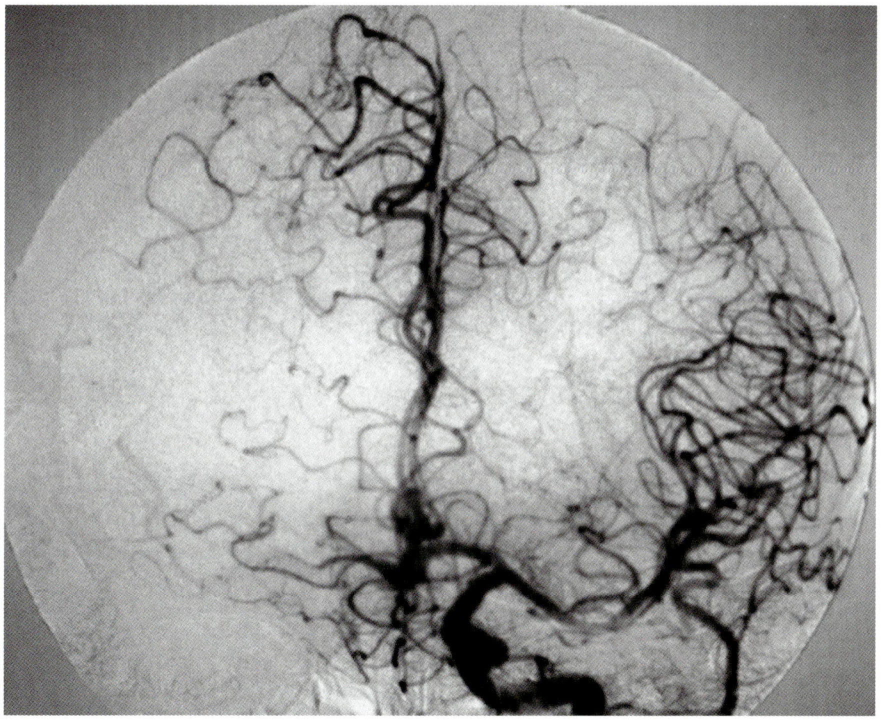

Fig. 6.1c Anteroposterior angiogram of the left CCA shows substantial cross filling to the right ACA but minimal filling of the right MCA via the leptomeningeal collaterals.

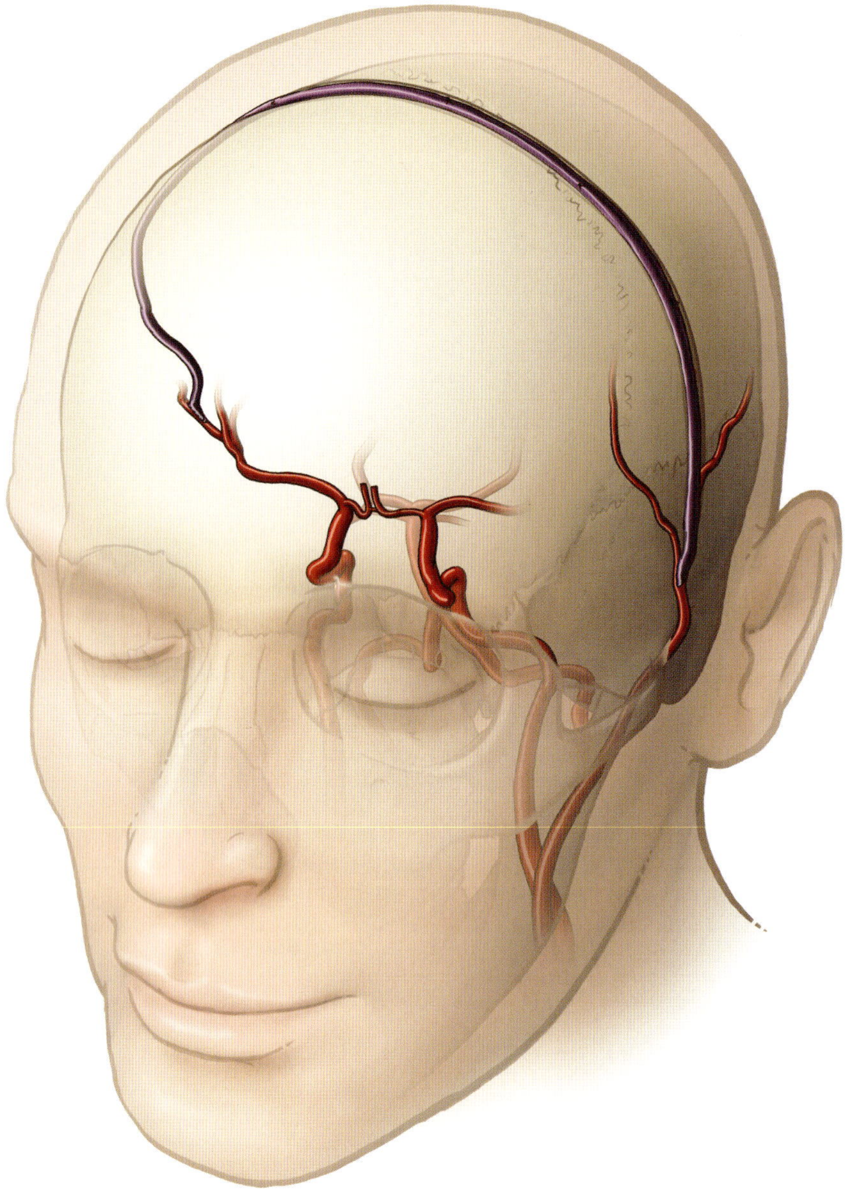

Fig. 6.1d Illustration shows a bonnet bypass running from the left STA bifurcation to the right MCA to bypass the right neck. Either a radial artery or saphenous vein graft can be used. The graft can be sewn between any two suitable vessels on either side of midline.

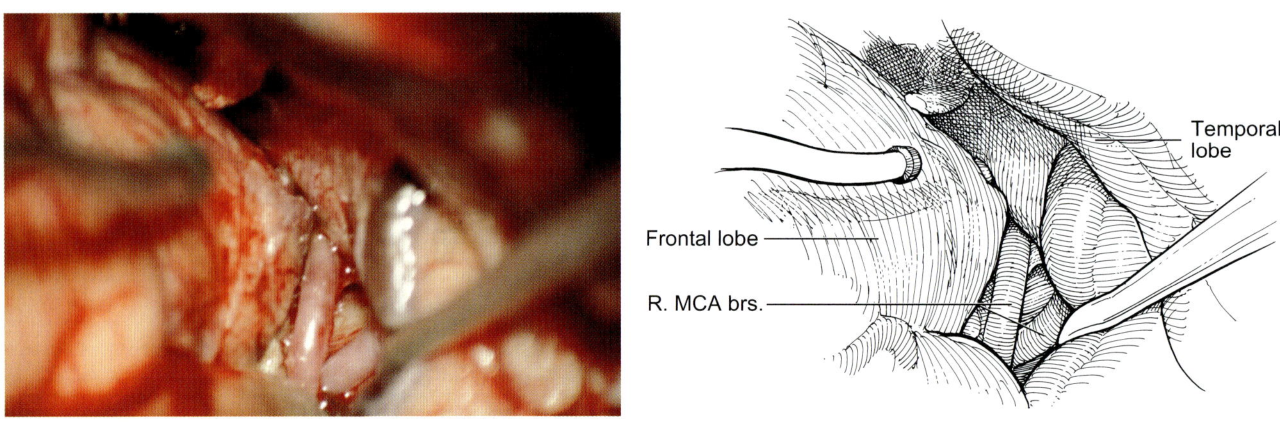

Fig. 6.1e A right pterional craniotomy is performed. The sylvian fissure is split widely to expose a branch of the proximal MCA to serve as a graft recipient.

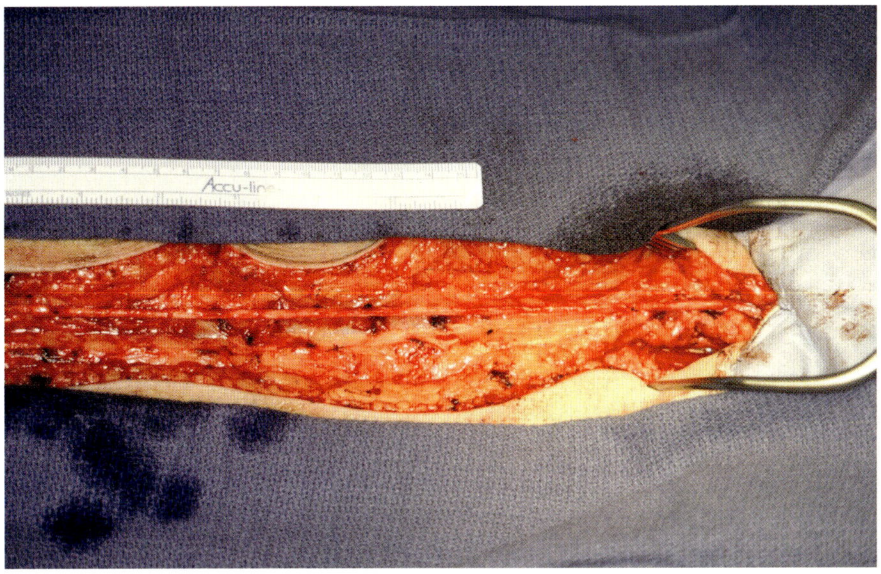

Fig. 6.1f The saphenous vein is exposed in the right thigh from the knee to its junction with the deep femoral vein.

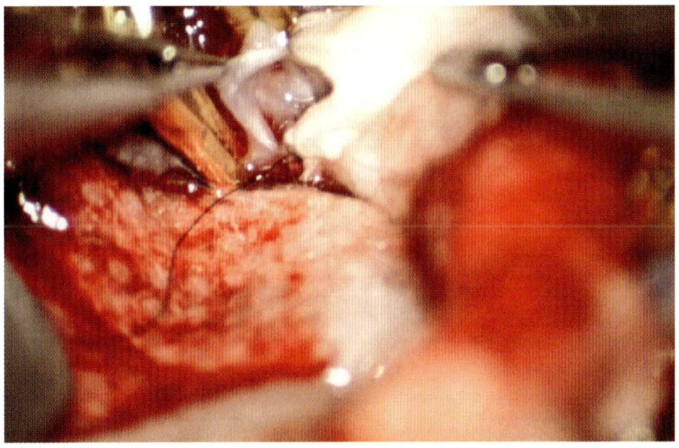

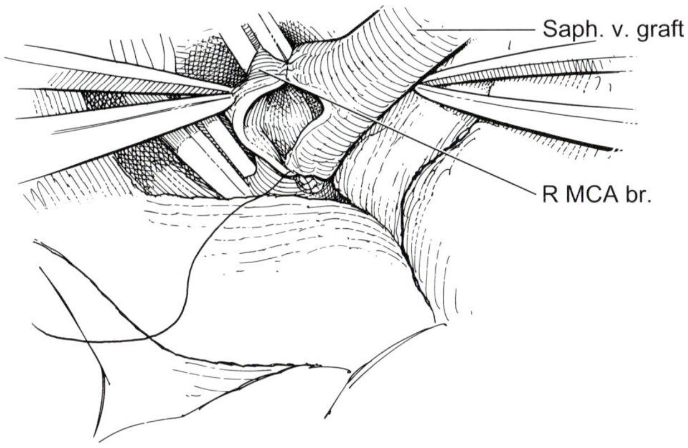

Fig. 6.1g The vein graft is sutured to the MCA branch. The back side is completed.

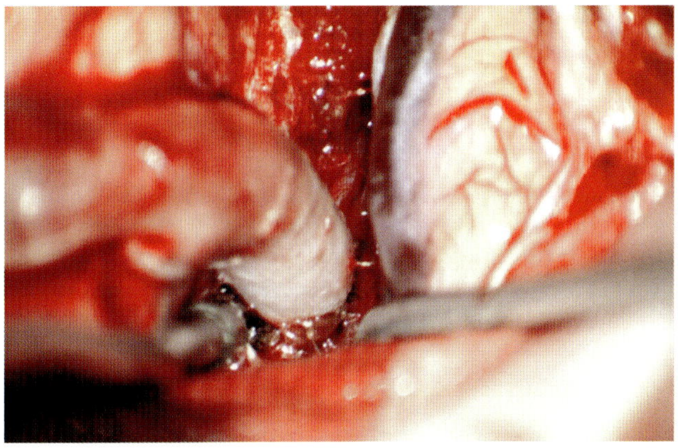

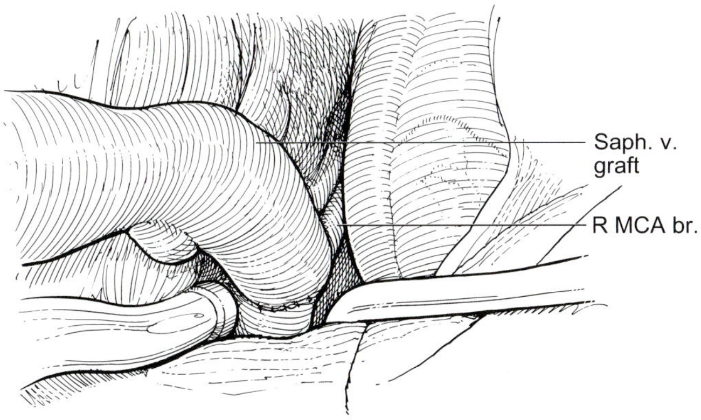

Fig. 6.1h The distal end of the bypass is completed, and the graft backfills. The anastomosis is checked for hemostasis.

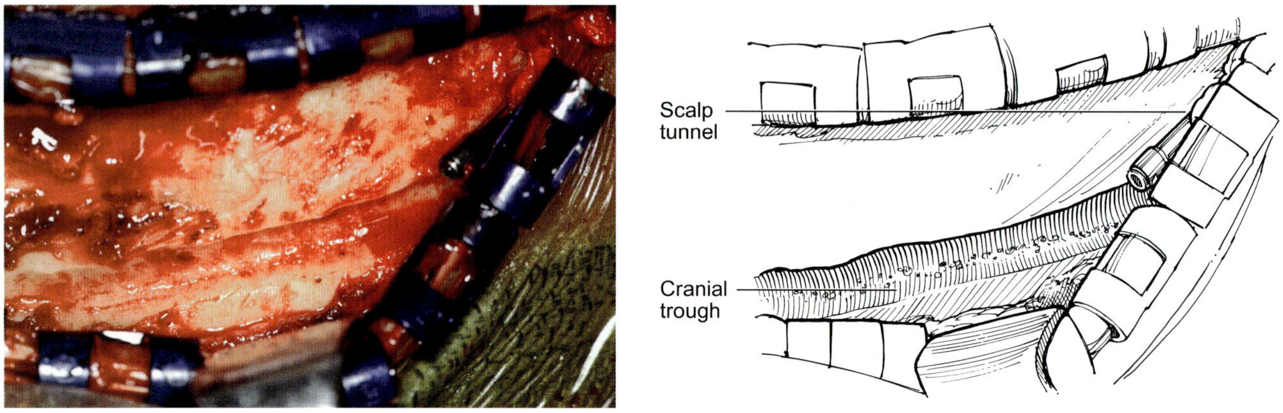

Fig. 6.1i A linear scalp incision proceeds from the roof of the left zygoma up toward the peak of the right-sided craniotomy incision. A shallow trough cut in the cranium allows the vein graft to be passed from left to right over the top of the head without being compressed by the scalp.

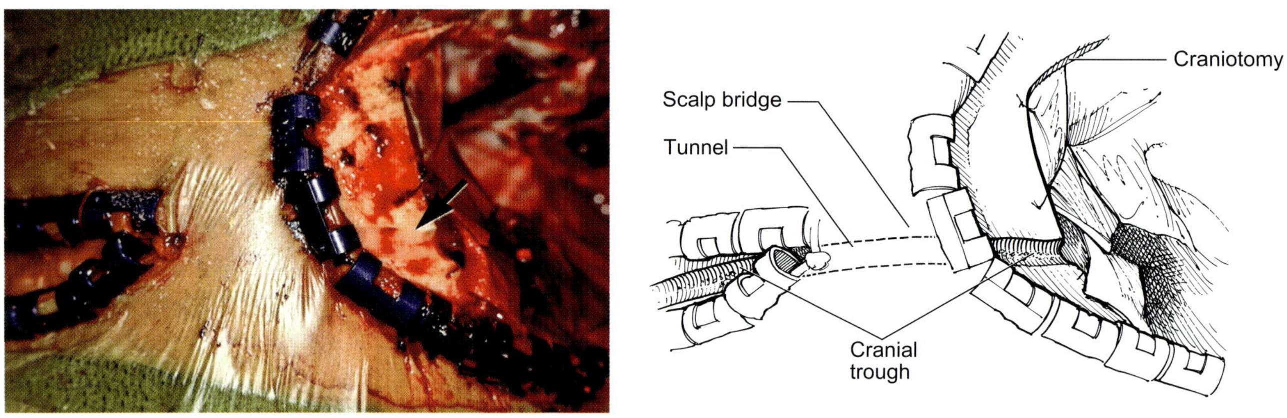

Fig. 6.1j The cranial trough is passed under a bridge of intact scalp to the edge of the craniotomy on the right (*arrow*).

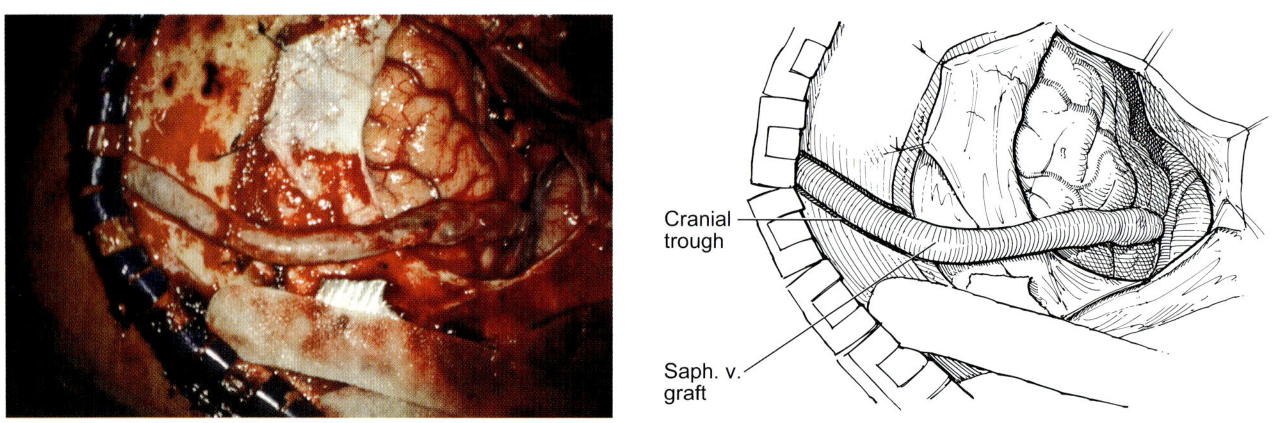

Fig. 6.1k The saphenous vein graft is laid in the cranial trough across the midline.

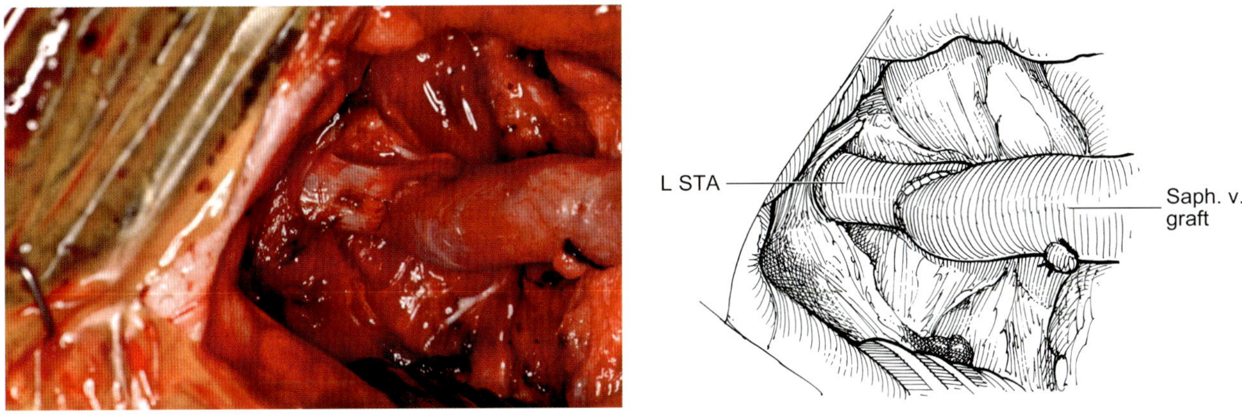

Fig. 6.1l The proximal end of the graft is anastomosed to the trunk of the left STA just below the root of the zygoma.

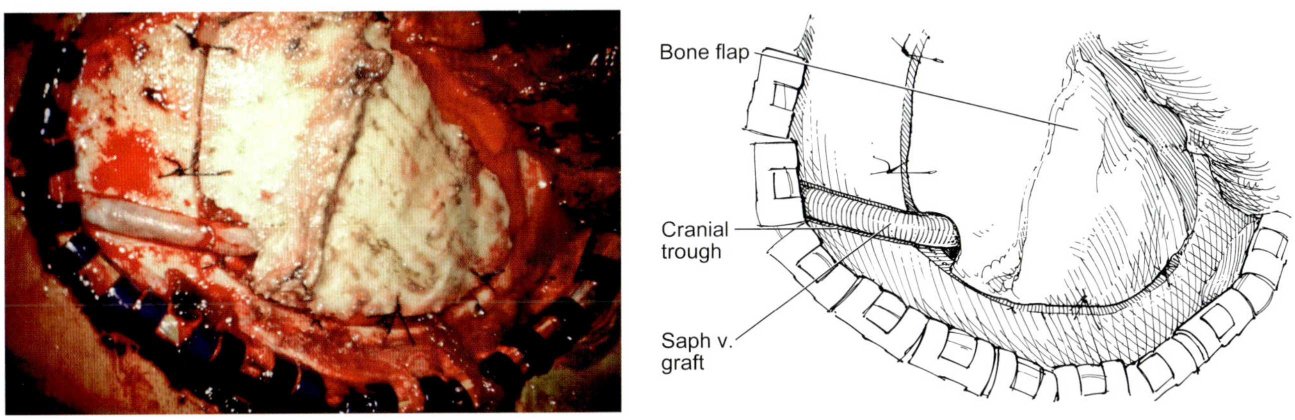

Fig. 6.1m The craniotomy bone flap is replaced and fixed into position on the right side. During closure care is exerted to assure that the vein graft is not compromised along its course.

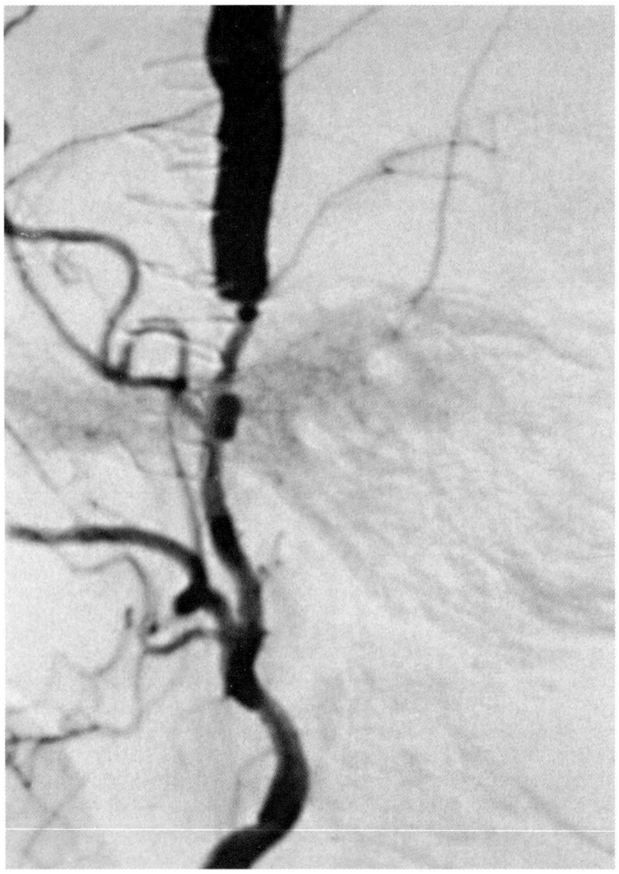

Fig. 6.1n Lateral angiographic view of the proximal anastomosis.

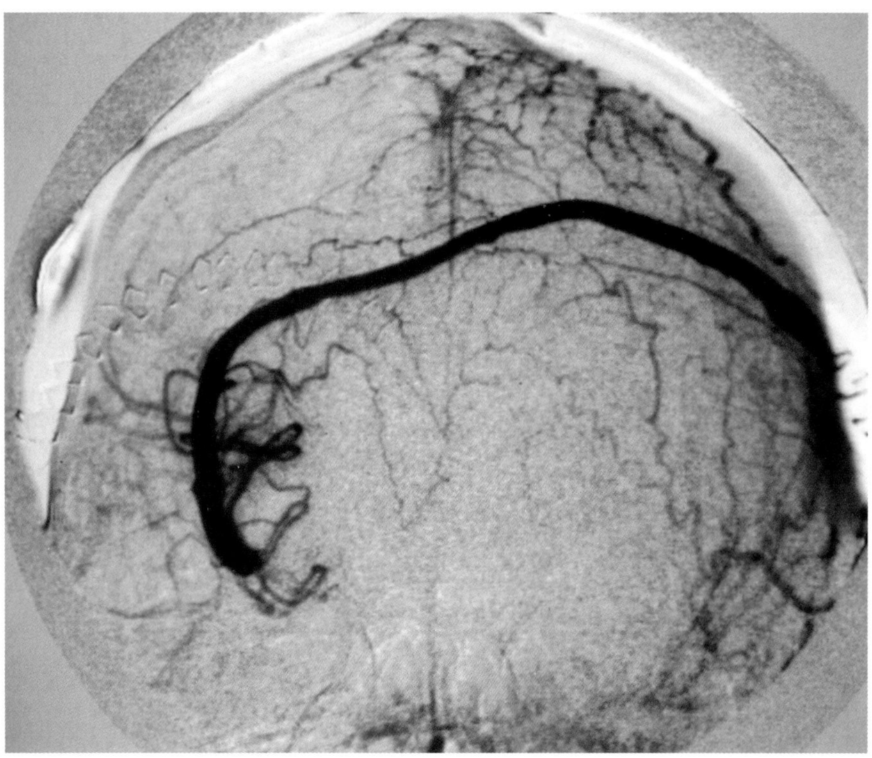

Fig. 6.1o Left ECA angiogram shows robust filling of the bonnet bypass and good filling of the branches of the MCA. After the bypass was completed, the right carotid artery in the neck was sacrificed without difficulty.

7 High-Flow Cervical Carotid Artery–to–MCA Bypass

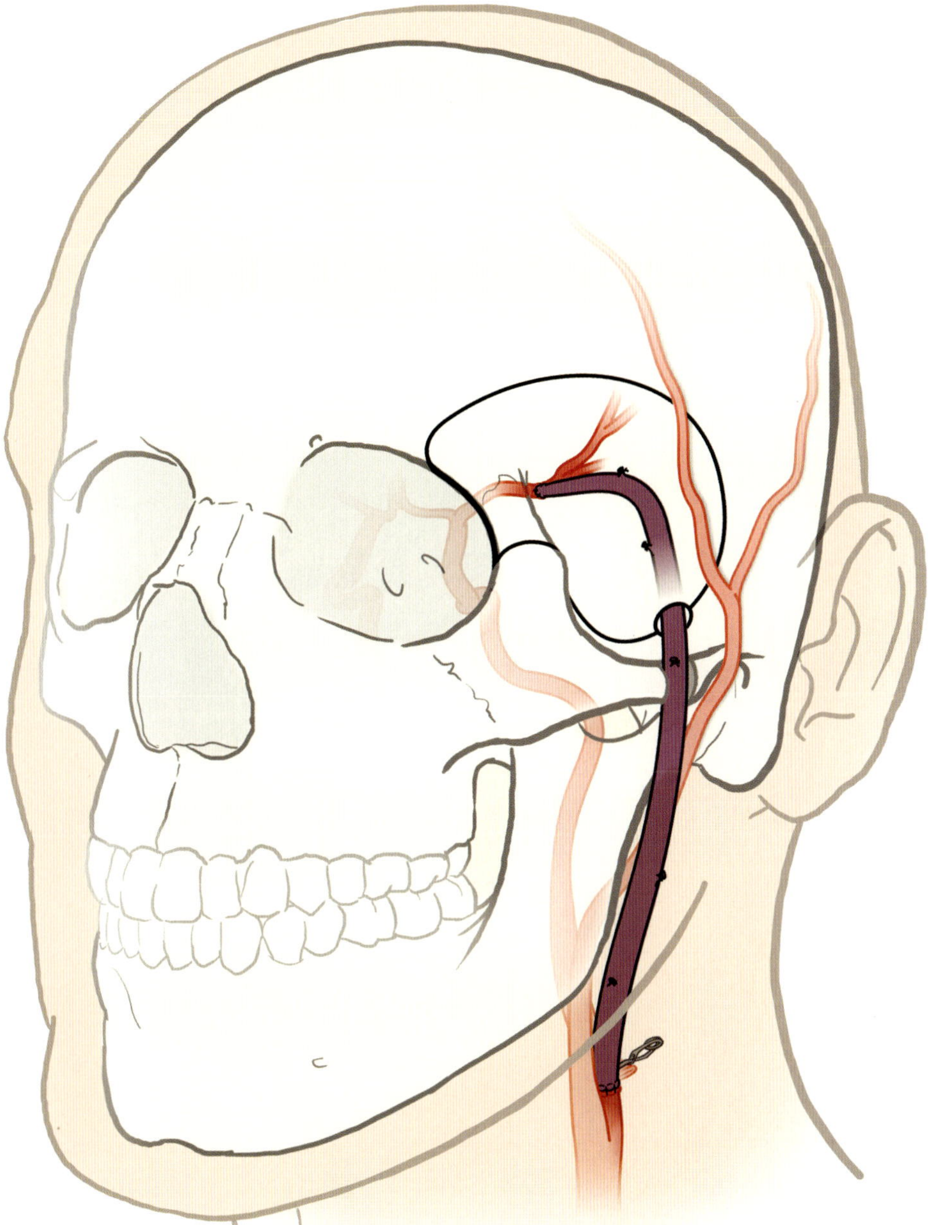

The high-flow cervical carotid artery–to–MCA bypass can replace the flow of one ICA entirely. The graft can arise from the side of the ECA, ICA, or CCA or from the stump of one of these vessels if it is being sacrificed as part of the same procedure. The graft travels from the neck outside the skull base, subcutaneously and in front of the ear, to the craniotomy that exposes the recipient vessel. Either the radial artery or saphenous vein can be used for this purpose. The radial artery, however, is a better match in terms of size and does not kink as easily as the vein. Over time we have used the radial artery for a graft more frequently than the saphenous vein. Both vessels are sufficiently long to reach the MCA from the neck.

The bifurcation of the cervical carotid artery is accessed through a transverse cervical incision. This incision provides adequate exposure of the CCA, ECA, and ICA and is cosmetically preferable to a vertical incision.

The graft is removed from the arm or leg. An M2 vessel is exposed in the sylvian fissure. The M2 anastomosis is performed first because mobility of the graft makes this anastomosis easier.

A small chest tube is passed subcutaneously from the neck to the cranial incision and cut lengthwise so that the graft can be placed into the tubing. The graft is then gently passed into the neck incision. Before the bypass is completed, the graft and anastomosis are flushed with pure heparin solution to clear them of blood and air.

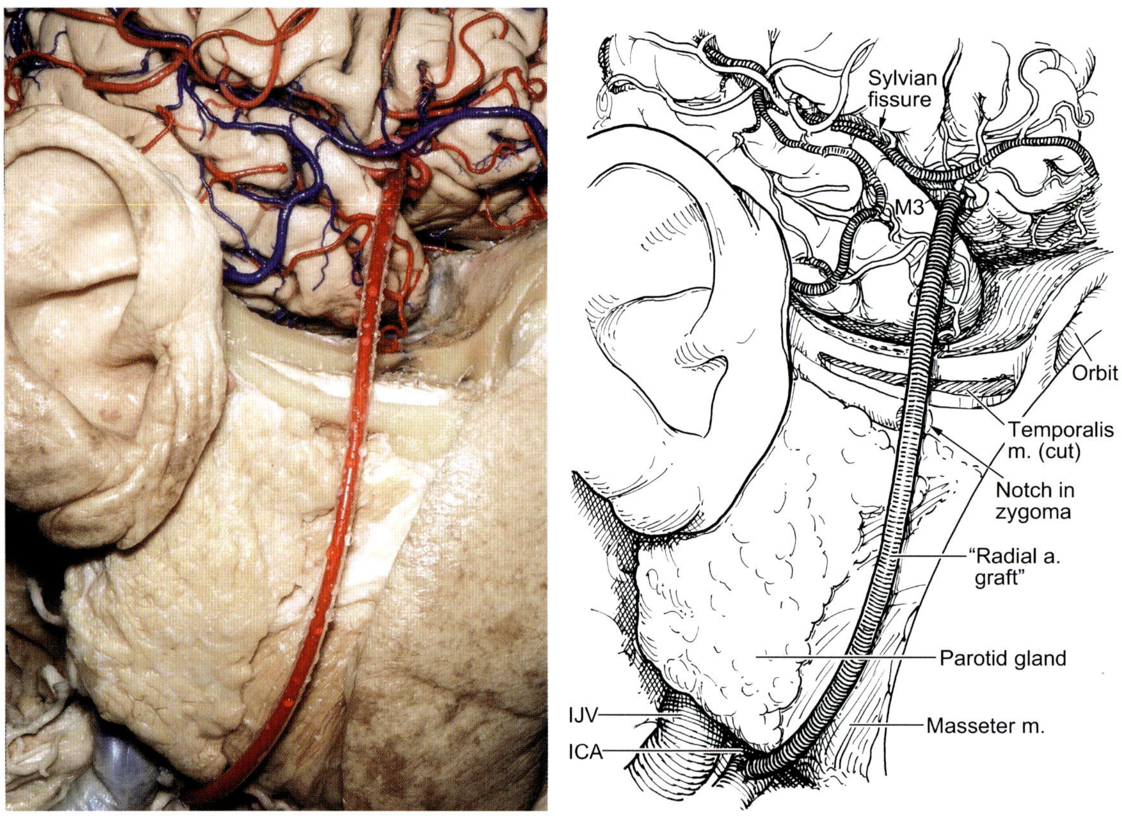

Fig. 7.0a A polyethylene tube simulates a radial artery graft from the base of the ICA to an M3 branch in the sylvian fissure. The zygoma is notched to allow the graft to lie flat.

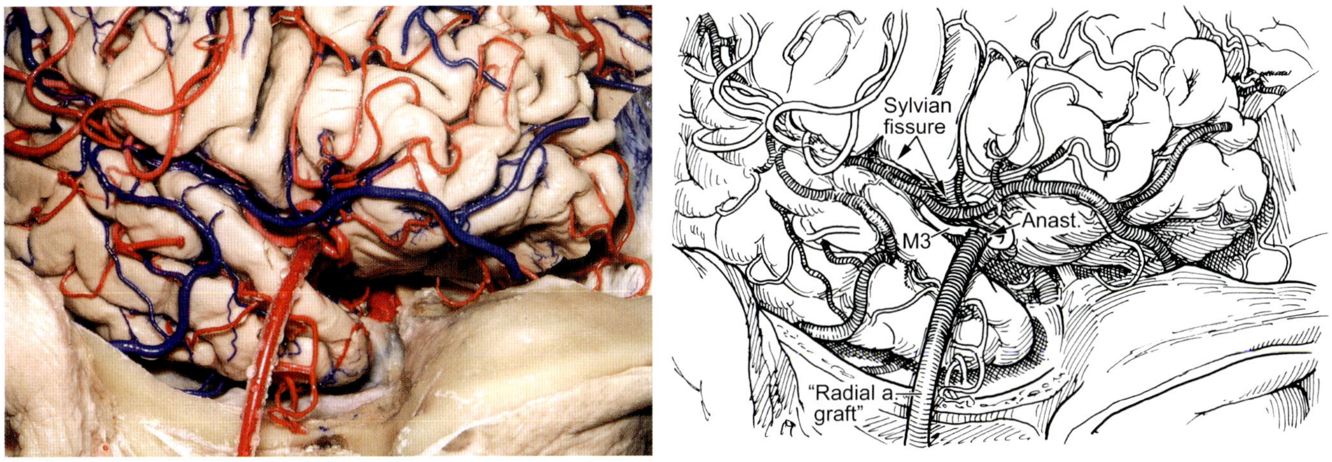

Fig. 7.0b The distal anastomosis is made to an M3 vessel in the sylvian fissure. With a radial artery graft, it may be necessary to use the M2 branch to achieve an acceptable match in size.

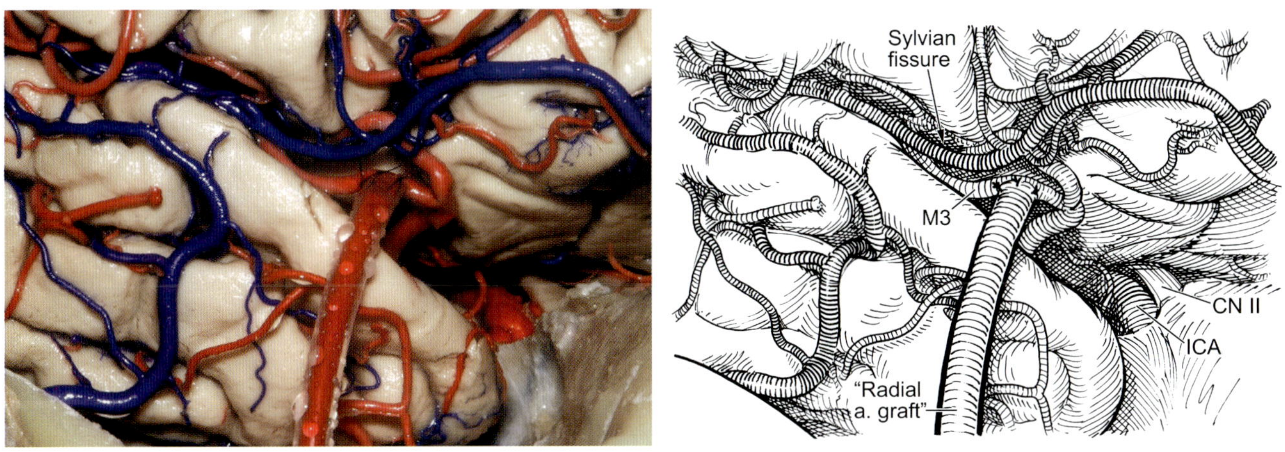

Fig. 7.0c Close-up view of the anastomosis. In a living patient, the anastomosis is typically fashioned flush along the vessel rather than perpendicular to it.

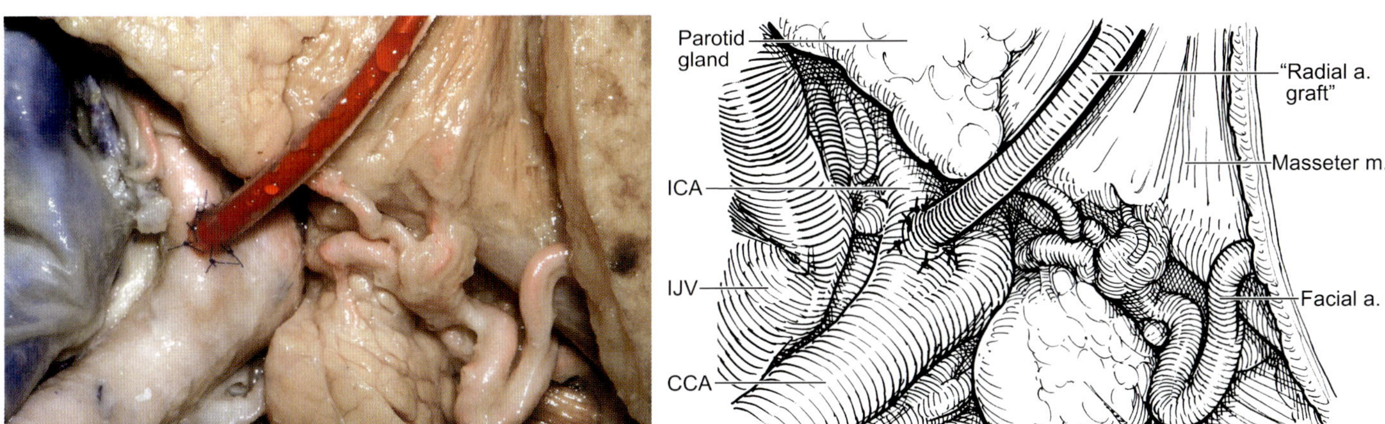

Fig. 7.0d The proximal anastomosis can be attached end-to-side to the base of the cervical segment of the ICA just above the carotid bifurcation.

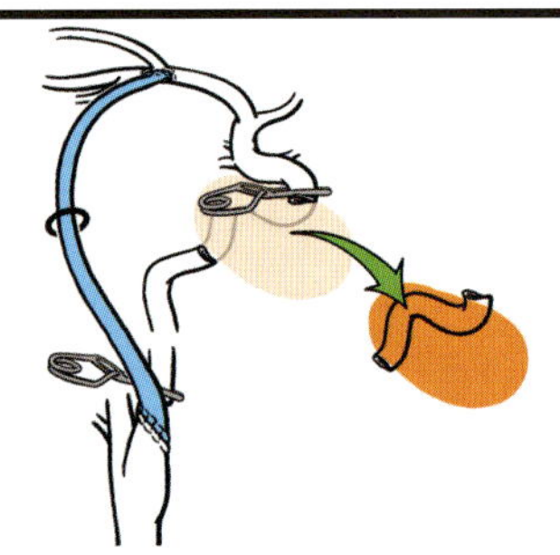

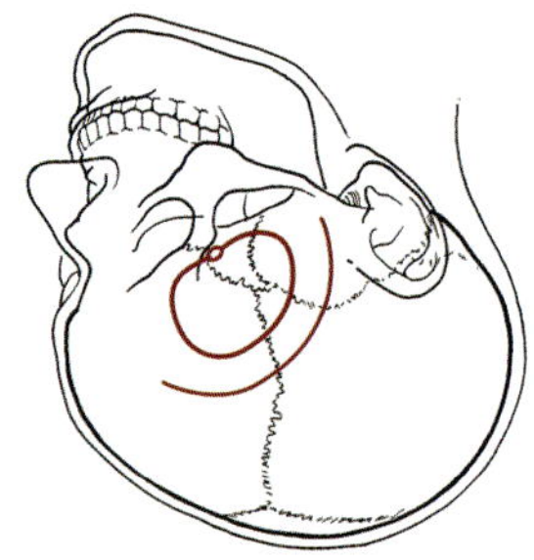

Case 7-1

Diagnosis: Right cavernous sinus malignant tumor

Bypass: Cervical ICA-to-MCA with vein graft

Approach: Right pterional

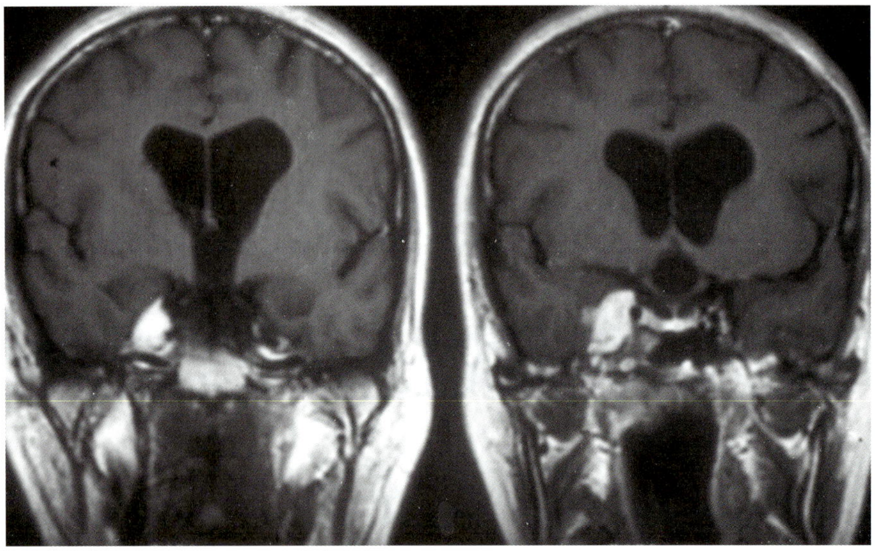

Fig. 7.1a Coronal T1-weighted MR images with gadolinium enhancement show a malignant tumor in the right cavernous sinus.

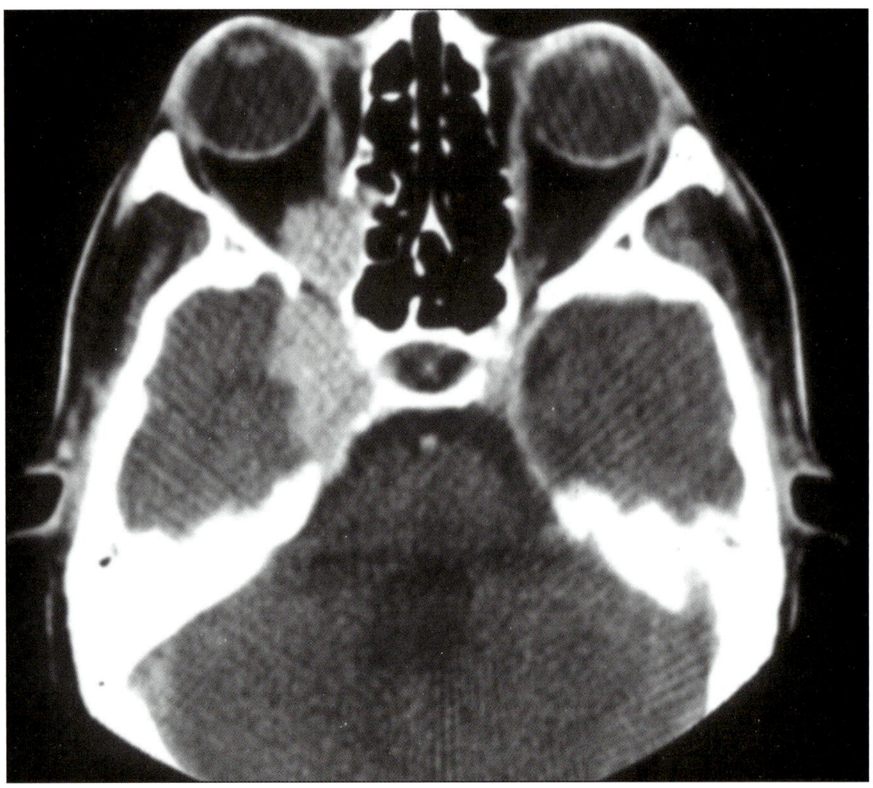

Fig. 7.1b Axial CT with contrast shows the enhancing mass in the right cavernous sinus extending into the orbit.

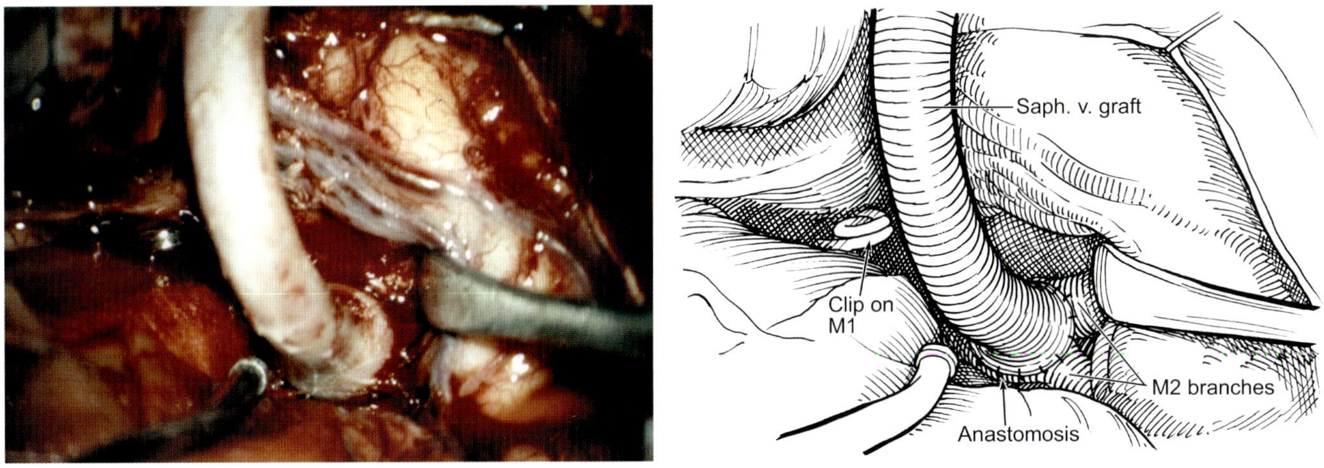

Fig. 7.1c A vein graft is anastomosed to the M1–M2 junction.

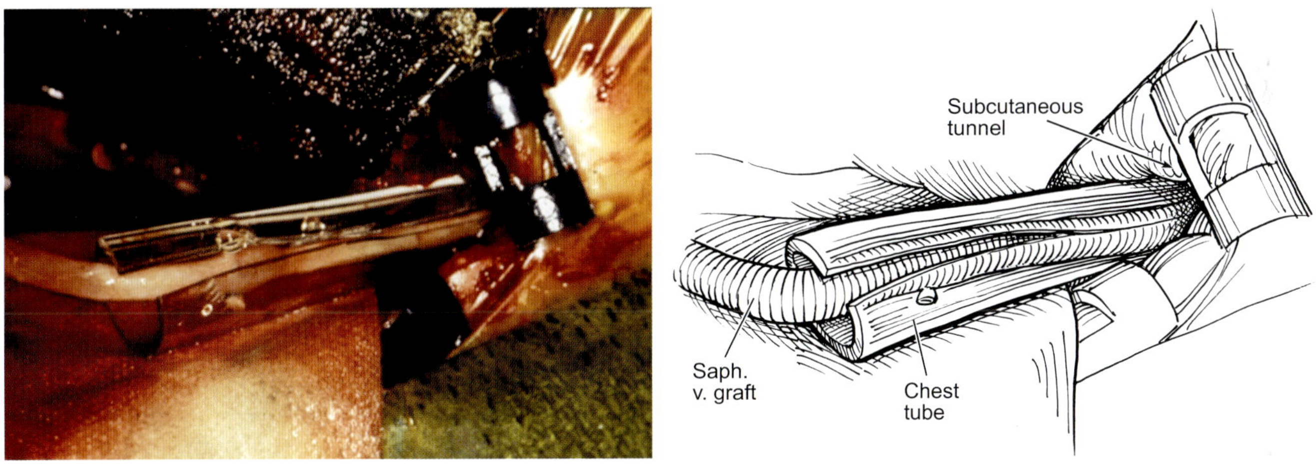

Fig. 7.1d A split length of chest tube is used to pass the graft to the neck.

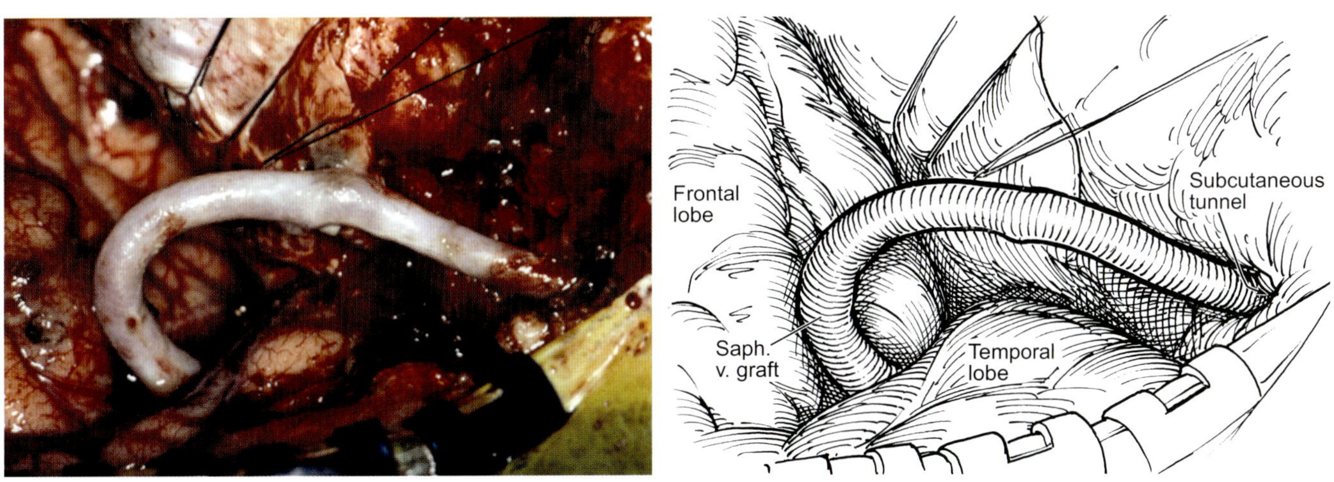

Fig. 7.1e The vein graft must be long enough so that it curves naturally without kinking.

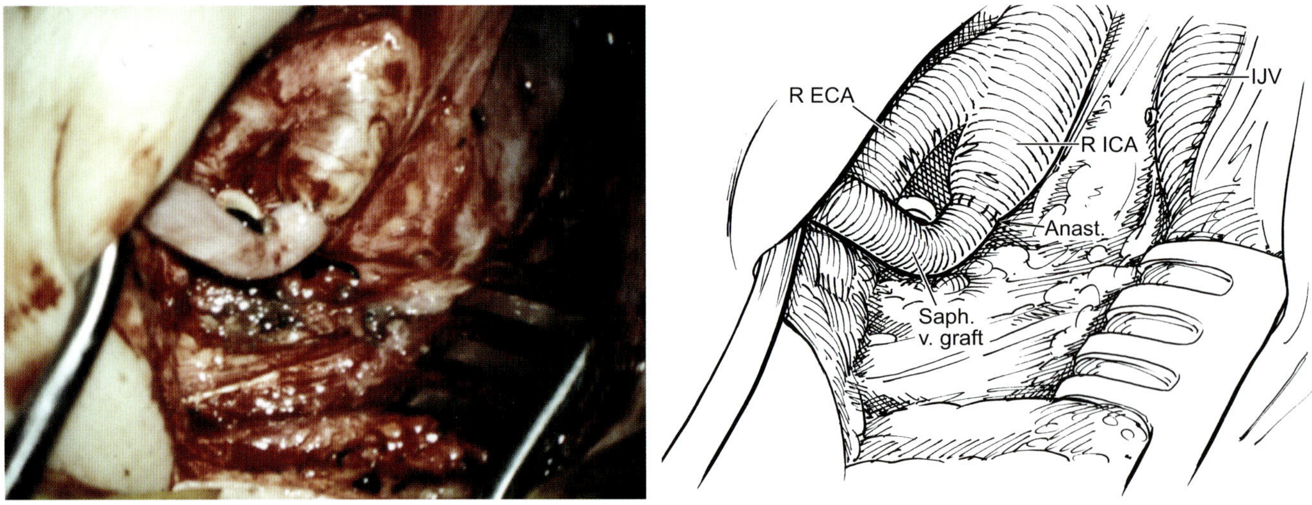

Fig. 7.1f The proximal end-to-end anastomosis between the stump of the ICA and the graft is completed.

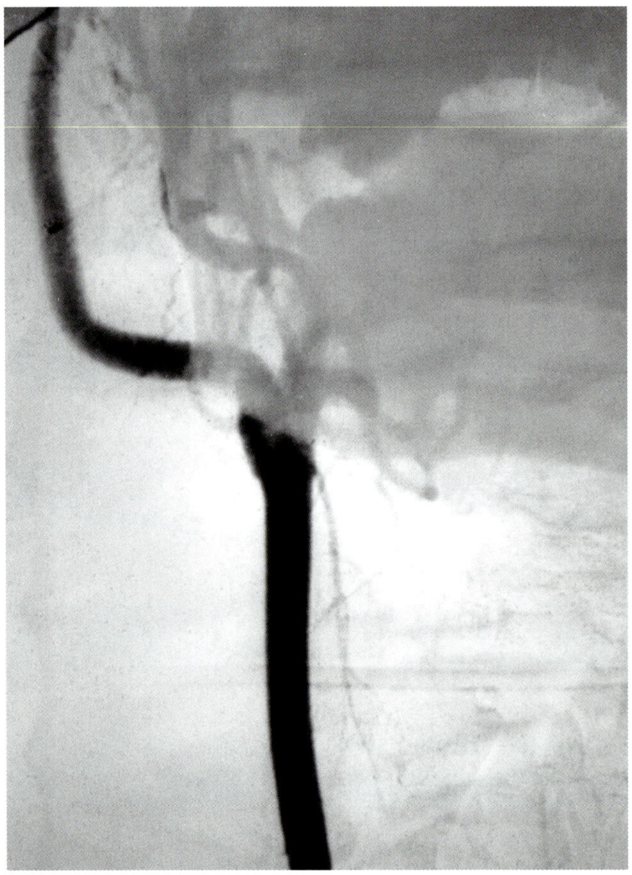

Fig. 7.1g Anteroposterior angiographic injection of the CCA shows the carotid bifurcation and course of the vein graft.

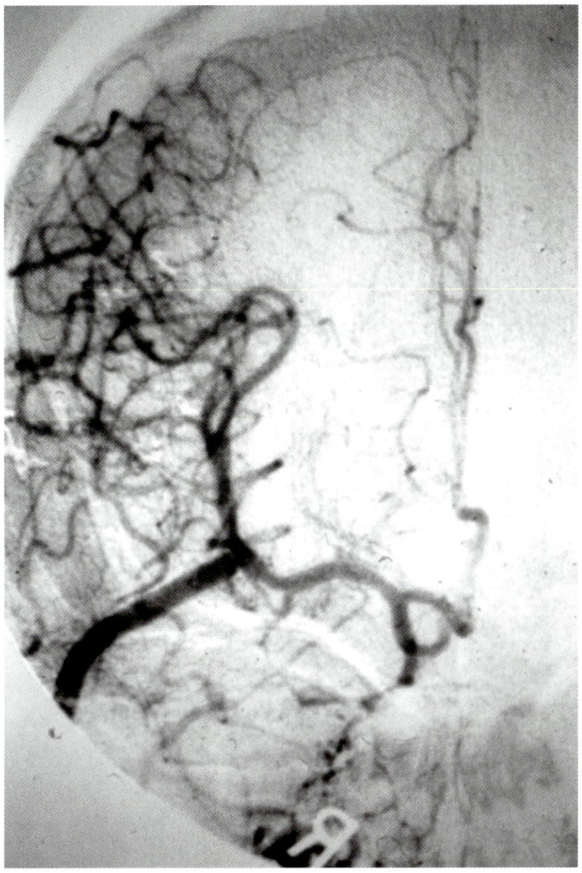

Fig. 7.1h The cranial portion of the same angiographic injection shows the anastomosis to the M1–M2 junction and filling of the ICA and ACA through the bypass.

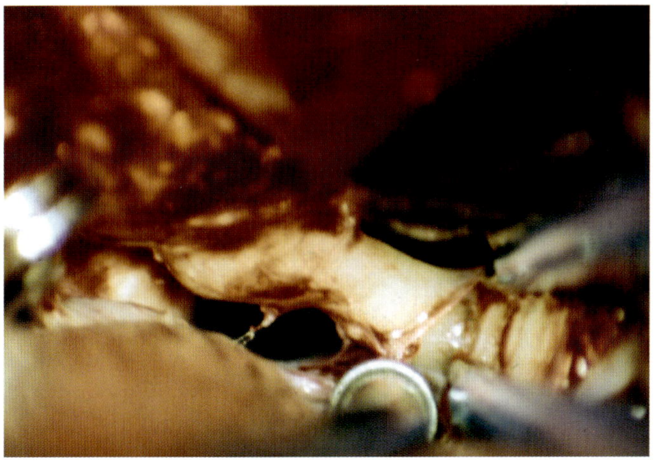

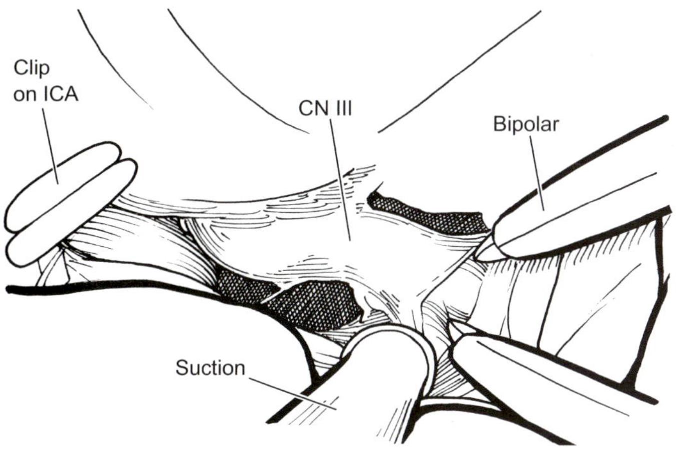

Fig. 7.1i CN III is exposed prior to being sacrificed.

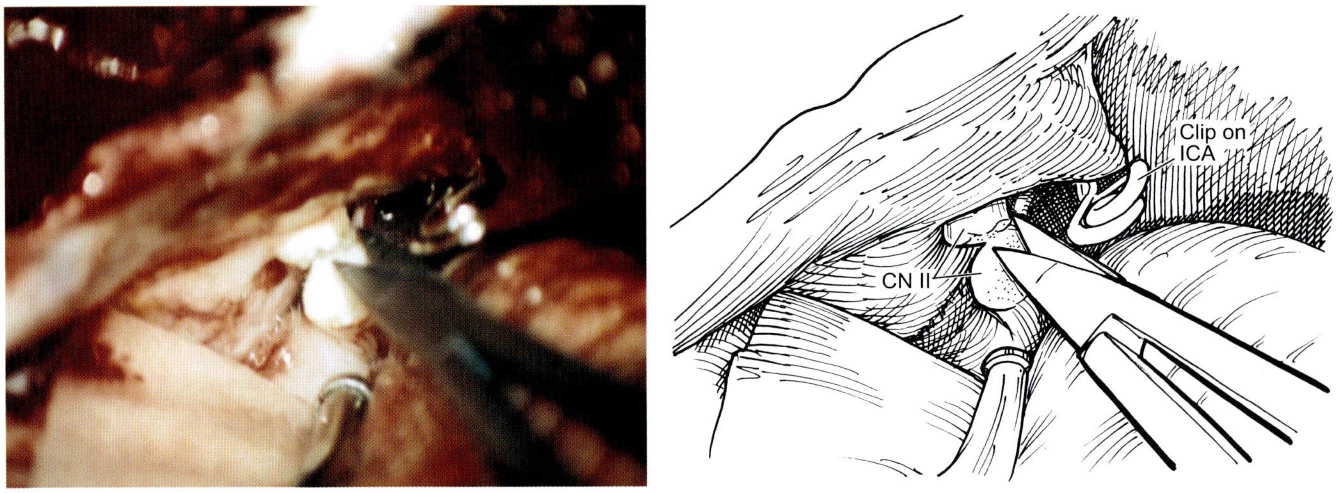

Fig. 7.1j CN II has been cut in preparation for removing the cavernous sinus in one piece.

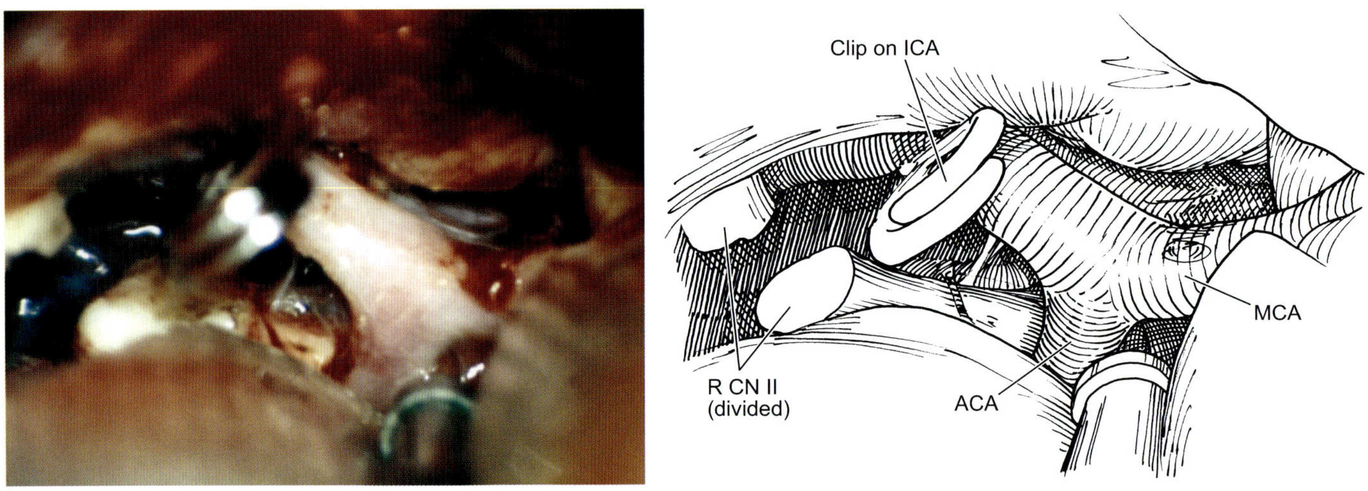

Fig. 7.1k The ICA is being prepared for sacrifice.

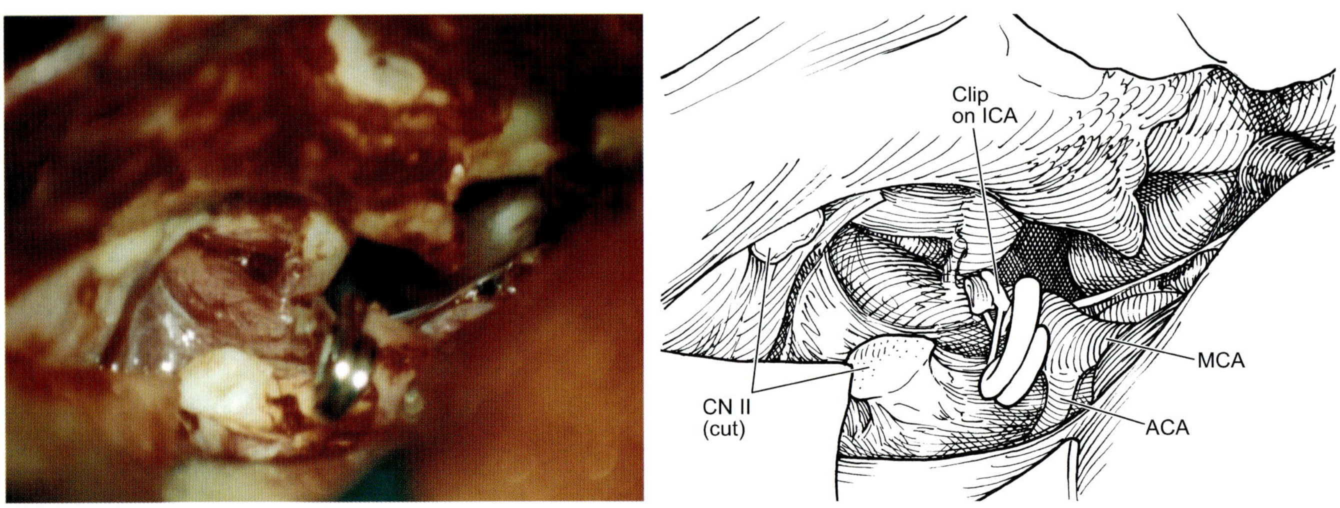

Fig. 7.1l After the orbit and the cavernous sinus have been removed, the site is prepared for the placement of a vascularized free flap.

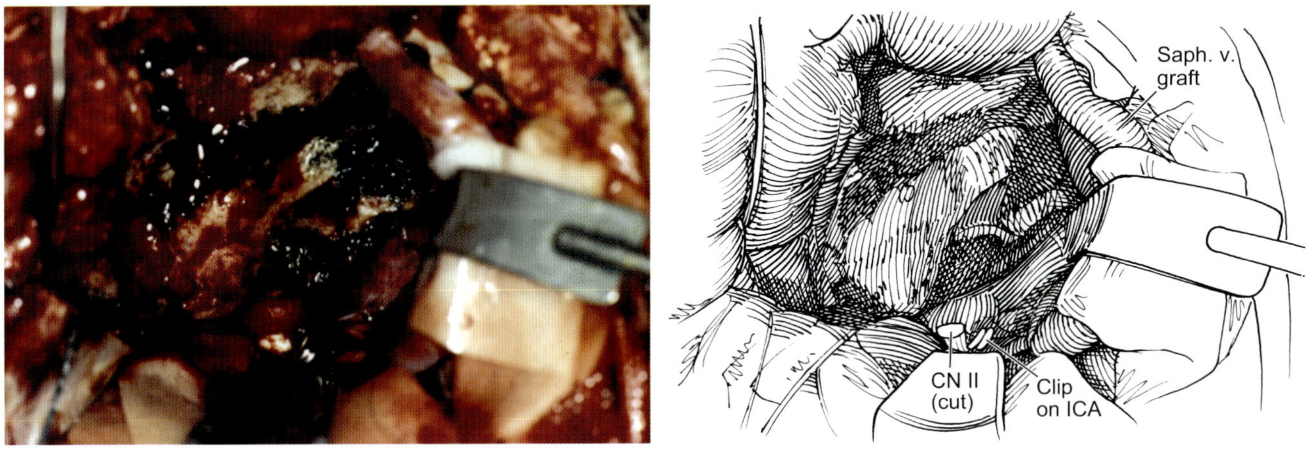

Fig. 7.1m Orbital exenteration and removal of the cavernous sinus create a large cavity.

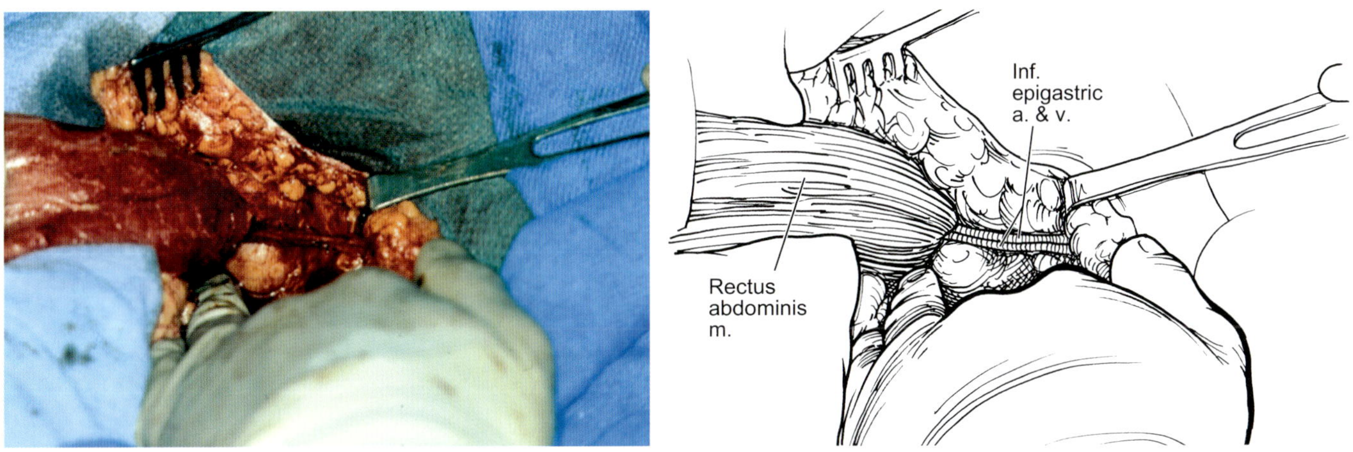

Fig. 7.1n A free flap is harvested from the rectus abdominis muscle.

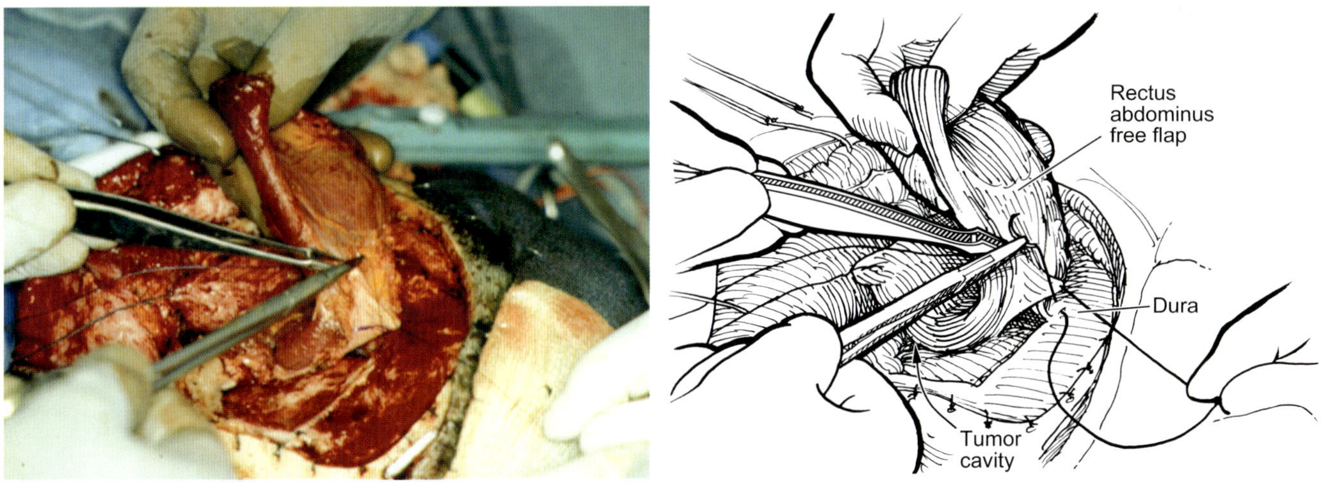

Fig. 7.1o The free graft flap is trimmed to fit the cavity. The artery and vein are anastomosed to the STA and vein.

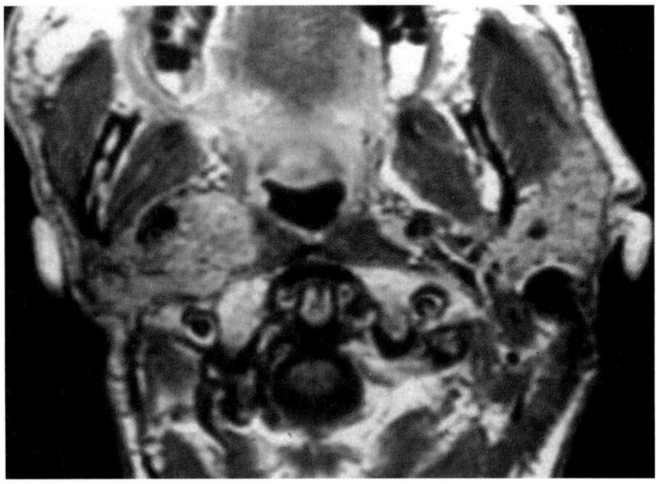

Fig. 7.1p Postoperative CT scan shows the vascularized pedicle.

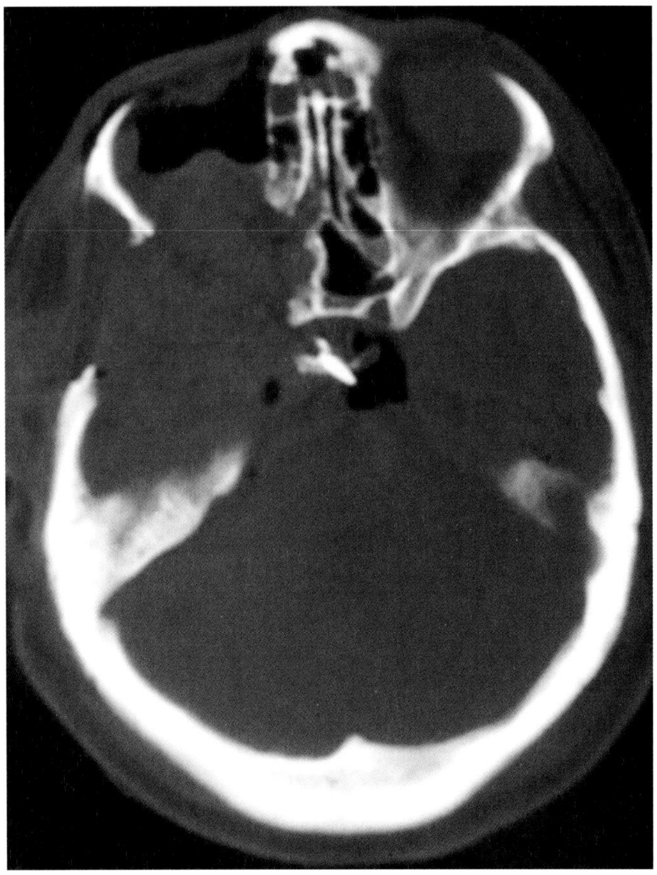

Fig. 7.1q Postoperative CT shows the size of the craniotomy, the absence of the cavernous sinus and orbit, and the placement of the clip on the distal ICA.

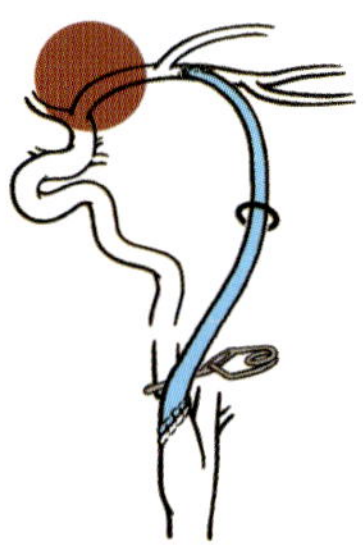

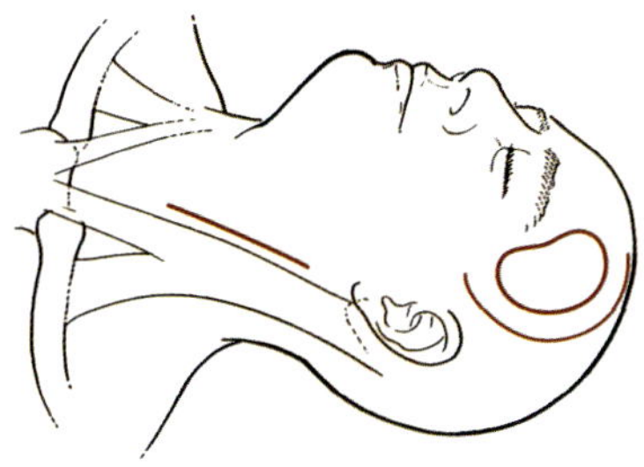

Case 7-2

Diagnosis: Left ICA bifurcation recurrent giant aneurysm

Bypass: Left cervical end-to-end ICA–to–MCA with saphenous vein graft with flow reversal

Approach: Left anterior cervical and left pterional

A 48-year-old woman suffered a sudden ictus. Eleven years earlier, she had undergone a craniotomy to treat an aneurysm.

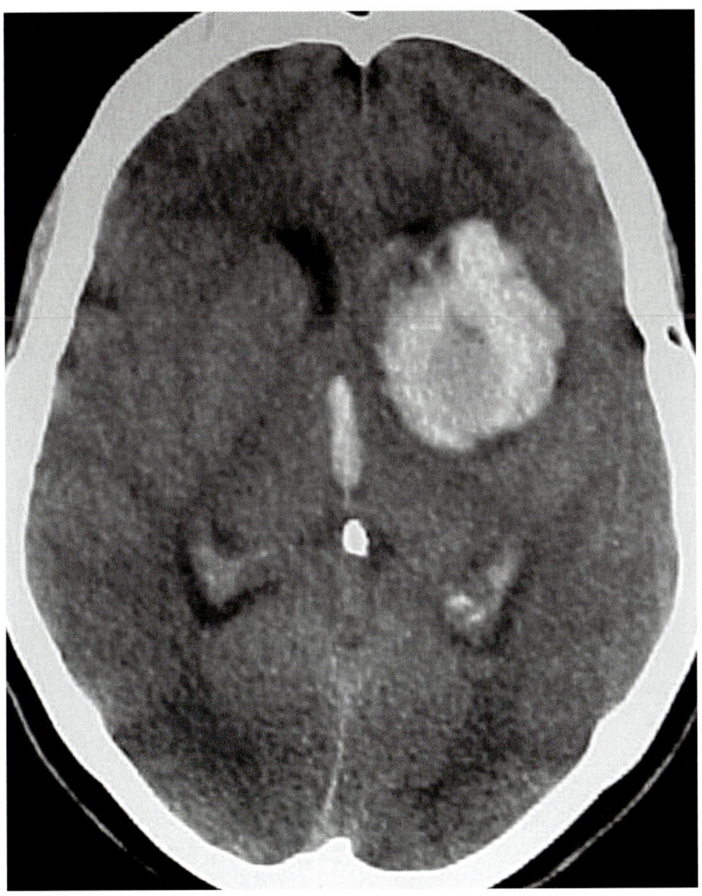

Fig. 7.2a Noncontrast axial CT scan shows a large left frontal intraparenchymal hemorrhage extending into the ventricles, especially into the third ventricle.

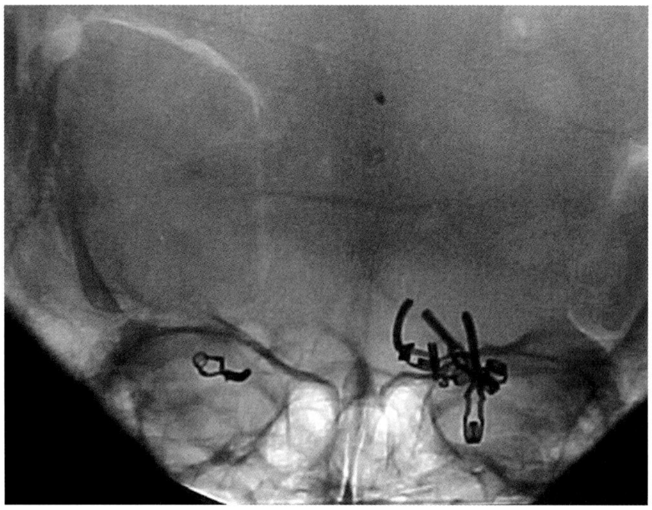

Fig. 7.2b Unsubtracted anteroposterior view of the skull base at the beginning of patient's preoperative angiogram shows evidence of earlier bilateral craniotomies. One aneurysm clip is on the right, and multiple clips are on the left.

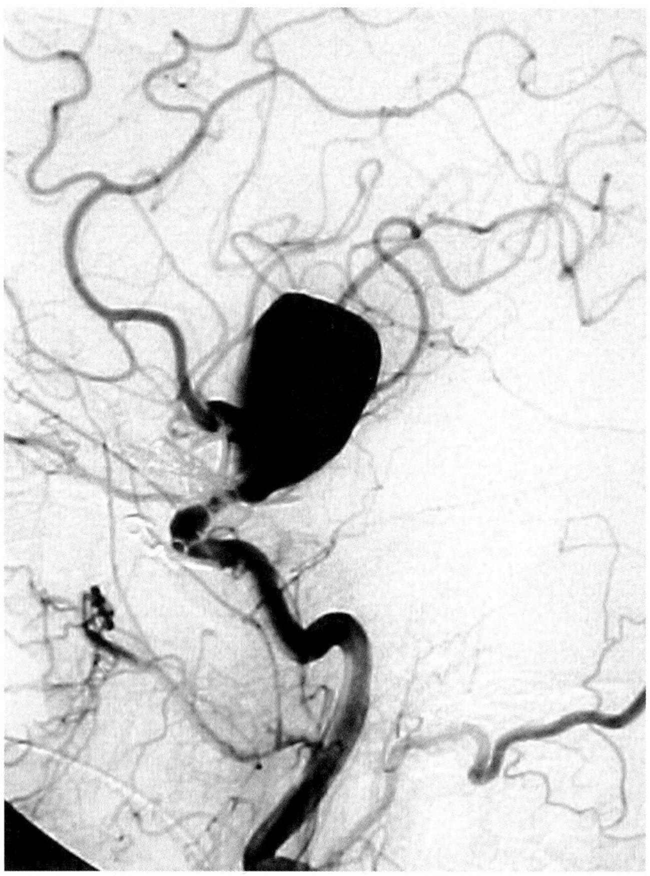

Fig. 7.2c Lateral left ICA angiogram shows a large recurrent aneurysm at the bifurcation of the ICA.

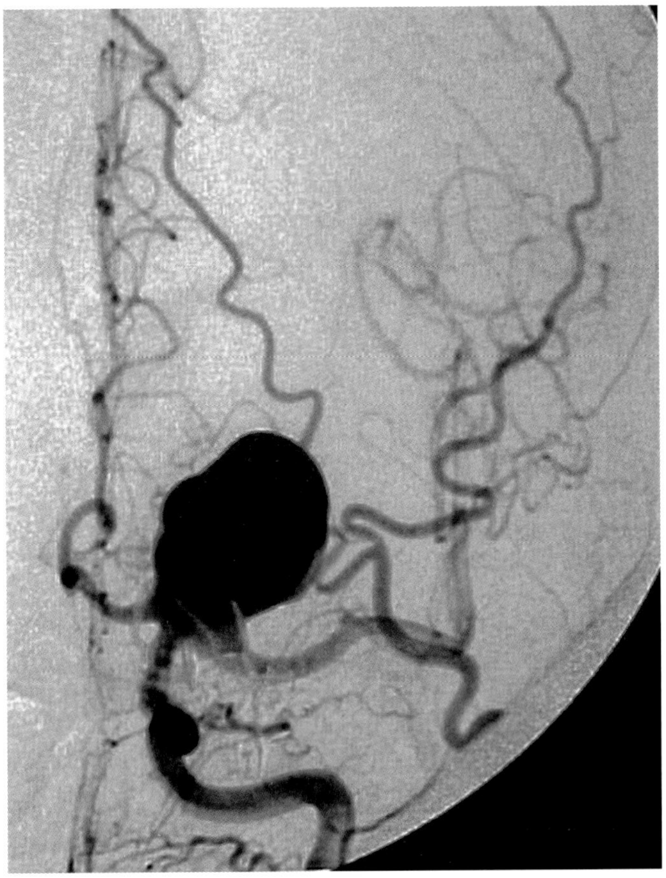

Fig. 7.2d Anteroposterior angiographic view shows that the aneurysm has a broad neck.

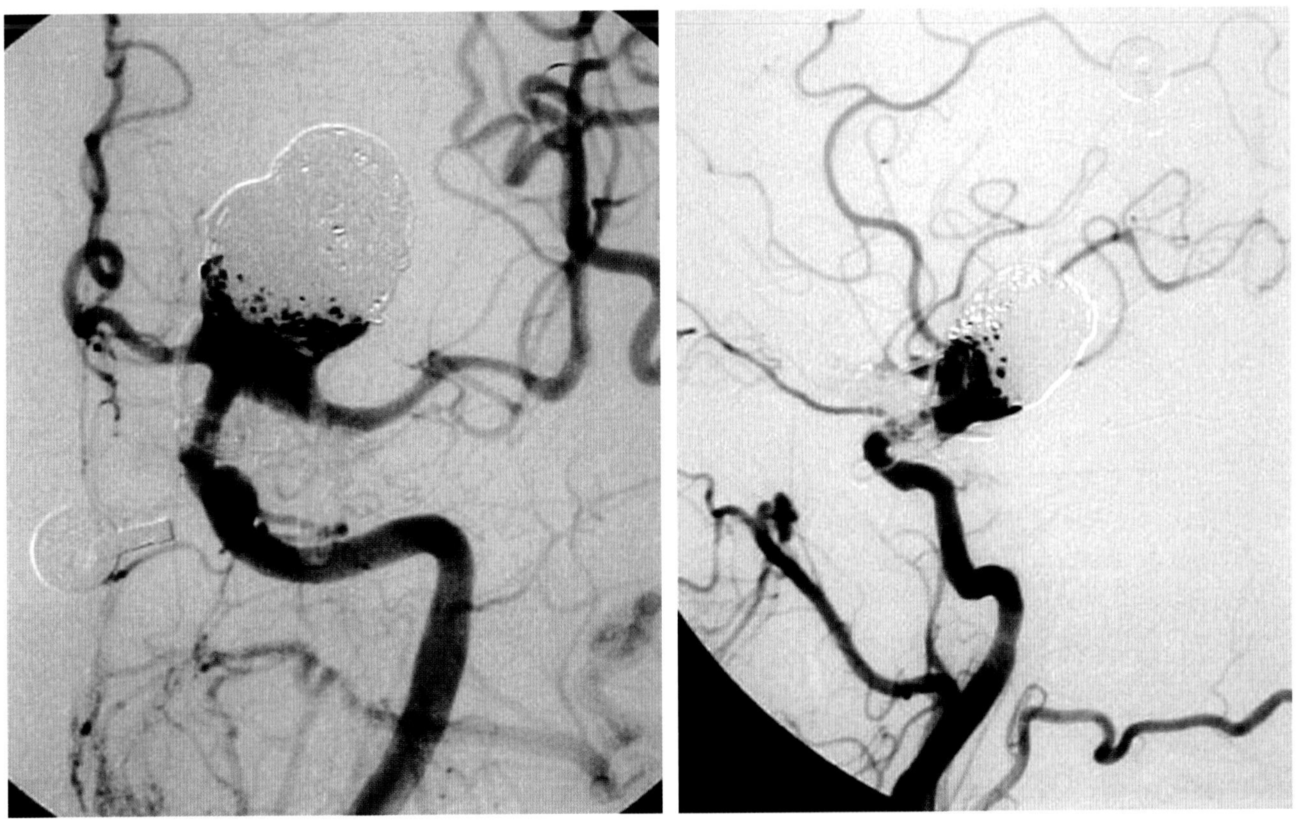

Fig. 7.2e, f Postoperative angiograms show the coils placed to minimize the risk of rebleeding after the patient's recent hemorrhage, which left her in a poor grade. Over several weeks she made a good recovery. An attempt at stent reconstruction failed. Because of the high risk of direct surgery with the old clips, a bypass was planned from the ICA to the MCA.

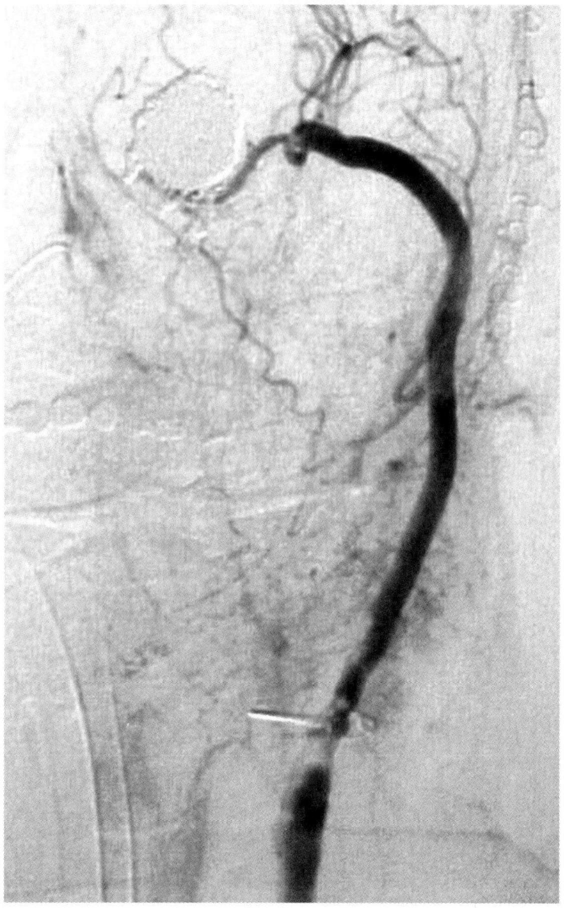

Fig. 7.2g Angiogram shows that after the bypass from the ICA in the neck to the M2 segment of the MCA was performed, the aneurysm disappeared completely. The change in blood flow eliminated any other filling of the aneurysmal neck.

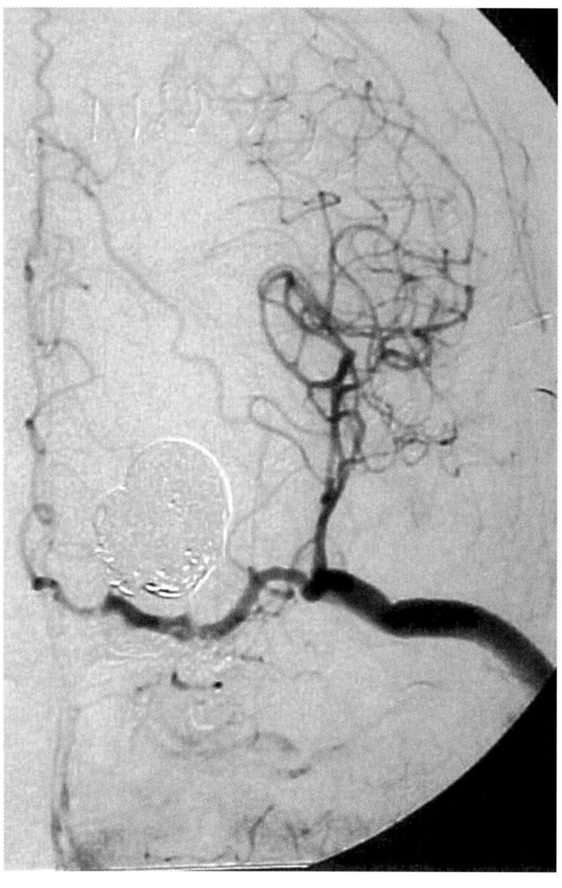

Fig. 7.2h Later phase angiogram shows filling of the MCA and ACA through the saphenous vein graft.

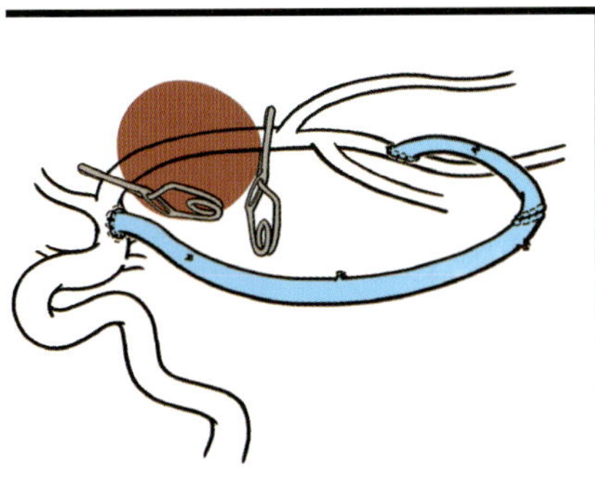

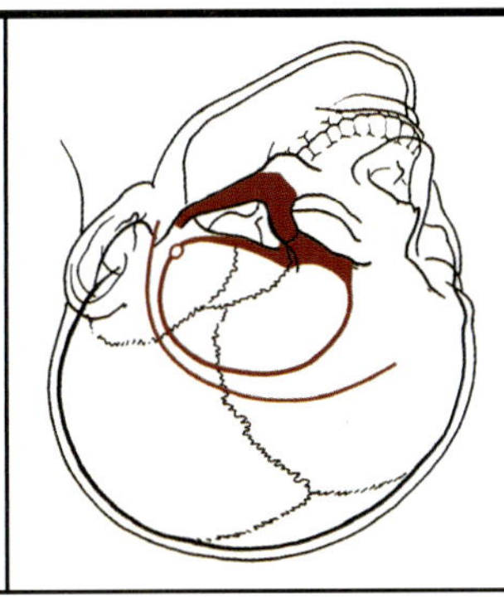

Case 7-3

Diagnosis: Giant left MCA aneurysm

Bypass: ICA to M2 with saphenous vein graft with ELANA anastomosis

Approach: Left orbitozygomatic

Video

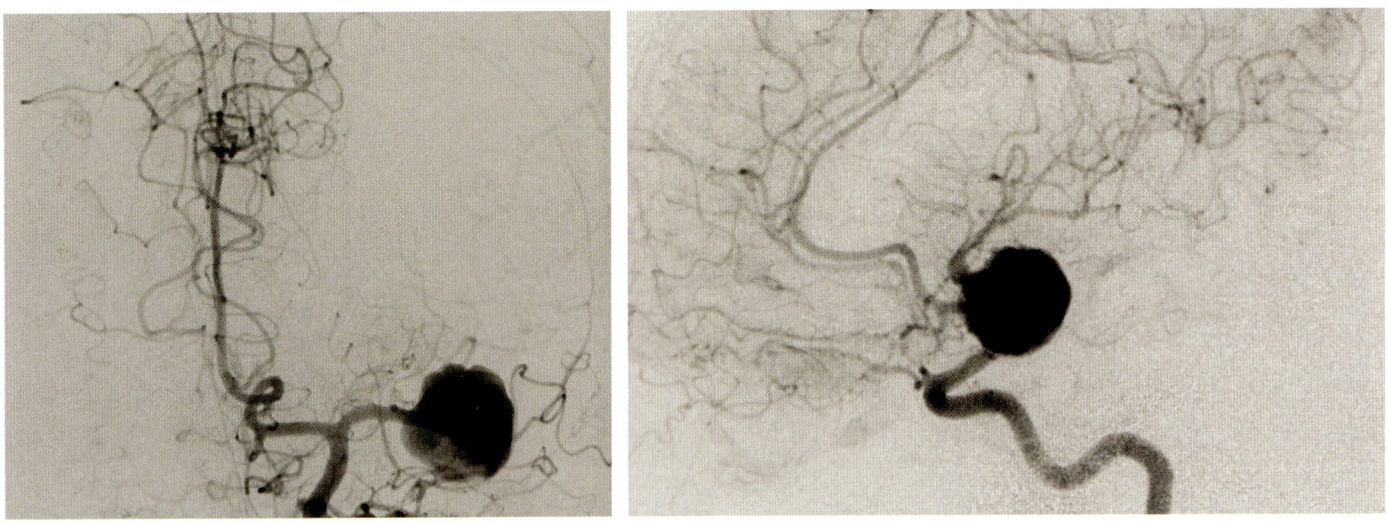

a b

Fig. 7.3a, b Preoperative anteroposterior and lateral angiograms show a giant left MCA aneurysm causing ischemic embolic events. (Courtesy of Albert van der Zwan, MD.)

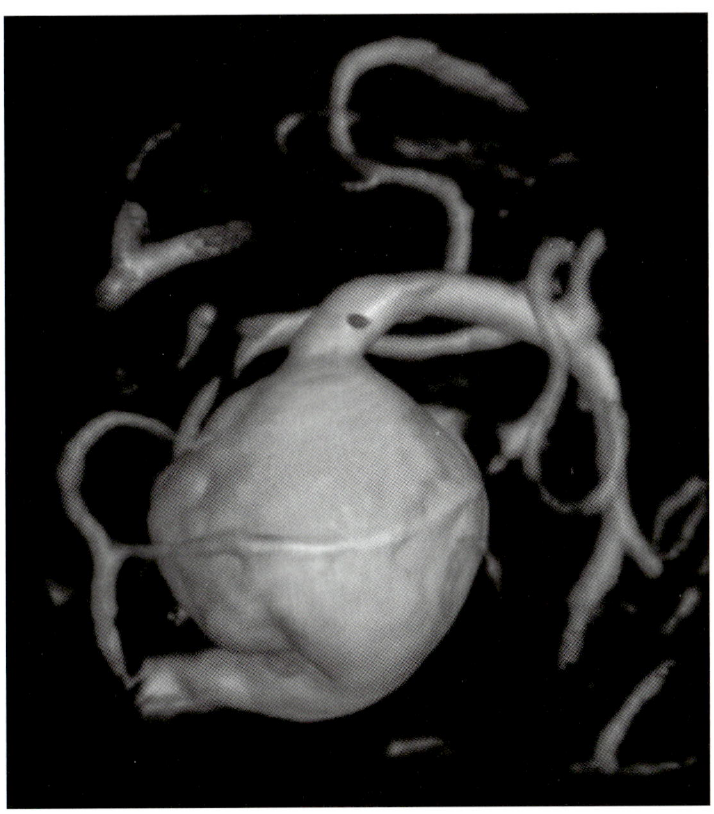

Fig. 7.3c Preoperative three-dimensional angiographic reconstruction shows the giant left MCA aneurysm. (Courtesy of Albert van der Zwan, MD.)

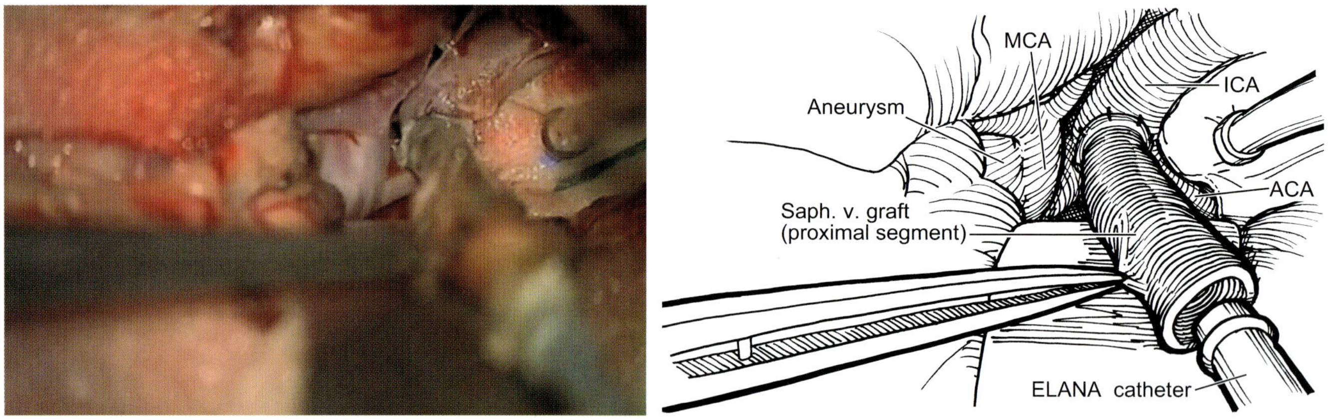

Fig. 7.3d A segment of the saphenous vein graft that will form the proximal half of the bypass has been sutured to the supraclinoid ICA. The ELANA catheter is then introduced into the saphenous vein graft and used to punch a hole through the wall of the ICA. (Photograph courtesy of Albert van der Zwan, MD.)

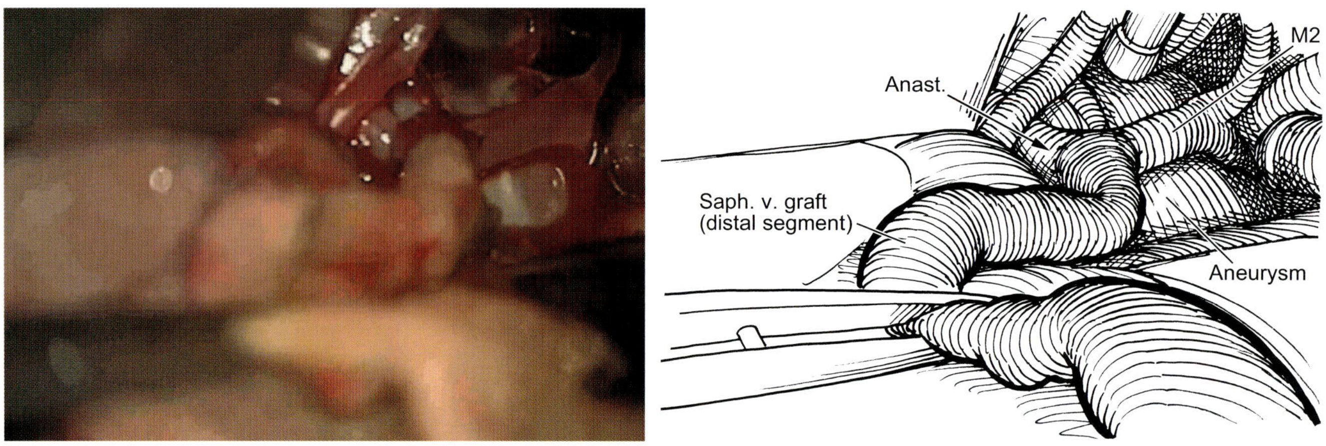

Fig. 7.3e The previous step is repeated with the segment of the saphenous vein graft that forms the distal half of the bypass, which is sutured to a distal MCA branch. The two segments of the saphenous vein graft are then anastomosed to complete the bypass. (Photograph courtesy of Albert van der Zwan, MD.)

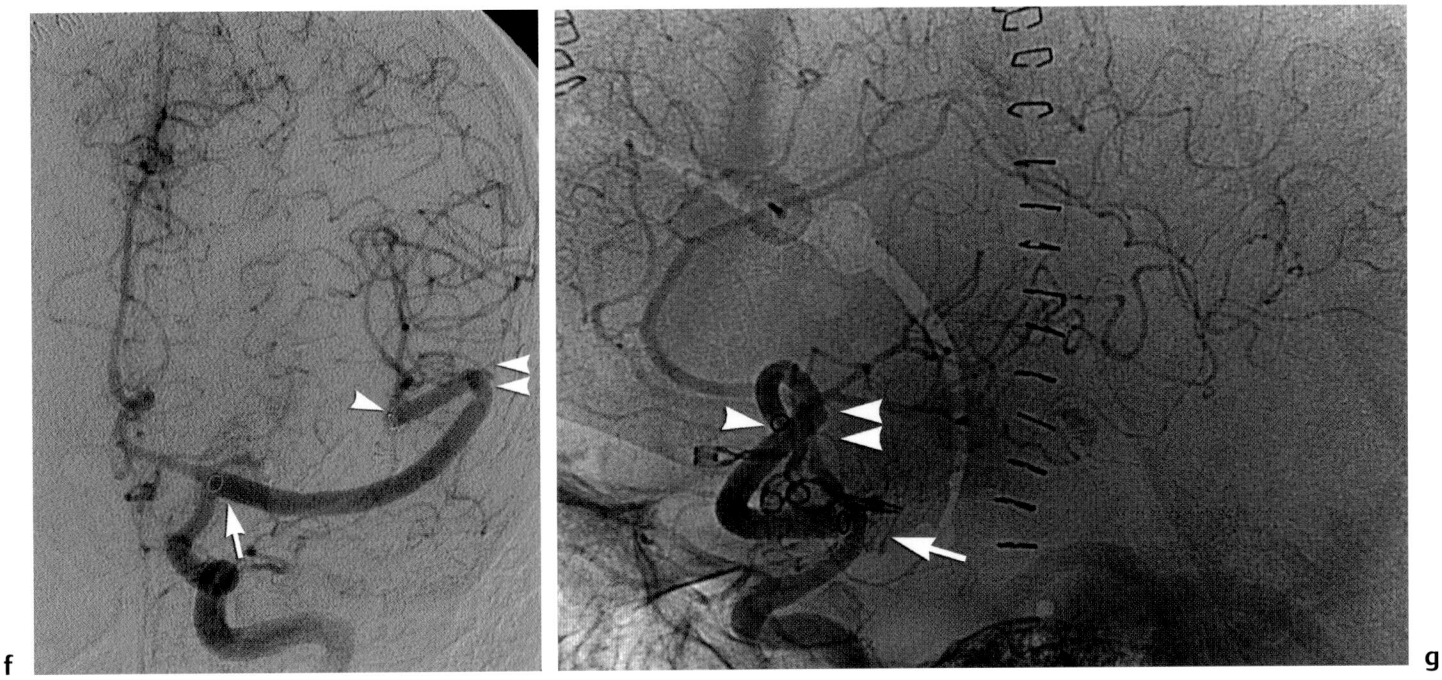

Fig. 7.3f, g Postoperative anteroposterior and lateral angiograms show the proximal (*arrow*) and distal (*arrowhead*) ELANA anastomosis as well as the end-to-end anastomosis (*double arrowheads*) of the two segments of the saphenous vein graft of the ICA-to-M2 bypass. (Courtesy of Albert van der Zwan, MD.)

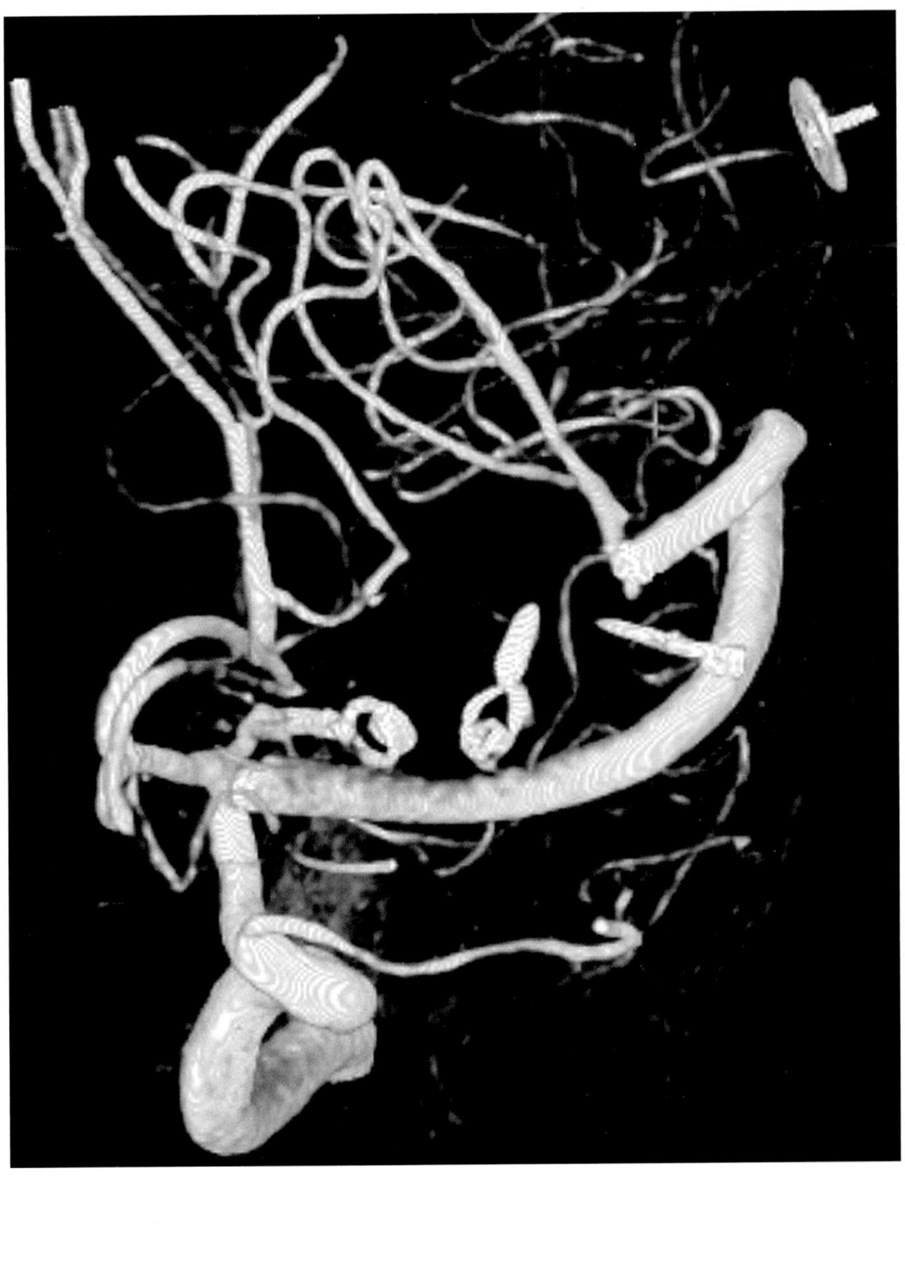

Fig. 7.3h Postoperative CT angiographic reconstruction shows the ELANA ICA-to-M2 bypass and the clips trapping the aneurysm. (Courtesy of Albert van der Zwan, MD.)

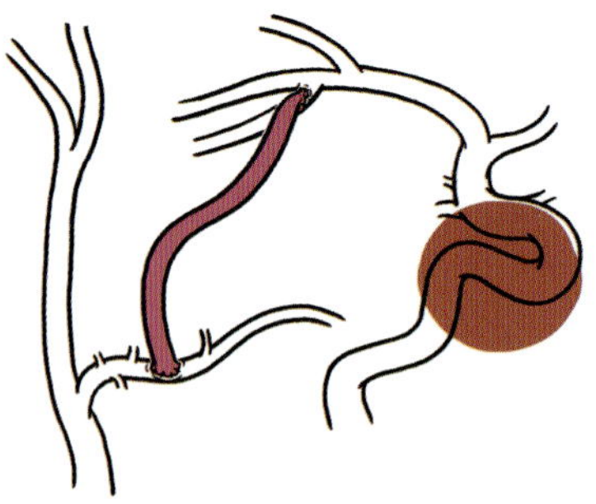

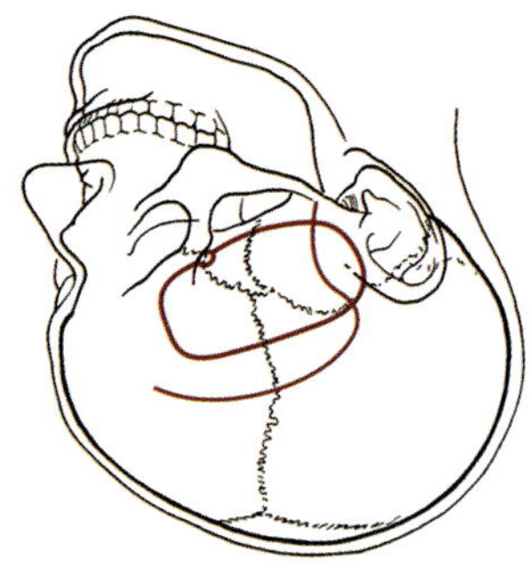

Case 7-4

Diagnosis: Giant cavernous sinus ICA aneurysm

Bypass: Abdulrauf IMA-to-MCA bypass

Approach: Right pterional with subtemporal extension

Video

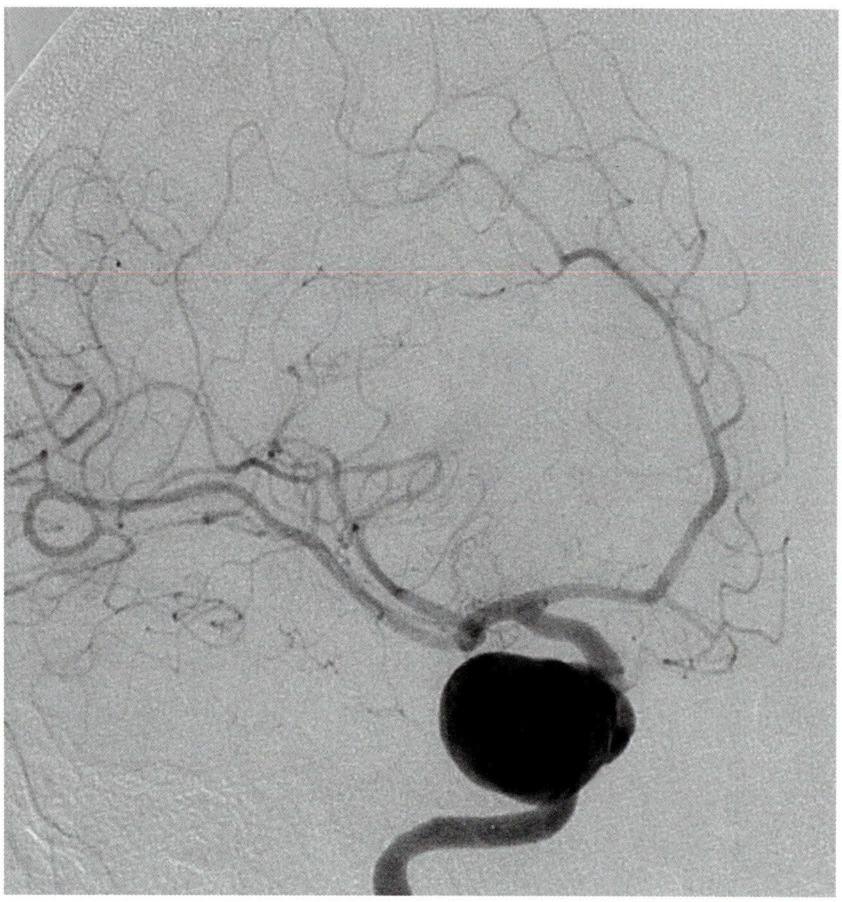

Fig. 7.4a A 57-year-old woman had progressive CN VI paresis on the right side. Right ICA angiogram shows a large cavernous sinus aneurysm. (Courtesy of Saleem I. Abdulrauf, MD, FACS.)

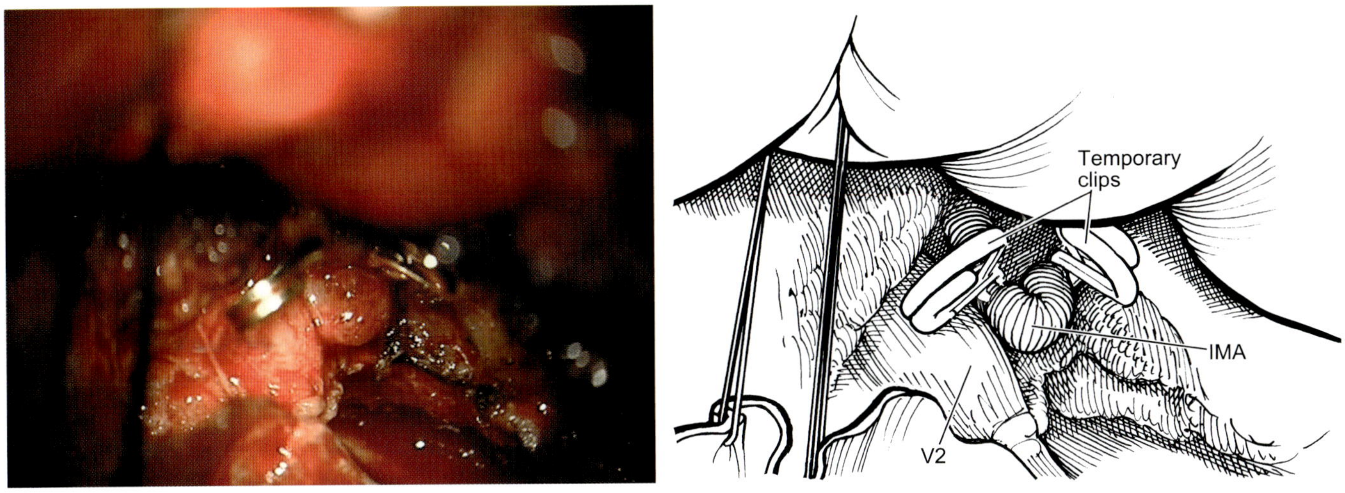

Fig. 7.4b Right-sided intraoperative view of the infratemporal fossa shows temporary clips on the anterior loop of the IMA adjacent to V2. (Photograph courtesy of Saleem I. Abdulrauf, MD, FACS.)

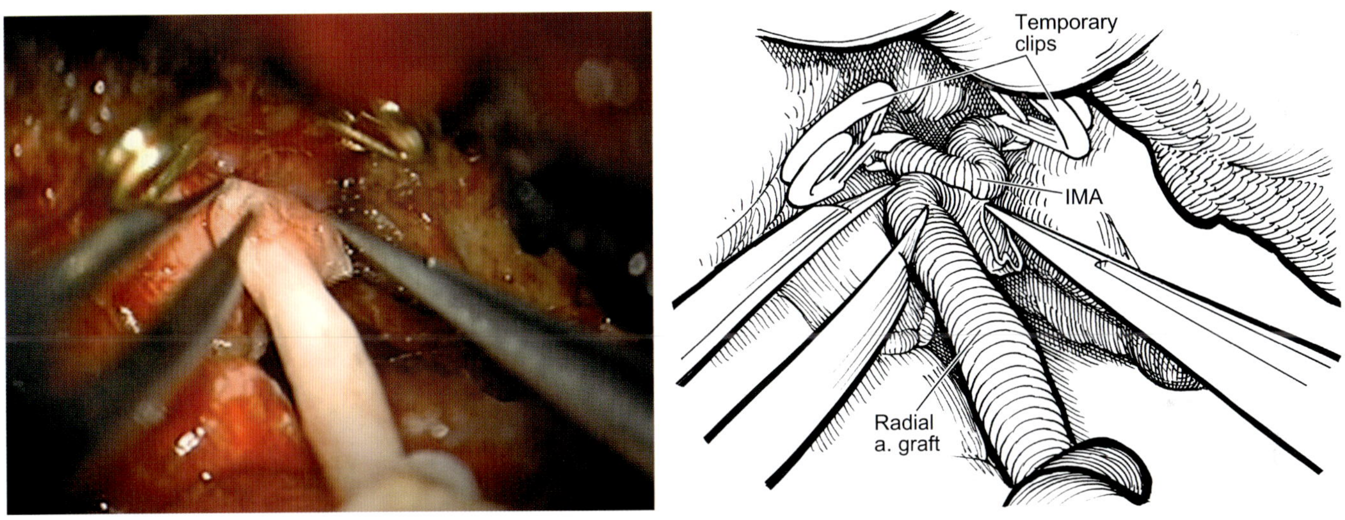

Fig. 7.4c Proximal end of the radial artery graft is anastomosed to the IMA. (Photograph courtesy of Saleem I. Abdulrauf, MD, FACS.)

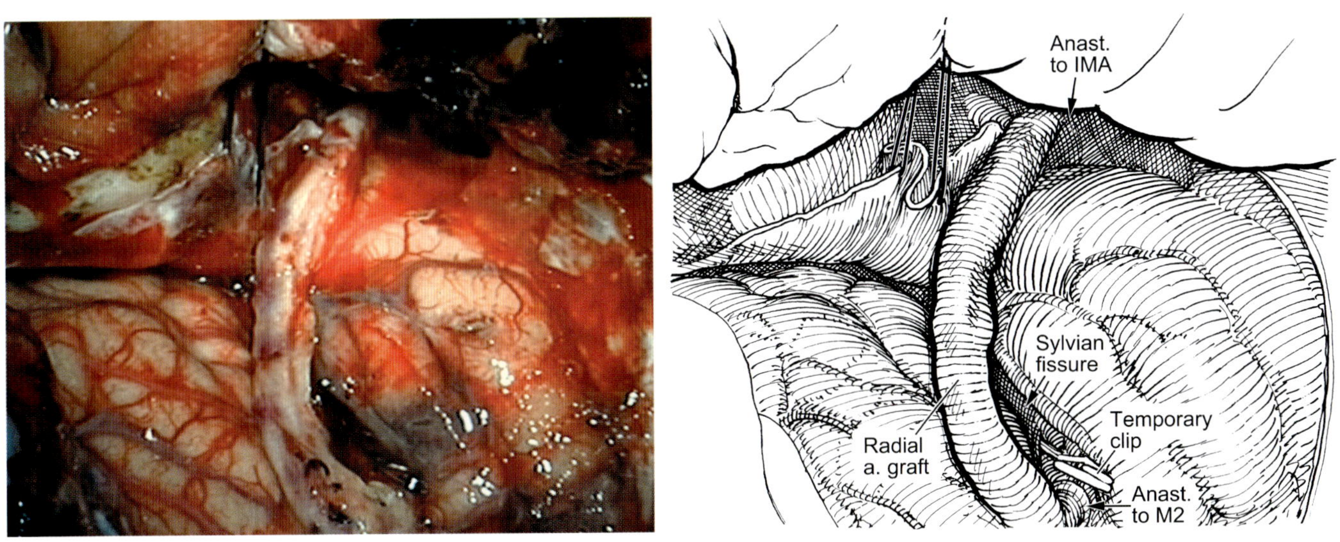

Fig. 7.4d Radial artery interposition graft is visible between the IMA and the M2 segment of the MCA. (Photograph courtesy of Saleem I. Abdulrauf, MD, FACS.)

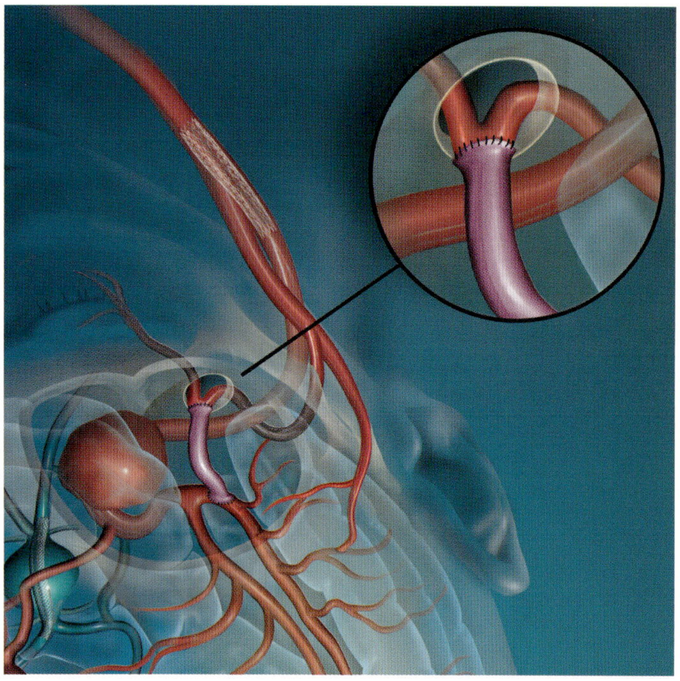

Fig. 7.4e Artist's rendering of Abdulrauf bypass. The interposition radial artery graft is anastomosed from the IMA, side-to-end, and to the M2, end-to-side. (Courtesy of Saleem I. Abdulrauf, MD, FACS.)

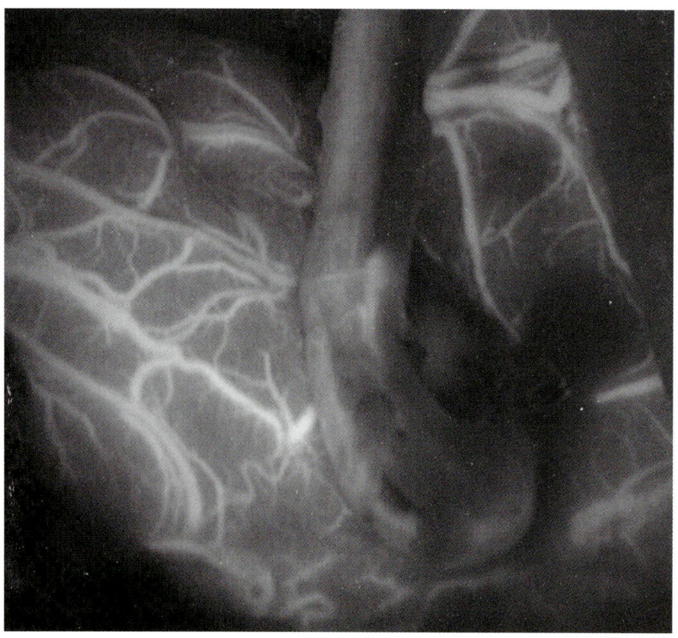

Fig. 7.4f Intraoperative ICG angiogram confirms patency of the radial artery graft. (Courtesy of Saleem I. Abdulrauf, MD, FACS.)

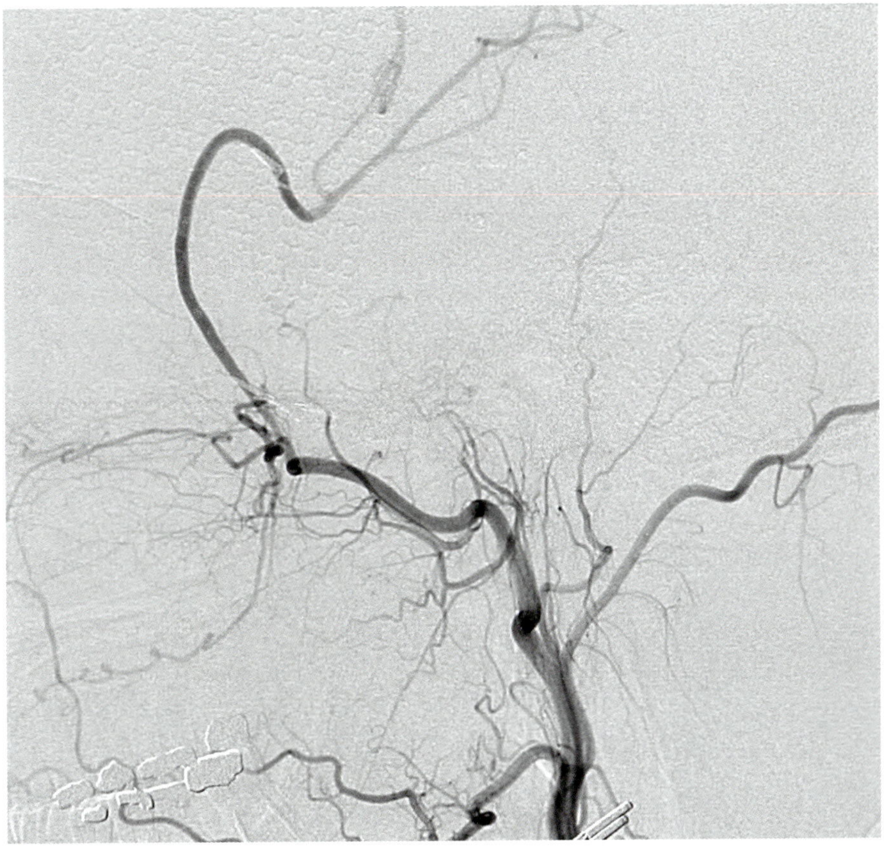

Fig. 7.4g Intraoperative angiogram shows the bypass formed by the interposition radial artery graft from the IMA to M2. (Courtesy of Saleem I. Abdulrauf, MD, FACS.)

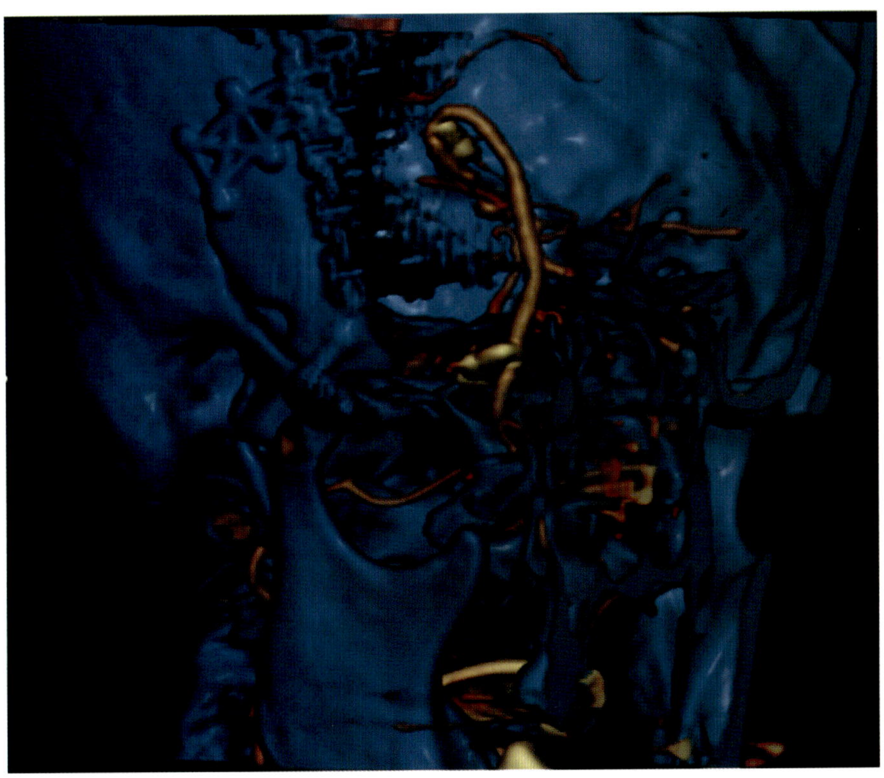

Fig. 7.4h Postoperative three-dimensional reconstruction CT angiogram shows the patent radial artery bypass graft between the IMA and M2. (Courtesy of Saleem I. Abdulrauf, MD, FACS.)

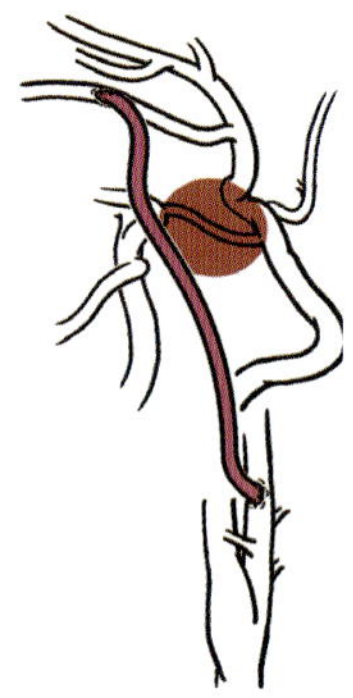

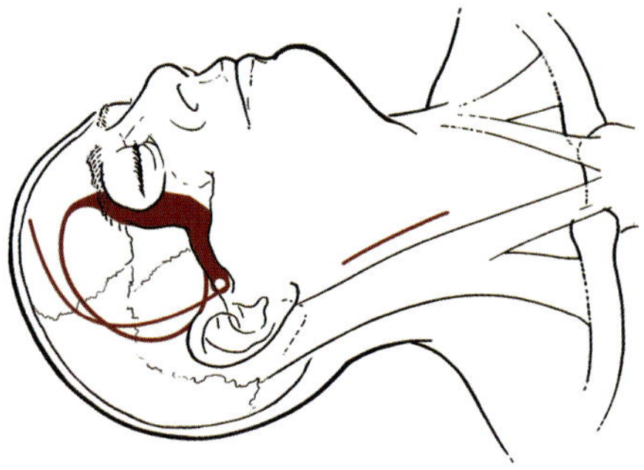

Case 7-5

Diagnosis: Giant right PCoA aneurysm after previous coiling

Bypass: Right ECA-to-MCA with radial artery graft

Approach: Right orbitozygomatic and anterior cervical

Video

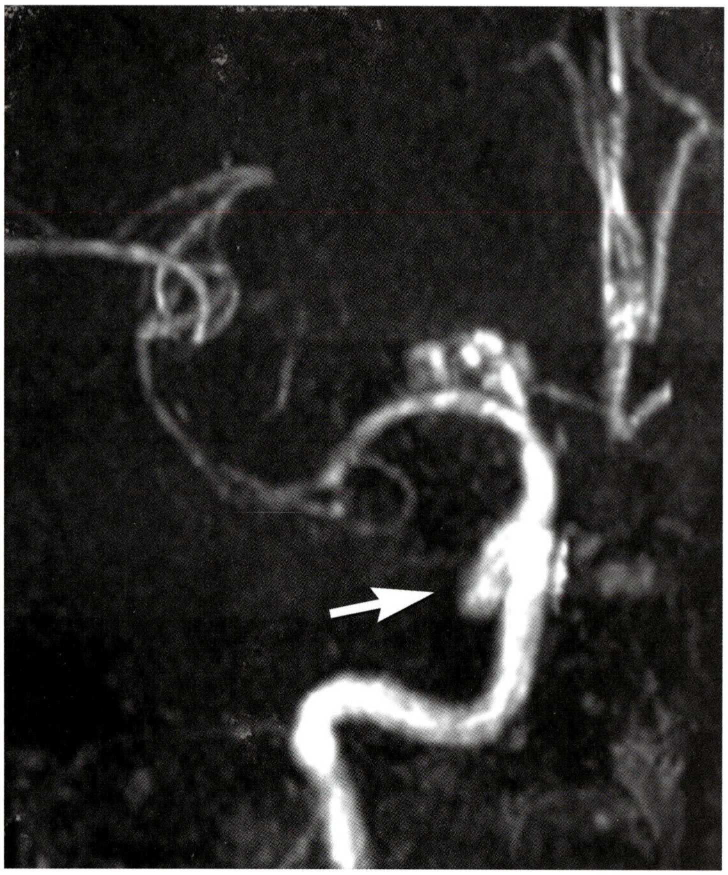

Fig. 7.5a Anteroposterior MR angiogram shows a complex, partially thrombosed aneurysm (*arrow*) in the region of the right PCoA.

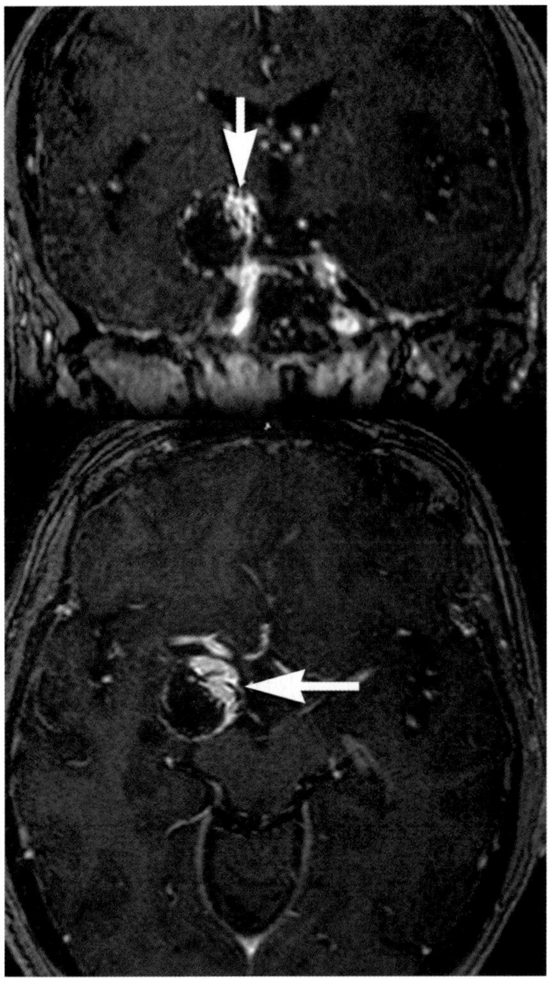

Fig. 7.5b Coronal and axial MR images demonstrate the size of the aneurysm (*arrows*). (Axial image used with permission from *Journal of Neurosurgery*.)

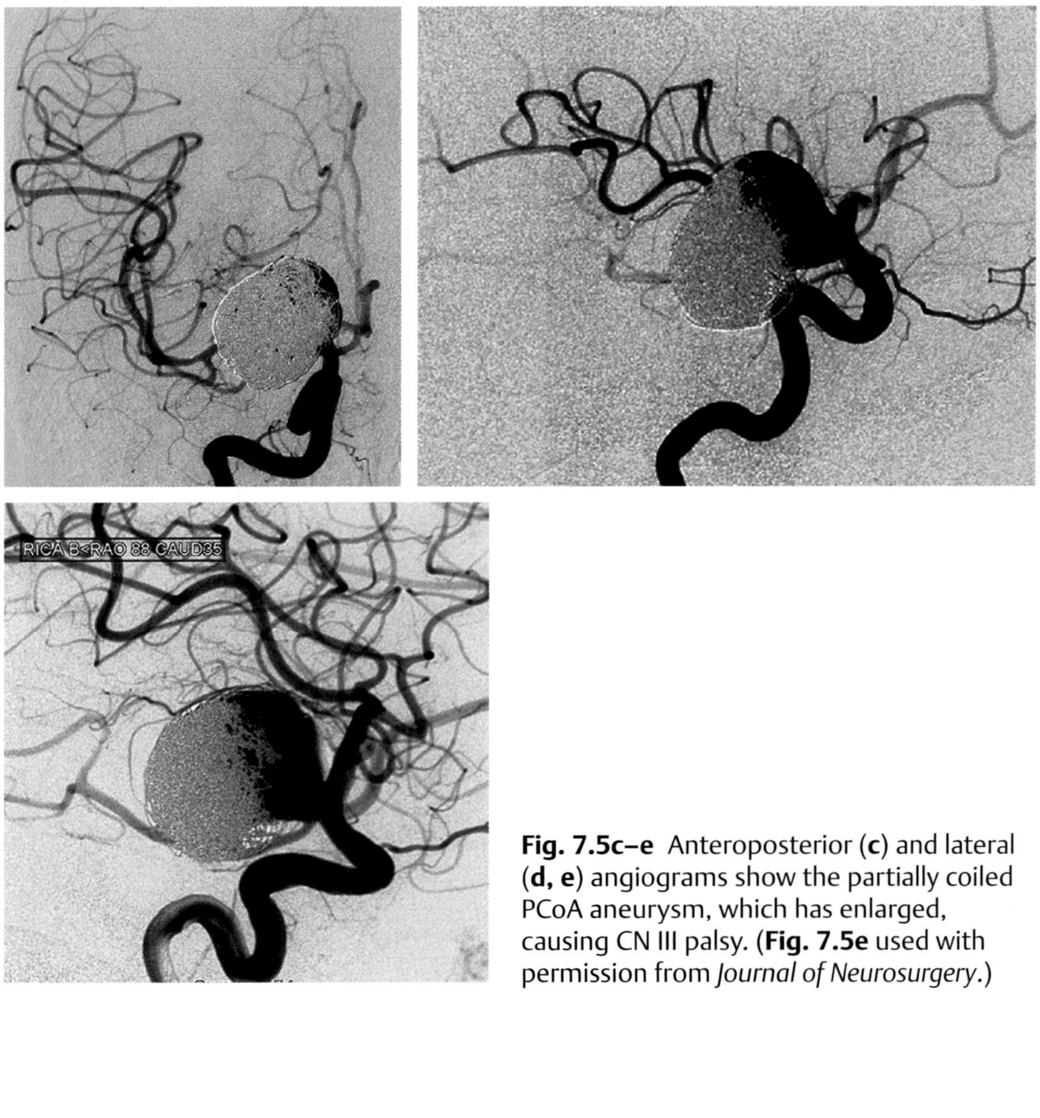

c d e

Fig. 7.5c–e Anteroposterior (**c**) and lateral (**d, e**) angiograms show the partially coiled PCoA aneurysm, which has enlarged, causing CN III palsy. (**Fig. 7.5e** used with permission from *Journal of Neurosurgery*.)

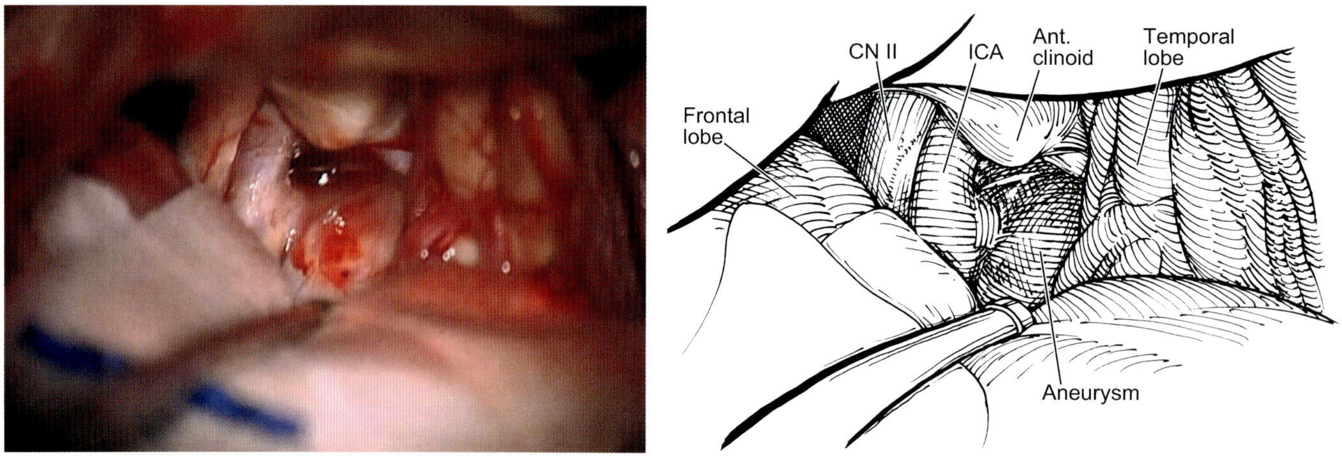

Fig. 7.5f Intraoperative photograph shows the right ICA with a large PCoA aneurysm. Because of the wide neck of the aneurysm and the presence of the stent and coils, the patient had been prepared for a radial artery graft.

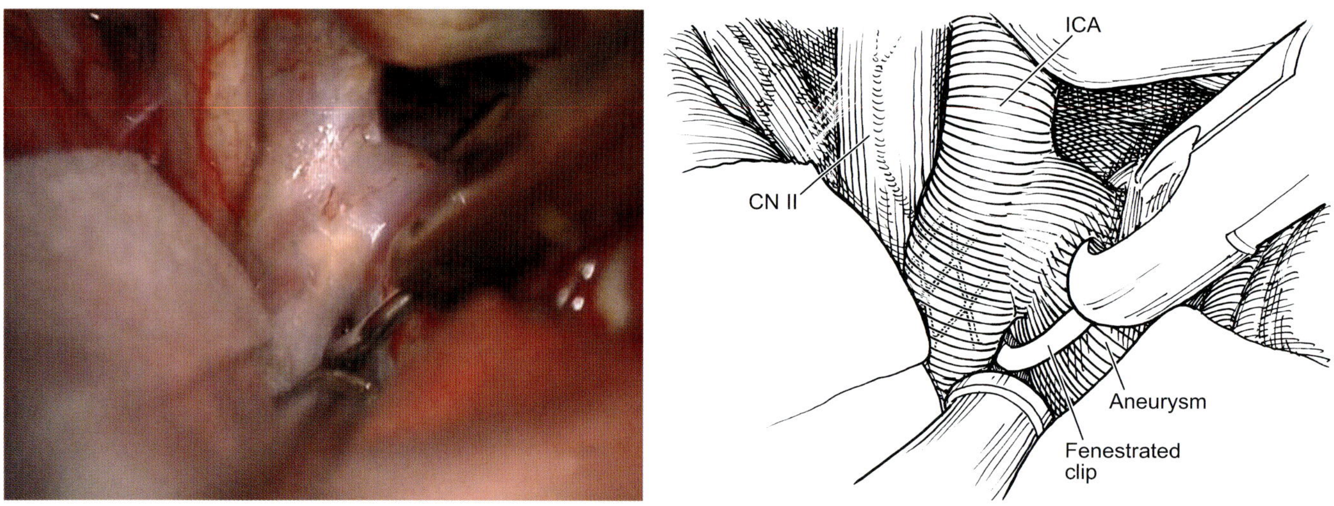

Fig. 7.5g A fenestrated clip has been placed on the neck of the aneurysm with the goal of occluding the most distal part of its neck. Then a straight clip would have been placed to close the opening of the fenestration.

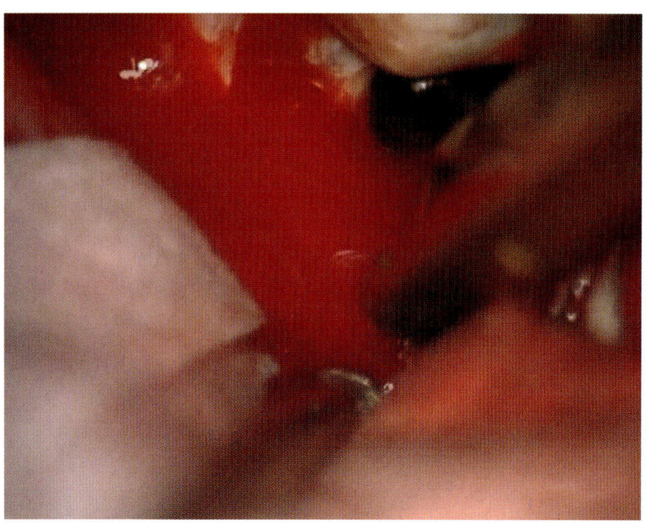

Fig. 7.5h The neck of the aneurysm has ruptured.

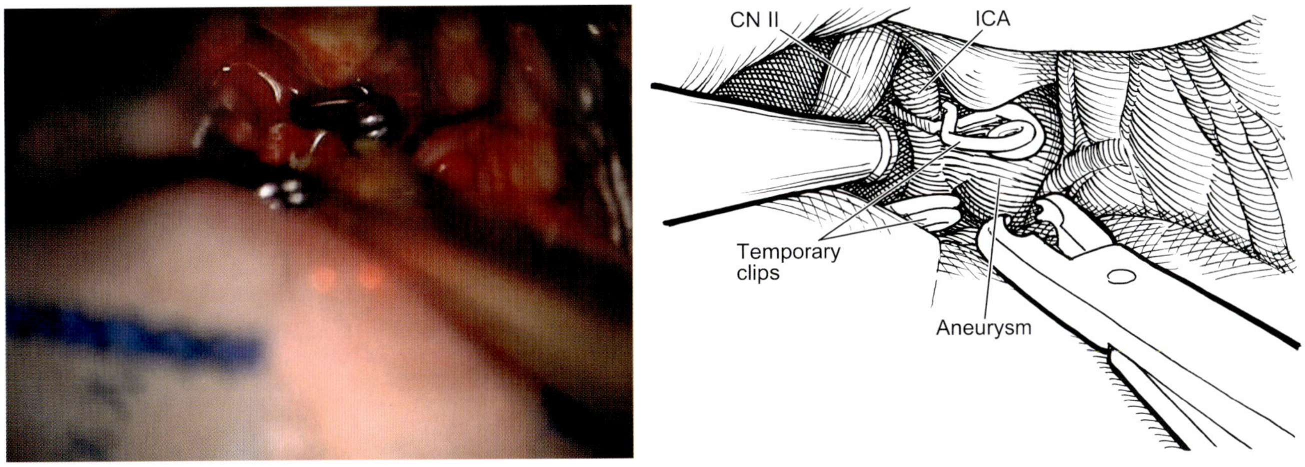

Fig. 7.5i Temporary clips are placed proximally and distally on the ICA to control the hemorrhage.

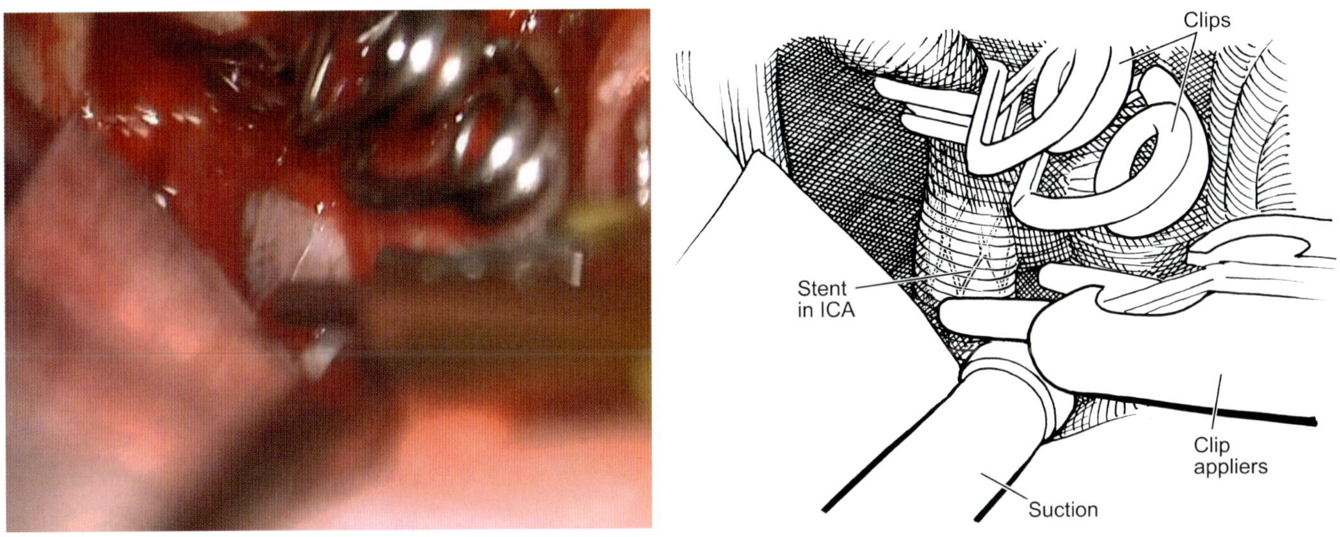

Fig. 7.5j Multiple clips have been placed on the ICA to occlude the neck of the aneurysm. The prongs of the stent are visible.

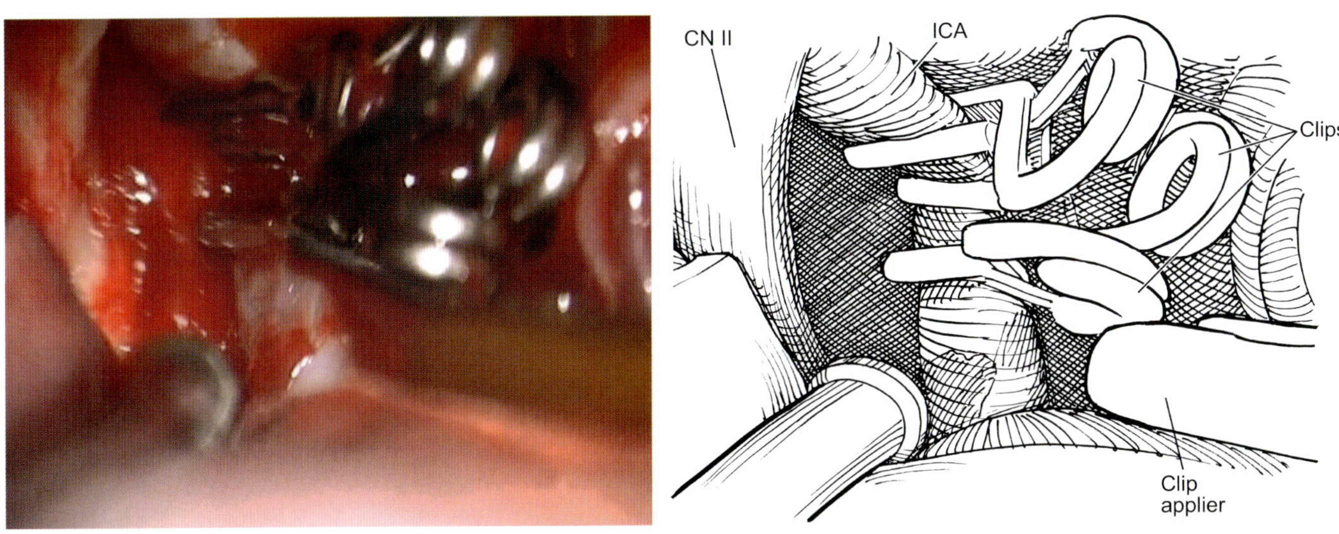

Fig. 7.5k After the multiple clips were placed on the ICA, the bleeding is controlled. Every attempt was made to preserve the origin of the AChoA.

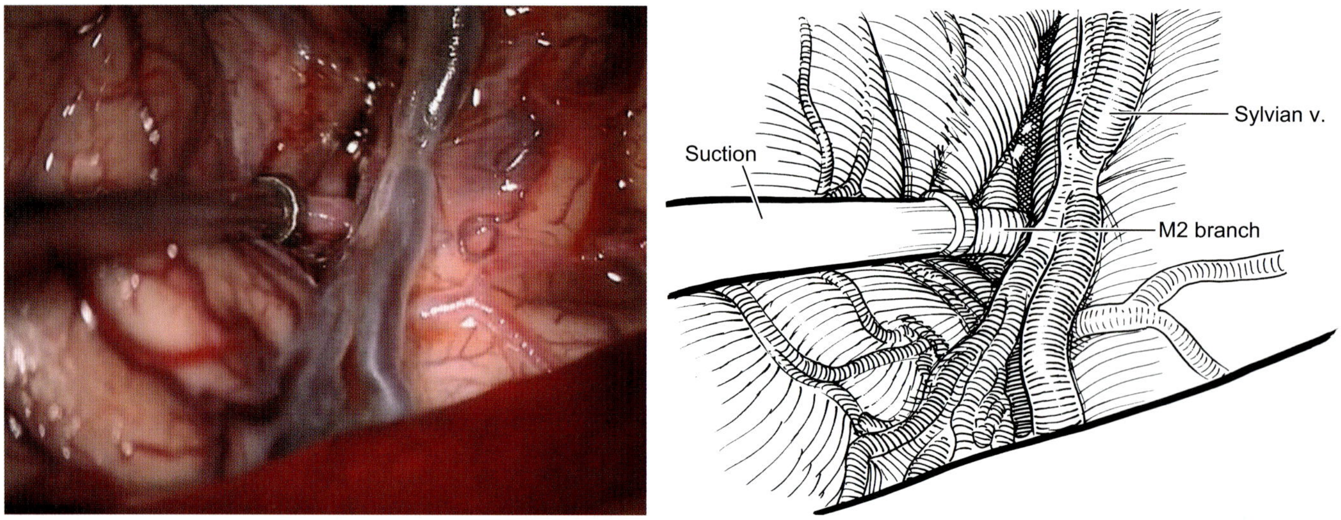

Fig. 7.5l The right M2 branch is prepared for a bypass.

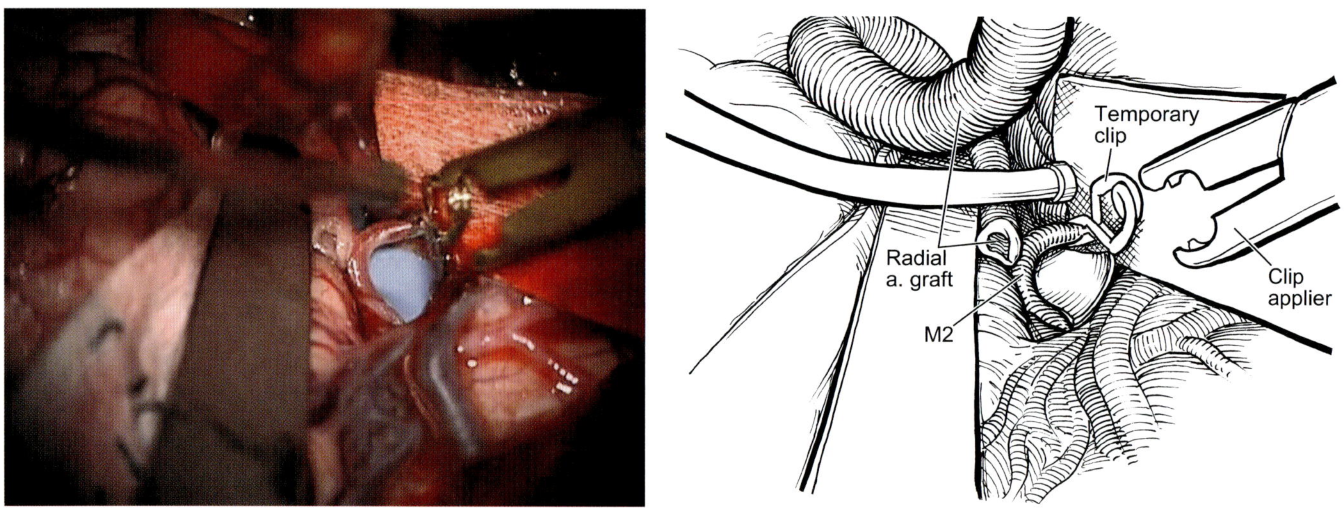

Fig. 7.5m A temporary clip is placed on the M2 branch selected for the bypass.

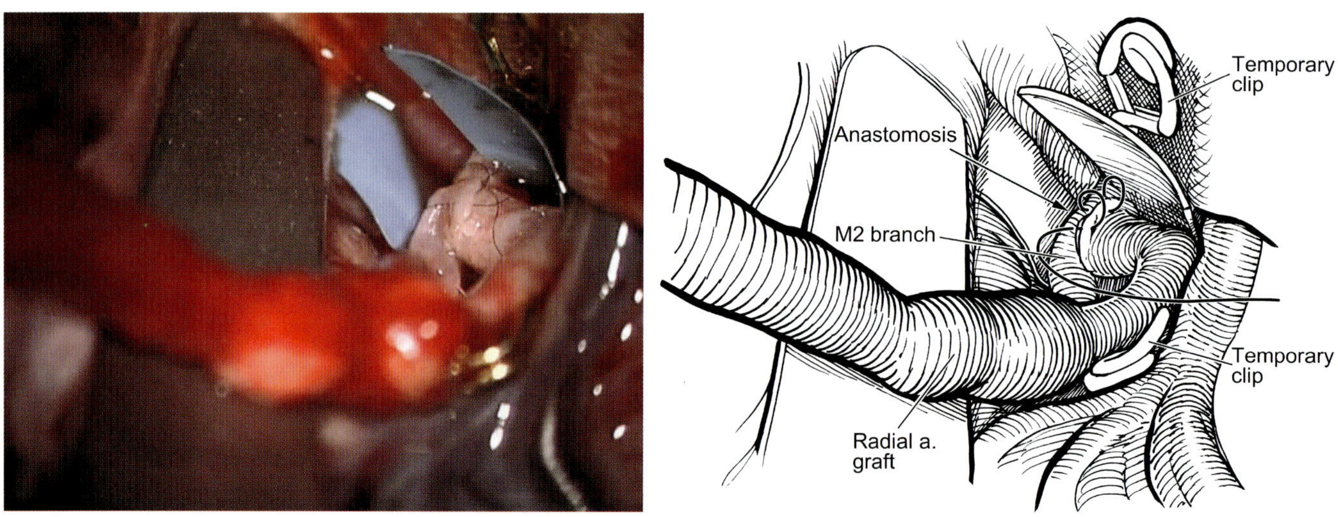

Fig. 7.5n The radial artery graft is being anastomosed end-to-side to the recipient MCA vessel.

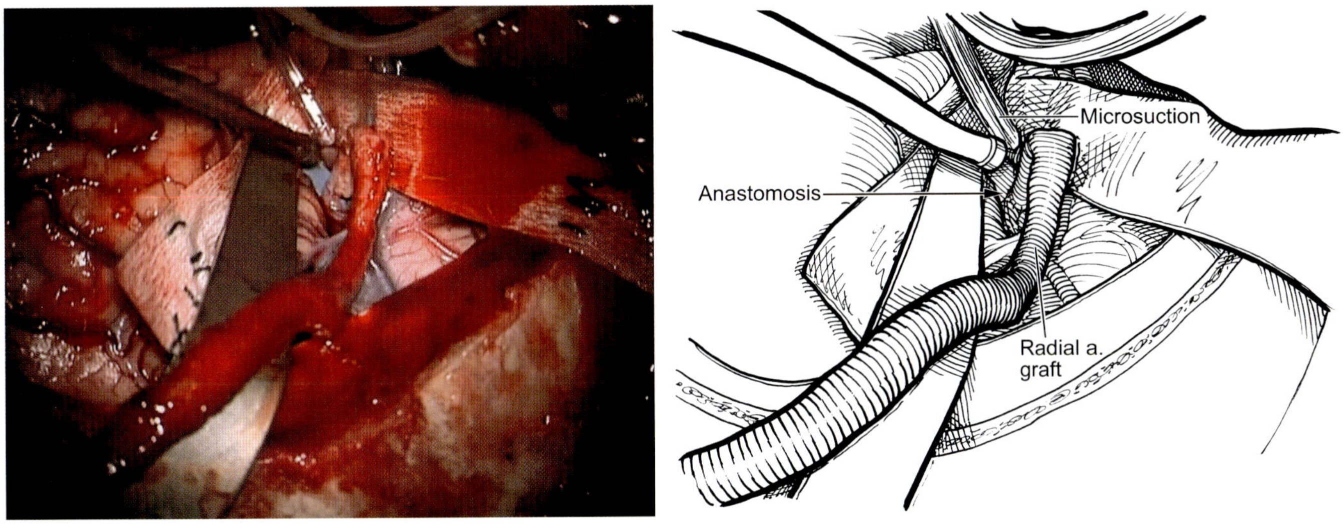

Fig. 7.5o The anastomosis is completed.

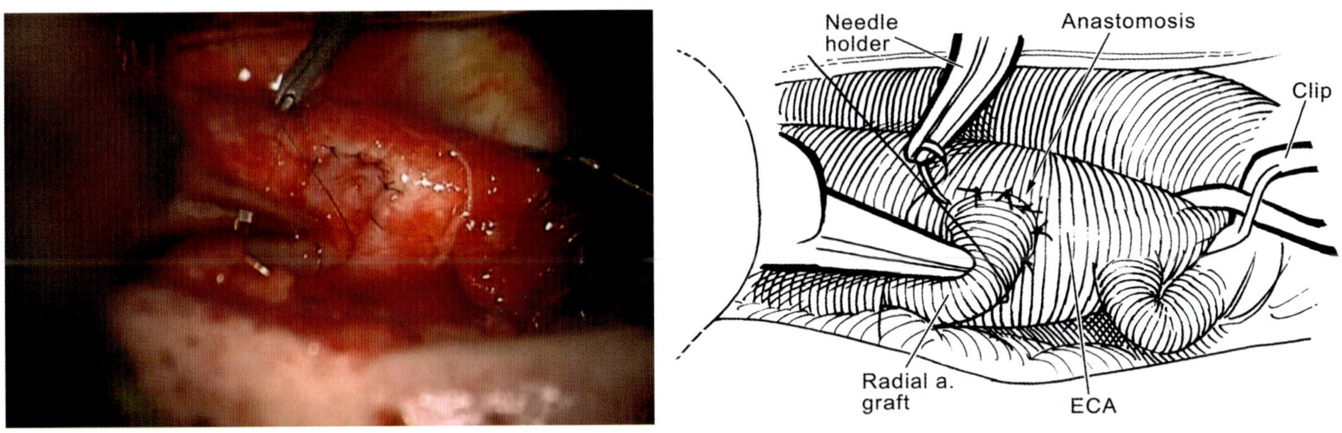

Fig. 7.5p After the radial artery graft was tunneled subcutaneously, it is anastomosed end-to-side to the ECA.

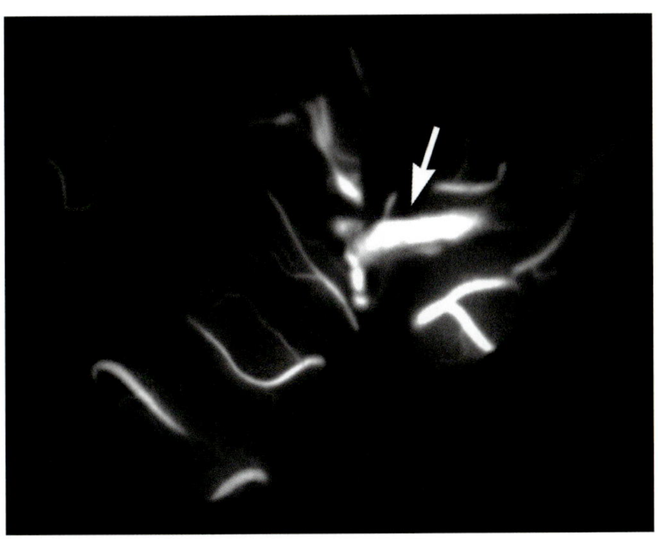

Fig. 7.5q ICG angiogram confirms patency of the bypass (*arrow*).

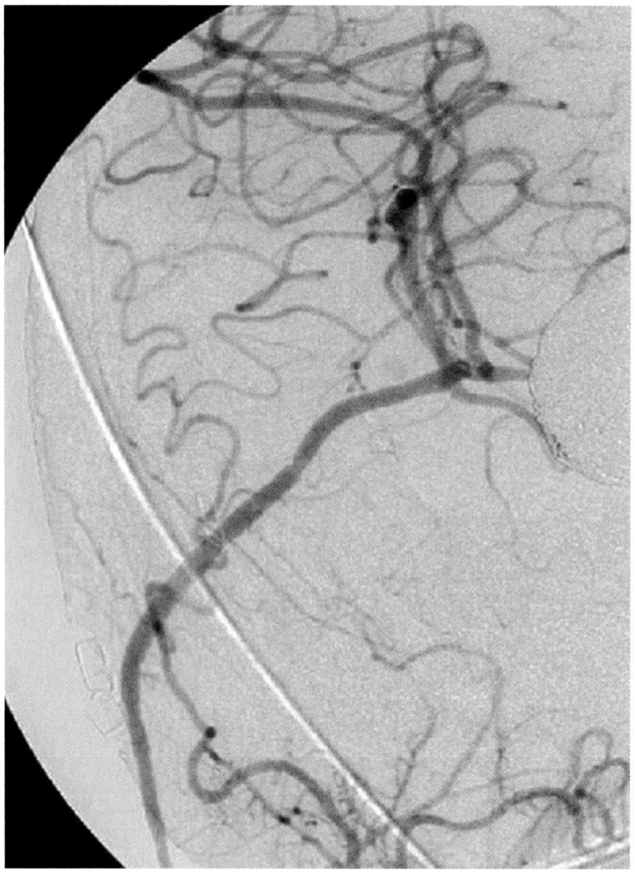

Fig. 7.5r Intraoperative angiogram confirms excellent patency of the radial artery graft bypass. From the start of the procedure, the patient was placed in a barbiturate coma to EEG burst suppression.

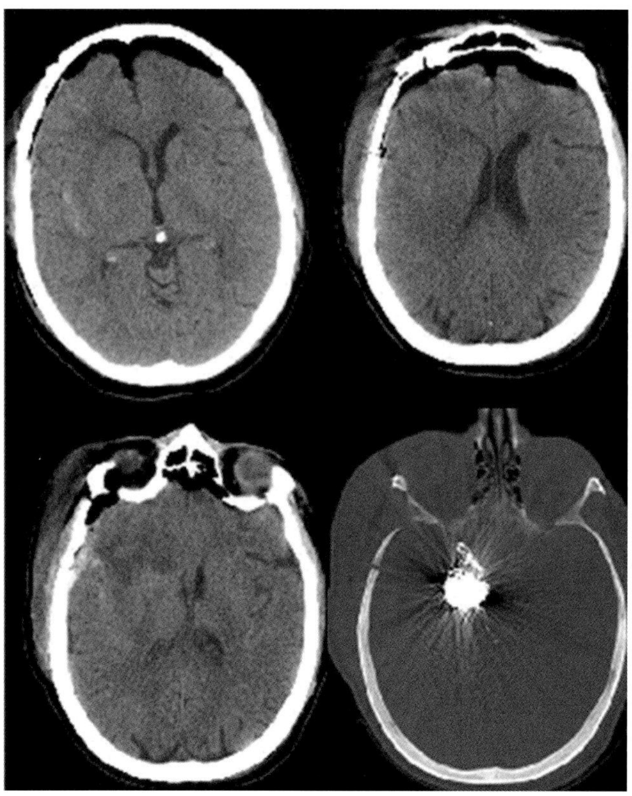

Fig. 7.5s Postoperative CT scans show no infarction.

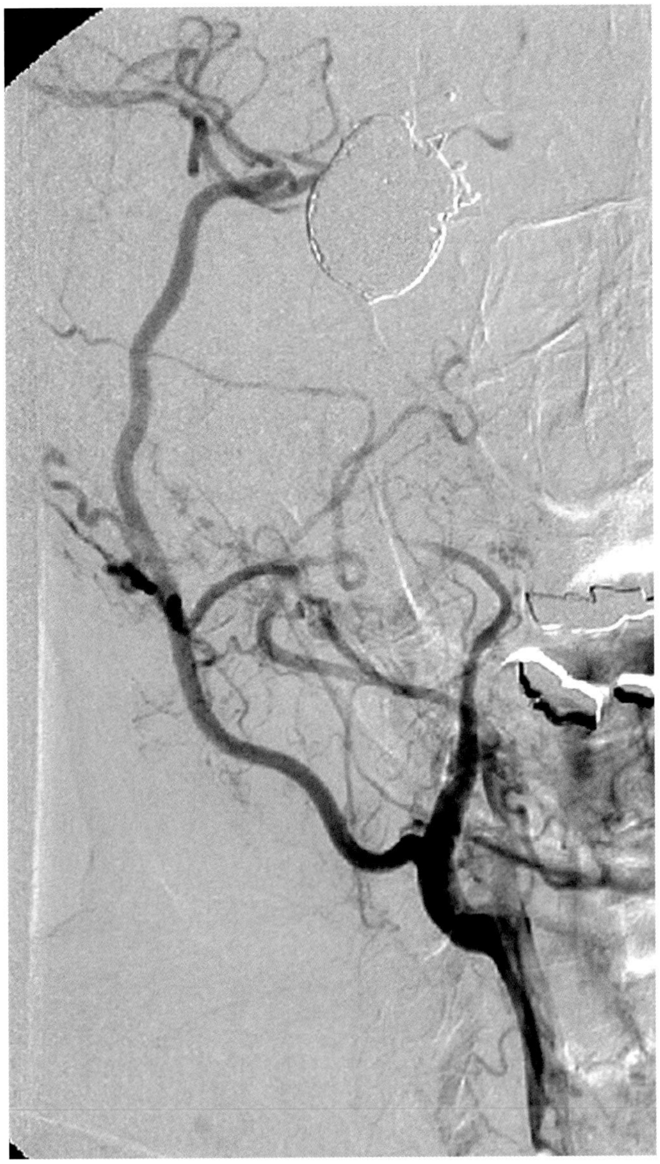

Fig. 7.5t Postoperative anteroposterior angiographic projection shows the radial artery graft from the ECA to the recipient MCA. (Used with permission from *Journal of Neurosurgery*.)

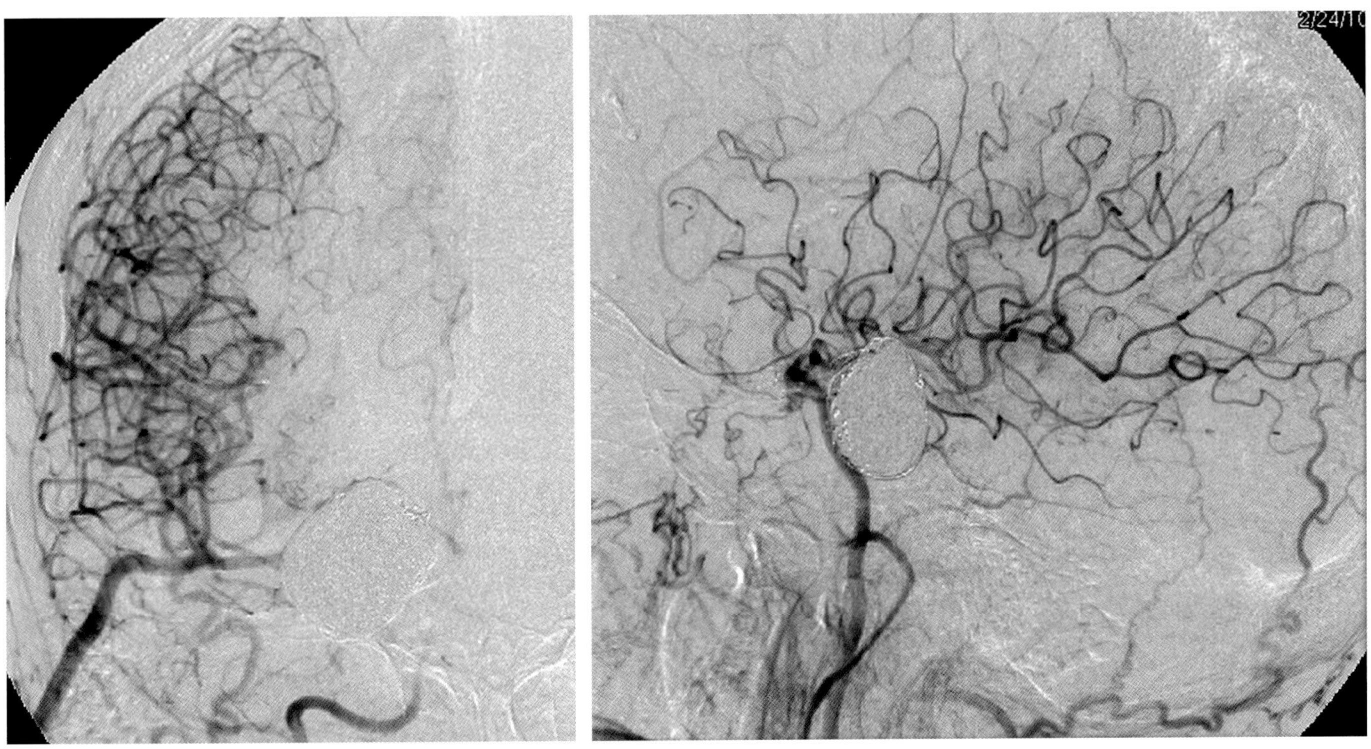

Fig. 7.5u, v Anteroposterior and lateral angiographic views of the bypass formed with the radial artery graft. Postoperatively, the patient had no neurological deficits.

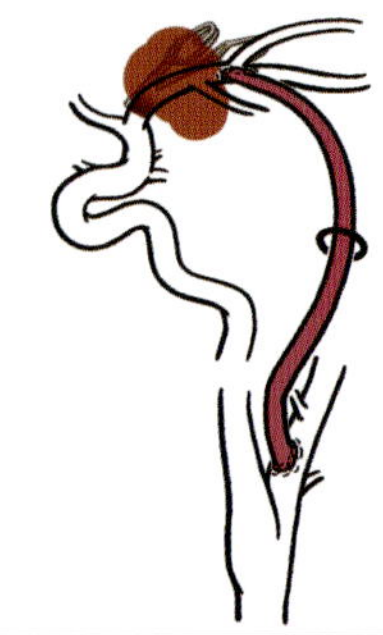

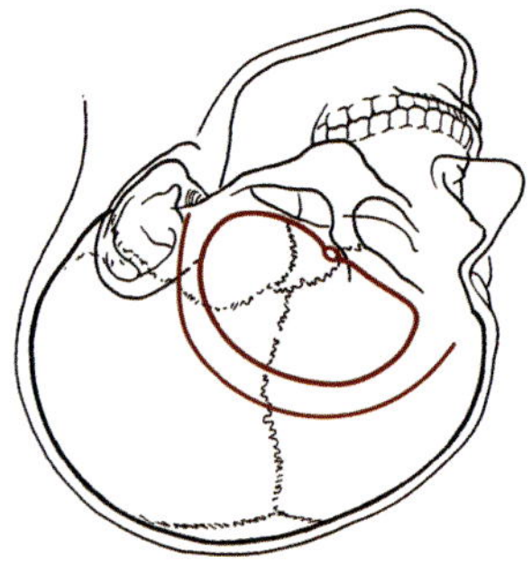

Case 7-6

Diagnosis: Recurrent MCA complex aneurysm

Bypass: ECA-to-MCA with radial artery graft and subsequent spontaneous occlusion of proximal MCA

Approach: Left frontotemporal

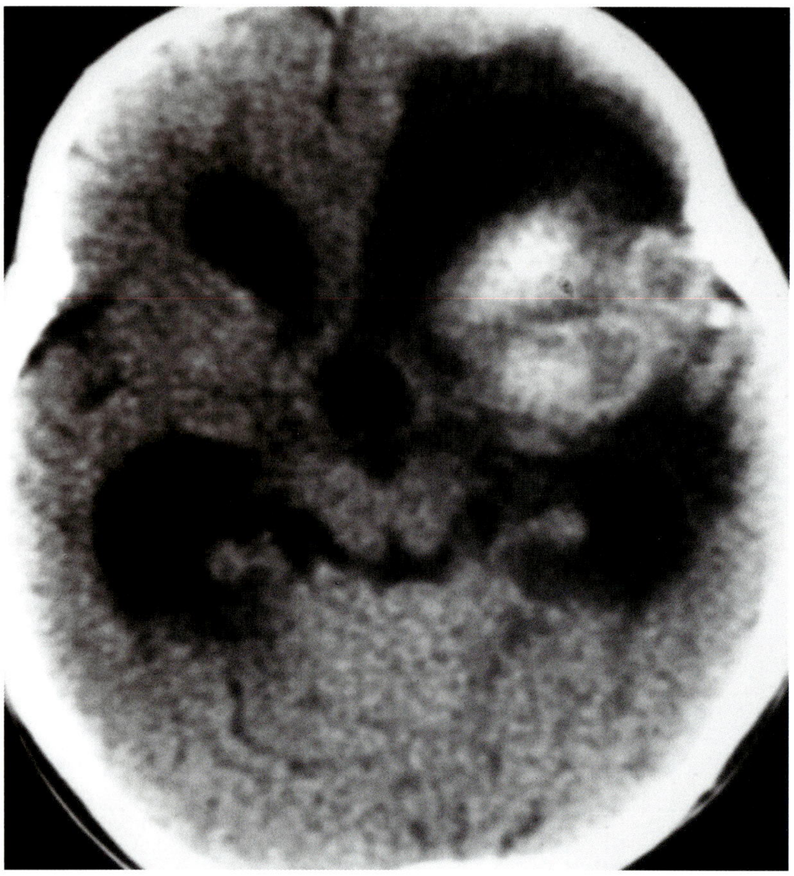

Fig. 7.6a Axial MR shows an MCA aneurysm that hemorrhaged in a 7-month-old boy. The patient was treated and made a good recovery.

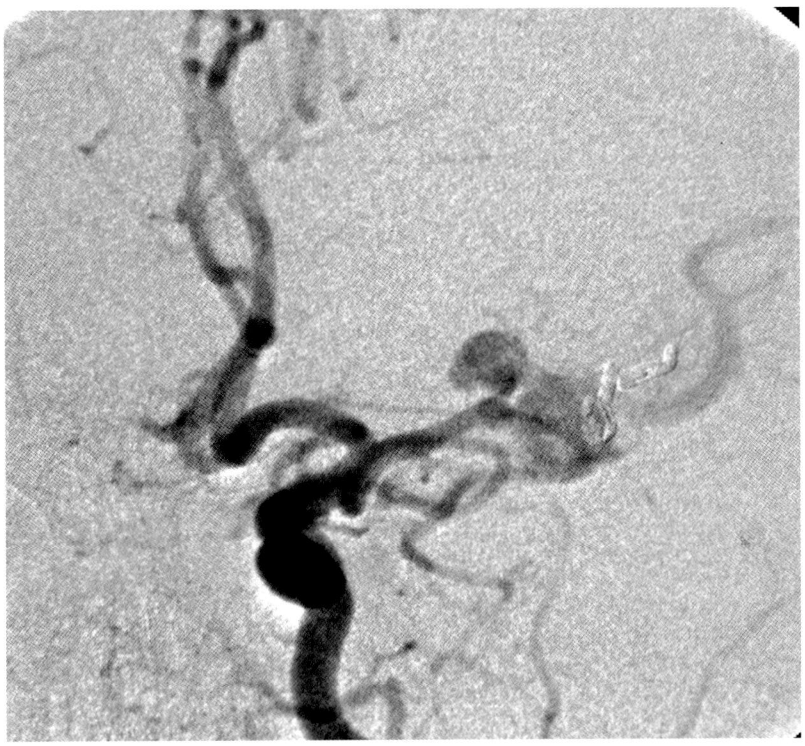

Fig. 7.6b Twelve years later the patient returned with a new onset of headache. Anteroposterior angiogram shows the old clips and a multilobulated dissecting M2–M3 aneurysm.

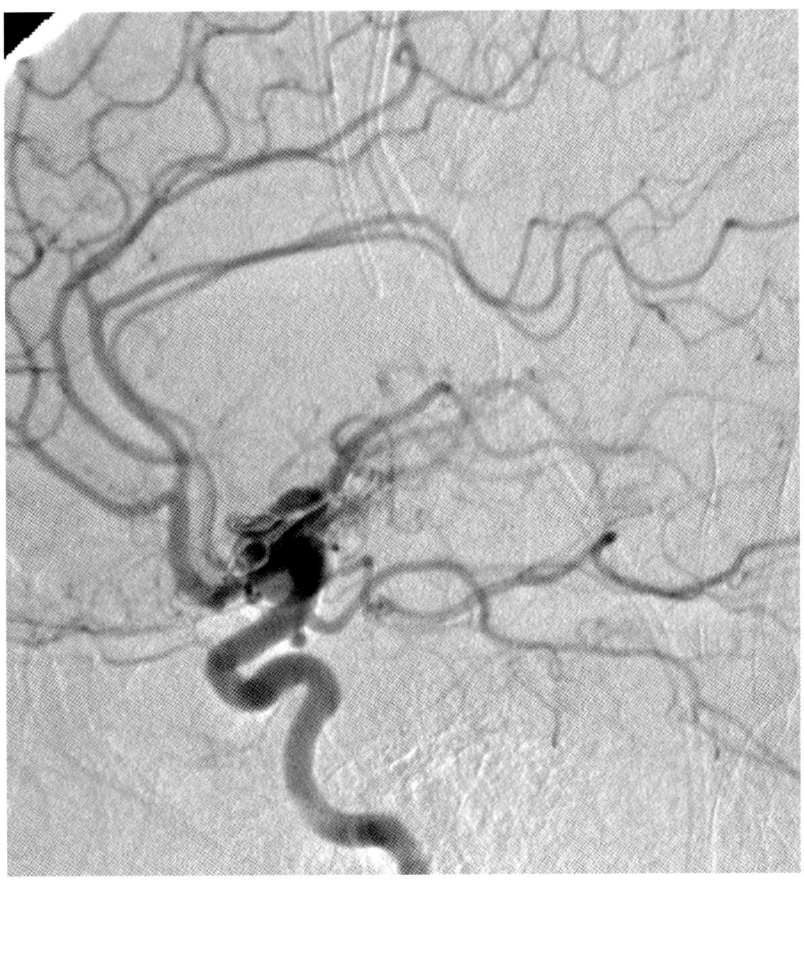

Fig. 7.6c Lateral angiographic projection shows the complex aneurysm and poor filling of some of the branches of the MCA.

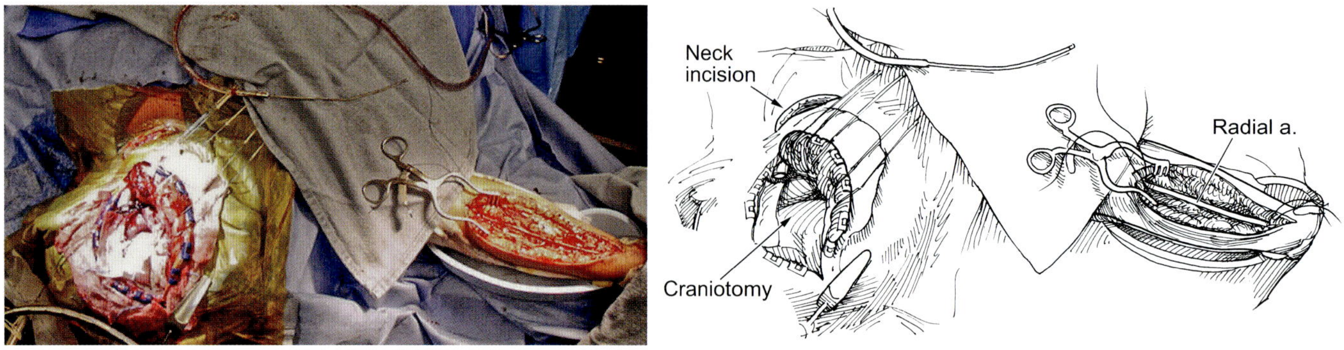

Fig. 7.6d Overview shows the craniotomy, neck incision, and exposed radial artery.

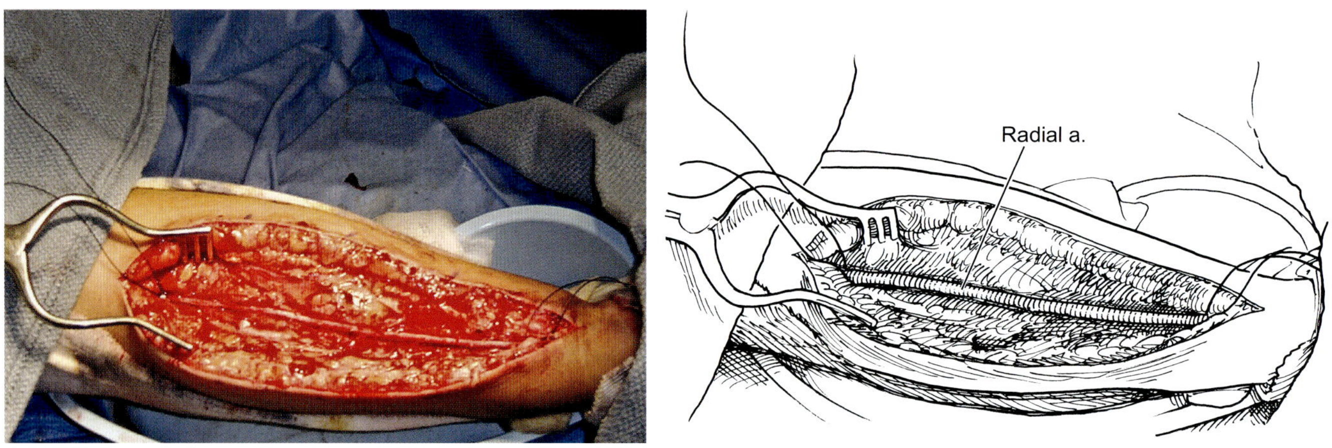

Fig. 7.6e Close-up of the exposed radial artery. Although this artery can be harvested endoscopically, we believe that an open approach is less traumatic to the donor vessel.

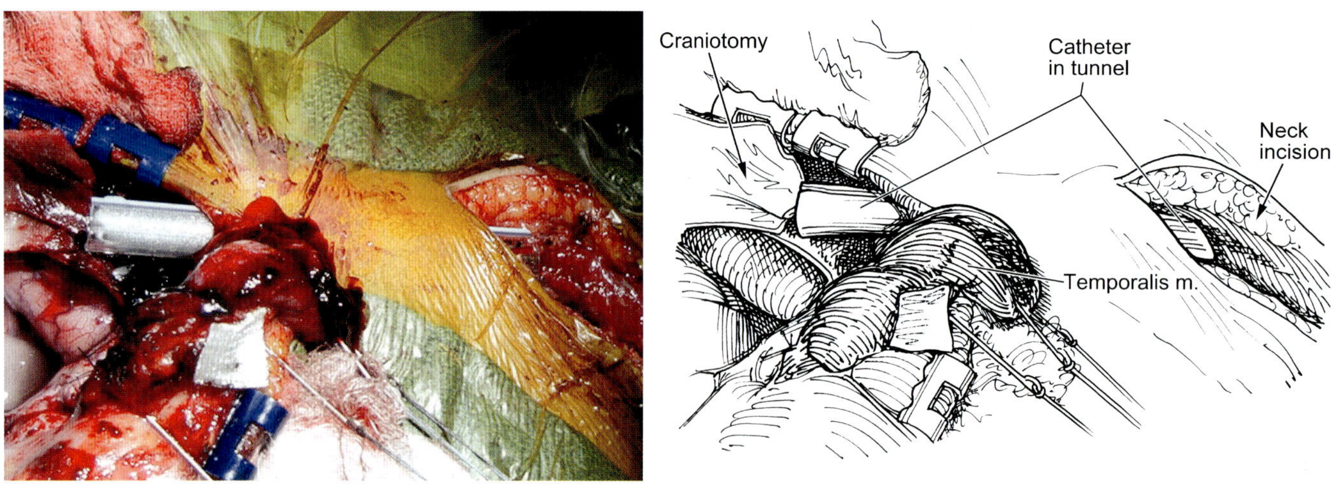

Fig. 7.6f The catheter is tunneled subcutaneously from the neck incision to the cranial incision. The radial artery graft is then passed through its lumen.

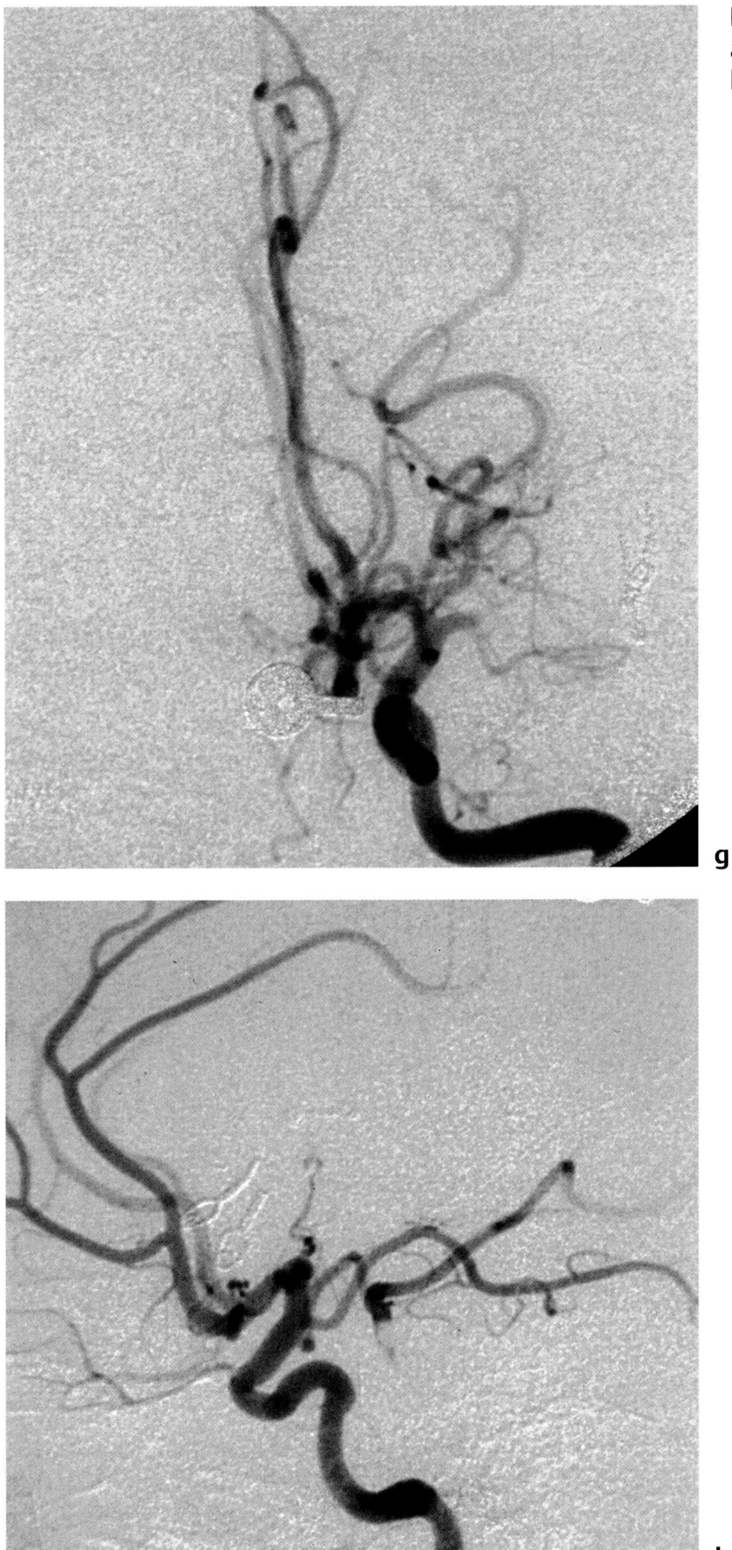

Fig. 7.6g, h Anteroposterior and lateral left ICA angiograms show that the MCA flow to the aneurysm has been eliminated.

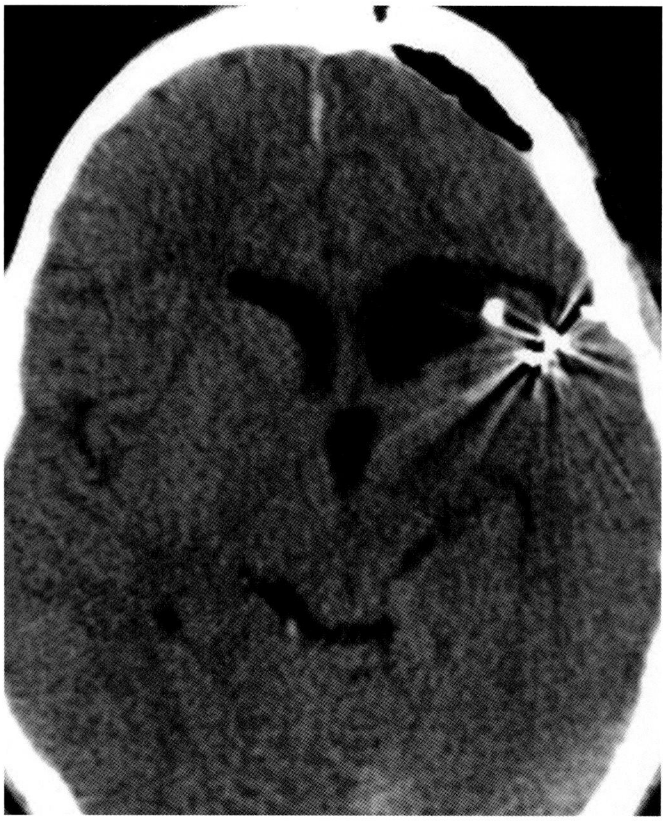

Fig. 7.6i Postoperative axial CT shows evidence of the old hemorrhage that the patient suffered as an infant but no further damage.

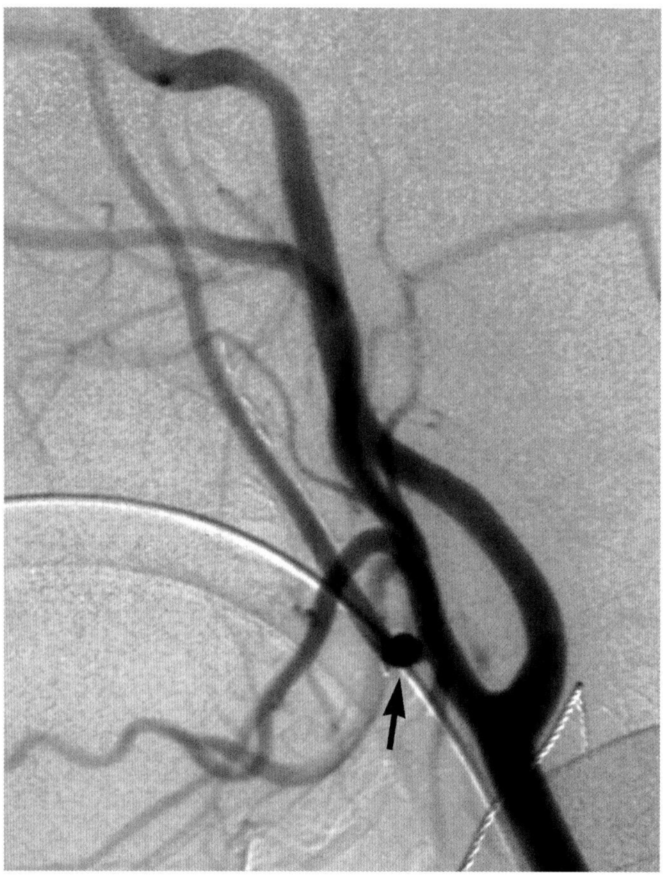

Fig. 7.6j Postoperative lateral left CCA angiographic injection shows the radial artery graft arising from the ECA (*arrow*).

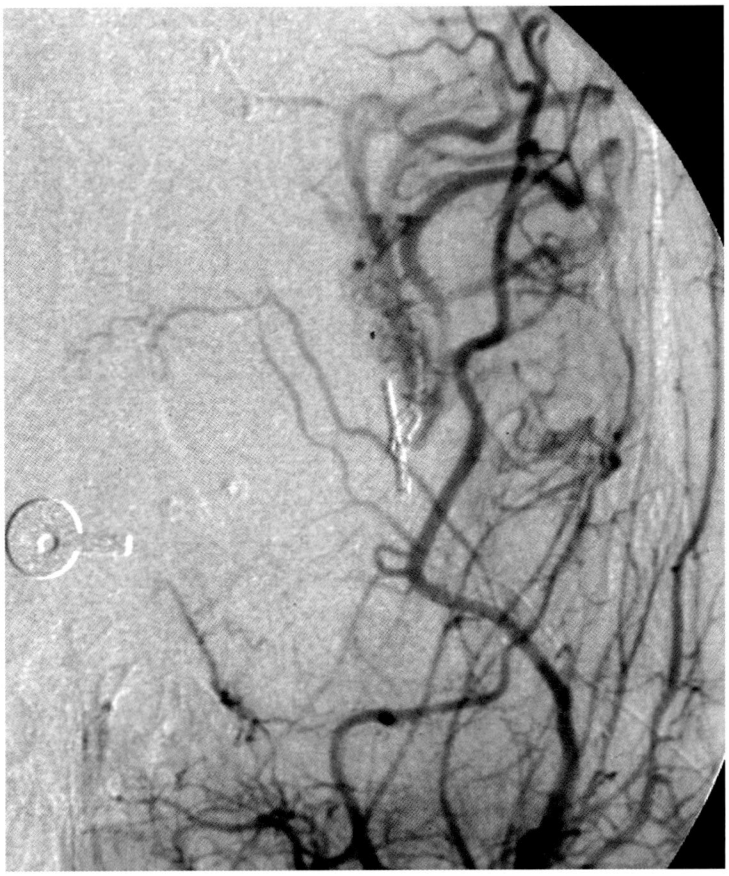

Fig. 7.6k Anteroposterior angiographic view shows the filling of MCA territory via the graft.

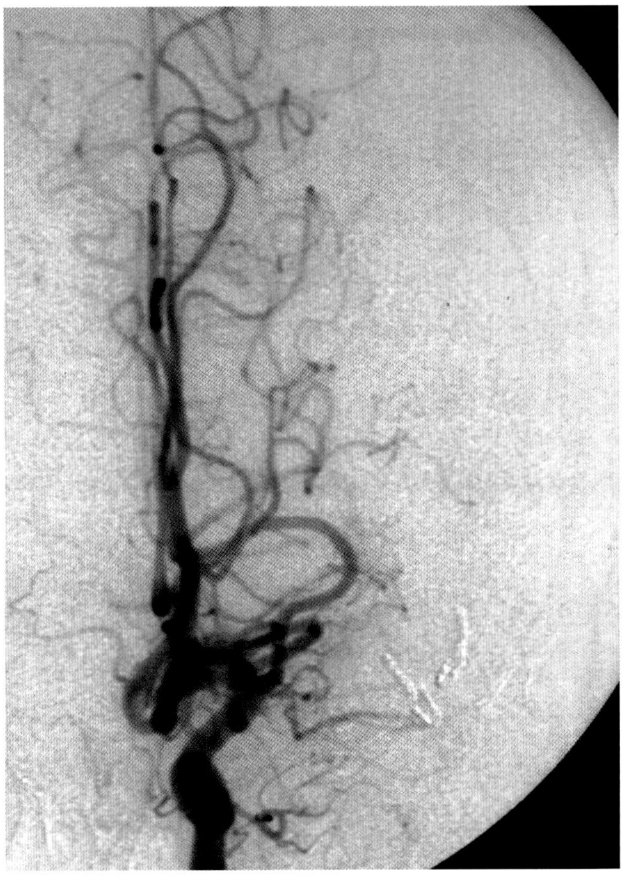

Fig. 7.6l Early anterior oblique angiogram of the left ICA injection shows complete occlusion of the MCA, from which the original aneurysm had arisen. This spontaneous occlusion of the MCA again emphasizes the importance of redirecting flow around an aneurysm.

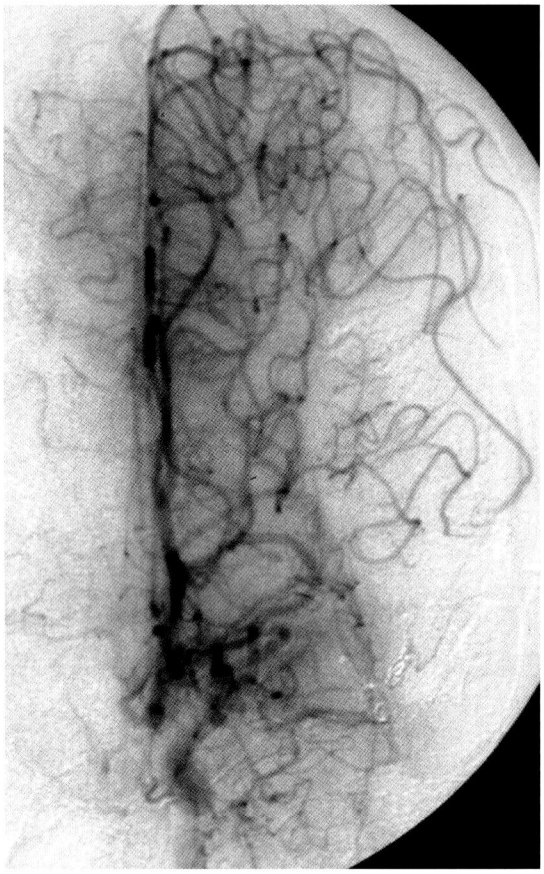

Fig. 7.6m Late phase angiogram of the ICA injection shows collateral circulation to MCA branches that had failed to fill previously.

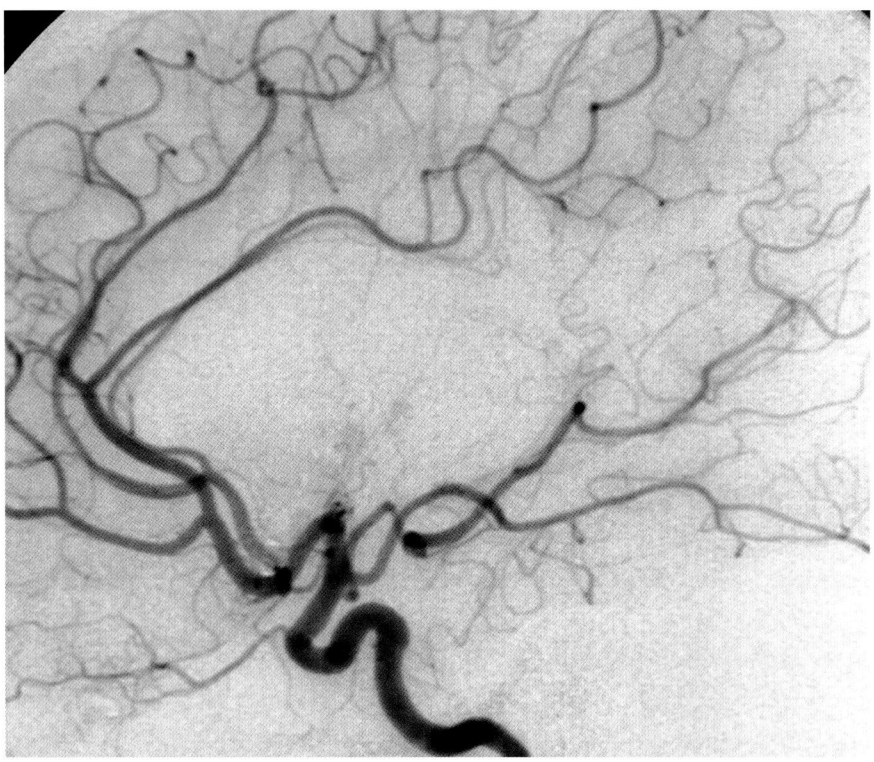

Fig. 7.6n Lateral angiogram of the ICA injection shows the lack of flow in the MCA territory.

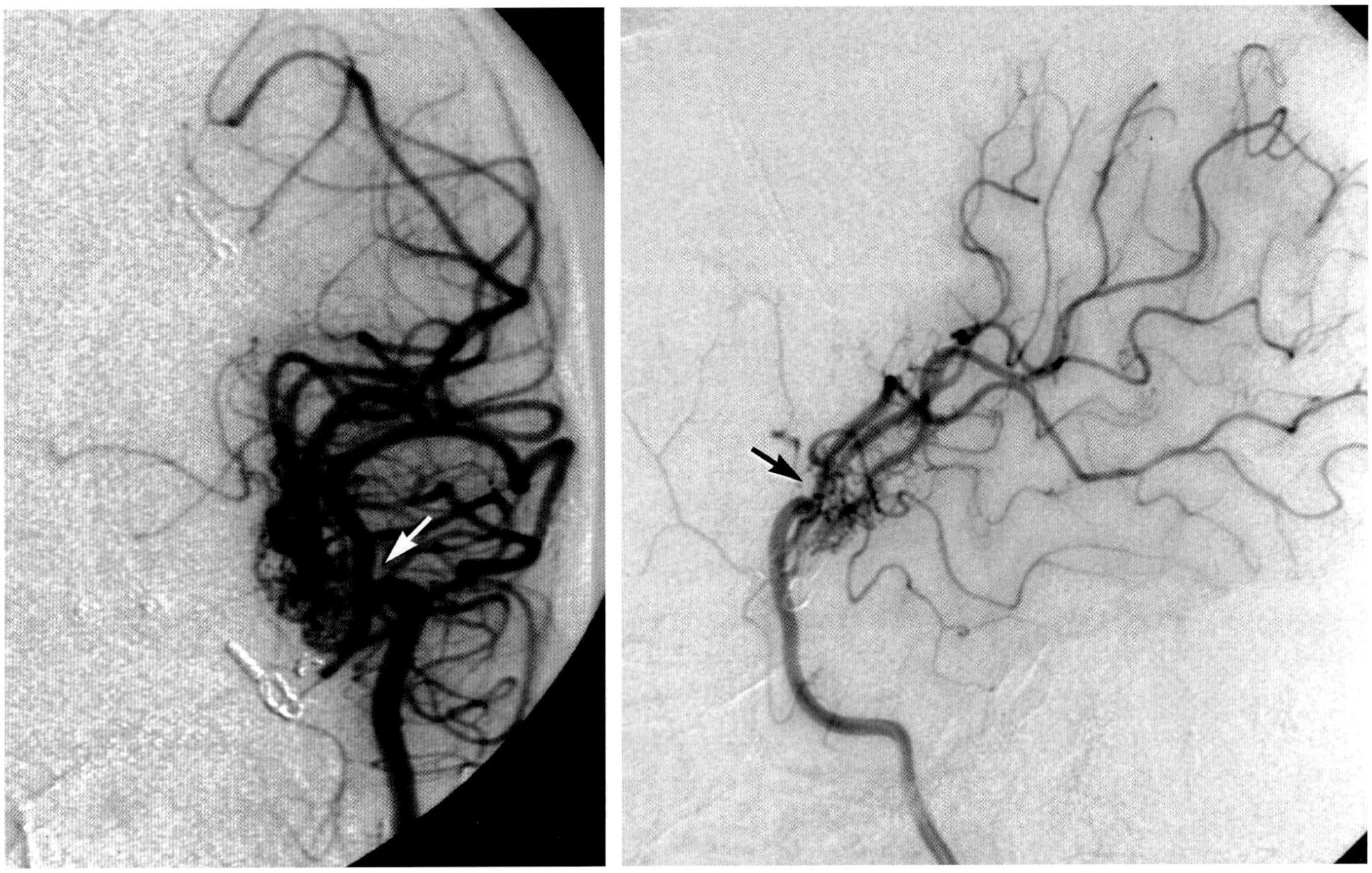

o p

Fig. 7.6o, p Anterior oblique and lateral angiograms obtained 3 months after surgery show the anastomosis (*arrows*) and confirm excellent filling of the MCA territory through the bypass.

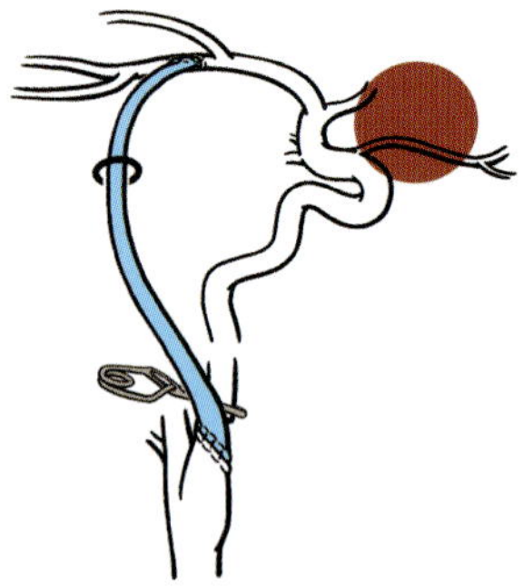

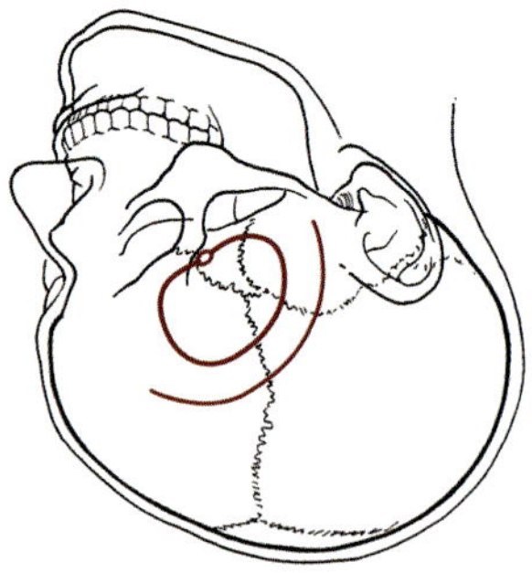

Case 7-7

Diagnosis: Right ophthalmic artery giant aneurysm

Bypass: Cervical ICA-to-MCA with saphenous vein graft

Approach: Right pterional

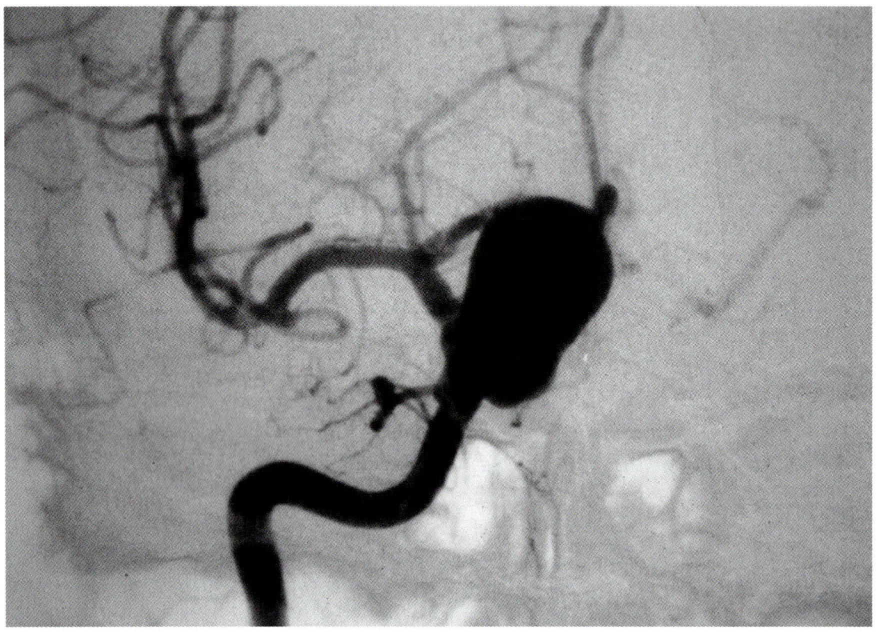

Fig. 7.7a Anteroposterior angiographic projection shows a giant calcified aneurysm with associated thrombosis. The patient did not tolerate BTO.

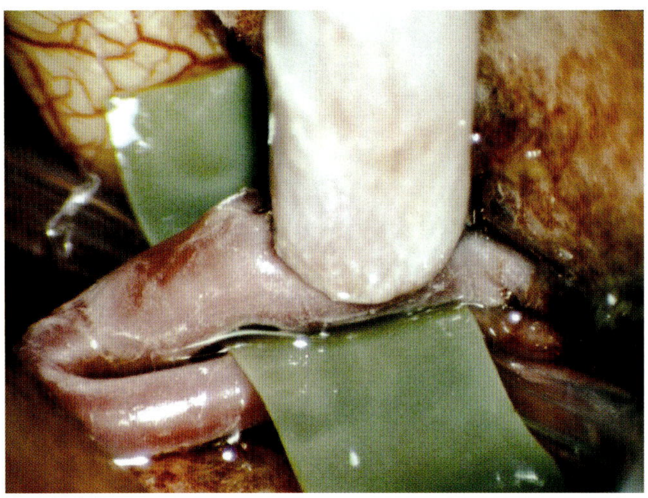

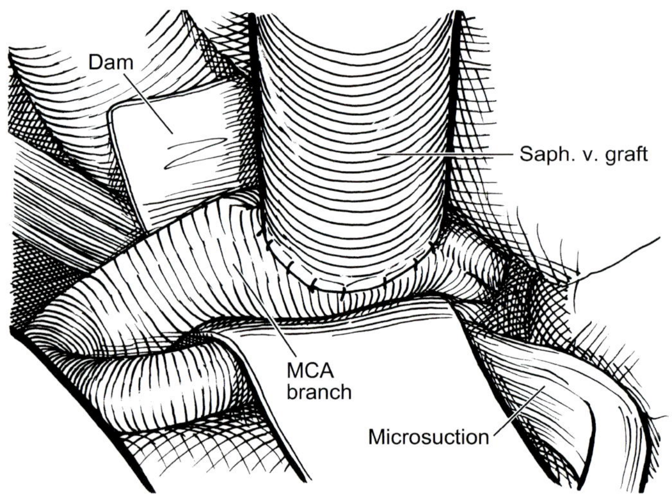

Fig. 7.7b A saphenous vein has been anastomosed to a branch of the MCA in an end-to-side fashion.

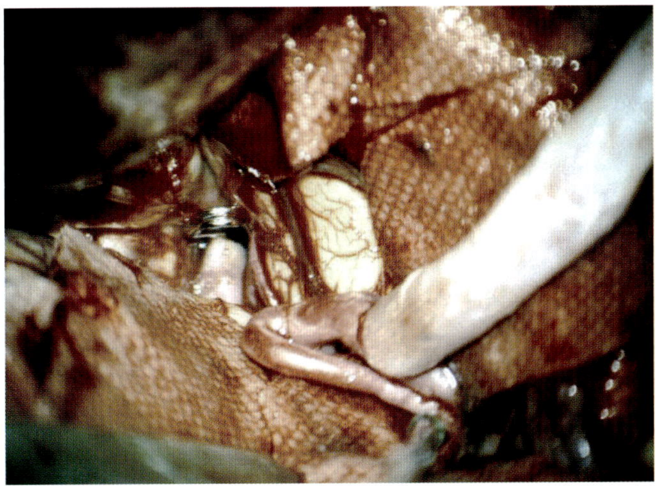

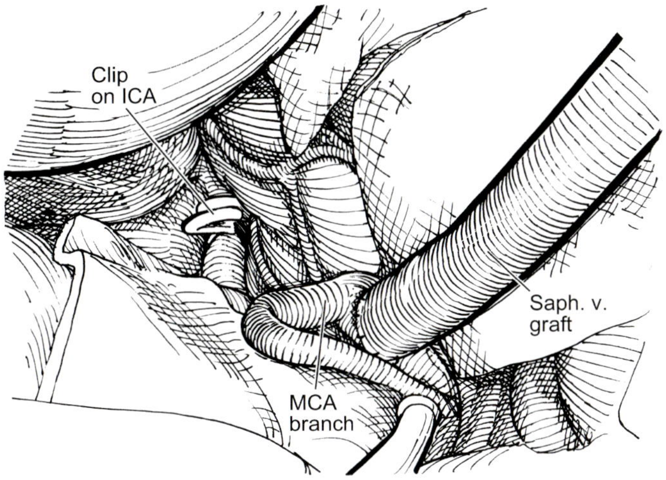

Fig. 7.7c Overview of the vein graft distended with back bleeding.

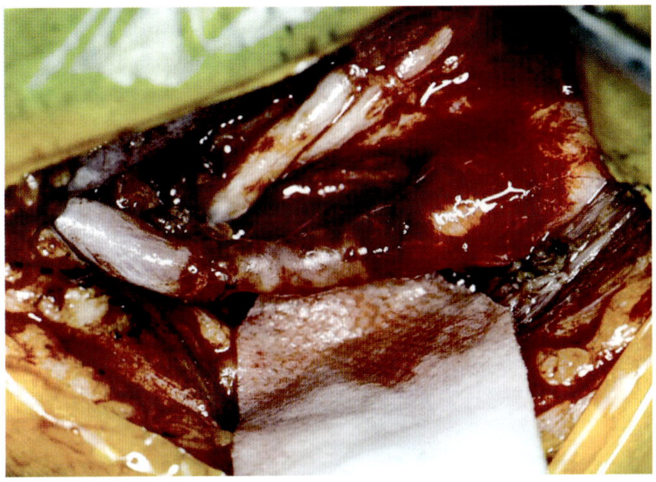

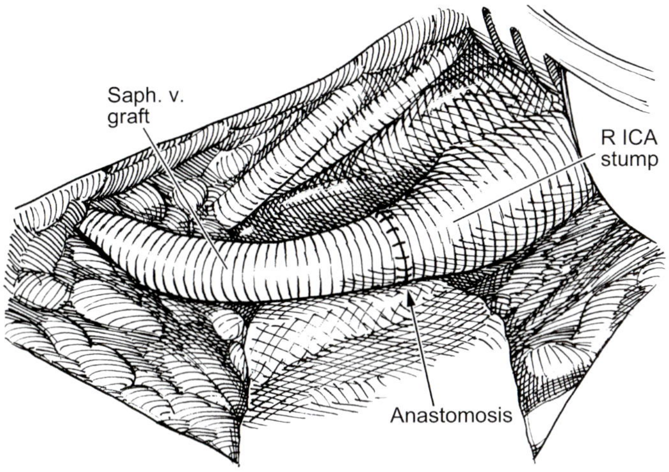

Fig. 7.7d The graft has been anastomosed to the stump of the ICA in the neck.

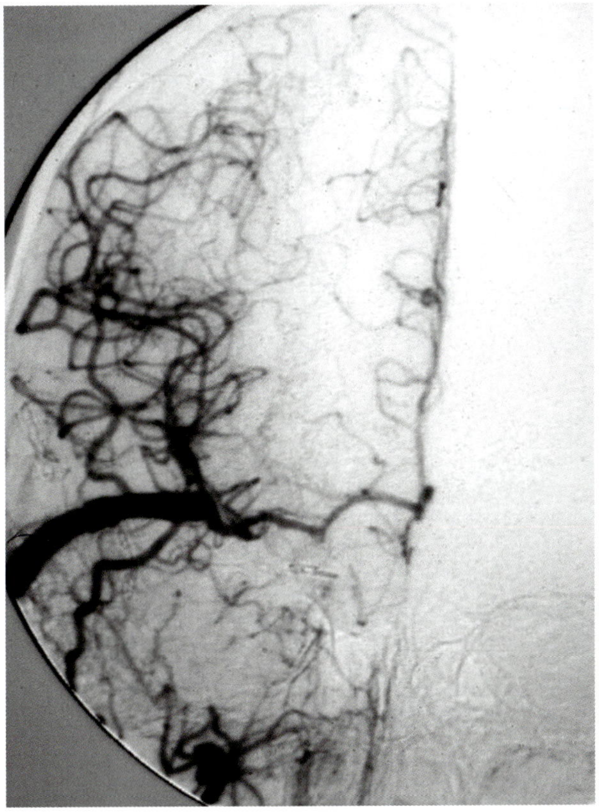

e

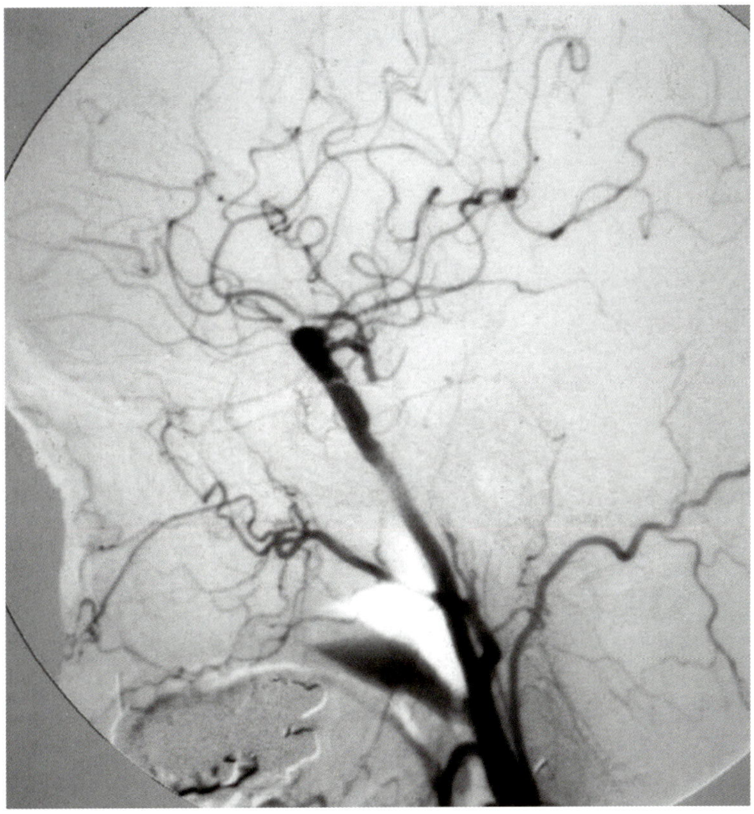

f

Fig. 7.7e, f Right anteroposterior and lateral angiographic projections confirm excellent feeding of the MCA and ACA territory through the saphenous vein bypass graft.

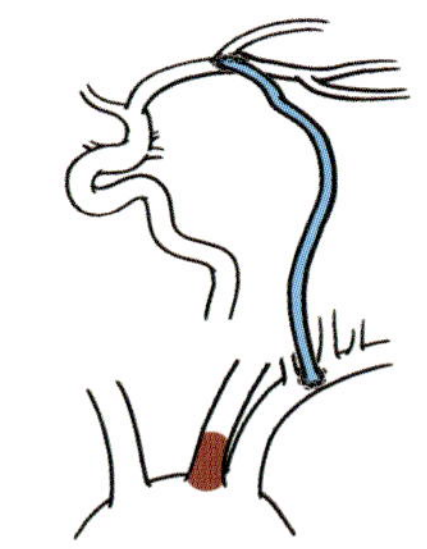

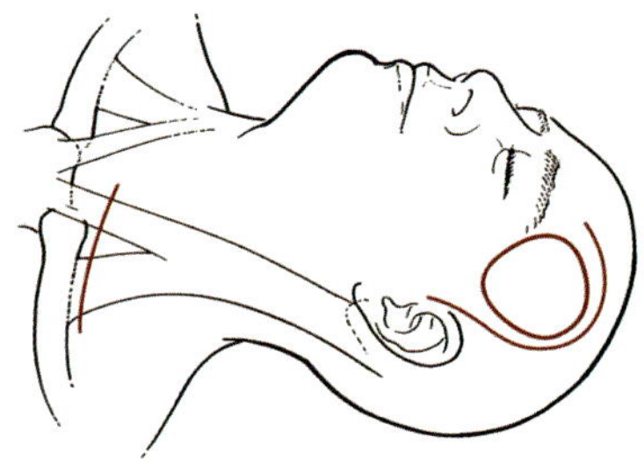

Case 7-8

Diagnosis: Left CCA occlusion

Bypass: Subclavian artery–to–MCA with saphenous vein graft

Approach: Left pterional and left transverse supraclavicular

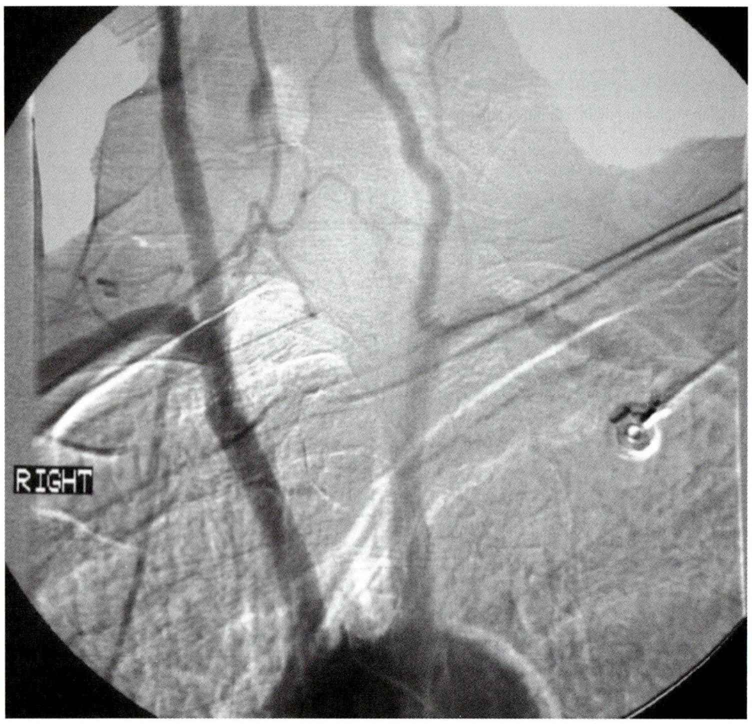

Fig. 7.8a Left anterior oblique arch angiogram shows complete occlusion of the left CCA at its origin.

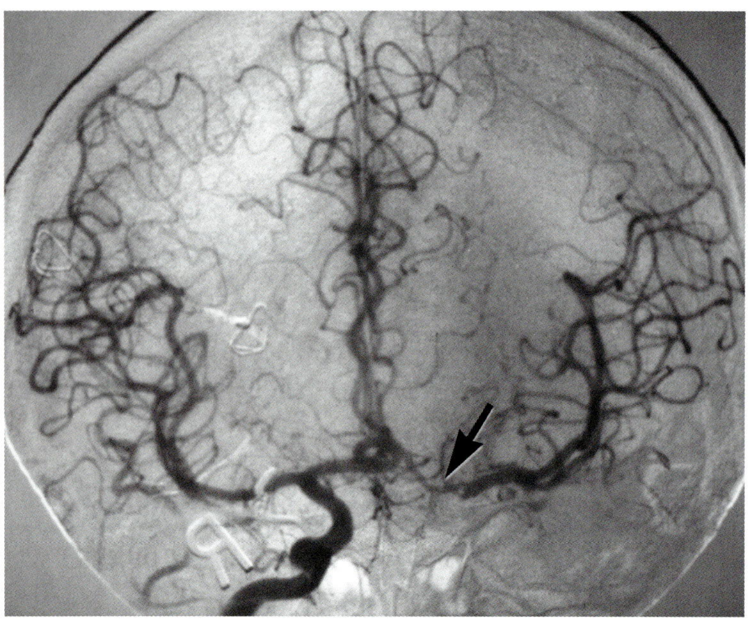

Fig. 7.8b Right anteroposterior CCA angiogram shows cross filling through the ACoA complex of the left MCA territory. The left A1 segment (*arrow*), which must carry the collateral blood flow to the left hemisphere, is quite small compared to the normal right side.

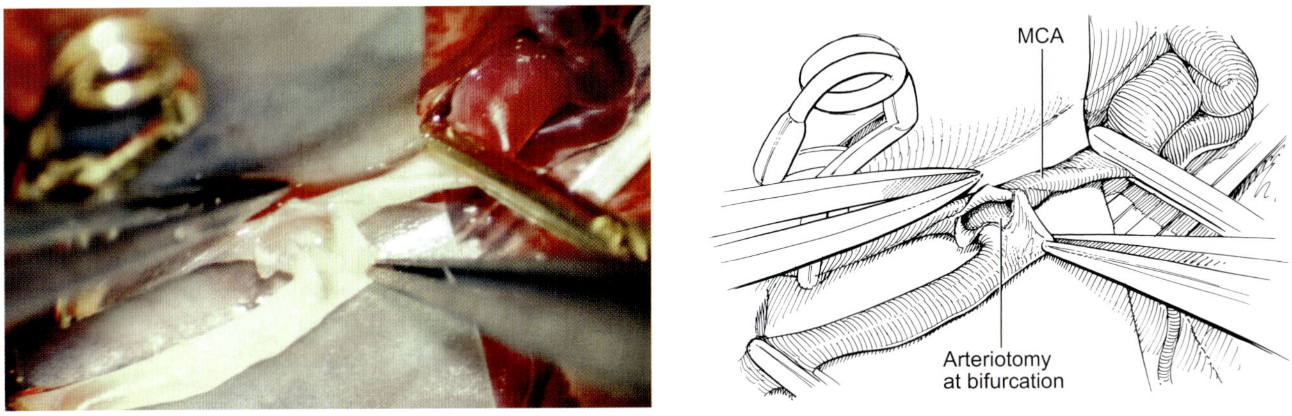

Fig. 7.8c A left pterional craniotomy has been performed and the sylvian fissure has been opened widely. The M2 segment is isolated between temporary aneurysm clips. An arteriotomy performed at the bifurcation provides a wide distal anastomotic site for the saphenous vein graft.

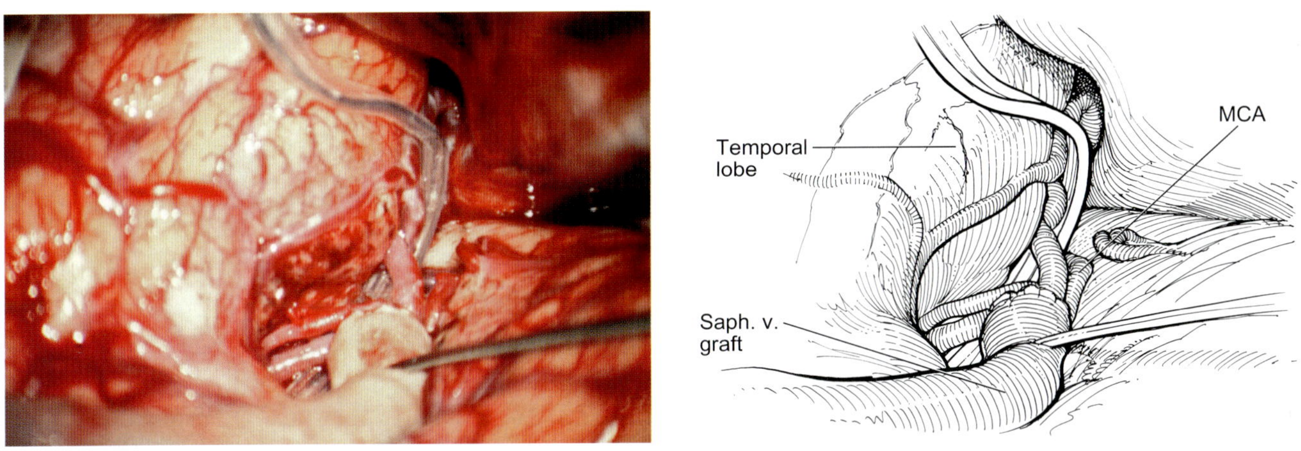

Fig. 7.8d The distal end of the saphenous vein graft is anastomosed to the M2 bifurcation. The temporary clips are removed and the anastomosis is inspected for hemostasis.

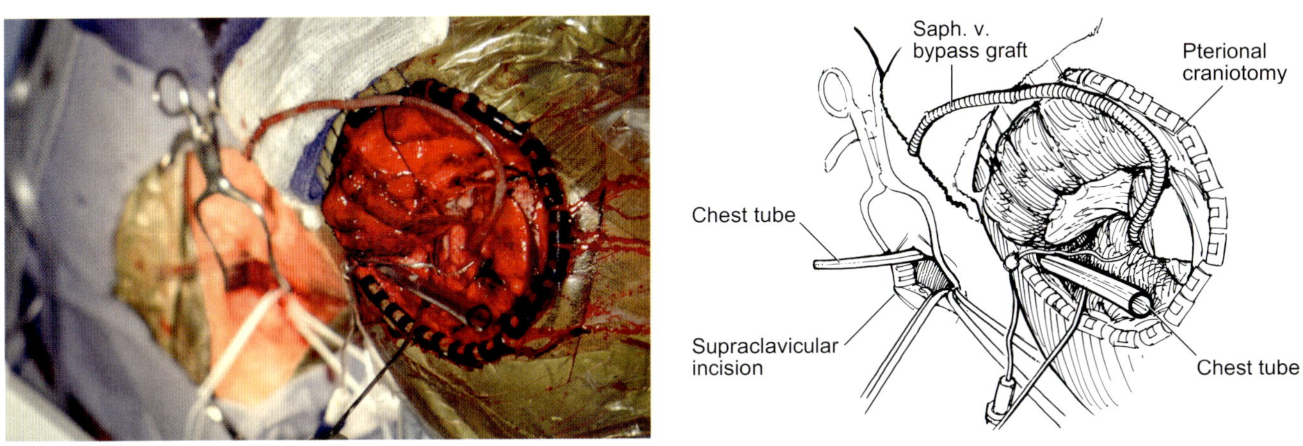

Fig. 7.8e Overview of the craniotomy site and supraclavicular incision used to isolate the subclavian artery. The long saphenous vein graft, which has been anastomosed to the MCA, is draped over the field.

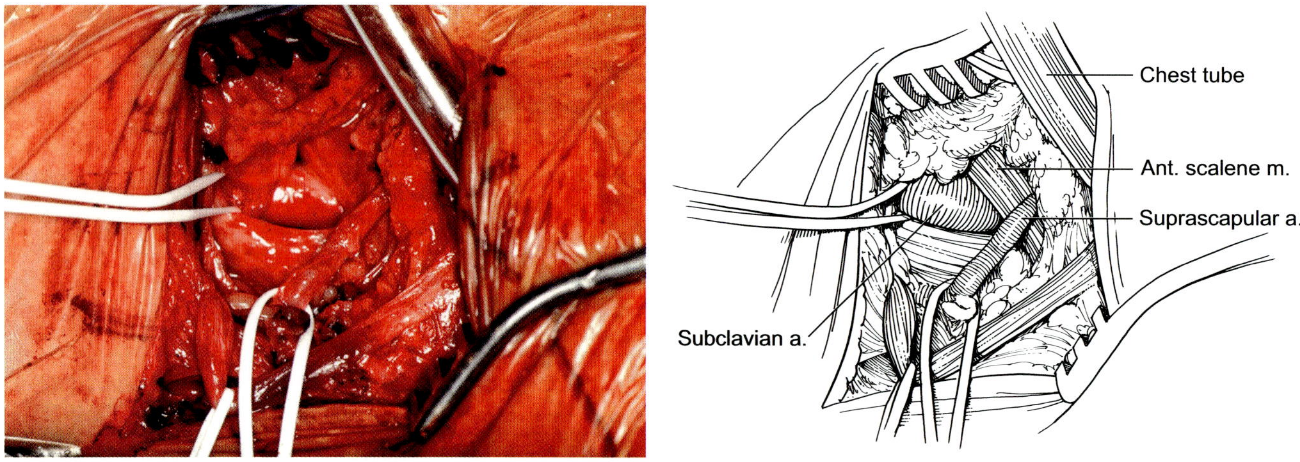

Fig. 7.8f The saphenous vein graft is tunneled subcutaneously from the craniotomy incision to the supraclavicular incision. One end of a 28-French chest tube exits along the upper margin of supraclavicular incision. After the chest tube is positioned, the vein graft can be readily passed through the tube by gentle irrigation. The graft is partially inflated to eliminate twisting or kinks before the chest tube is removed.

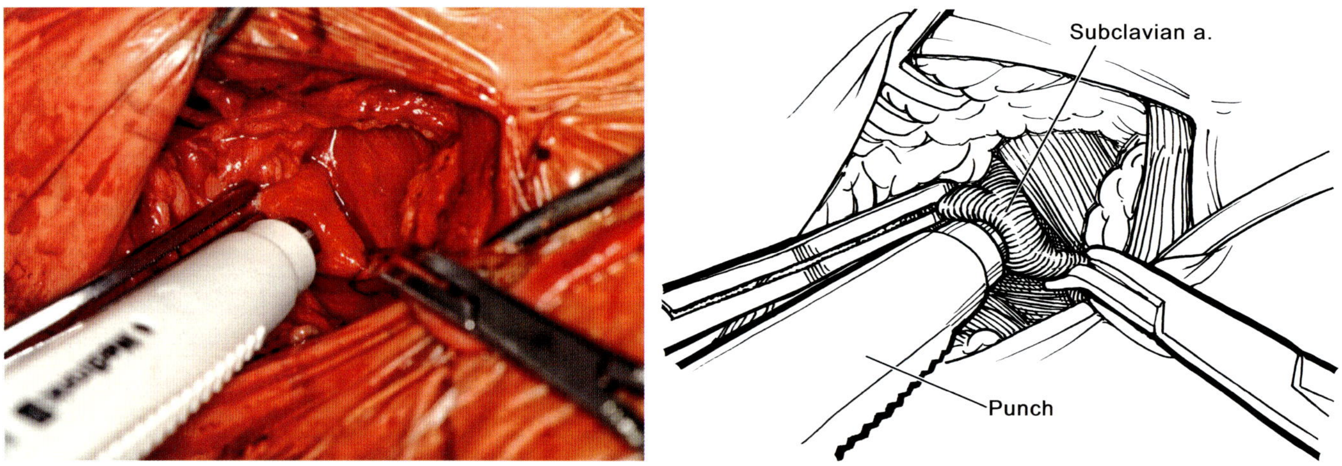

Fig. 7.8g A short segment of the subclavian artery is isolated between vascular clamps and an aortic punch is used to create a suitable proximal anastomotic site for the saphenous vein graft.

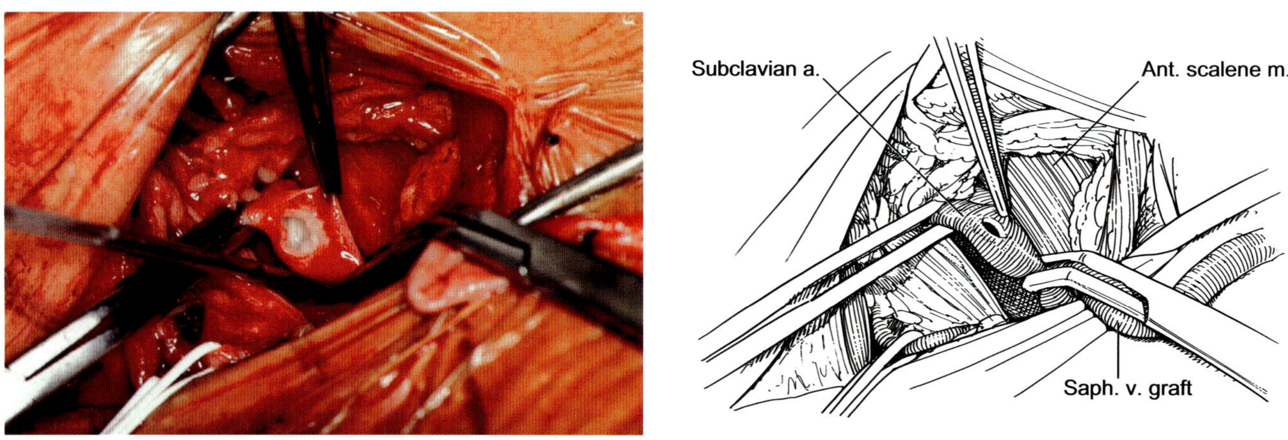

Fig. 7.8h Immediately before the anastomosis is begun, the smooth arteriotomy is inspected. The anastomosis is completed with 6–0 Prolene (Ethicon, Somerville, NJ).

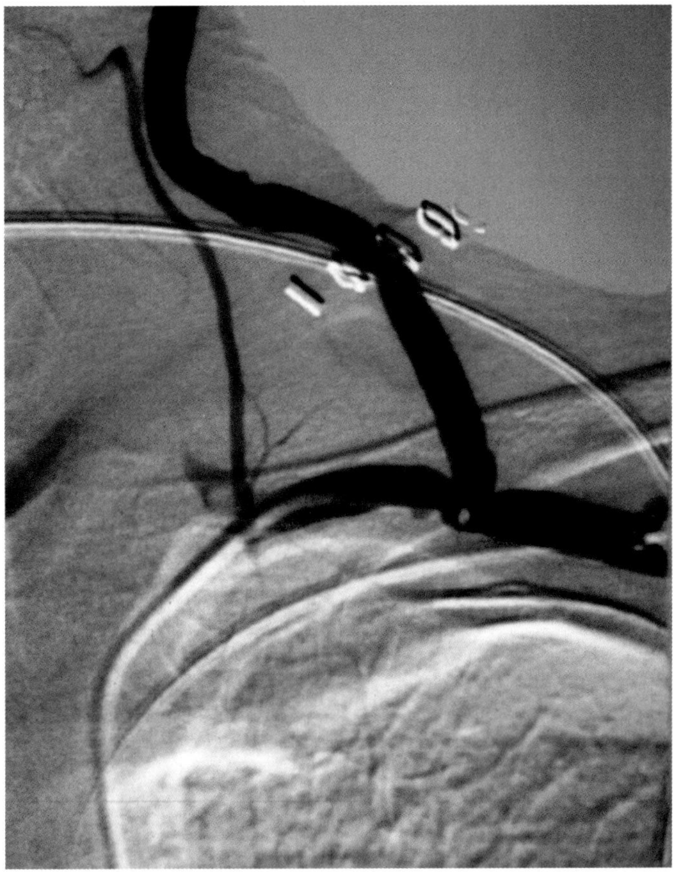

Fig. 7.8i Selective left subclavian artery angiogram obtained the day after surgery confirms that the proximal anastomosis is widely patent.

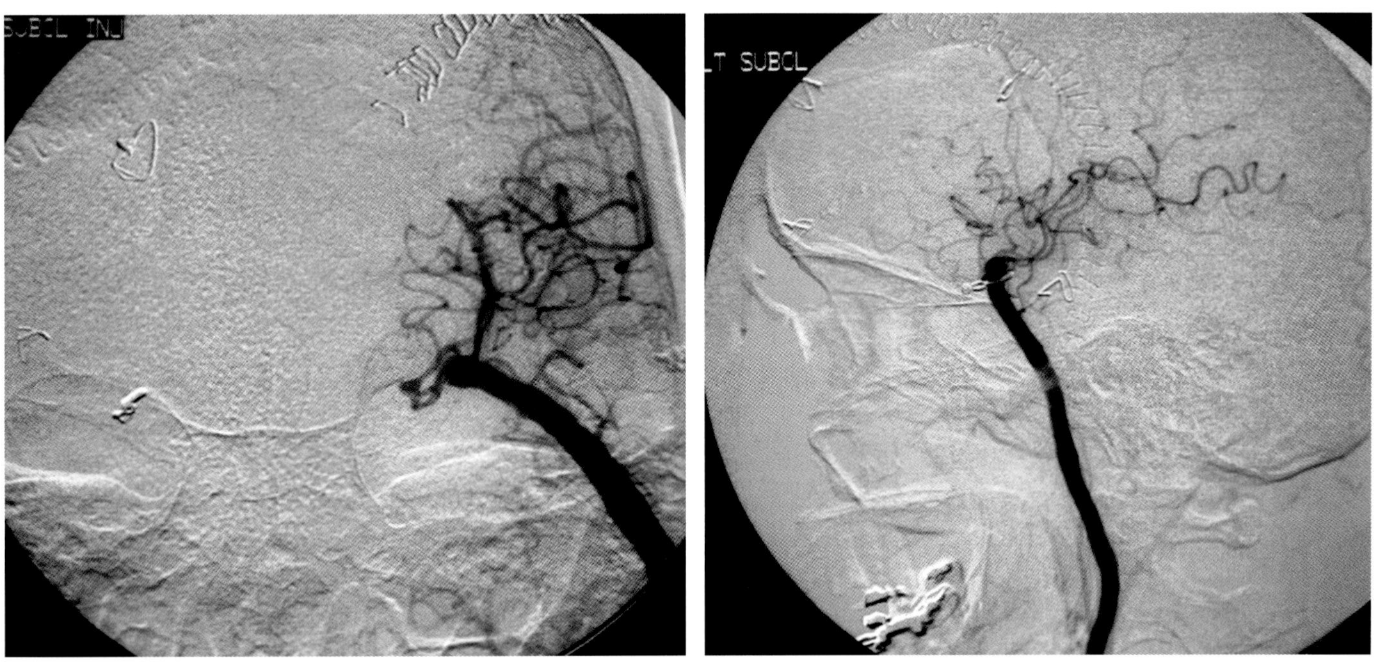

j

k

Fig. 7.8j, k Anteroposterior and lateral angiographic views of the cranium from the same injection show the brisk filling of the distribution of the MCA through the saphenous vein graft.

8 IMA–to–Cervical ICA Bypass

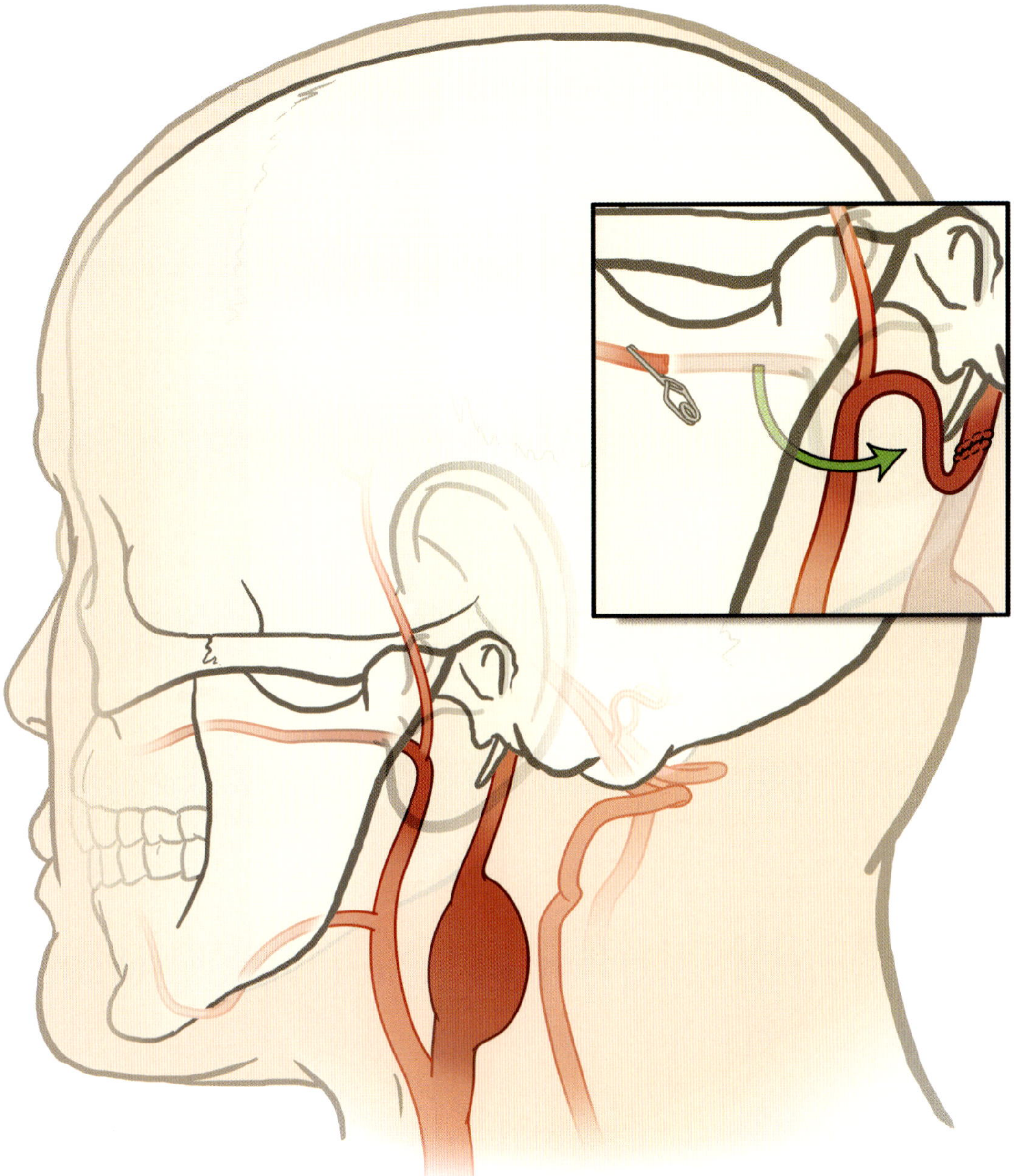

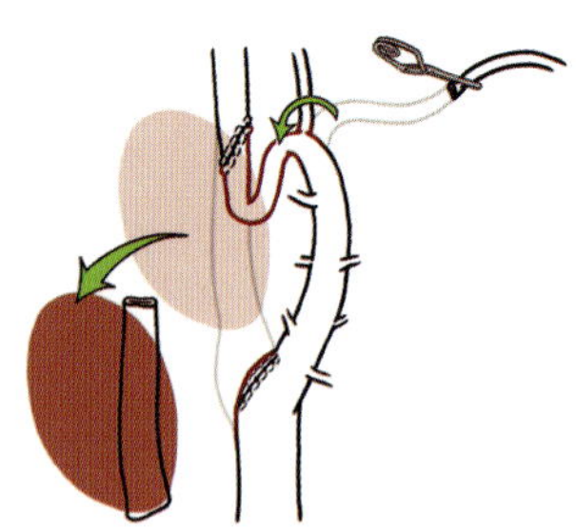

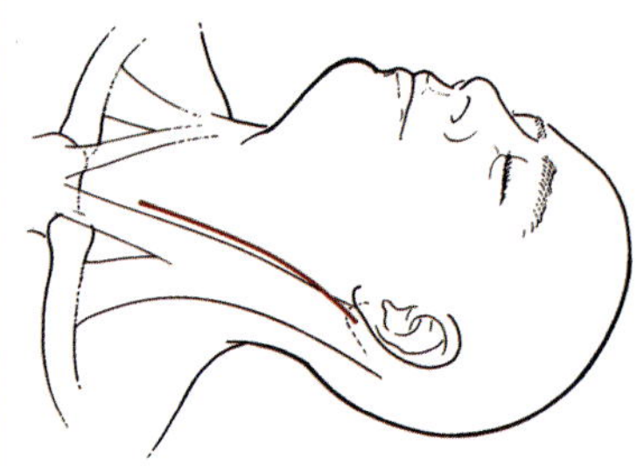

Case 8-1

Diagnosis: Left cervical ICA pseudoaneurysm

Bypass: IMA-to-ICA

Approach: Left anterior cervical

Video

A 70-year-old woman with renal insufficiency had undergone a left carotid endarterectomy 5 years earlier. She now presented with swallowing difficulty and an expanding, pulsatile mass in the left neck.

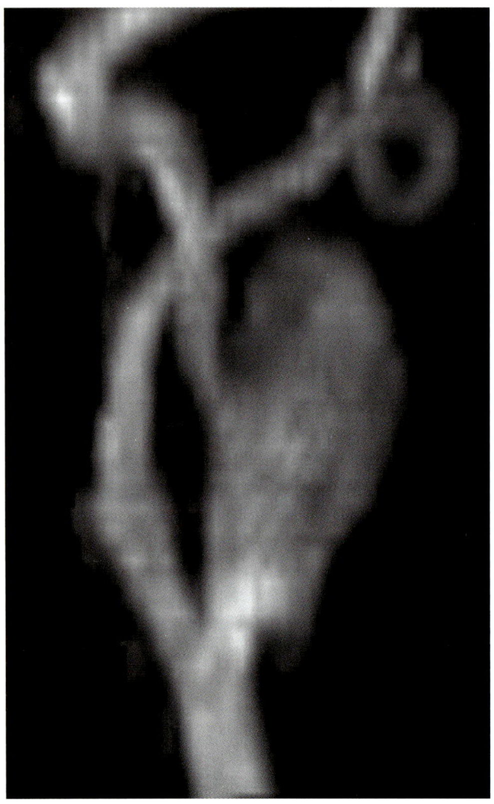

Fig. 8.1a MR angiogram shows a large pseudoaneurysm arising from the cervical portion of the ICA.

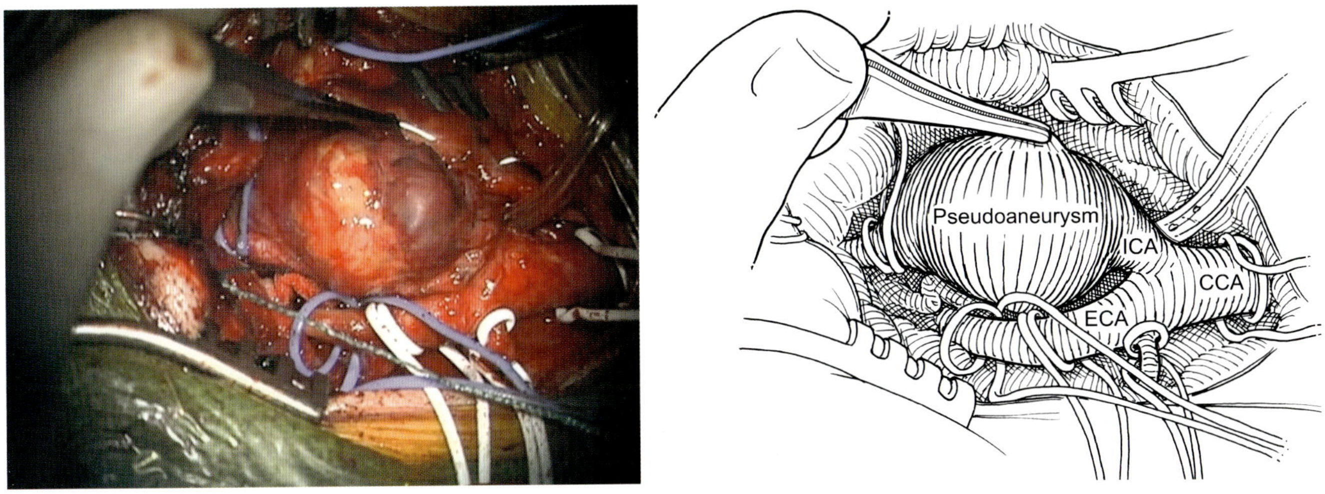

Fig. 8.1b The mass is exposed and all of the branches are identified.

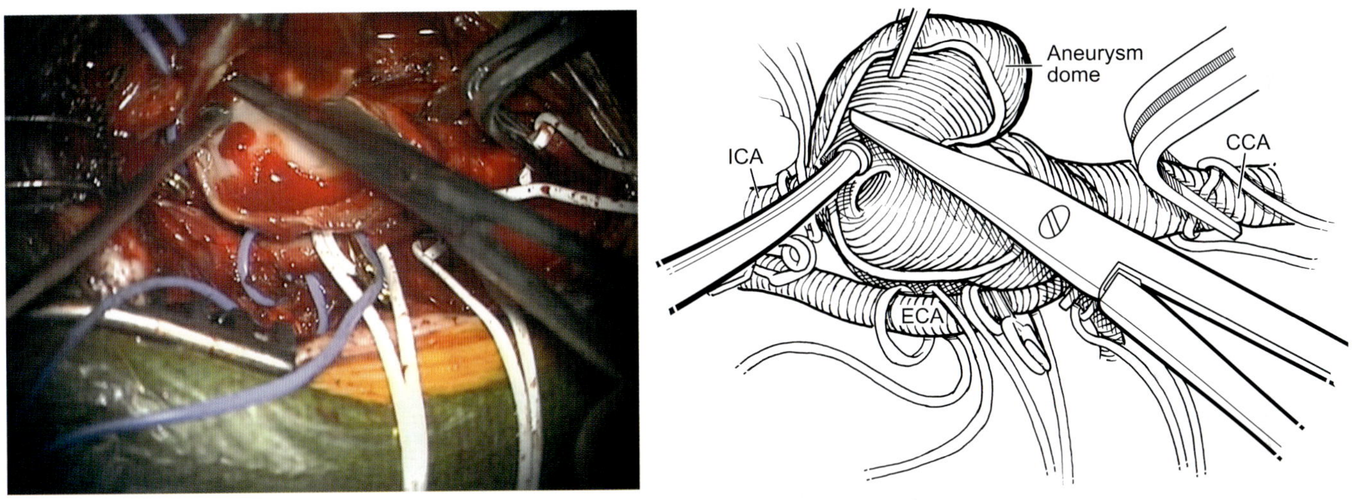

Fig. 8.1c The aneurysm dome is cut away. The old patch is found within the wall.

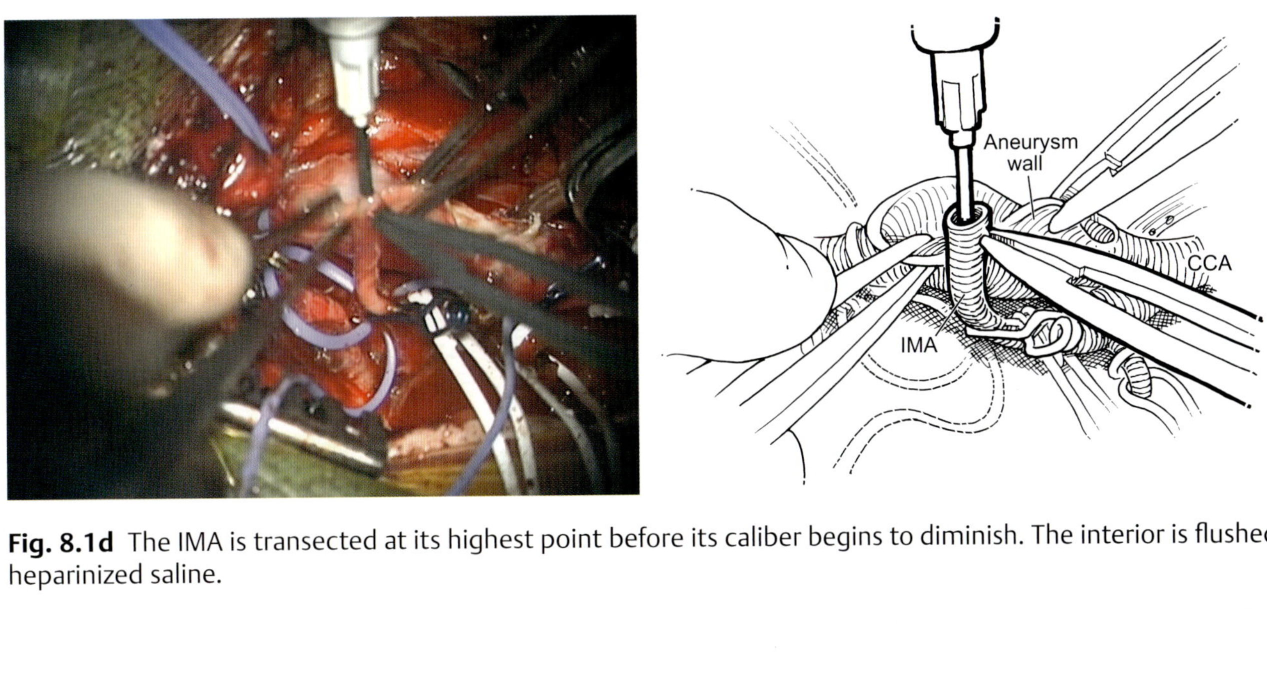

Fig. 8.1d The IMA is transected at its highest point before its caliber begins to diminish. The interior is flushed with heparinized saline.

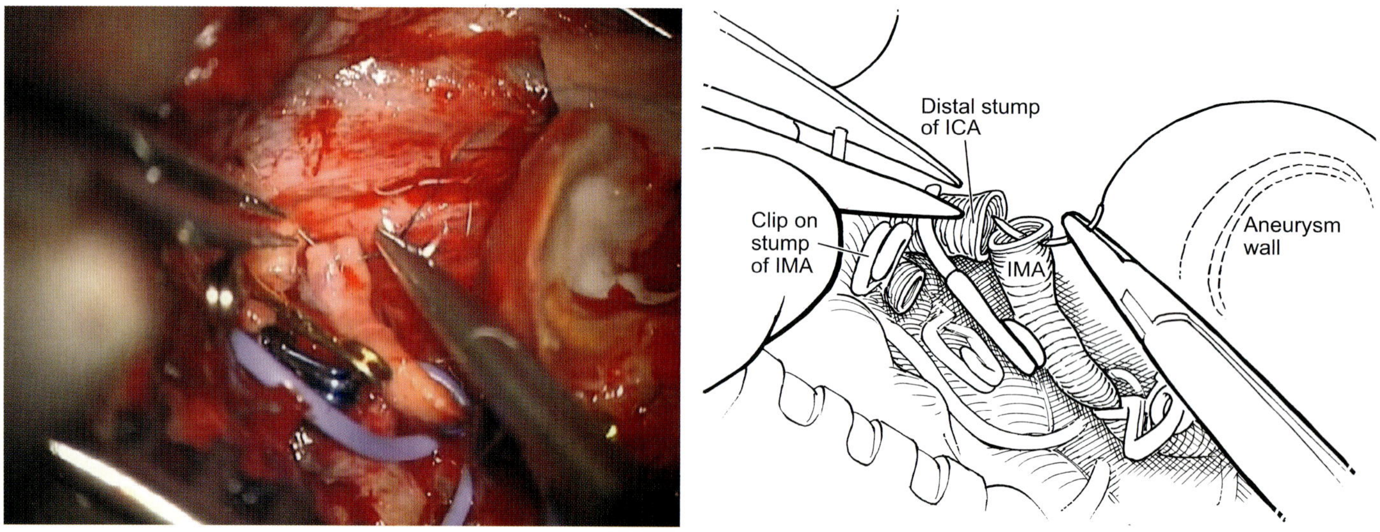

Fig. 8.1e The IMA is sewn to the stump of the ICA.

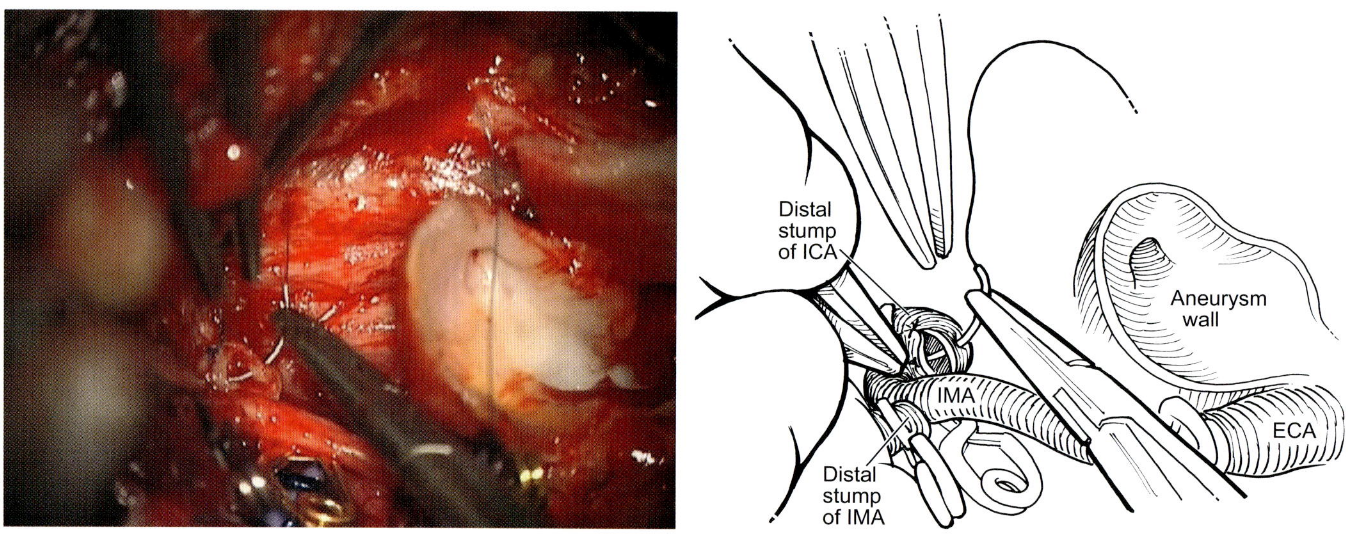

Fig. 8.1f Interrupted sutures are placed at intervals around the circumference of the anastomosis.

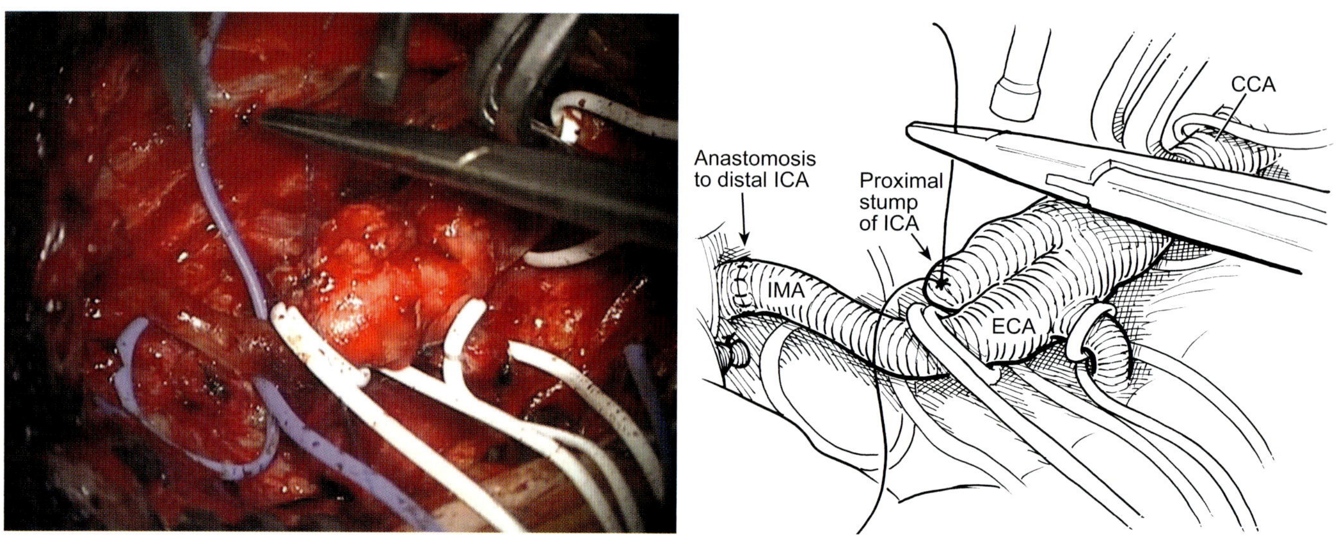

Fig. 8.1g The stump of the ICA is oversewn at the bulb.

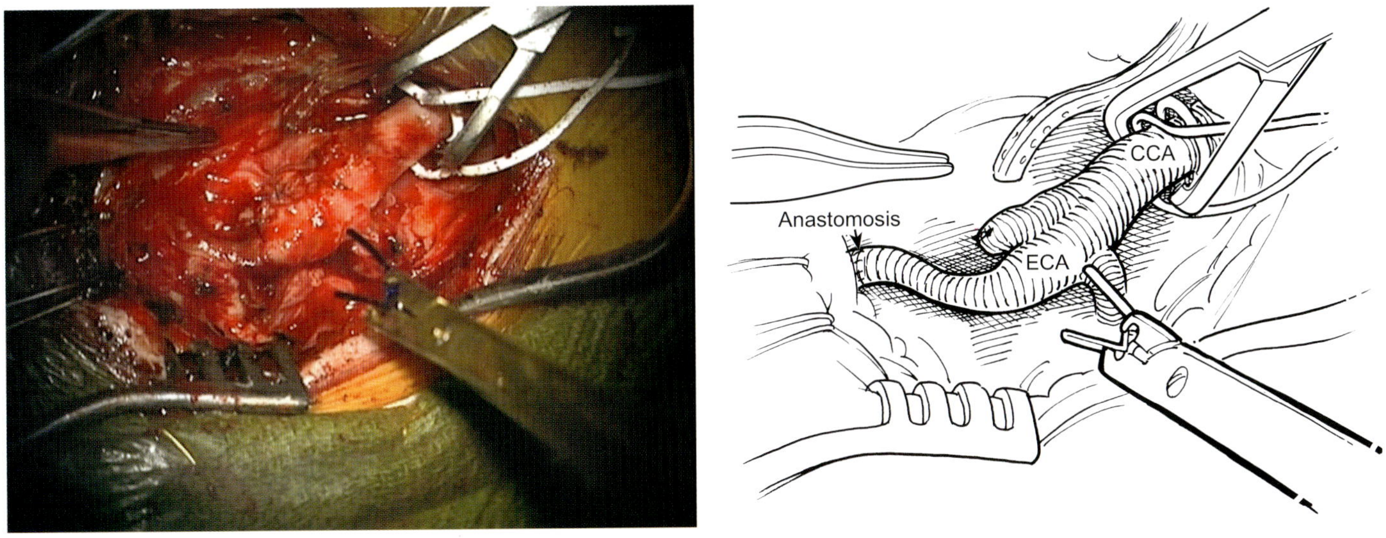

Fig. 8.1h All temporary clips were removed and good hemostasis was achieved. There was good pulsation of the carotid artery and the Doppler signal confirmed blood flow.

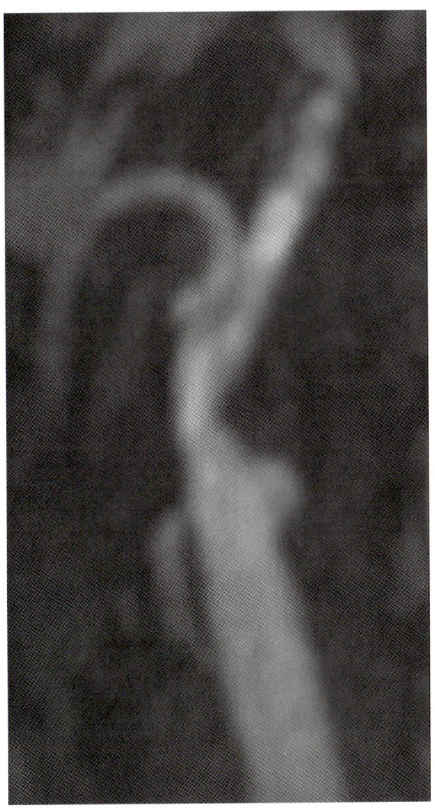

Fig. 8.1i Postoperative MR angiogram shows the IMA filling the ICA.

9 Petrous ICA Bypass

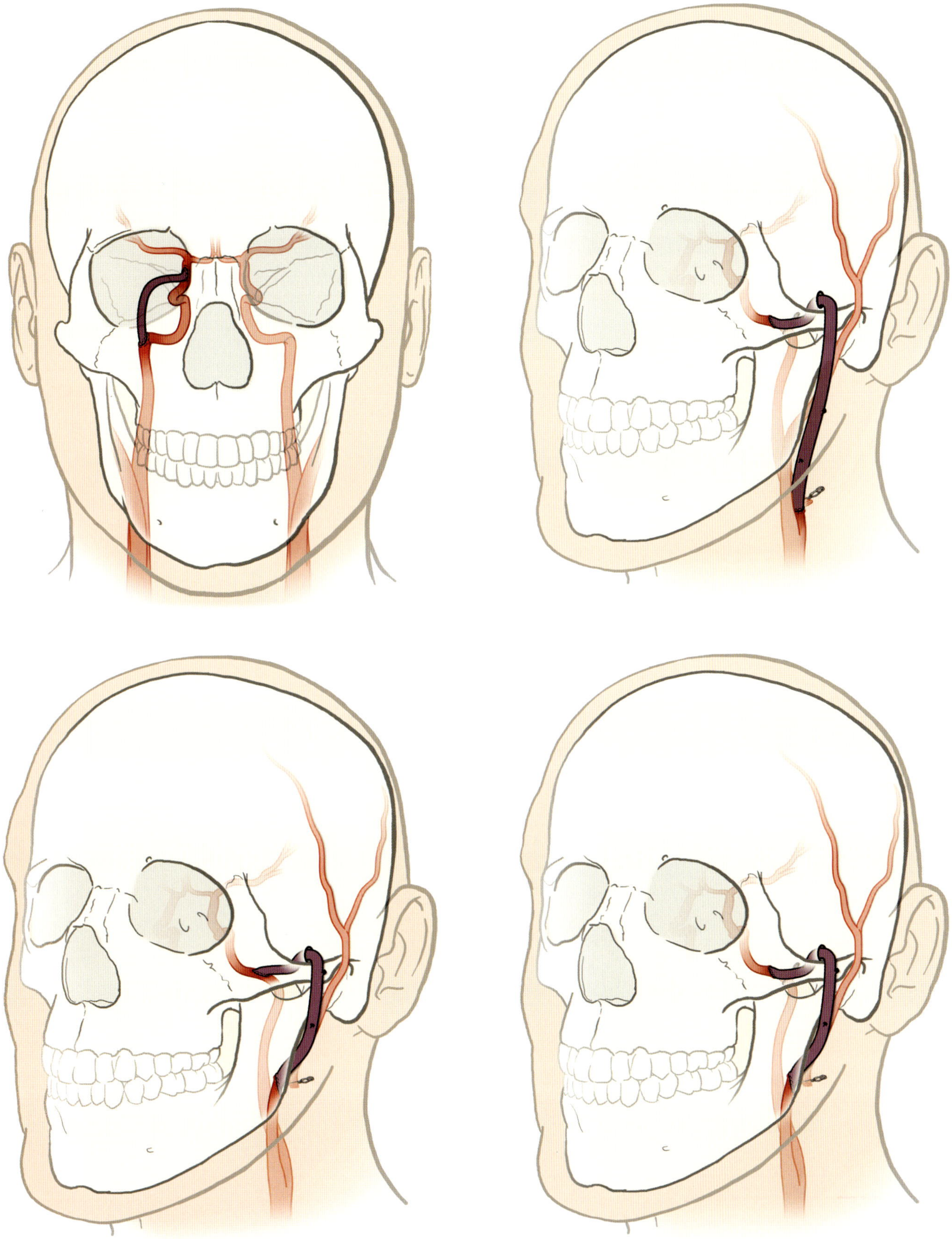

The petrous segment of the ICA can be used as a donor or recipient vessel. The petrous ICA can be exposed in one of two ways. The more common method is to access Glasscock's triangle by elevating the dura on the floor of the middle fossa. The ICA, which lies just posterior and medial to the foramen ovale, may or may not be covered by a thin rim of bone. The ICA is exposed by drilling the bone medially and posteriorly to the curve of the ICA. To avert injury to CN VII during exposure of the ICA, great care must be exerted to avoid traction on the GSPN arising from the geniculate ganglion. The GSPN can be cut or carefully dissected free and elevated with the dura. The second method of exposing the ICA is from the intradural route. In this case, the ICA is identified through the dura with image guidance or Doppler ultrasonography. Once the artery is identified, the dura is opened directly over the ICA, which is then exposed in the usual manner.

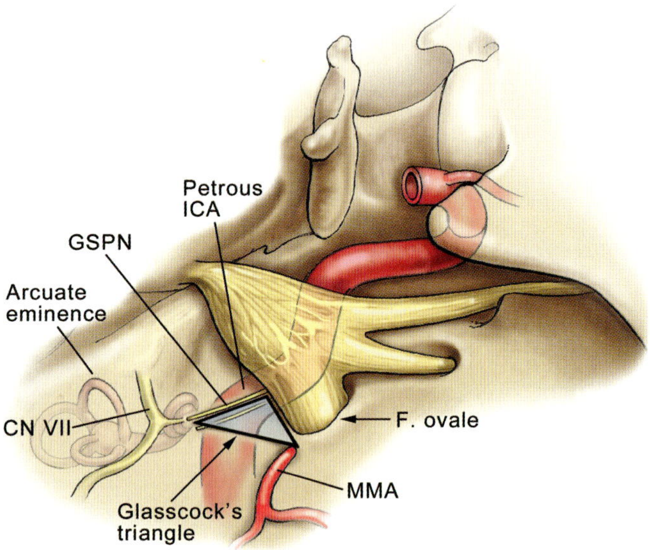

Fig. 9.0a Anatomic orientation shows Glasscock's triangle demonstrating the relationship of the ICA to the foramen ovale, MMA, and arcuate eminence.

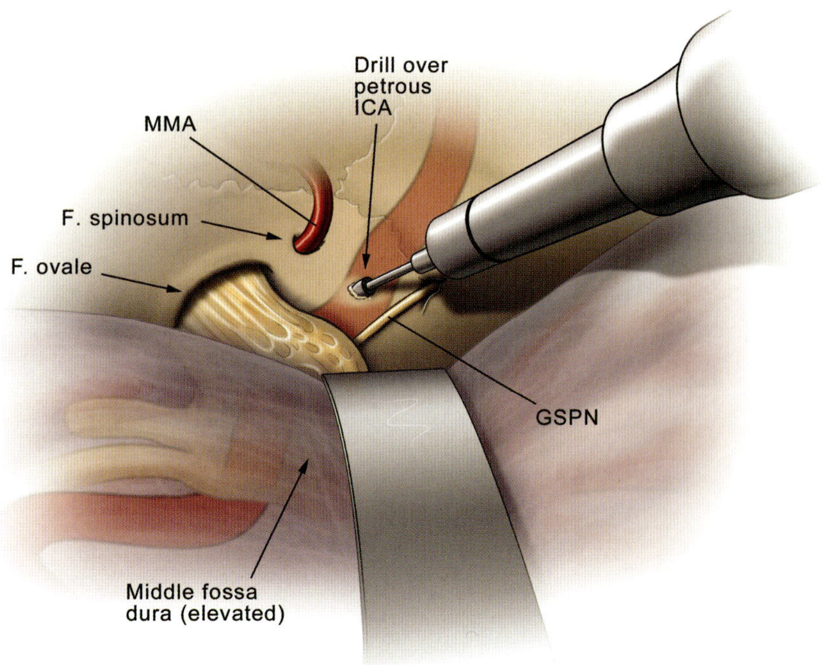

Fig. 9.0b Surgical orientation shows exposure of the floor of the middle fossa in preparation for drilling the carotid canal.

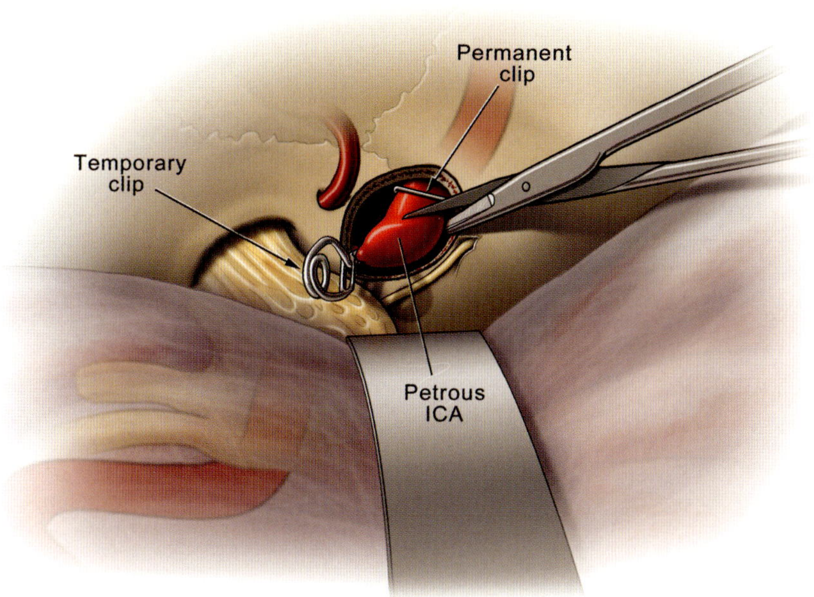

Fig. 9.0c A temporary clip has been applied to the ICA as it enters the cavernous sinus. A permanent clip has been placed on the ICA proximally, and the artery is about to be cut.

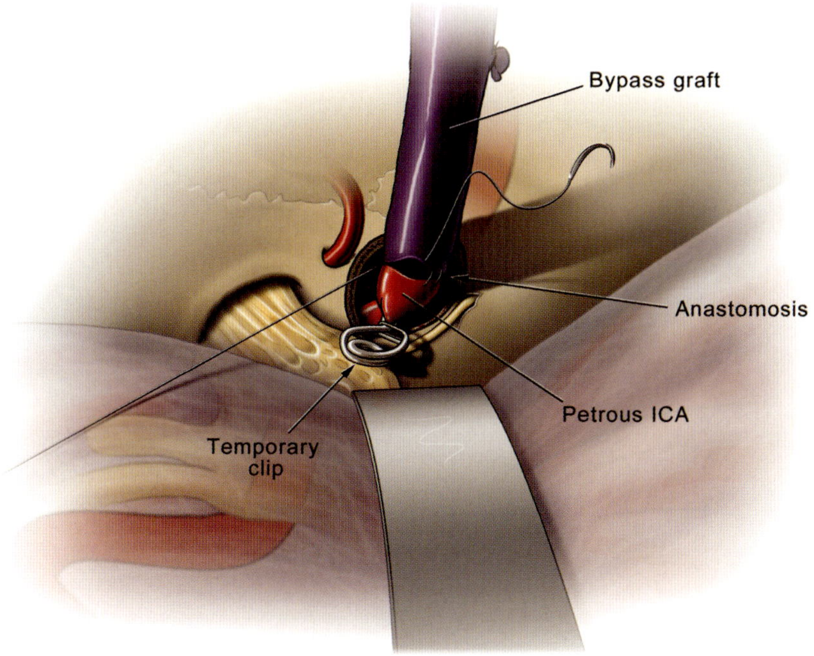

Fig. 9.0d An anastomosis is being performed between the graft and the distal ICA.

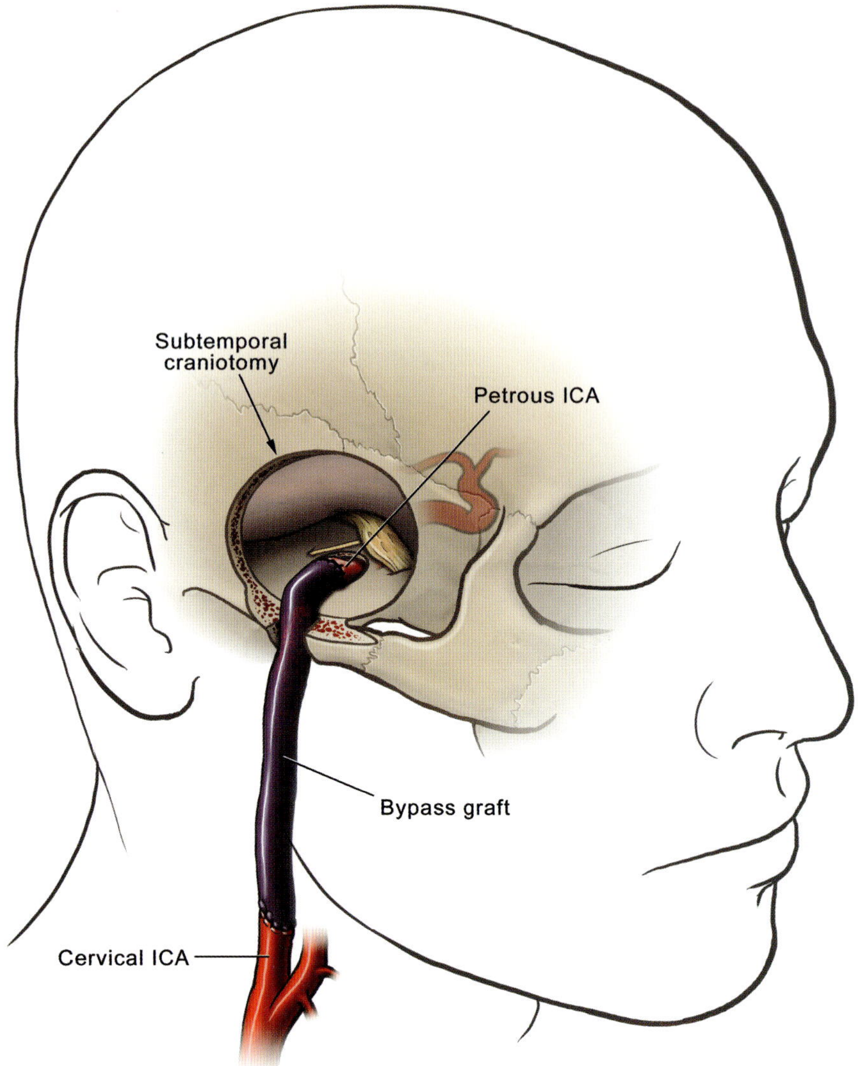

Fig. 9.0e Completed bypass from the ICA in the neck to the ICA in the petrous bone.

Anatomy of the Petrous ICA–to–Supraclinoid ICA Bypass

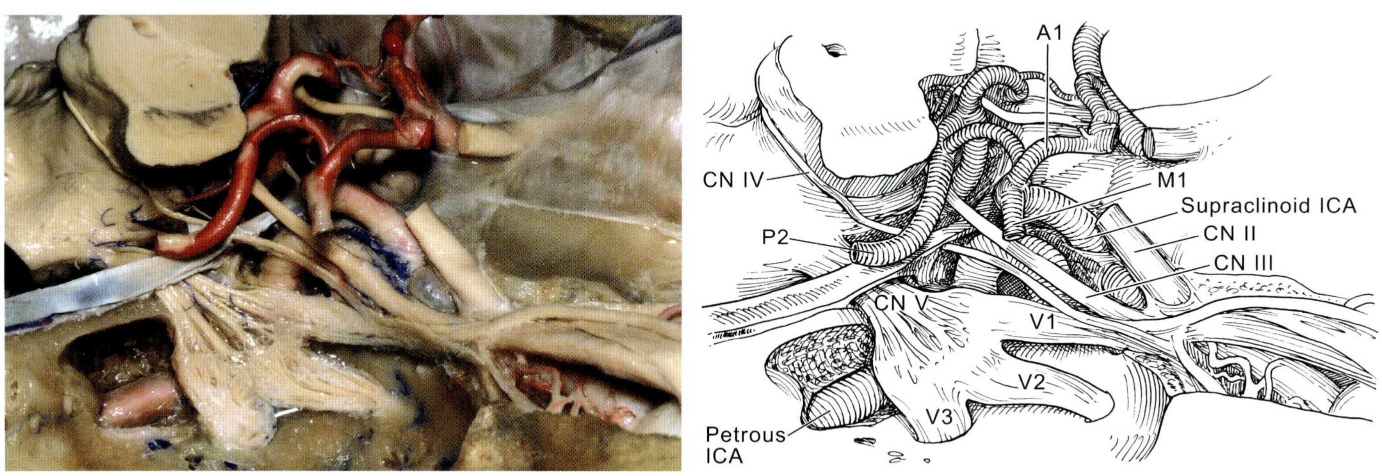

Fig. 9.0f This anatomical preparation shows the floor of the middle fossa with the dura removed and the petrous bone drilled to expose the carotid canal. The petrous ICA is visible as it enters below CN V into the cavernous sinus. (Photograph used with permission from *Journal of Neurosurgery*.)

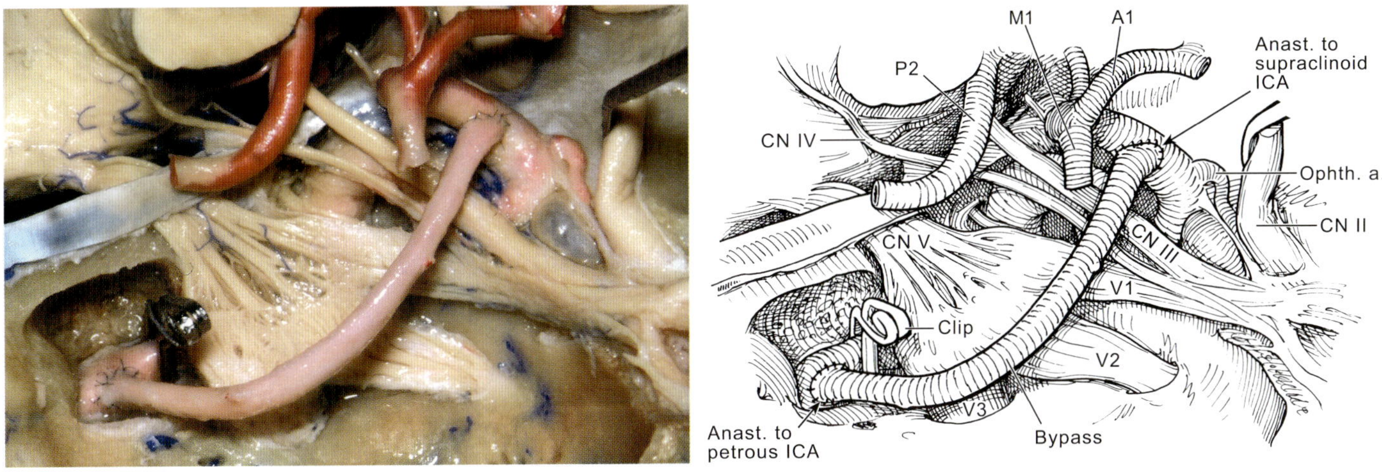

Fig. 9.0g A completed bypass using a radial artery graft between the petrous ICA and the ICA in the subarachnoid space proximal to the PCoA. (Photograph used with permission from *Journal of Neurosurgery*.)

Anatomy of Cervical ICA–to–Petrous ICA Bypass

The cervical carotid artery–to–petrous ICA bypass allows a short-segment bypass for the treatment of lesions of the cervical ICA or skull base. The carotid artery is exposed in the neck, and the ICA, ECA, or even the CCA is prepared as the donor vessel. A radial artery or saphenous vein graft is harvested in the usual fashion.

The middle fossa craniotomy exposes the petrous ICA extradurally as described previously. It is worth reemphasizing that traction should not be placed on the GSPN to avoid injury to CN VII. The graft is anastomosed to the ICA in the petrous bone and then tunneled subcutaneously into the neck incision for its proximal anastomosis.

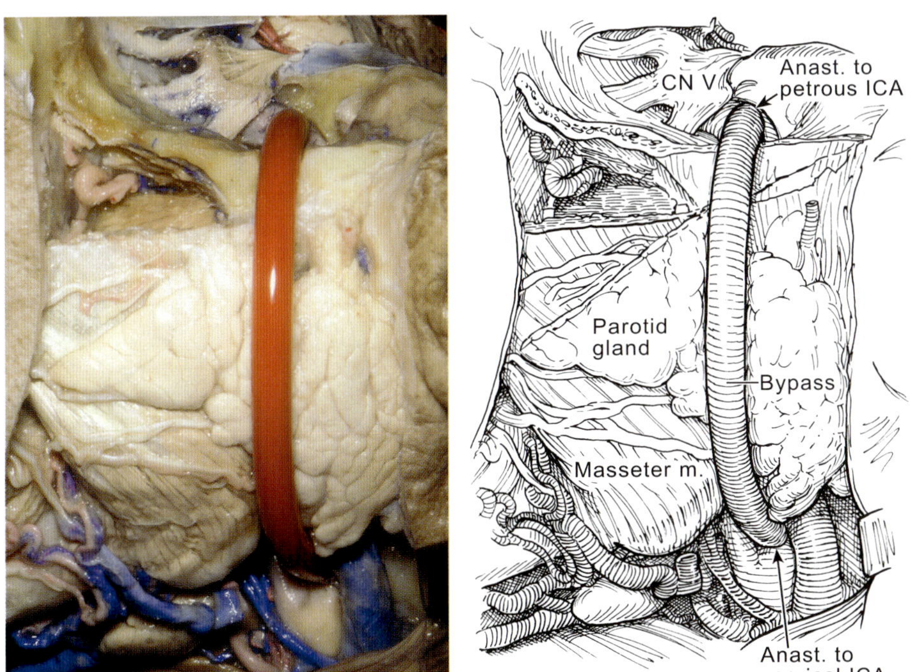

Fig. 9.0h Anatomical representation of a bypass from the ICA in the neck to the petrous ICA in the middle fossa.

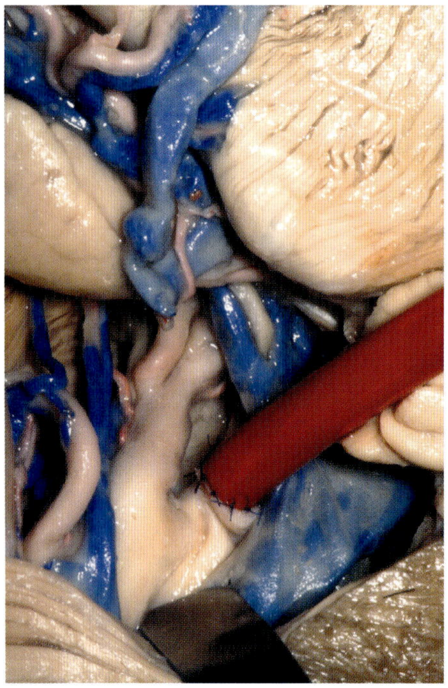

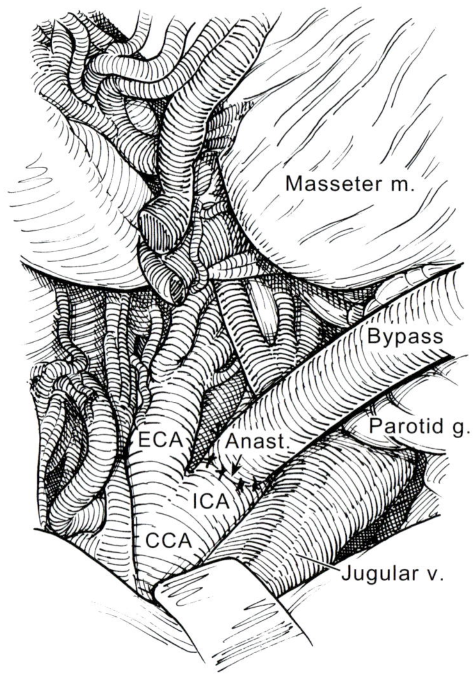

Fig. 9.0i Close-up view of the ICA-to-graft anastomosis.

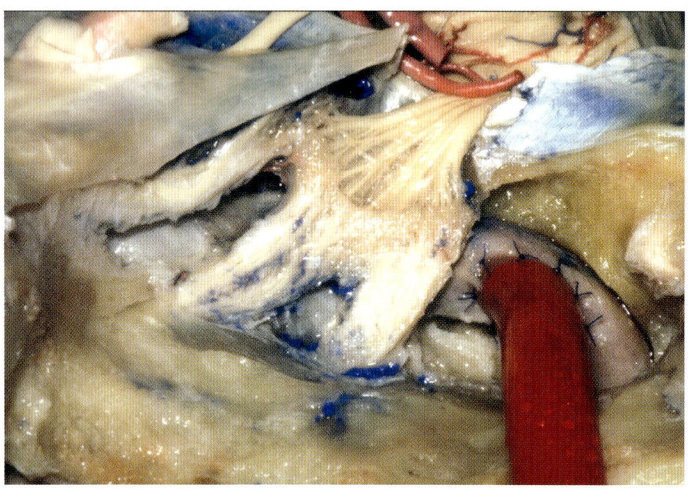

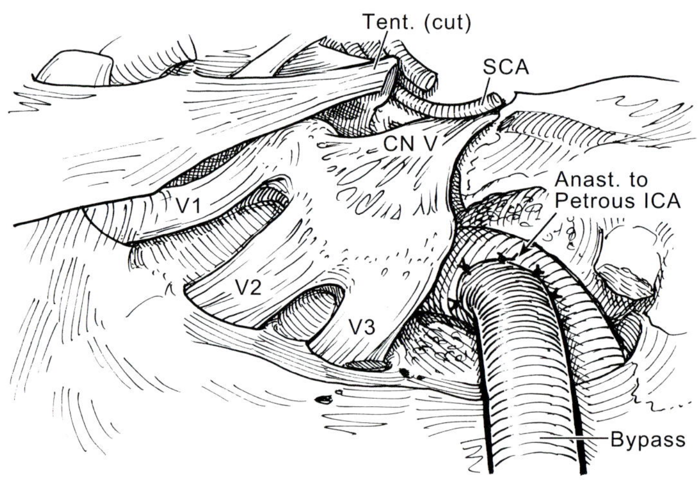

Fig. 9.0j The distal anastomosis between the graft and the petrous ICA.

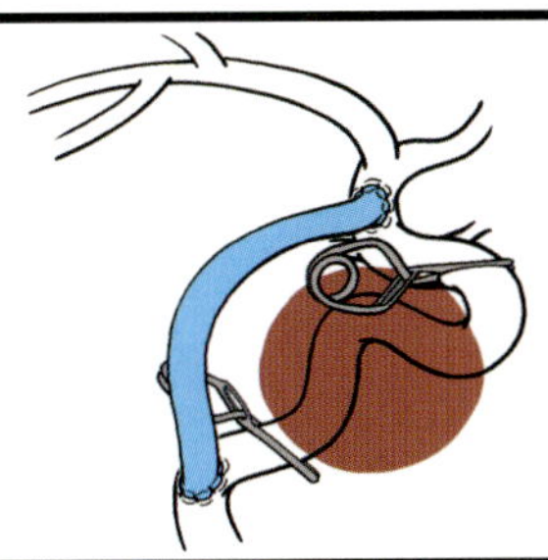

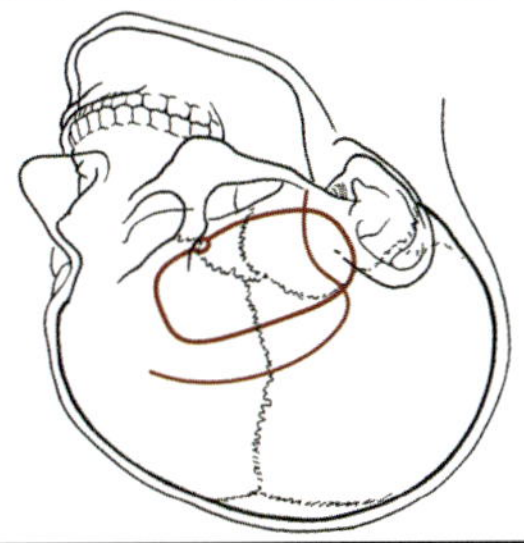

Case 9-1

Diagnosis: Bilateral intracavernous ICA aneurysms

Bypass: Right petrous ICA-to-supraclinoid ICA

Approach: Right pterional with subtemporal extension

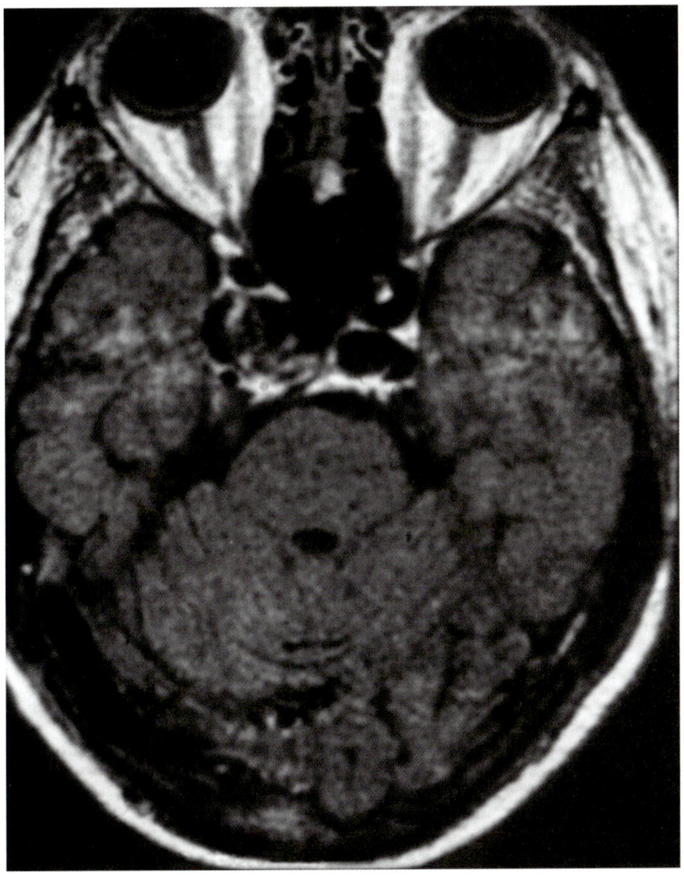

Fig. 9.1a Axial MR image of a patient with diplopia and progressive right ophthalmoparesis shows the flow voids of bilateral cavernous sinus aneurysms.

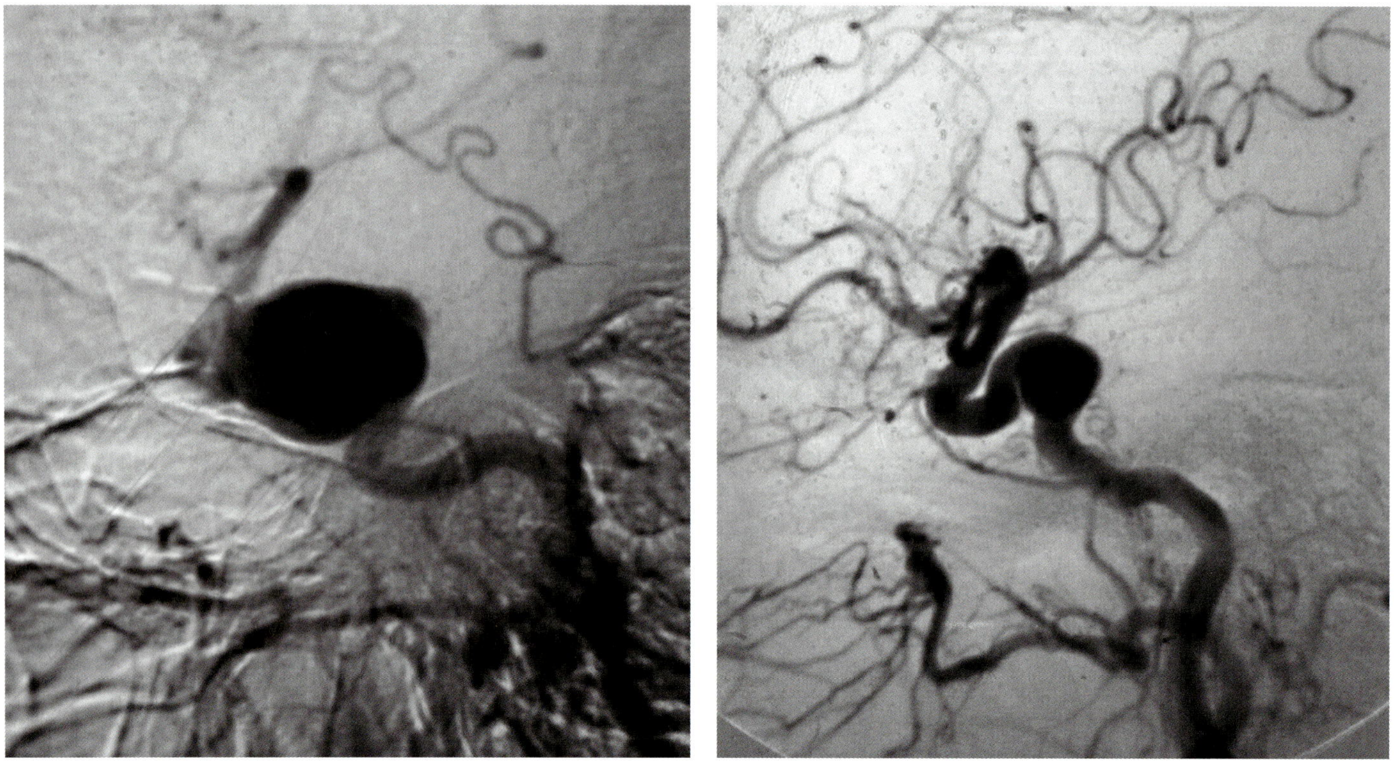

b c

Fig. 9.1b, c Right and left lateral CCA angiograms show a very large right cavernous ICA aneurysm and a smaller left cavernous ICA aneurysm.

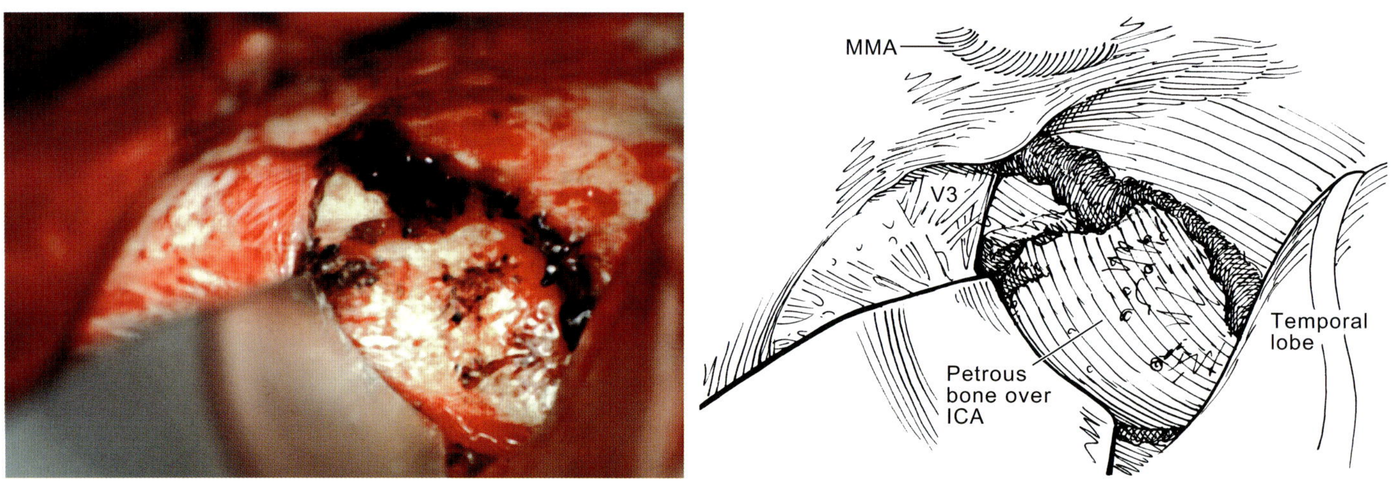

Fig. 9.1d A right pterional craniotomy generously extended on the temporal side allows a flat intradural approach to the temporal fossa. The dura at the temporal floor is opened medially and posteriorly to the MMA, along the posterolateral margin of the V3 division of CN V. A microDoppler probe can be used to locate the origin of the MMA, which is not clearly visible as it would be in an extradural exposure. The advantage of the intradural exposure is that the greater and lesser superficial petrosal nerves can be spared.

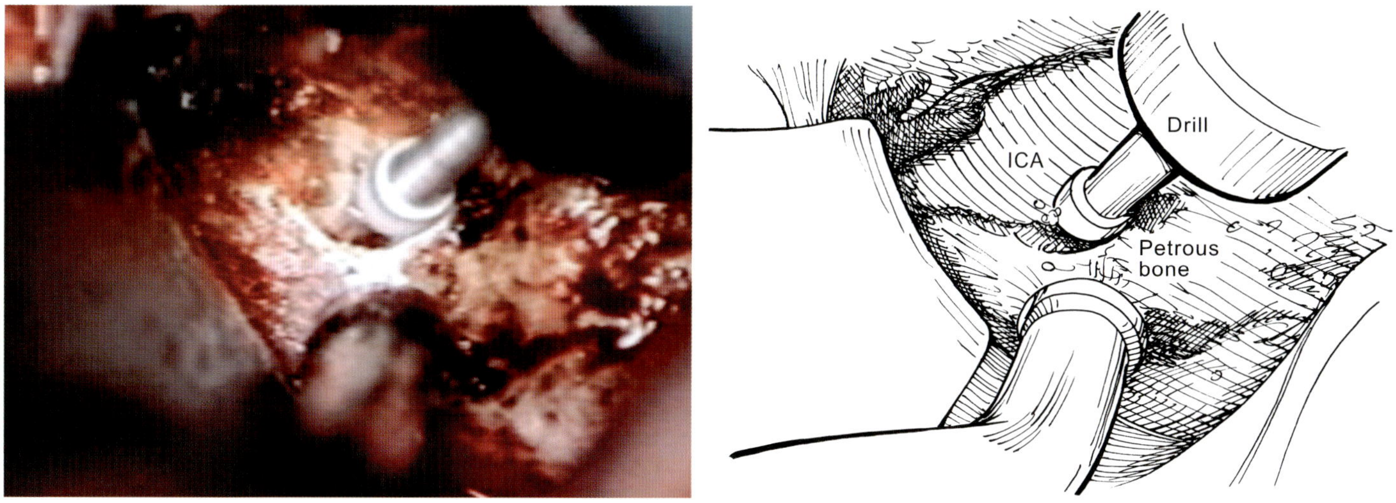

Fig. 9.1e A diamond bit is used to drill through Glasscock's triangle down to the petrous ICA.

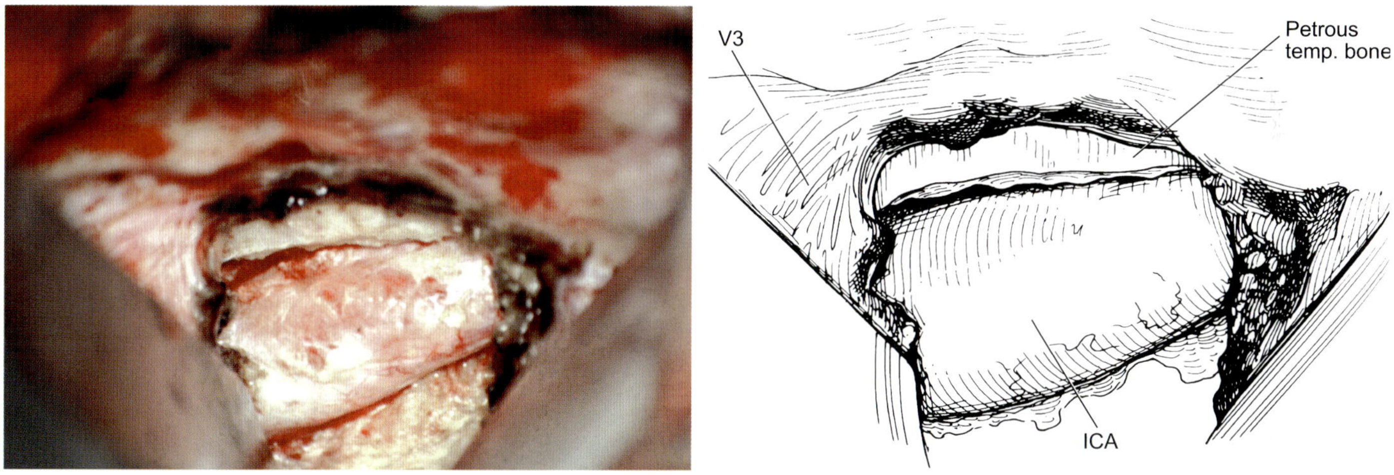

Fig. 9.1f The petrous bone has been removed, exposing the petrous ICA. The boundaries for drilling are the eustachian tube laterally and the cochlea posteriorly, violation of which causes hearing loss. Medially, extensive drilling provides excellent access to the petrous ICA. If air cells are encountered, they should be packed at the end of the procedure with muscle or fat and fibrin glue.

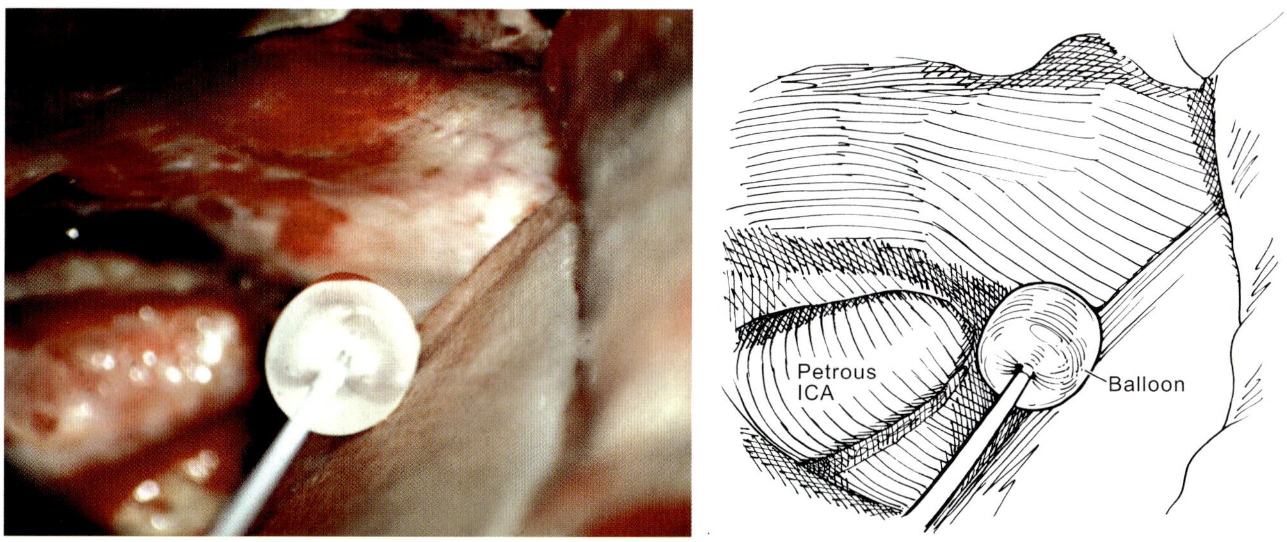

Fig. 9.1g A 2-French Fogarty balloon catheter can be inserted into the carotid canal to gain proximal control of the ICA.

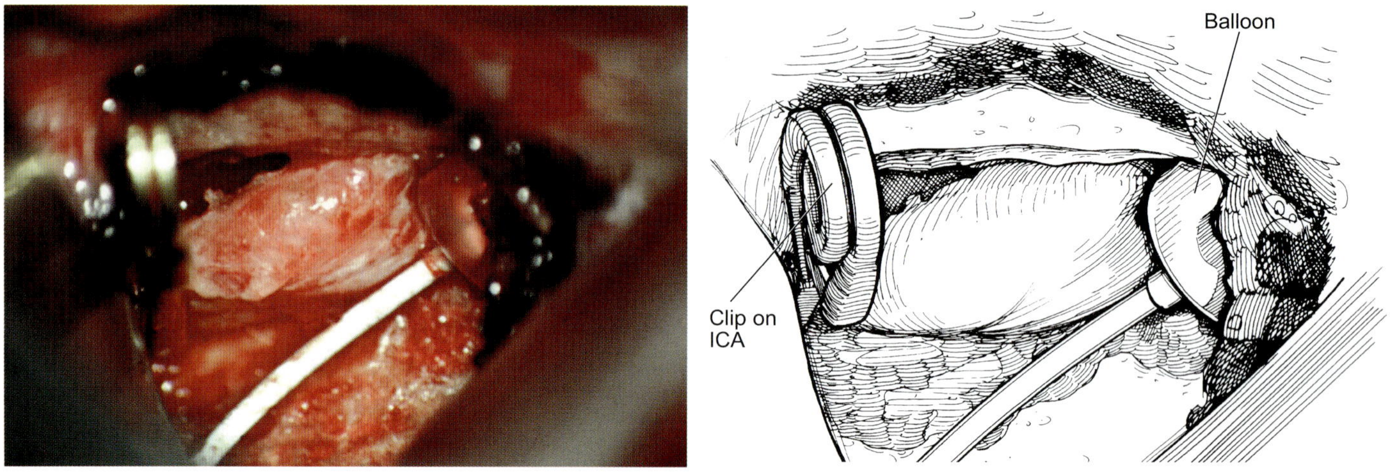

Fig. 9.1h The inflated balloon partially protrudes from the carotid canal, occluding the ICA. Using the balloon eliminates the need for a second clip to control the ICA proximally and allows more freedom of movement for performing the anastomosis. A permanent clip is placed distally on the exposed ICA.

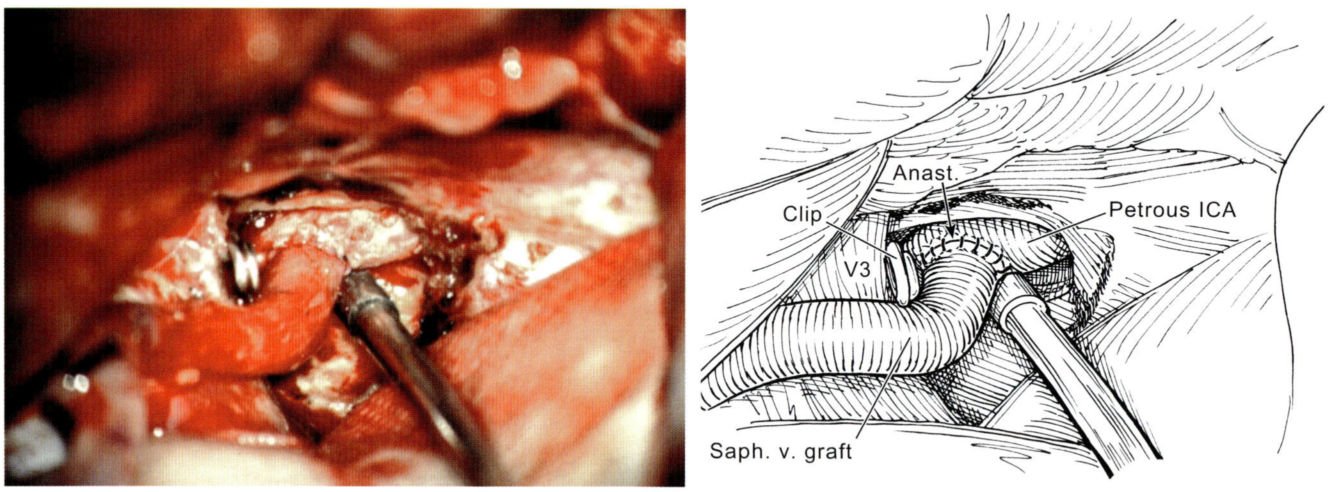

Fig. 9.1i A saphenous vein graft is anastomosed to the petrous ICA.

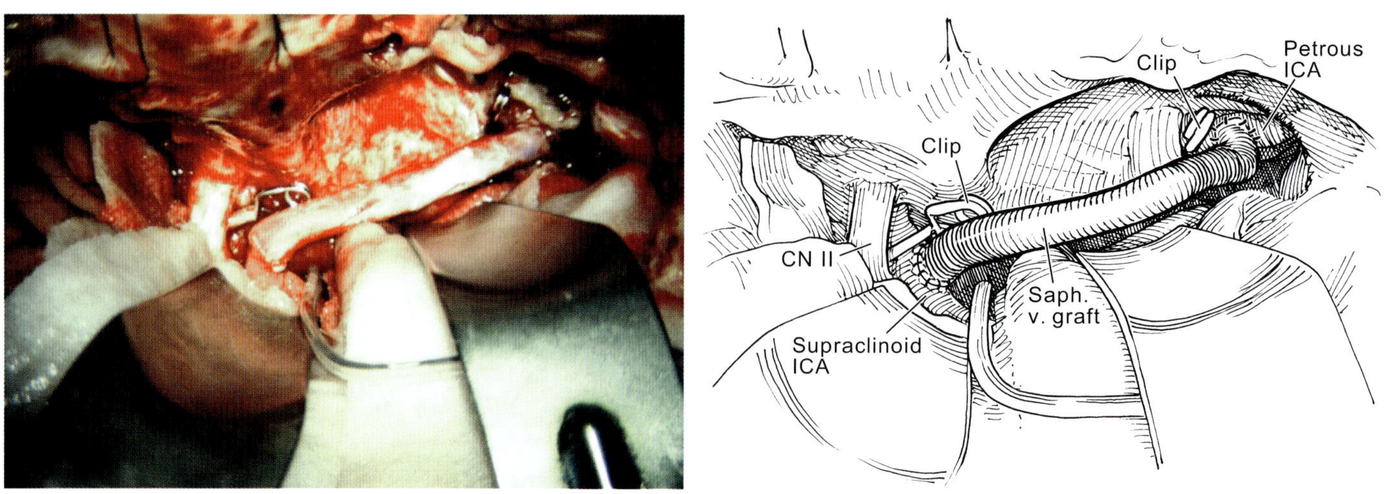

Fig. 9.1j An anterior clinoidectomy has been performed, and the distal end of the saphenous vein graft is anastomosed to the supraclinoid ICA. A clip placed on the ICA proximal to the ophthalmic artery traps the cavernous sinus aneurysm.

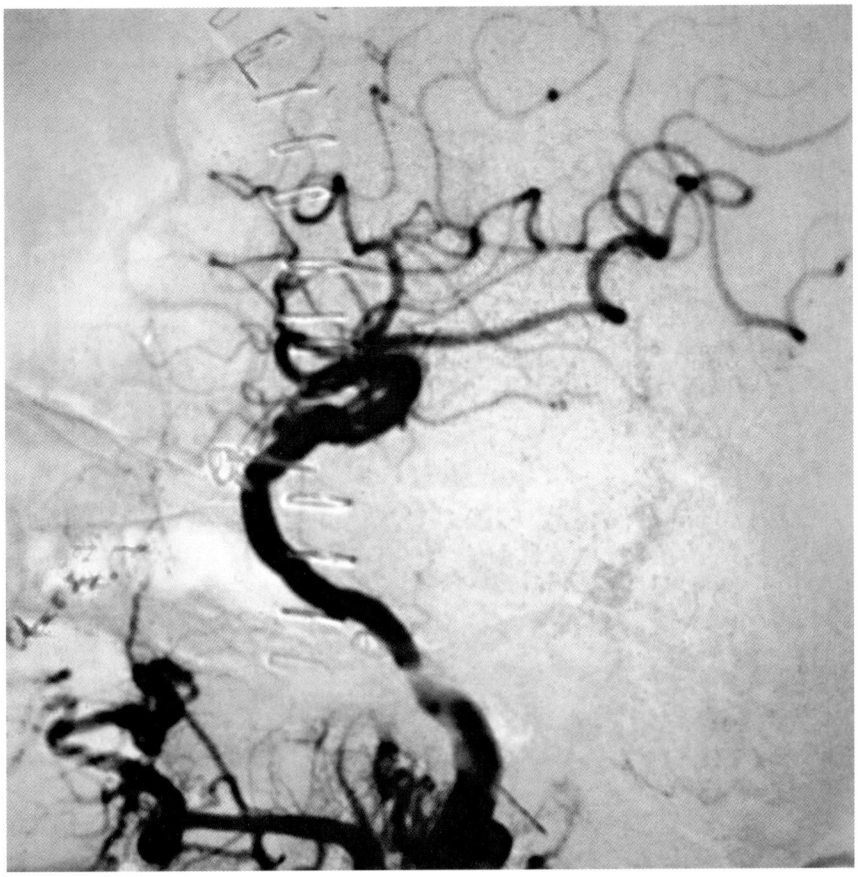

Fig. 9.1k Postoperative right lateral angiogram confirms elimination of the aneurysm with good flow through the saphenous vein graft.

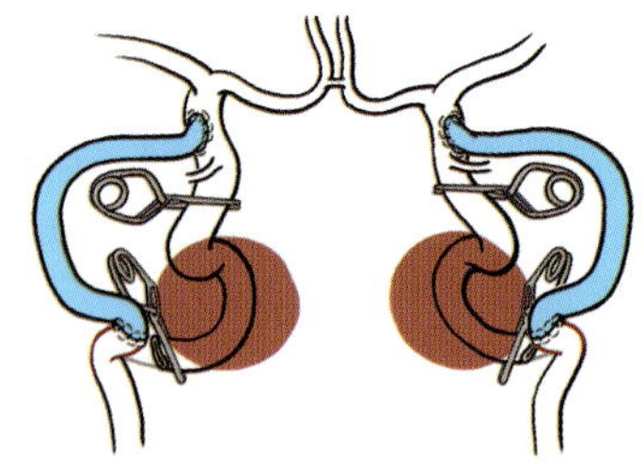

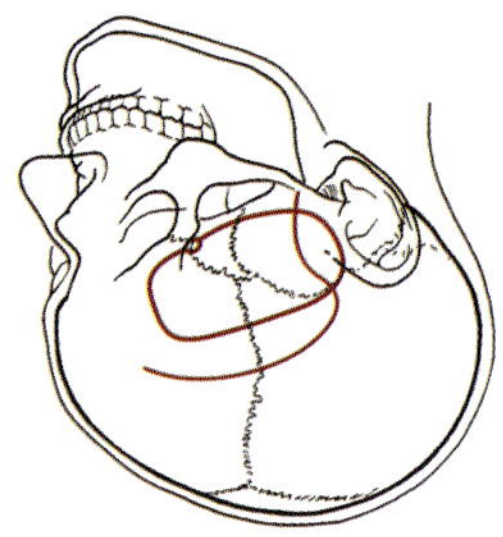

Case 9-2

Diagnosis: Bilateral traumatic ICA-cavernous sinus fistulas and aneurysms

Bypass: Bilateral petrous ICA–to–supraclinoid ICA with saphenous vein grafts

Approach: Bilateral pterional with subtemporal extension

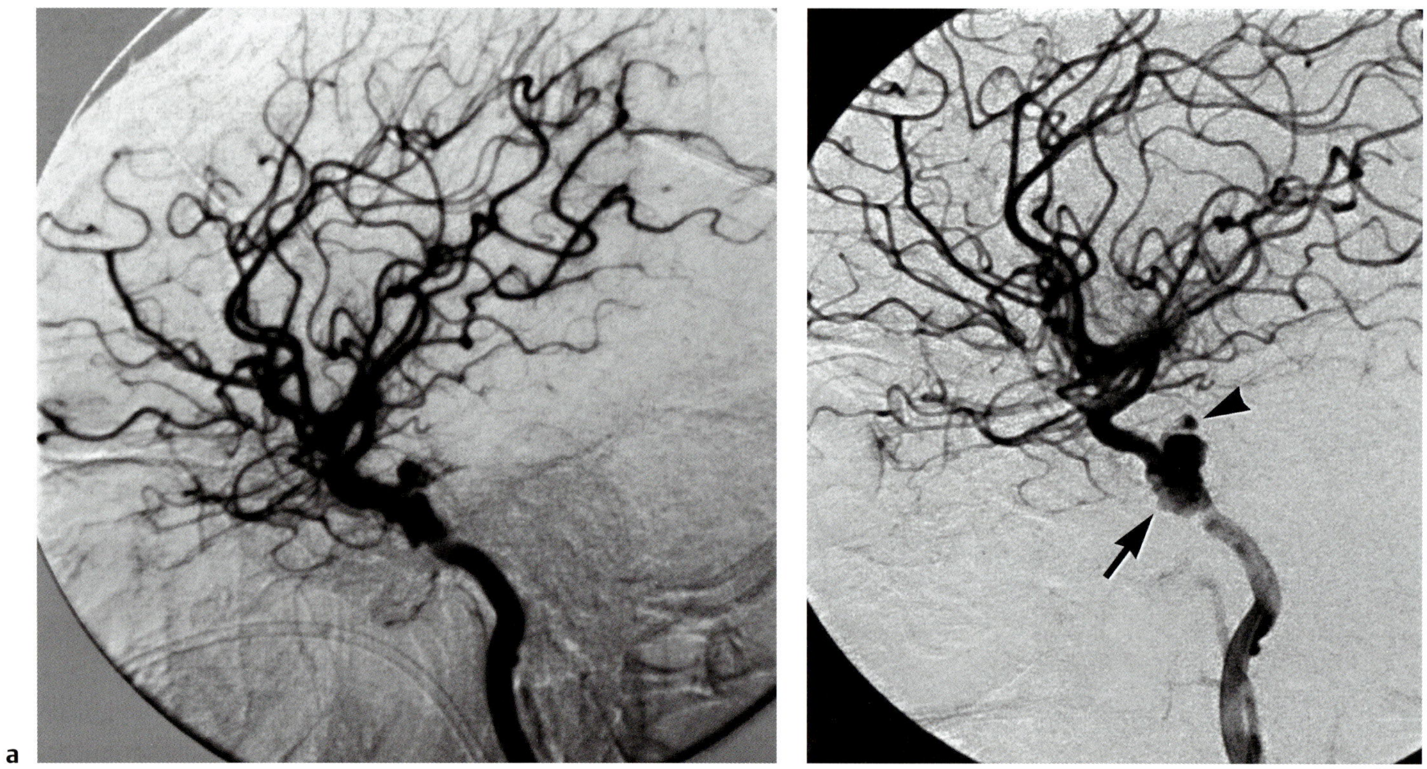

Fig. 9.2a, b Right lateral ICA angiograms show a cavernous sinus aneurysm (*arrow*) with a small fistulous component (*arrowhead*). The aneurysm continued to flow despite endovascular treatment.

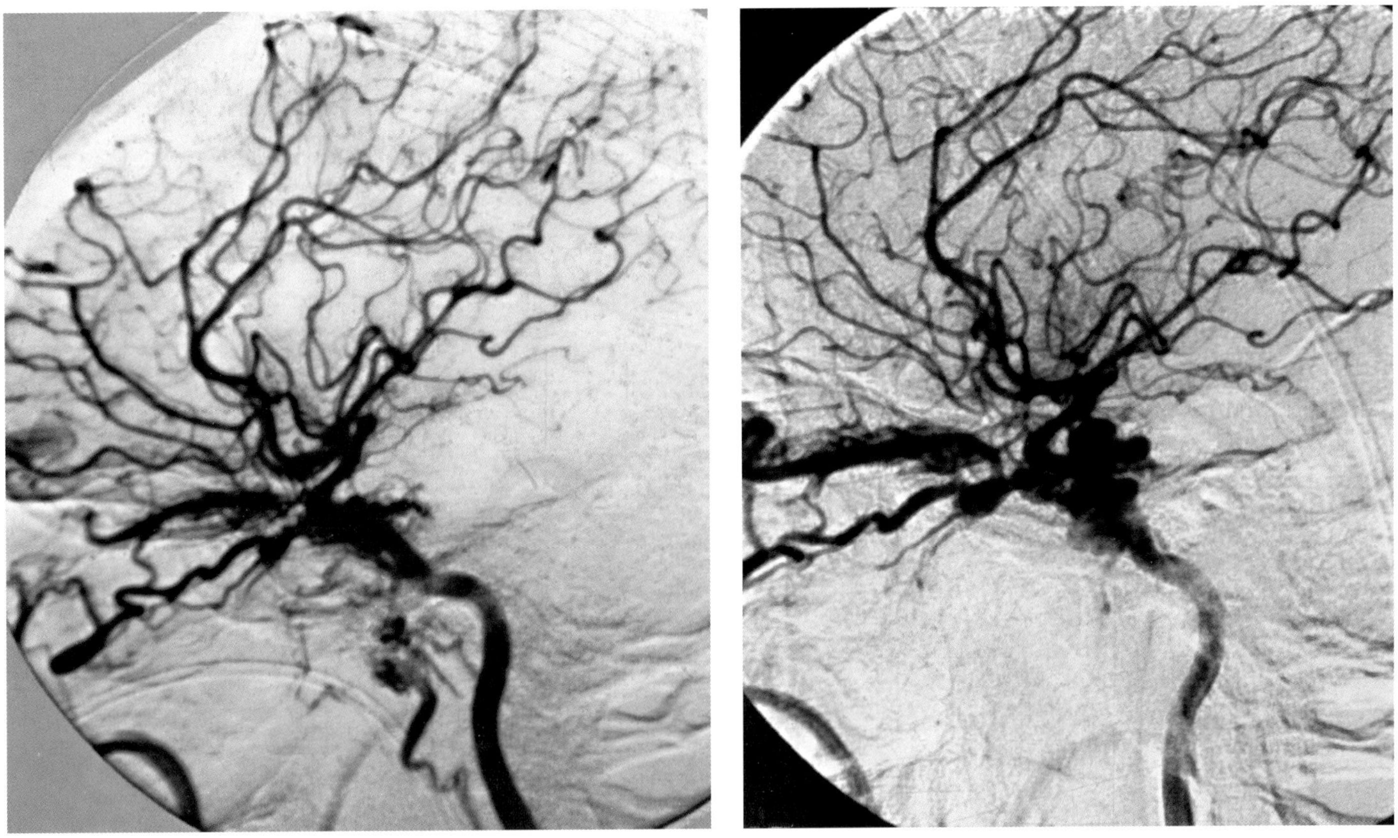

c d

Fig. 9.2c, d Left ICA angiograms show a cavernous sinus fistula with aneurysmal growth over time despite endovascular packing.

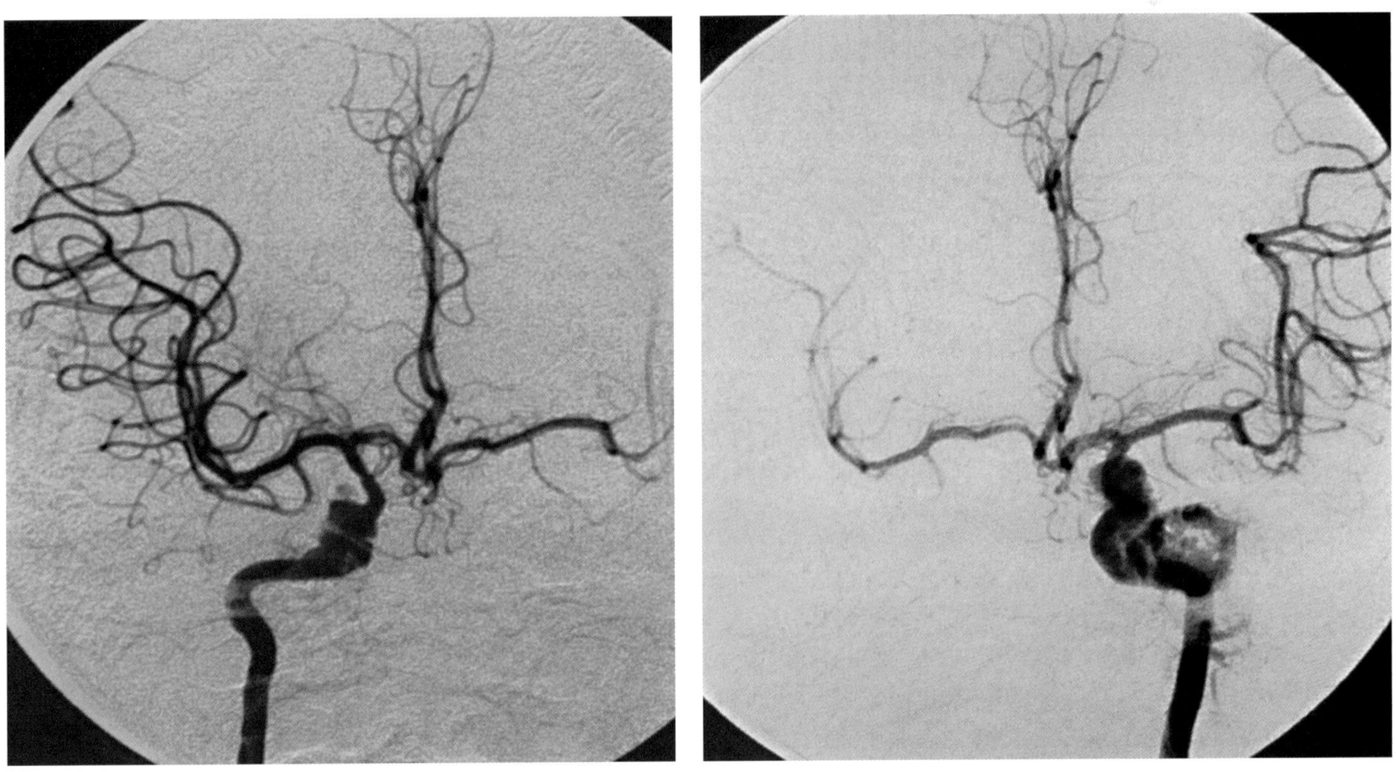

e f

Fig. 9.2e, f Right and left anteroposterior ICA injections show that embolization failed to obliterate the growing aneurysms despite repeated attempts.

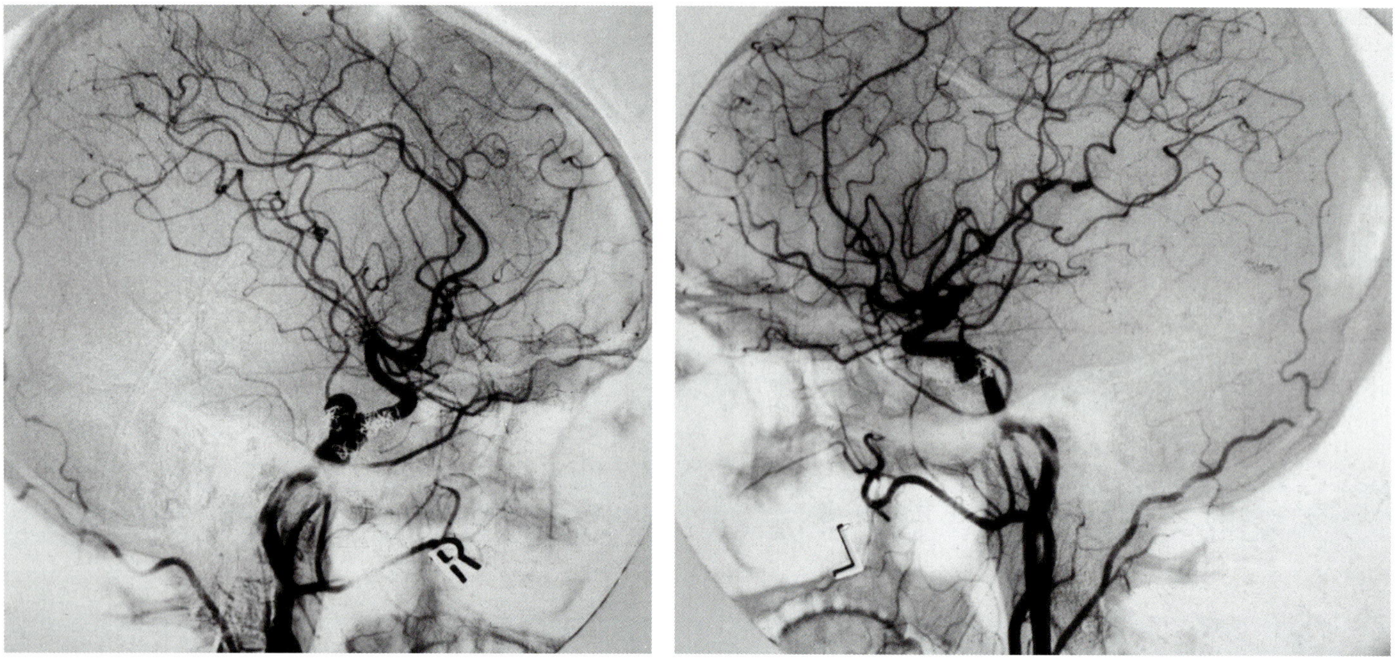

g h

Fig. 9.2g, h Right and left ICA injections demonstrate severe bilateral carotid artery stenosis resulting in ischemic symptoms.

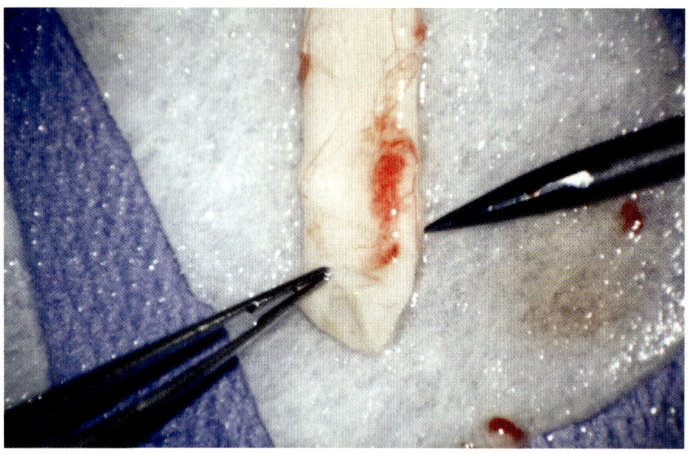

Fig. 9.2i The saphenous vein is prepared for a petrous ICA–to–supraclinoid ICA bypass.

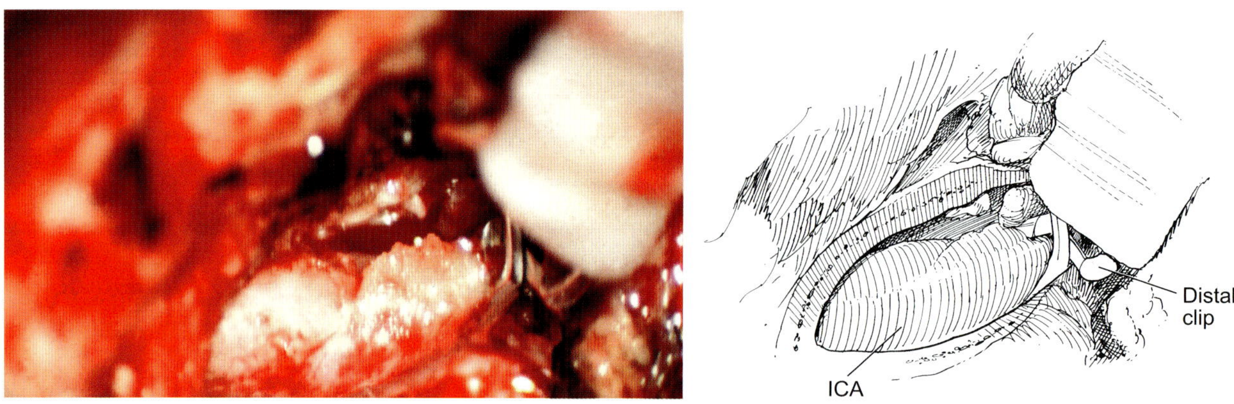

Fig. 9.2j The petrous portion of the left ICA is exposed. A permanent clip is placed on the ICA as it enters the cavernous sinus.

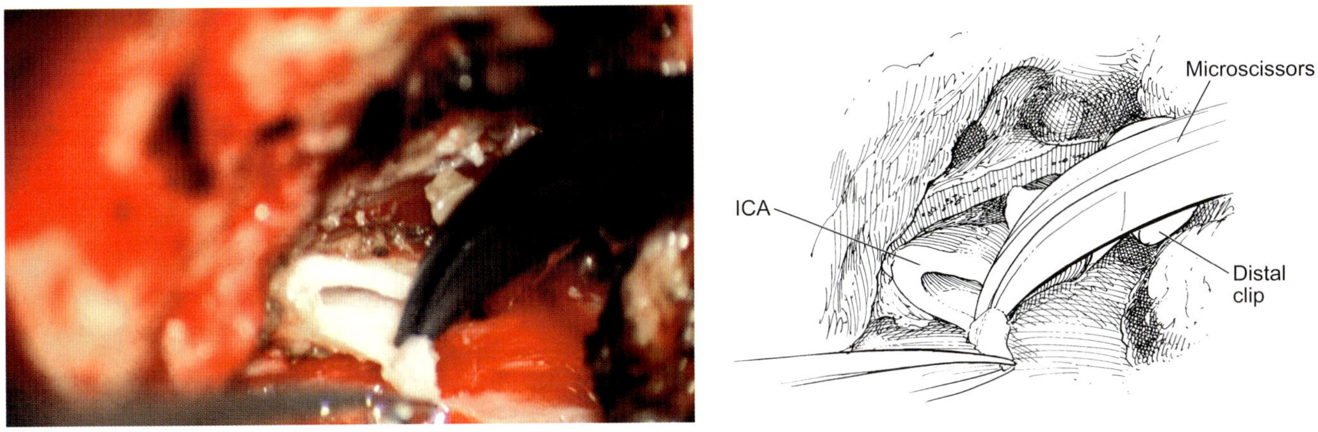

Fig. 9.2k The ICA is cut in preparation for an end-to-end anastomosis to the saphenous vein graft.

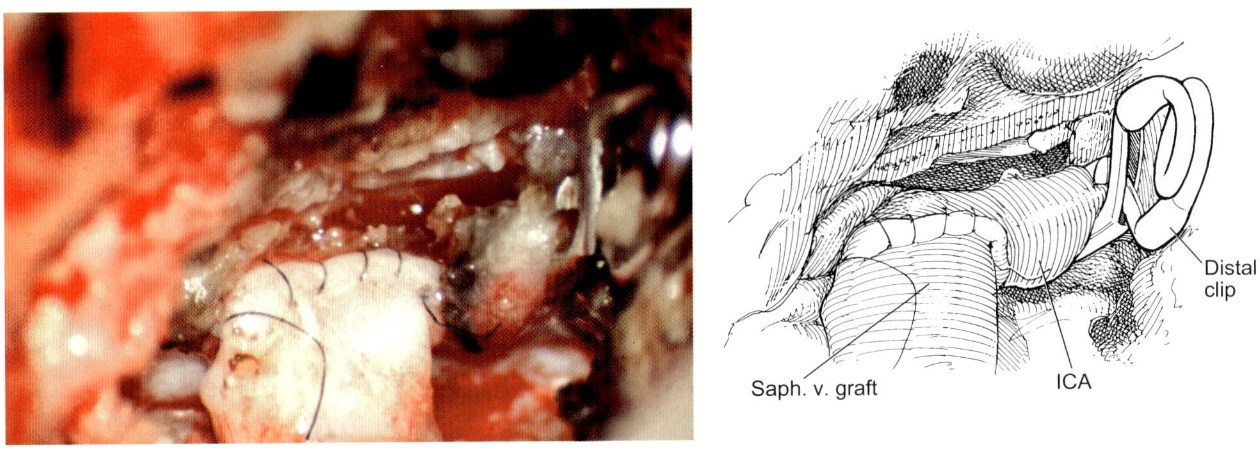

Fig. 9.2l The saphenous vein graft is being anastomosed to the petrous ICA.

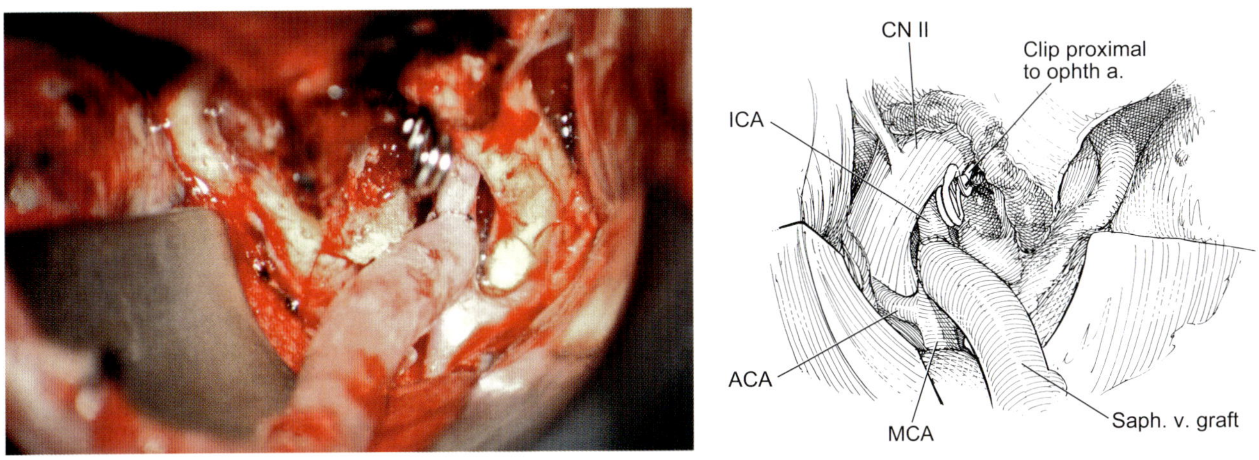

Fig. 9.2m The other end of the saphenous vein graft is anastomosed to the ICA below CN II.

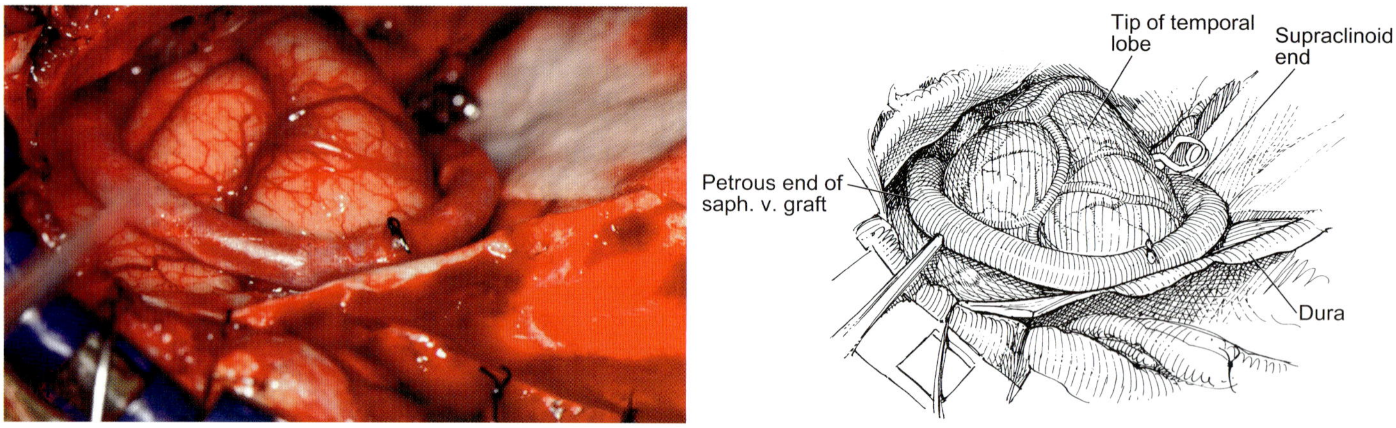

Fig. 9.2n Overview of the saphenous vein graft from the petrous ICA to the supraclinoid ICA.

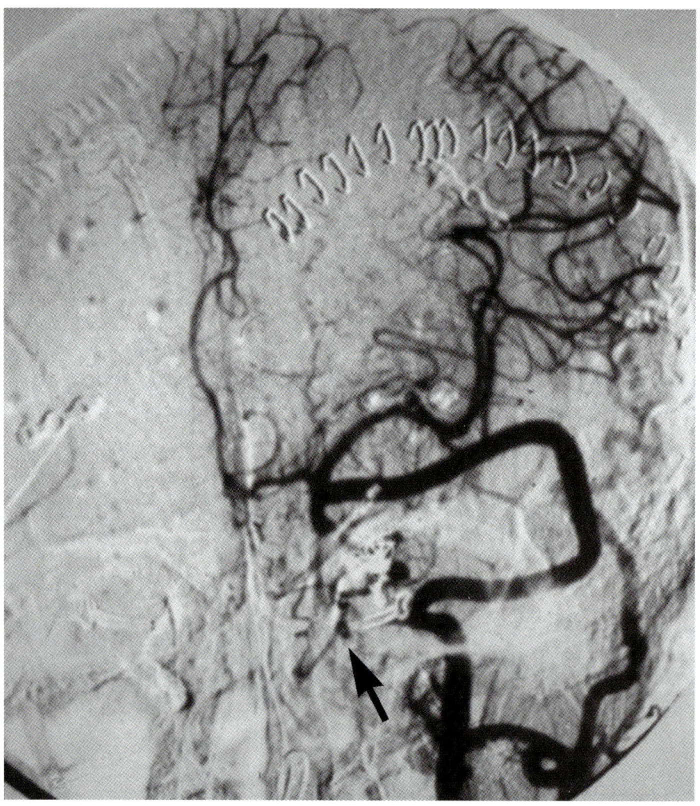

Fig. 9.2o After the first bypass is completed, good circulation is maintained in the ICA. Note the backflow to the ophthalmic artery (*arrow*).

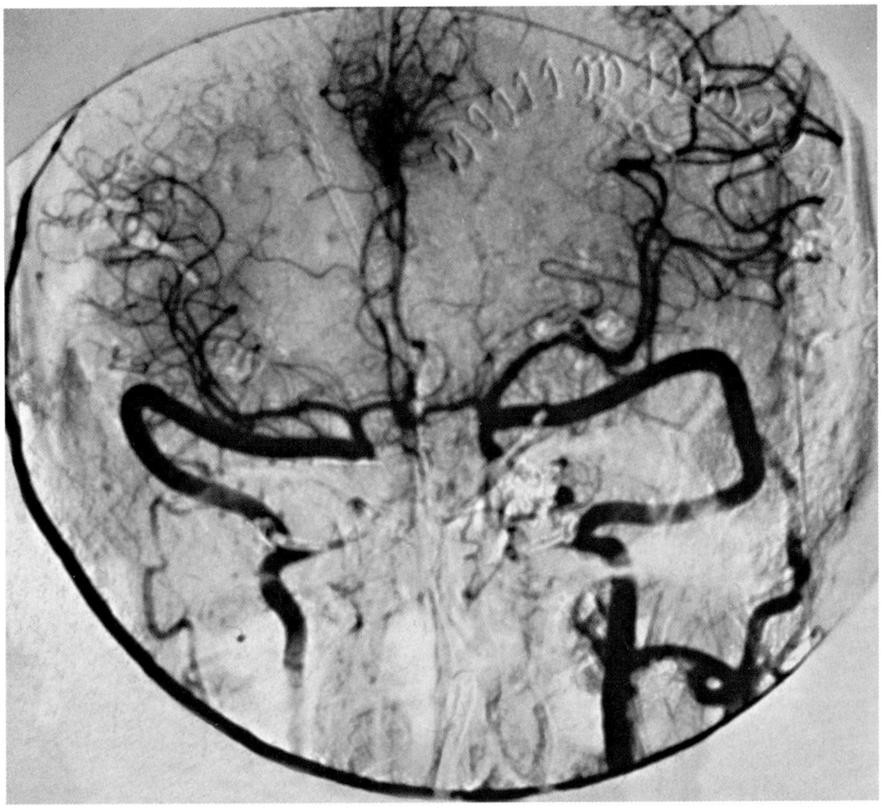

Fig. 9.2p One week after the first bypass the patient underwent a right petrous ICA–to–supraclinoid ICA saphenous vein graft bypass. Postoperative angiogram demonstrates filling of the supratentorial compartment through both ICA saphenous vein bypasses. The patient had no further ischemic events.

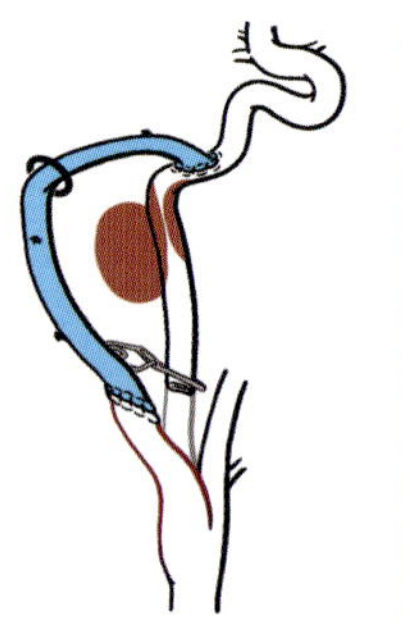

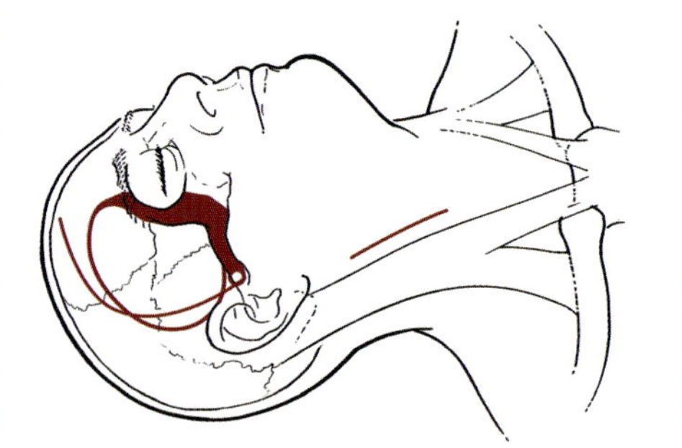

Case 9-3

Diagnosis: Bilateral traumatic dissection of ICAs with pseudoaneurysm formation

Bypass: Cervical ICA–to–petrous ICA with saphenous vein graft

Approach: Right anterior cervical and right orbitozygomatic

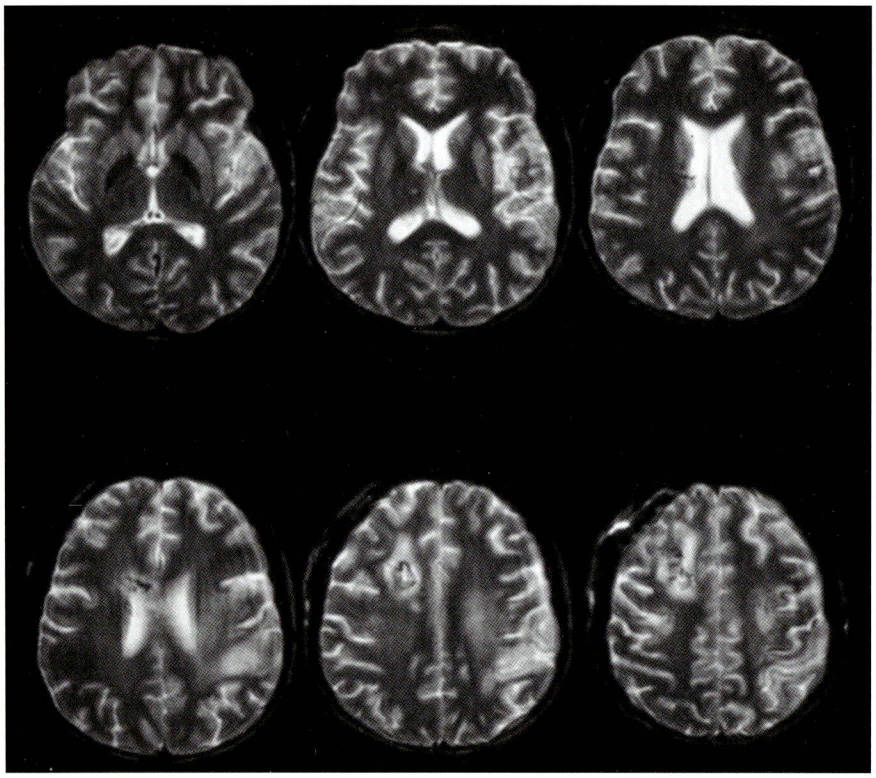

Fig. 9.3a MR images of a 17-year-old girl who was in a motor vehicle collision show bilateral ischemic disease of the cerebral hemisphere related to bilateral traumatic dissections of the carotid arteries. Despite anticoagulation therapy, the patient had recurrent episodes of ischemia. Repeat angiography demonstrated progressive arterial stenosis related to the dissections.

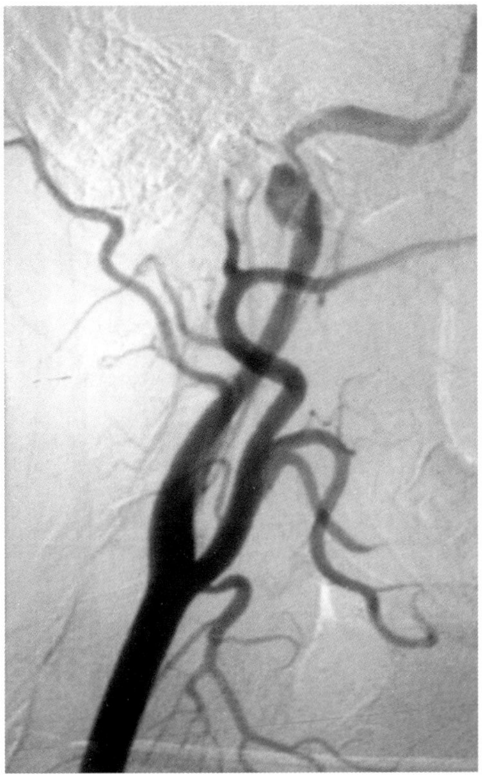

Fig. 9.3b Lateral angiogram of the right CCA demonstrates severe narrowing of the ICA just distal to the formation of a pseudoaneurysm.

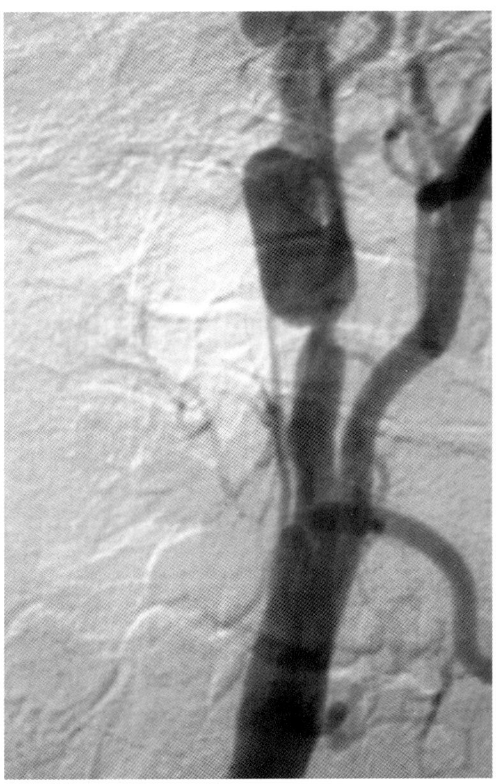

Fig. 9.3c Lateral angiogram of the left CCA demonstrates the dissection of the vessel with pseudoaneurysm formation.

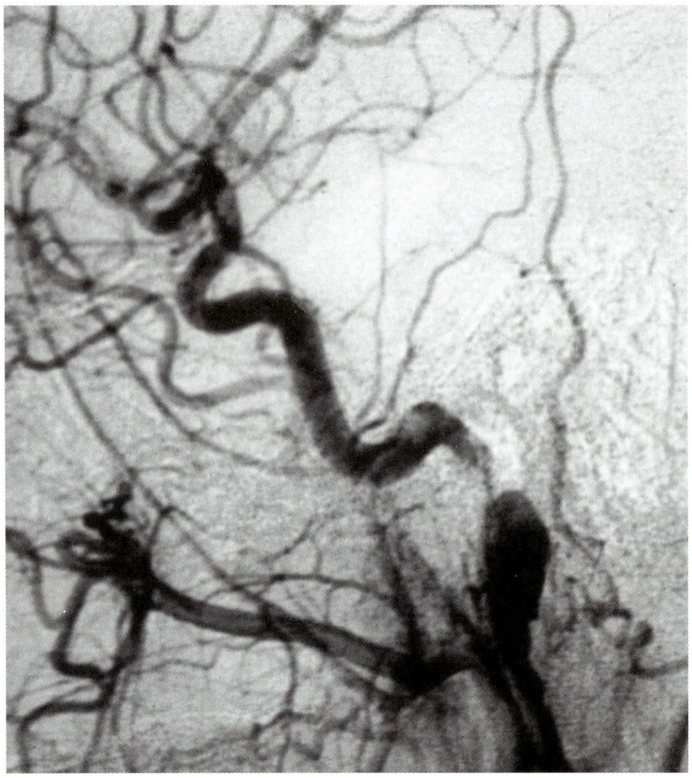

Fig. 9.3d After another ischemic episode, a repeat angiogram of the left lateral CCA demonstrates further narrowing of the ICA distal to the pseudoaneurysm.

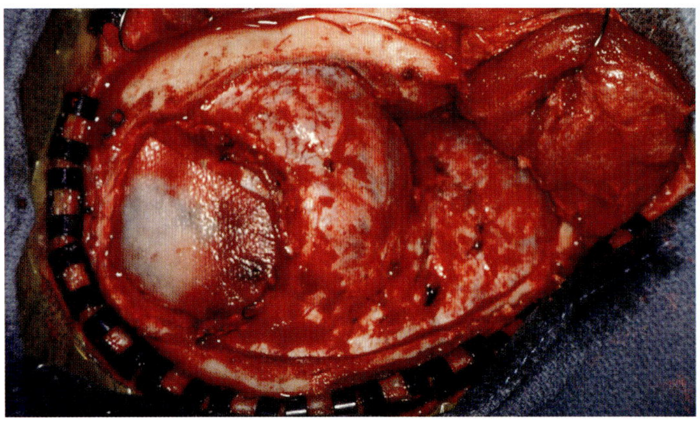

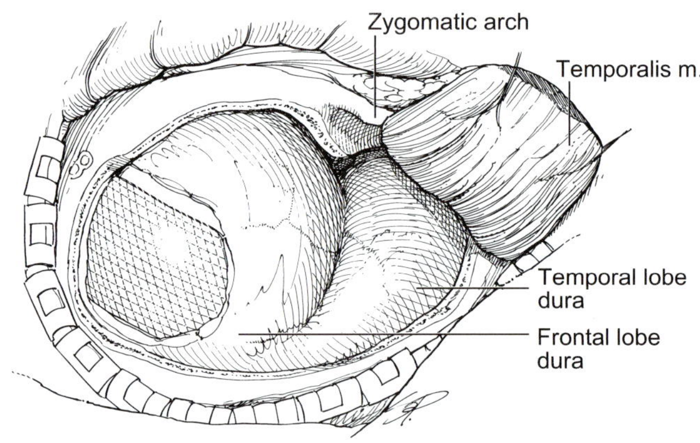

Fig. 9.3e An orbitozygomatic craniotomy is begun.

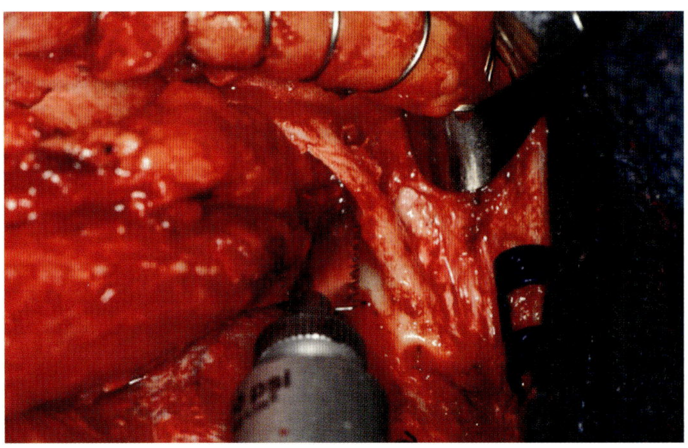

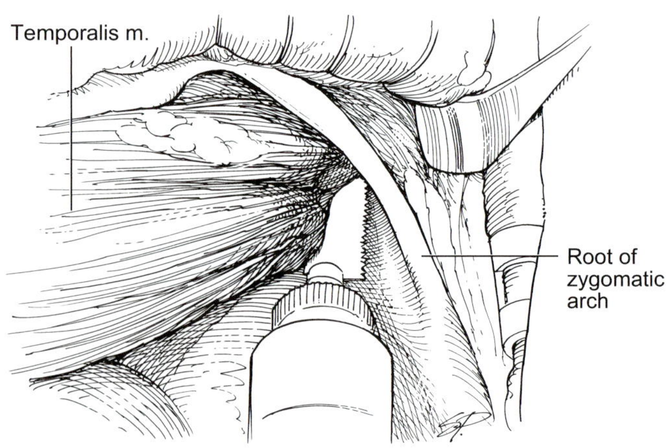

Fig. 9.3f The root of the zygomatic arch is cut.

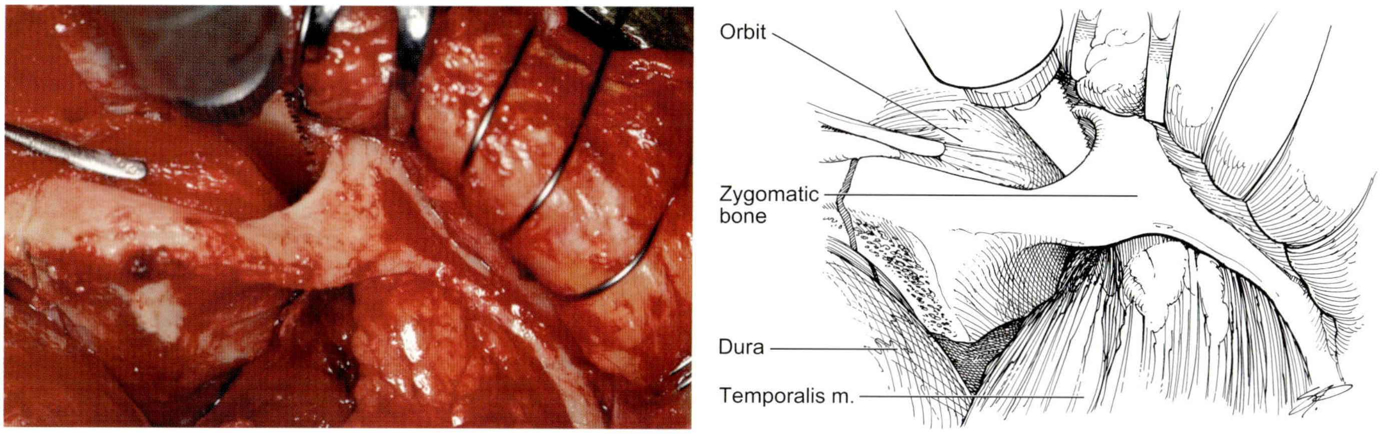

Fig. 9.3g With the orbit retracted, the orbitozygomatic osteotomy is begun.

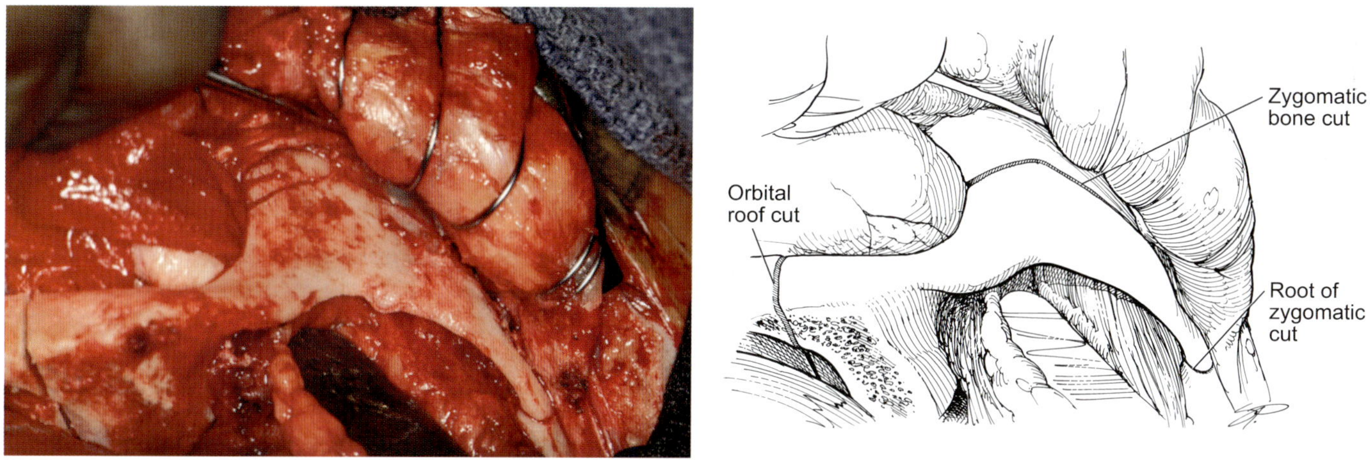

Fig. 9.3h Overview of the osteotomy cuts.

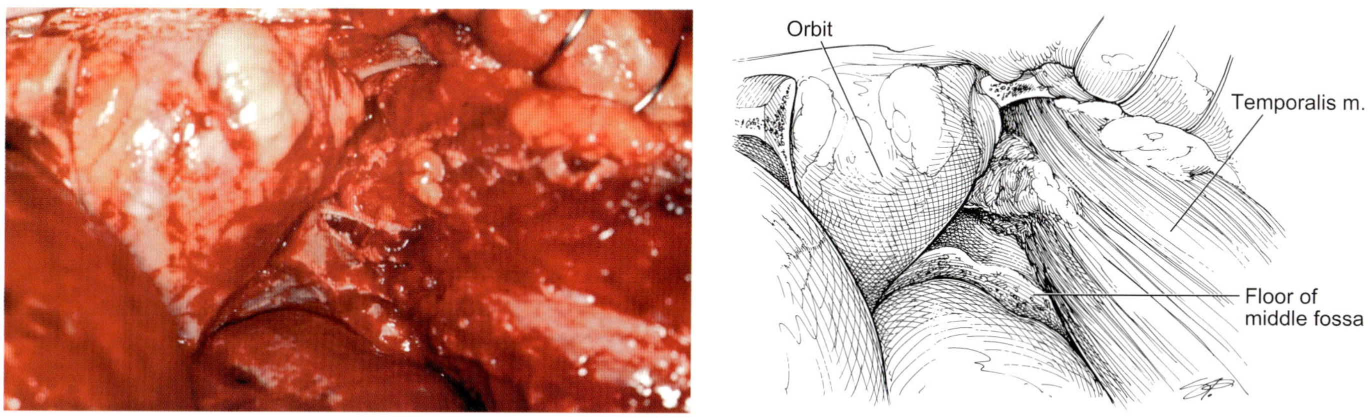

Fig. 9.3i The orbital contents are exposed after the orbitozygomatic bone is removed. This maneuver allows the temporalis muscle to be pulled anteriorly and inferiorly with fishhooks, greatly increasing exposure of the floor of the middle fossa.

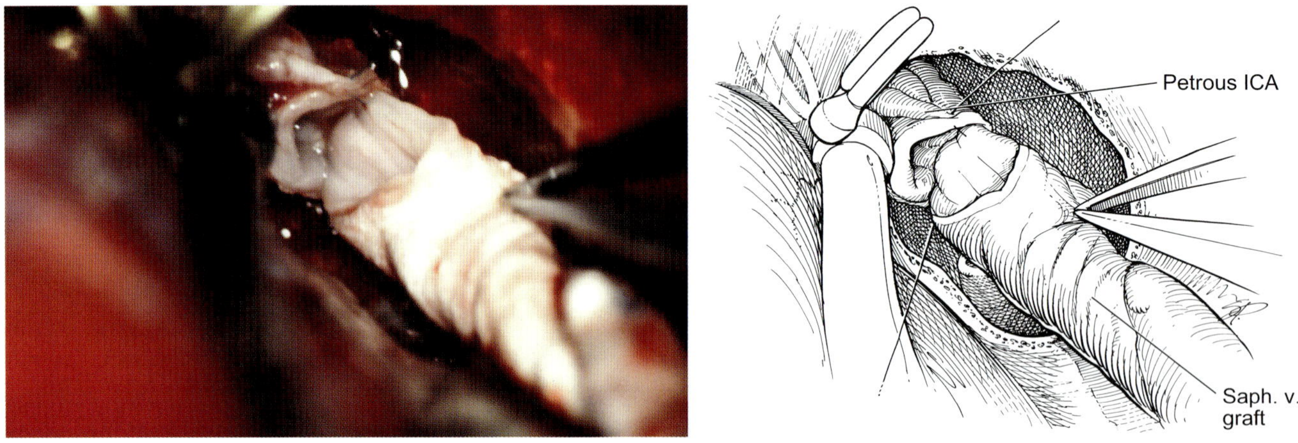

Fig. 9.3j The petrous ICA is isolated and opened. The back wall of the end-to-side anastomosis to the saphenous vein graft has been completed.

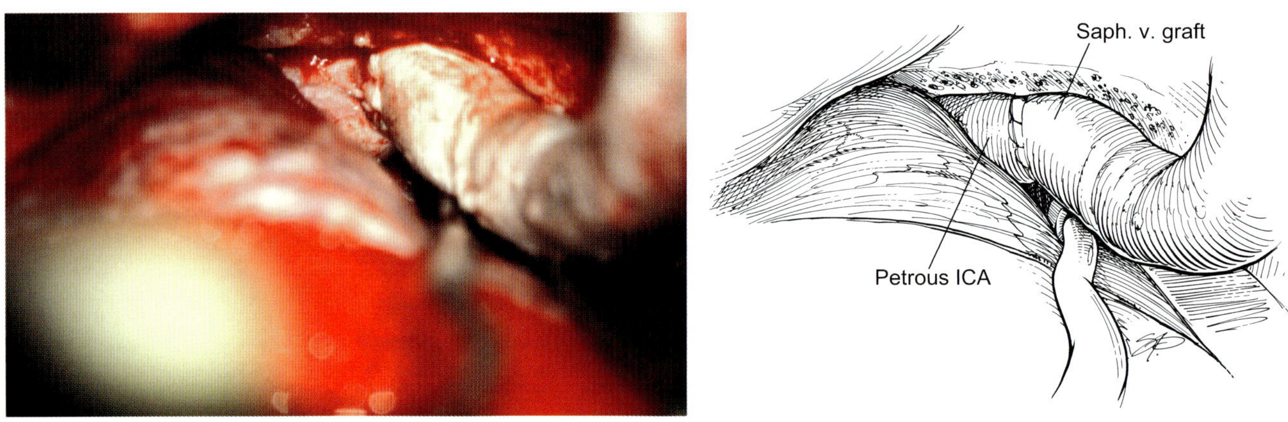

Fig. 9.3k The completed anastomosis is inspected for hemostasis.

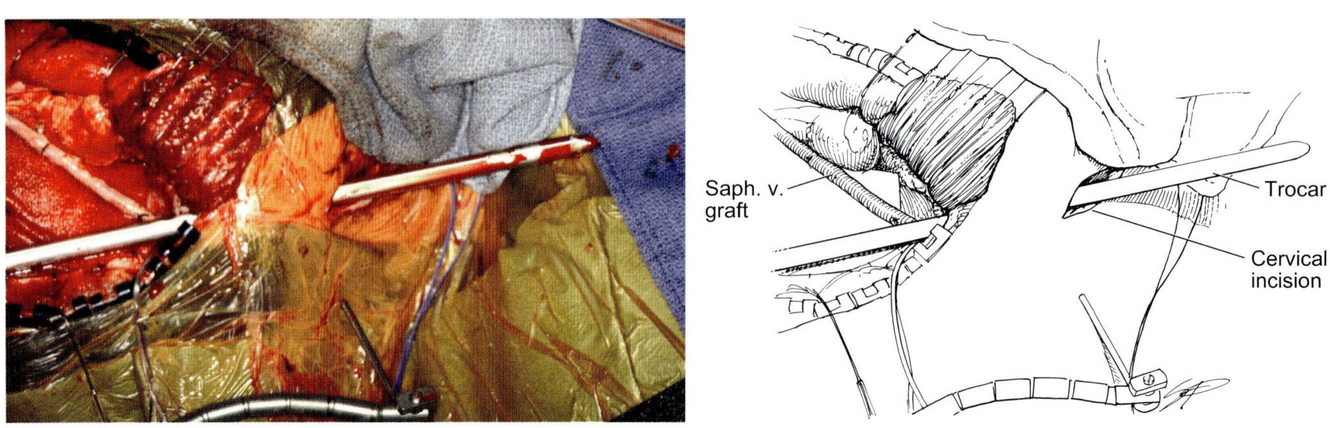

Fig. 9.3l A 28-French trocar is passed subcutaneously from the cranial to the cervical incision where the carotid bifurcation has been exposed.

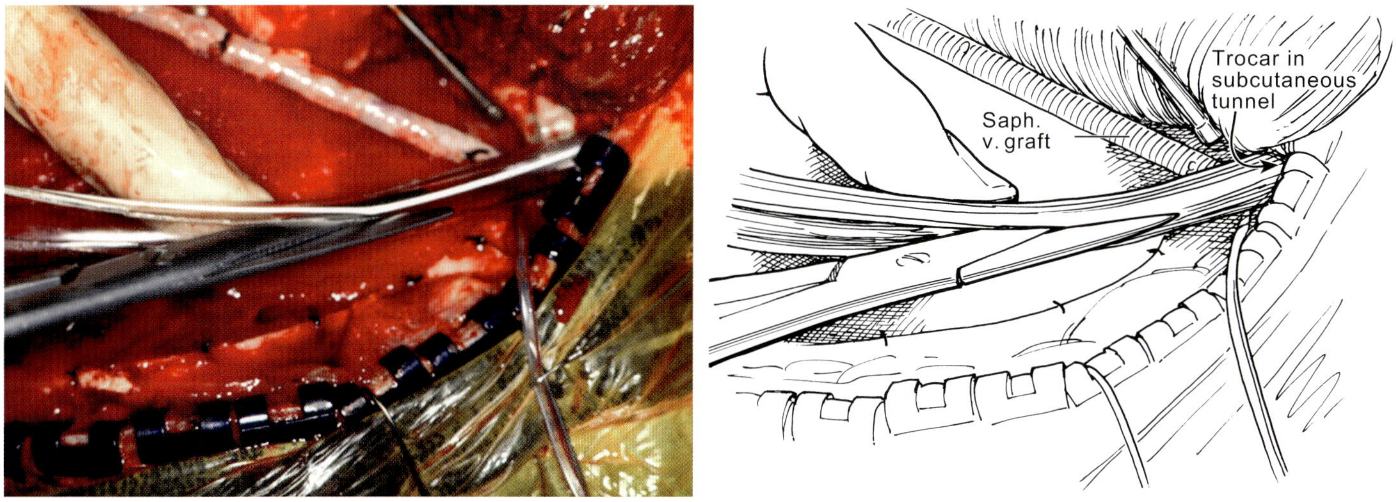

Fig. 9.3m After the metal stylet is withdrawn, the distal end of the trocar is cut longitudinally.

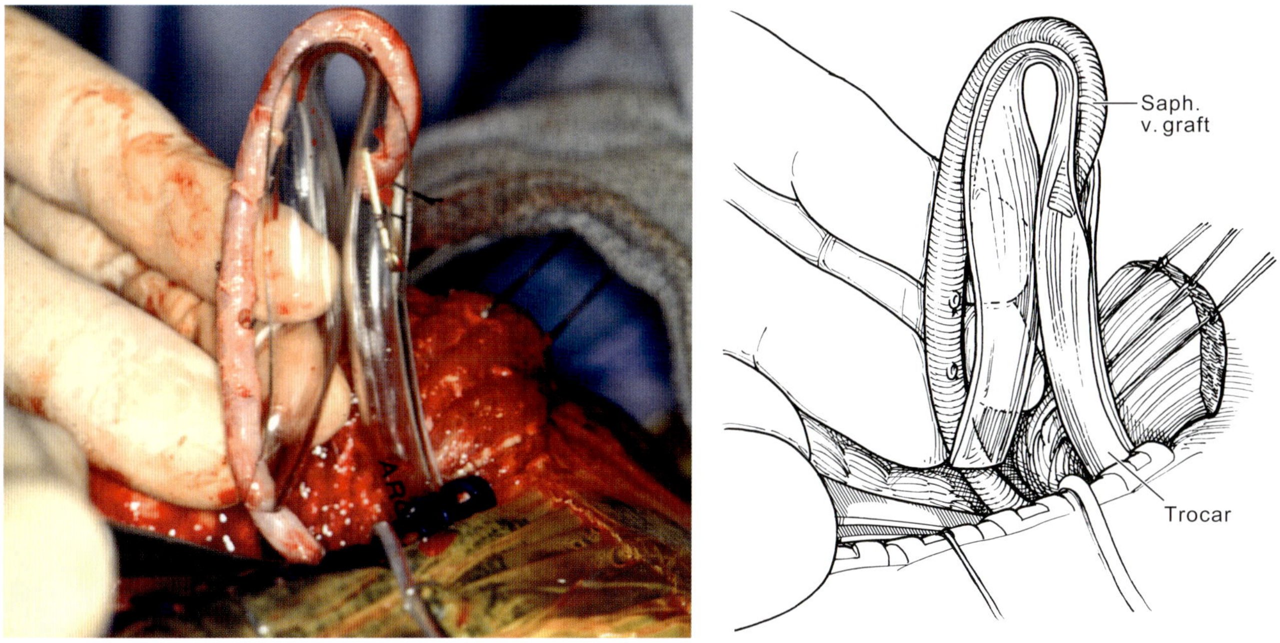

Fig. 9.3n The saphenous vein graft is placed inside the opened end of the trocar.

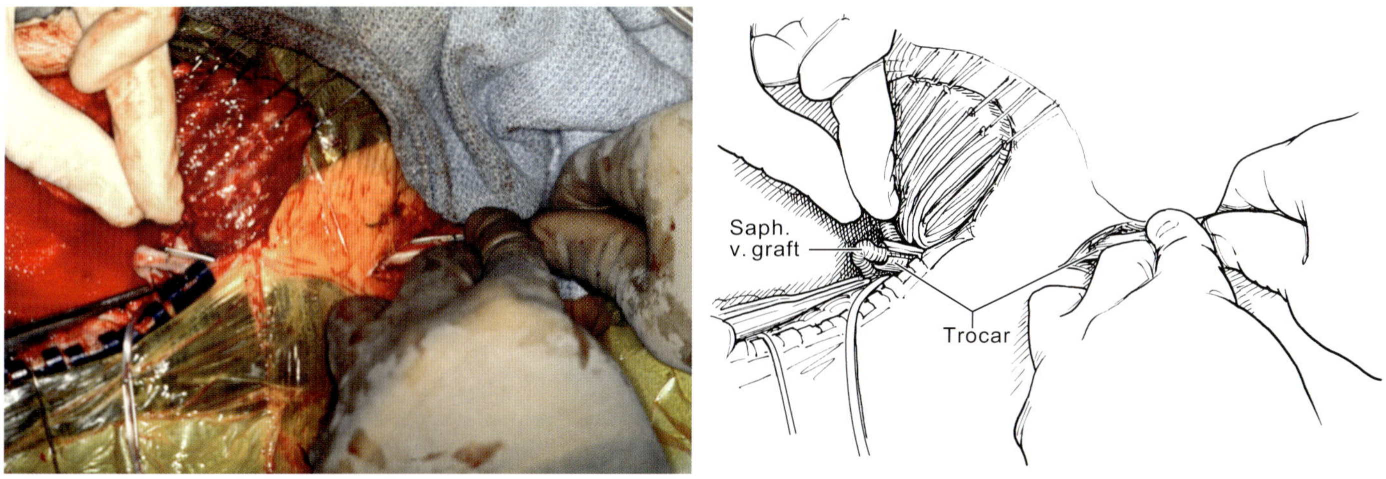

Fig. 9.3o While the surgeon holds the saphenous vein graft with vascular forceps to prevent traction on the anastomosis, the trocar is pulled through the subcutaneous tunnel.

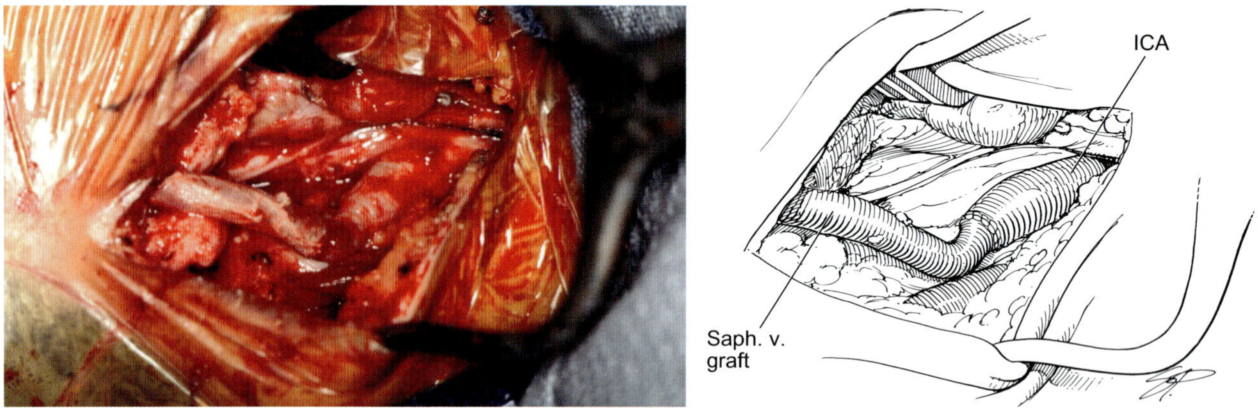

Fig. 9.3p The end-to-end anastomosis of the saphenous vein graft and ICA is completed.

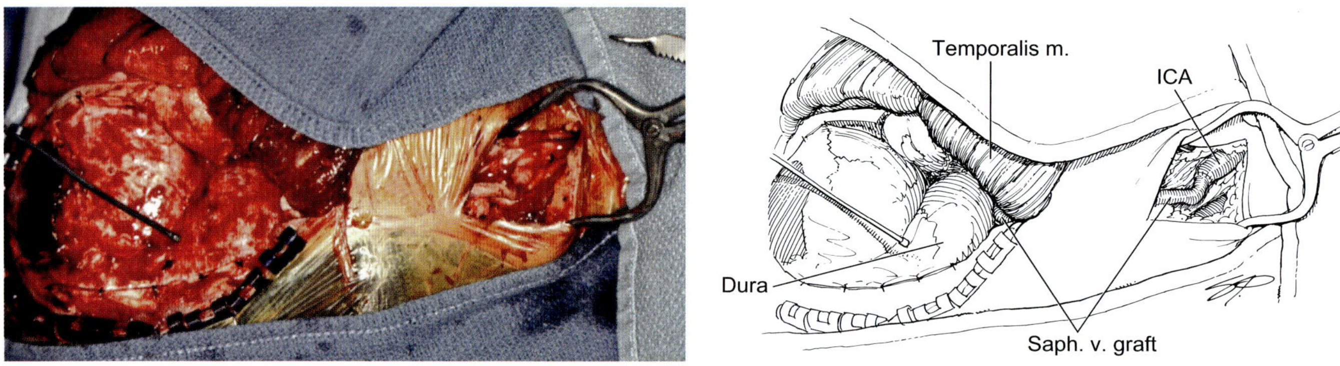

Fig. 9.3q Overview of operative sites demonstrates the saphenous vein graft extradurally and its anastomosis with the ICA.

r 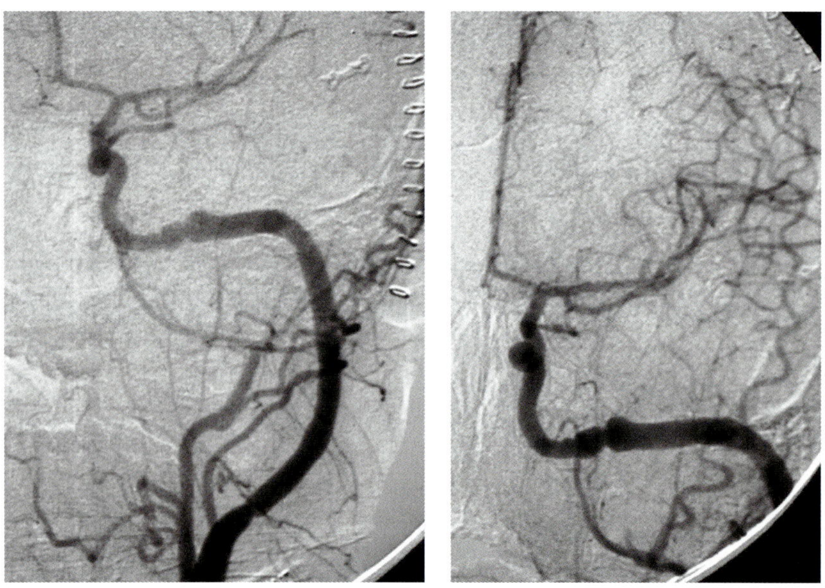 s

Fig. 9.3r, s Anteroposterior angiograms of the CCA demonstrate the widely patent saphenous vein graft bypass.

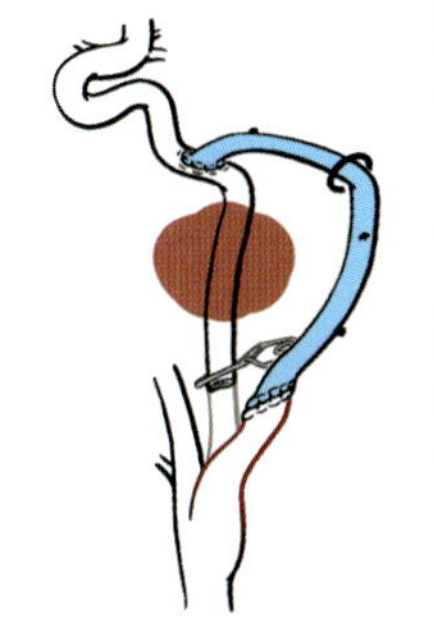

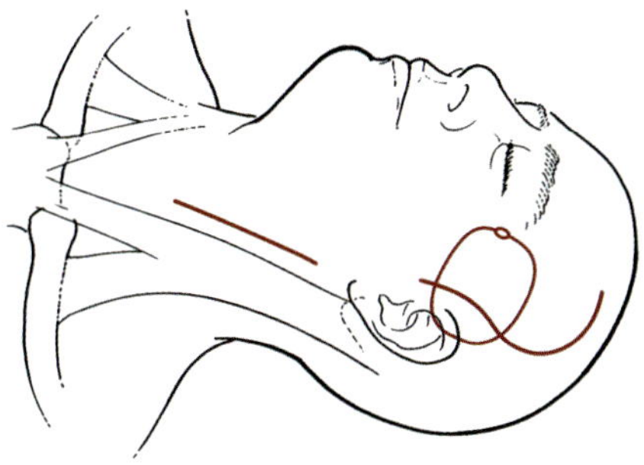

Case 9-4

Diagnosis: Large left cervical ICA pseudoaneurysm

Bypass: Cervical ICA-to-petrous ICA with saphenous vein graft

Approach: Left anterior cervical and left subtemporal

Video

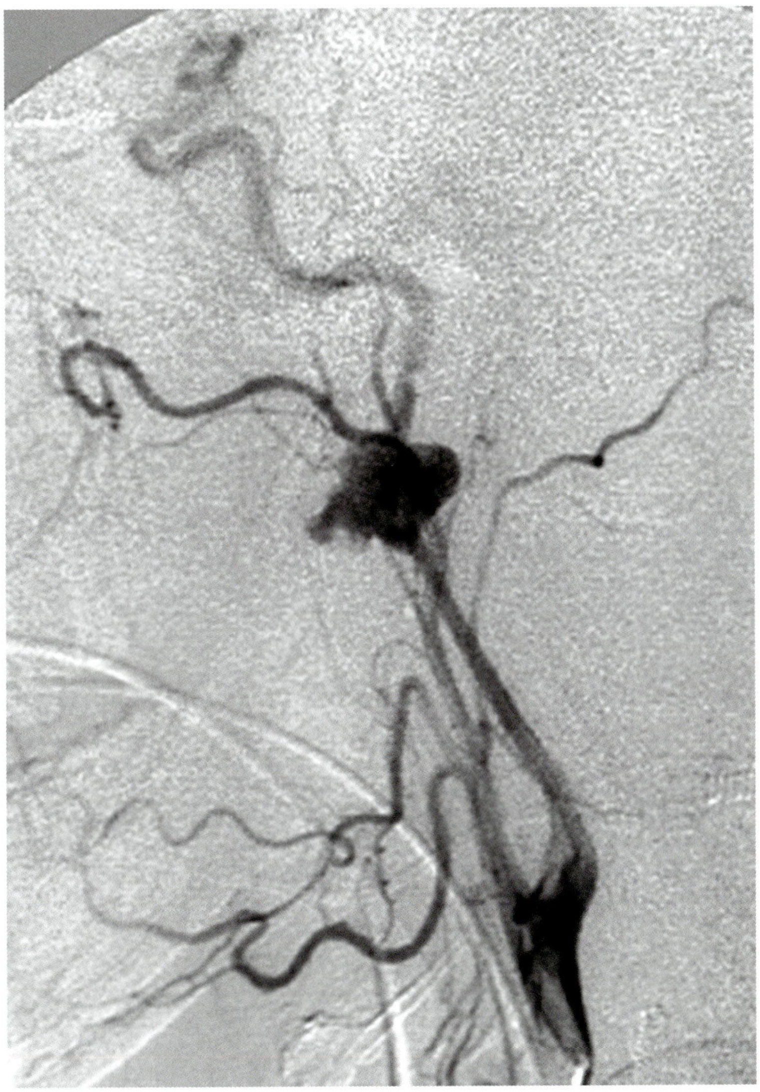

Fig. 9.4a Left lateral angiogram shows a large pseudoaneurysm of the cervical ICA. This patient presented with a severe intraoral hemorrhage after the identification of a lancinating mass. The patient was fortunate enough to have been intubated and transferred for acute care.

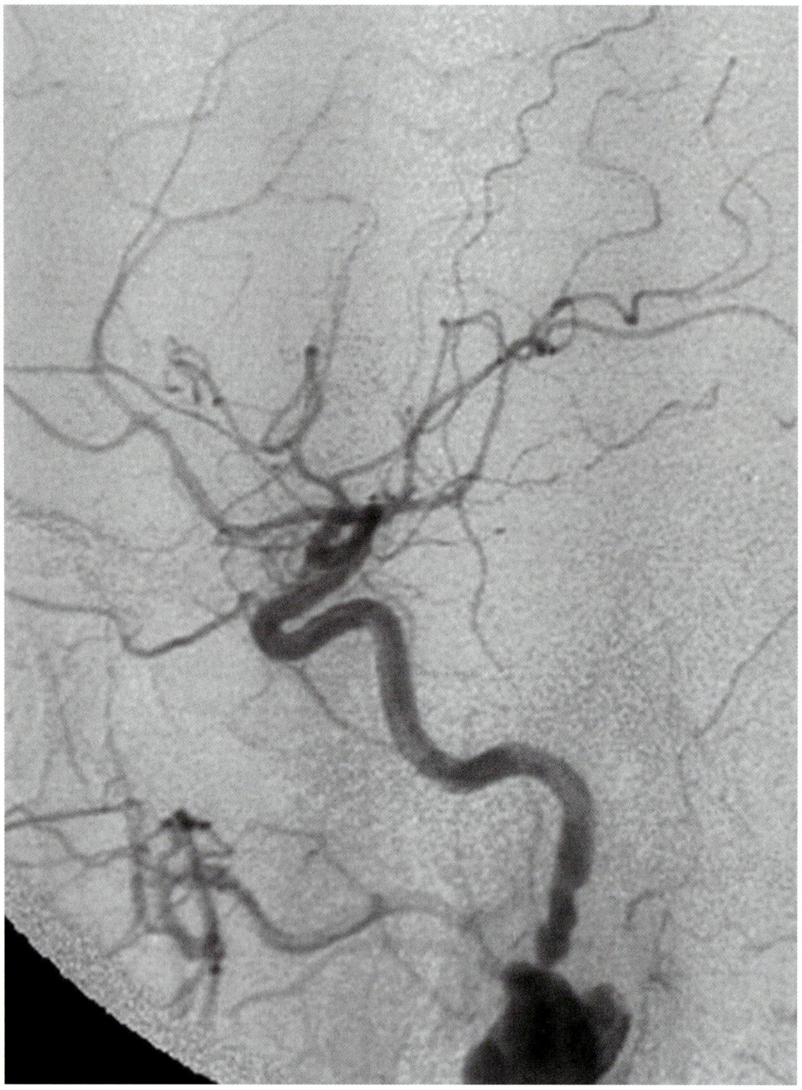

Fig. 9.4b Left CCA angiographic injection shows a pseudoaneurysm of the high cervical ICA.

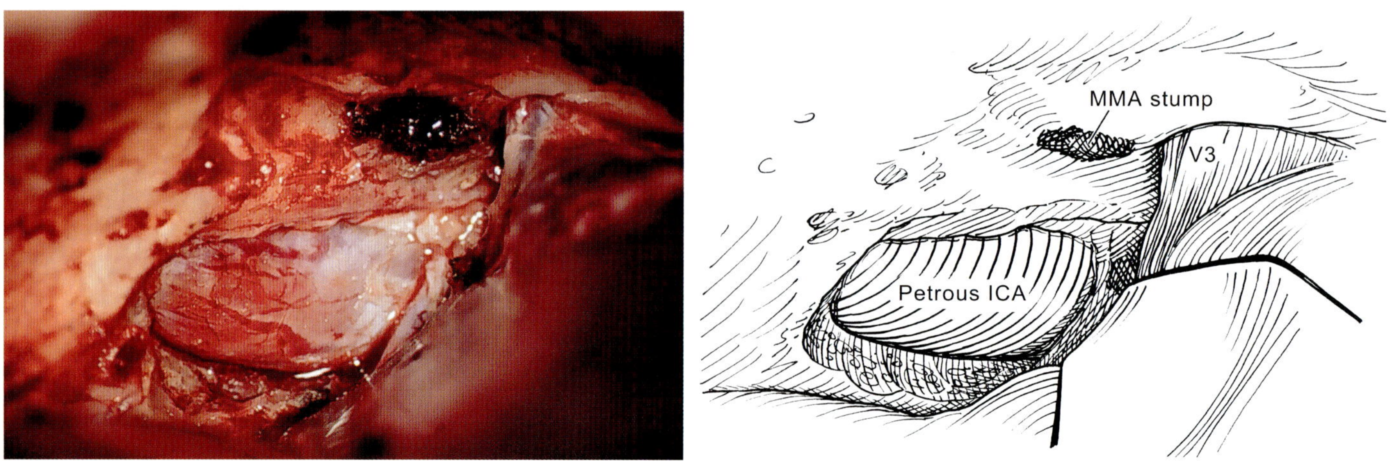

Fig. 9.4c After the patient had failed a balloon occlusion test of the ICA, the petrous ICA was exposed in the middle fossa.

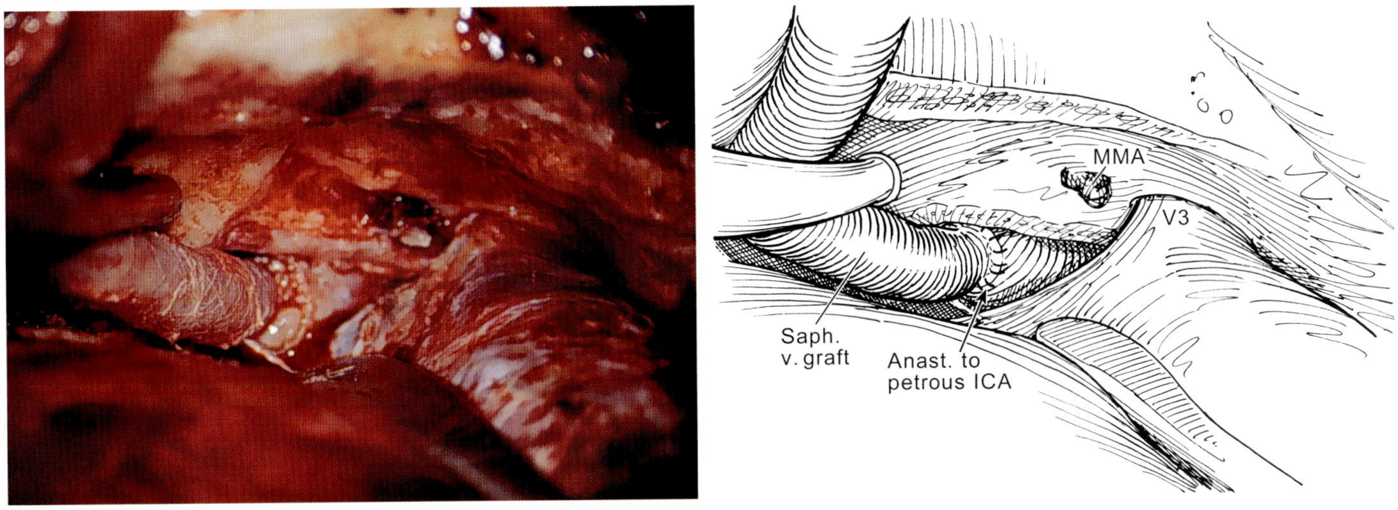

Fig. 9.4d The distal petrous ICA has been anastomosed to the saphenous vein graft.

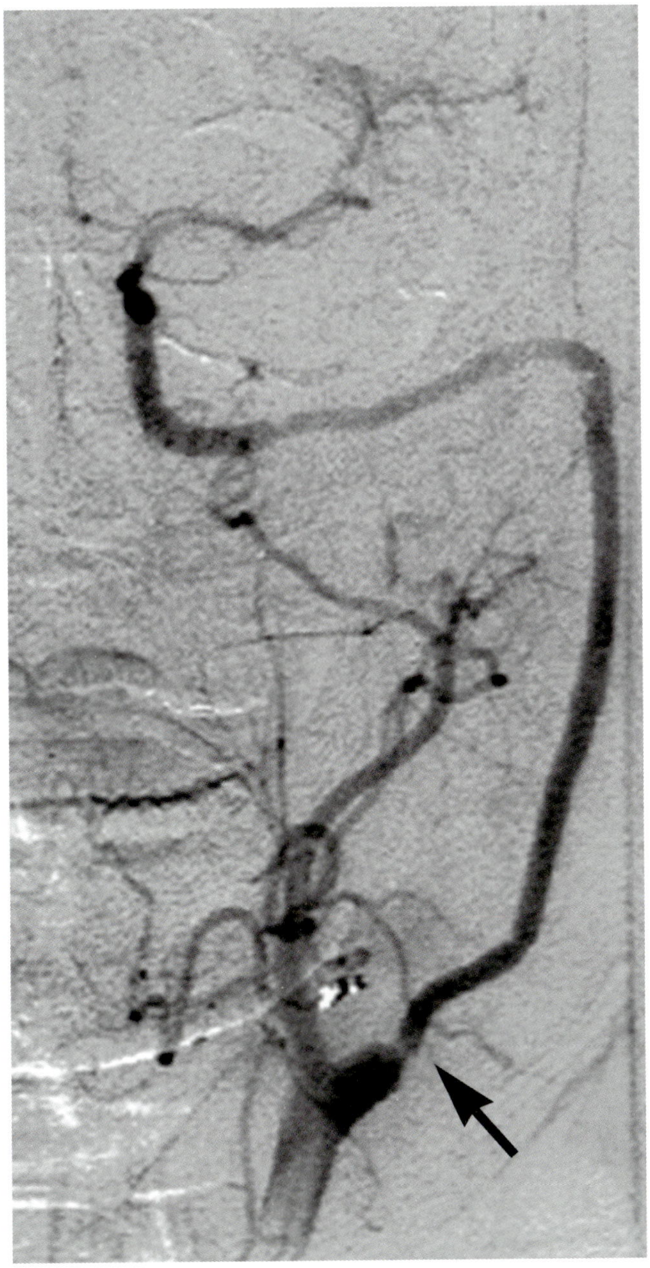

Fig. 9.4e Postoperative anteroposterior angiogram shows the large venous graft from the cervical ICA *(arrow)* to the petrous ICA.

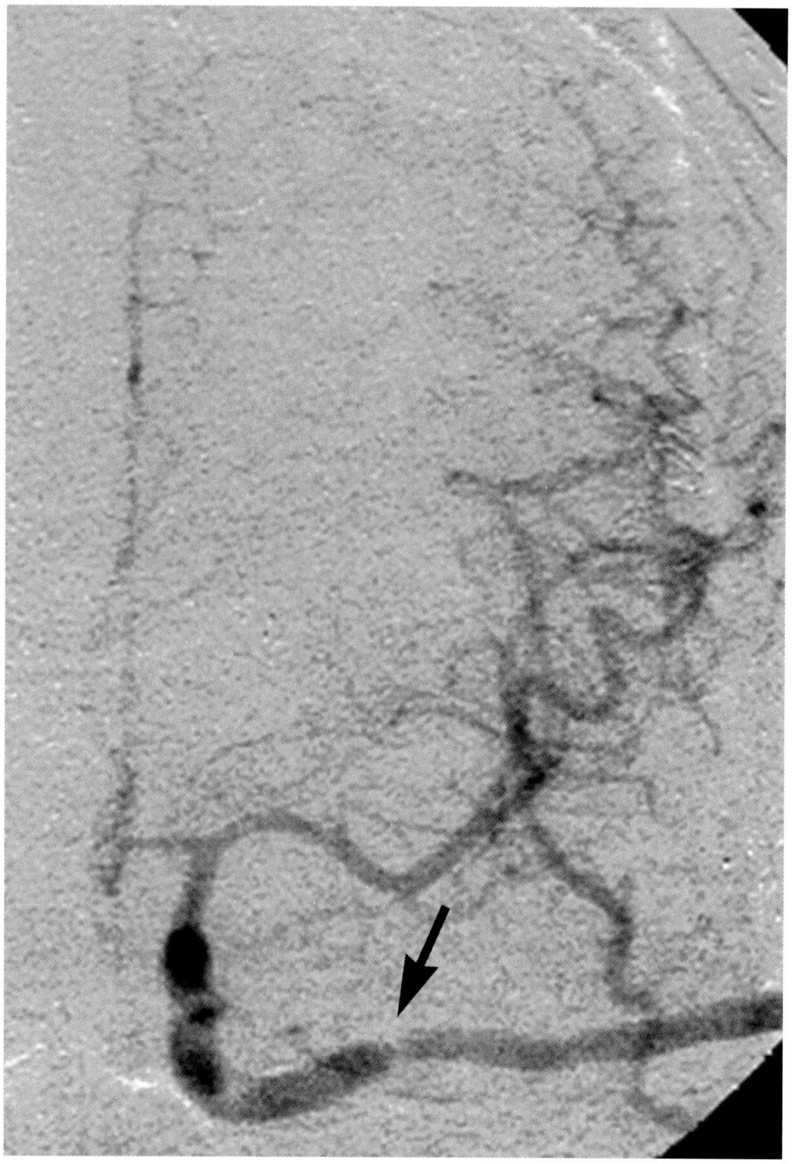

Fig. 9.4f Left anteroposterior angiographic view shows the distal anastomotic site *(arrow)*.

10 Cervical ICA–to–Cervical ICA Interposition Graft or Primary Reanastomosis

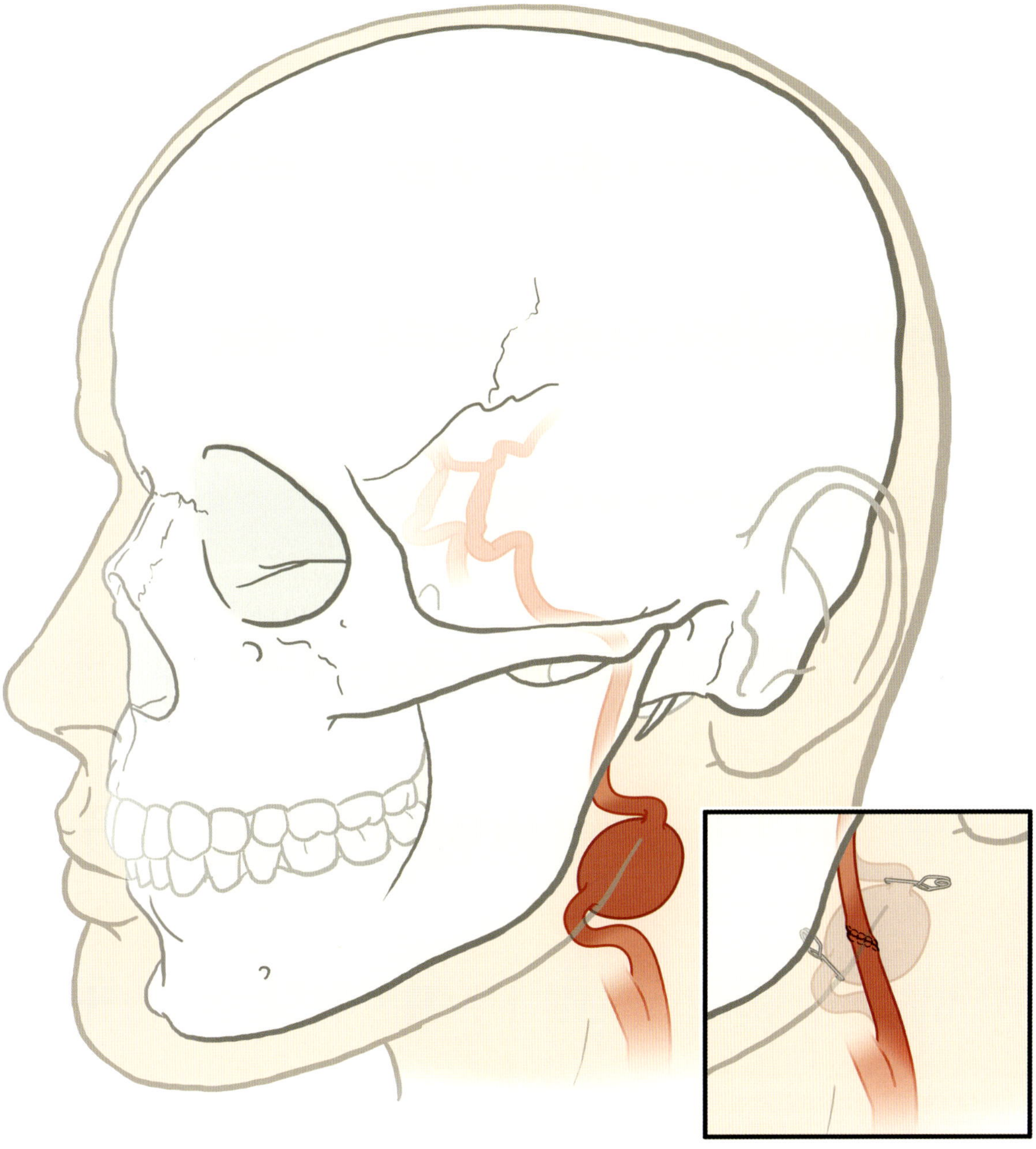

Lesions of the cervical carotid artery may require bypass. When a direct reanastomosis is feasible, however, it should be the preferred method for maintaining blood flow in the ICA.

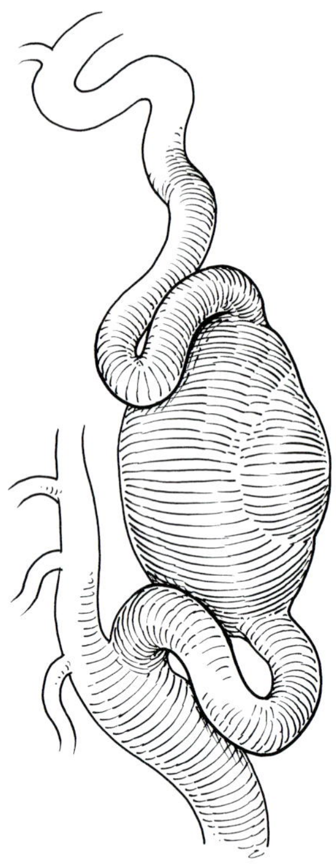

Fig. 10.0a The significant redundancy in the ICA allows excision of the aneurysm.

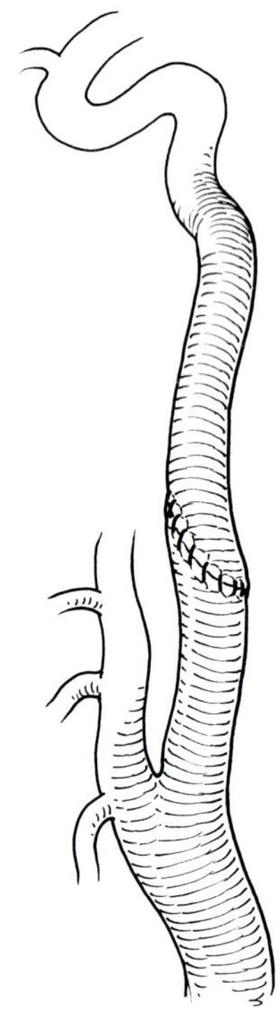

Fig. 10.0b Direct reanastomosis of the ICA.

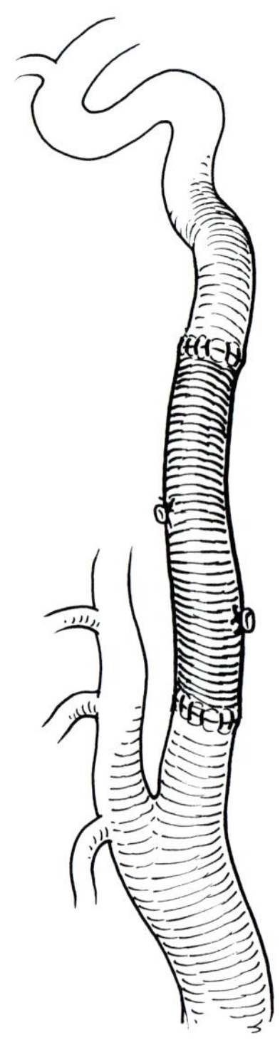

Fig. 10.0c In an alternative option, blood flow is maintained through the ICA with the use of an interposition graft.

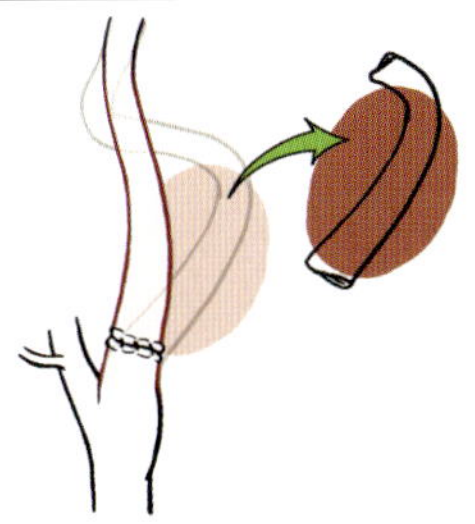

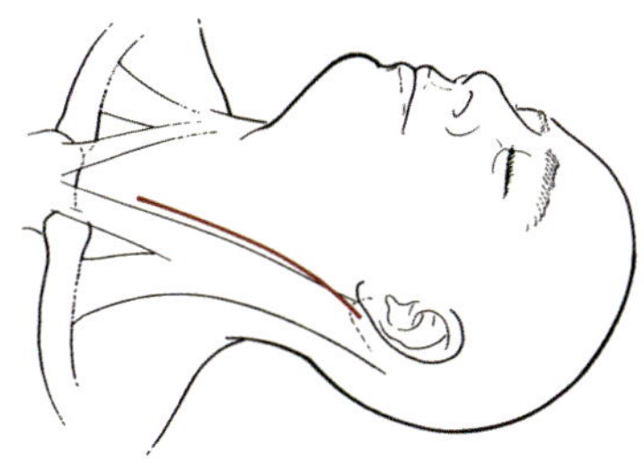

Case 10-1

Diagnosis: Complex left cervical ICA aneurysm

Bypass: Cervical ICA–to–cervical ICA primary end-to-end reanastomosis

Approach: Left anterior cervical

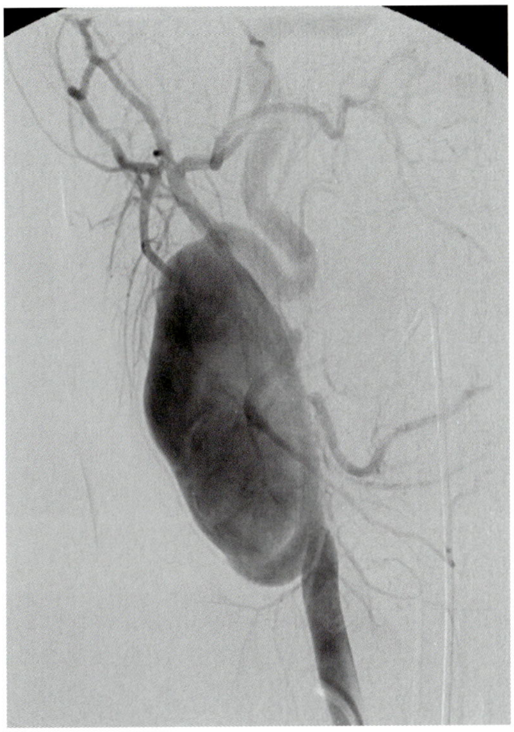

Fig. 10.1a Anteroposterior angiographic view shows the aneurysm and the redundant ICA above it.

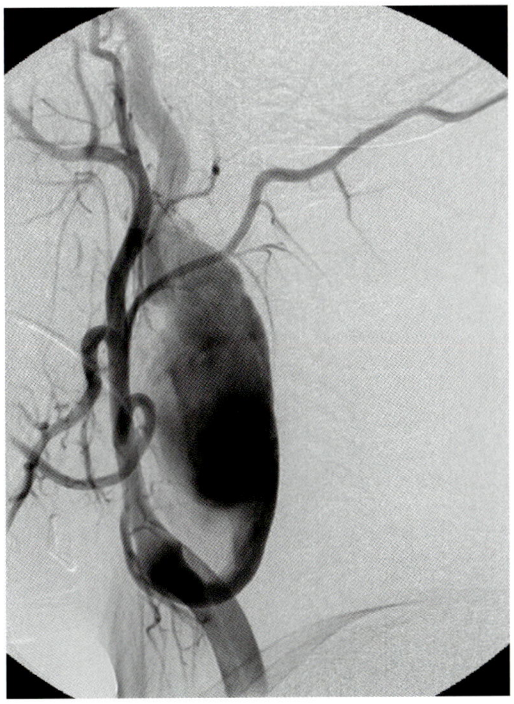

Fig. 10.1b Right anterior oblique angiographic view also shows some redundancy of the ICA proximal to the aneurysm.

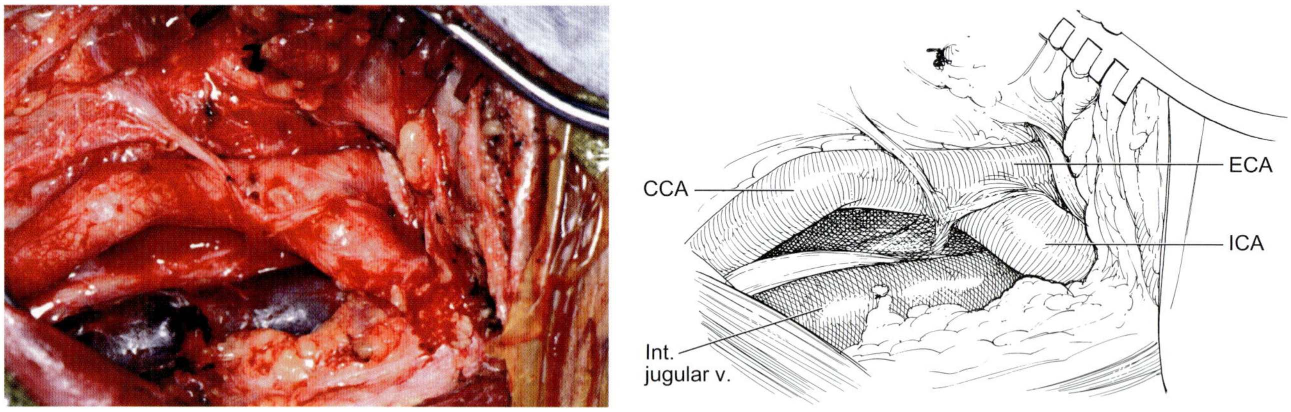

Fig. 10.1c Through a high anterolateral incision, the carotid artery bifurcation is exposed.

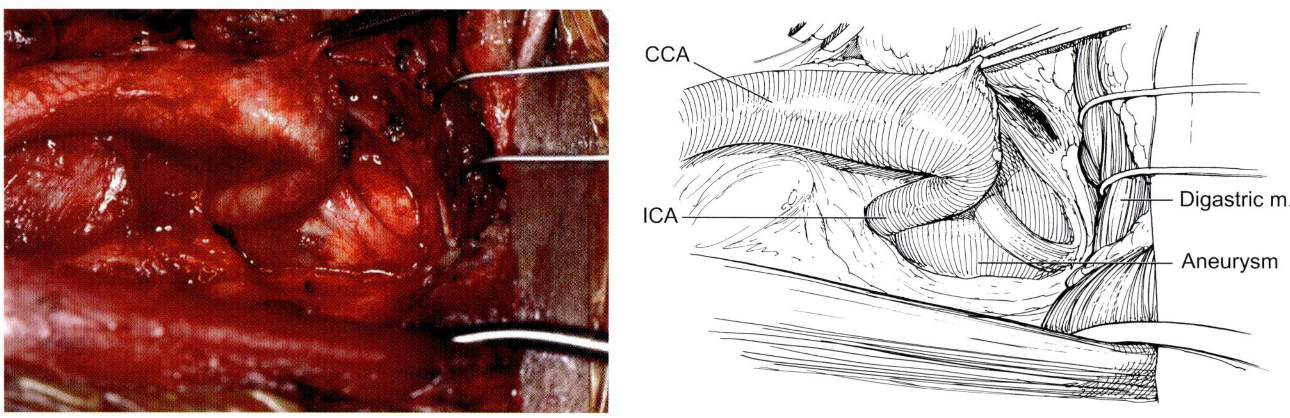

Fig. 10.1d With further dissection, the base of the aneurysm is exposed.

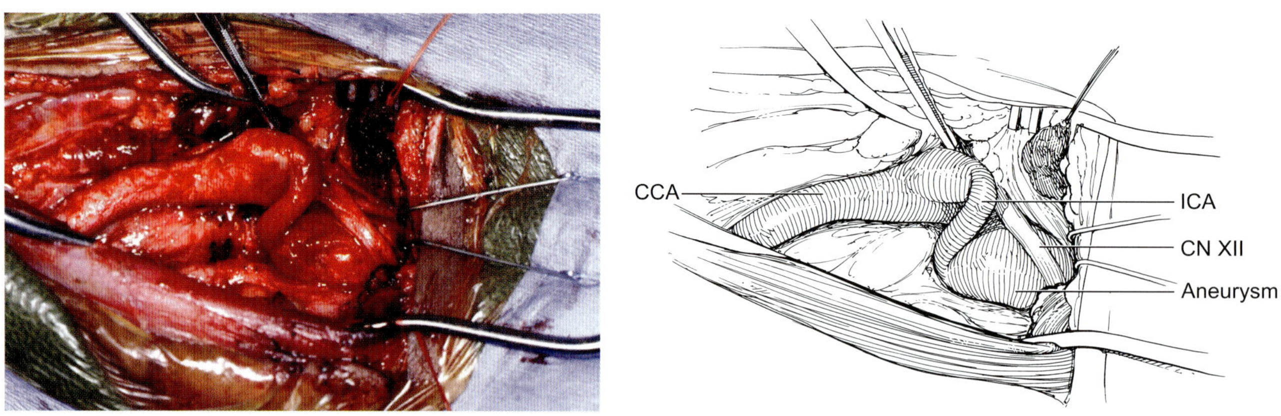

Fig. 10.1e Overview shows CN XII coursing over the aneurysm.

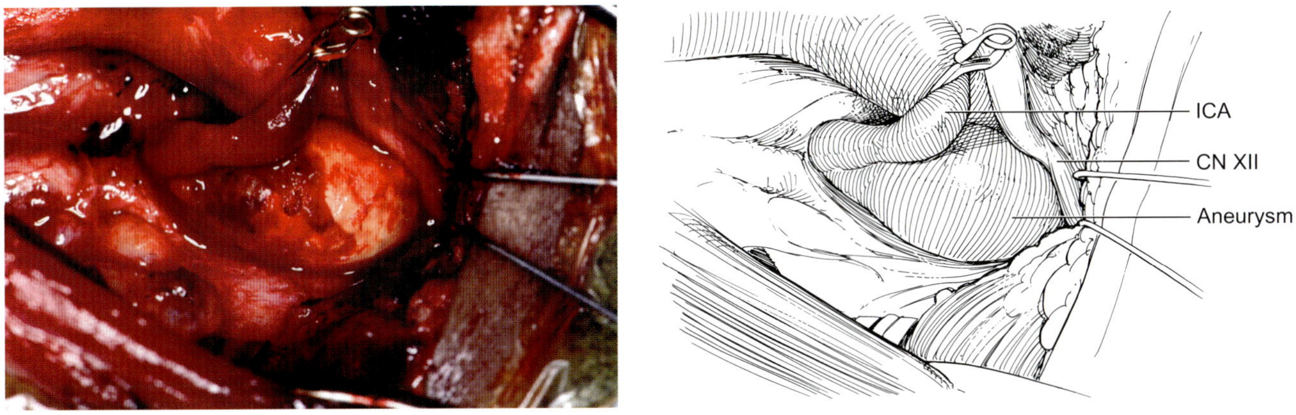

Fig. 10.1f As the dissection is extended superiorly, the top of the aneurysm becomes visible.

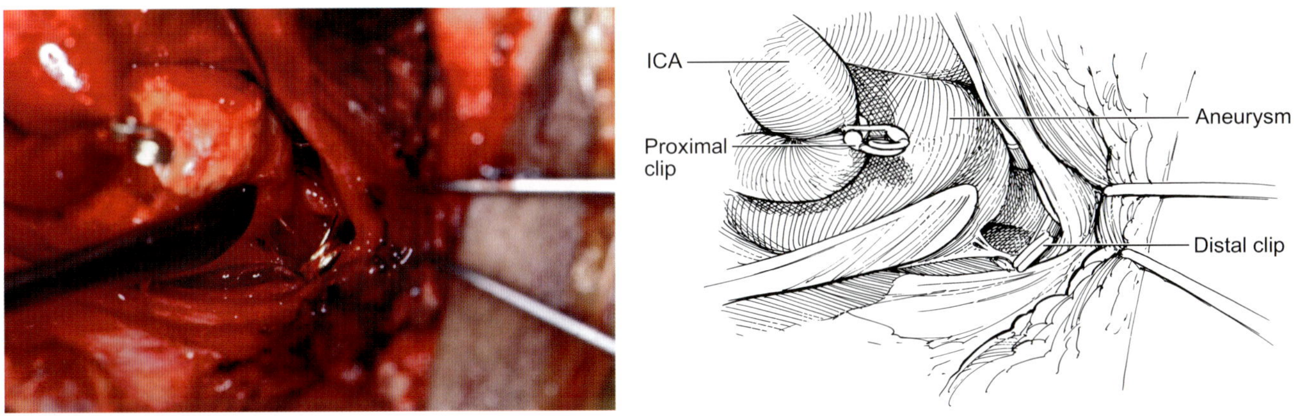

Fig. 10.1g With the patient placed under barbiturate anesthesia to burst suppression, the aneurysm is isolated between temporary aneurysm clips.

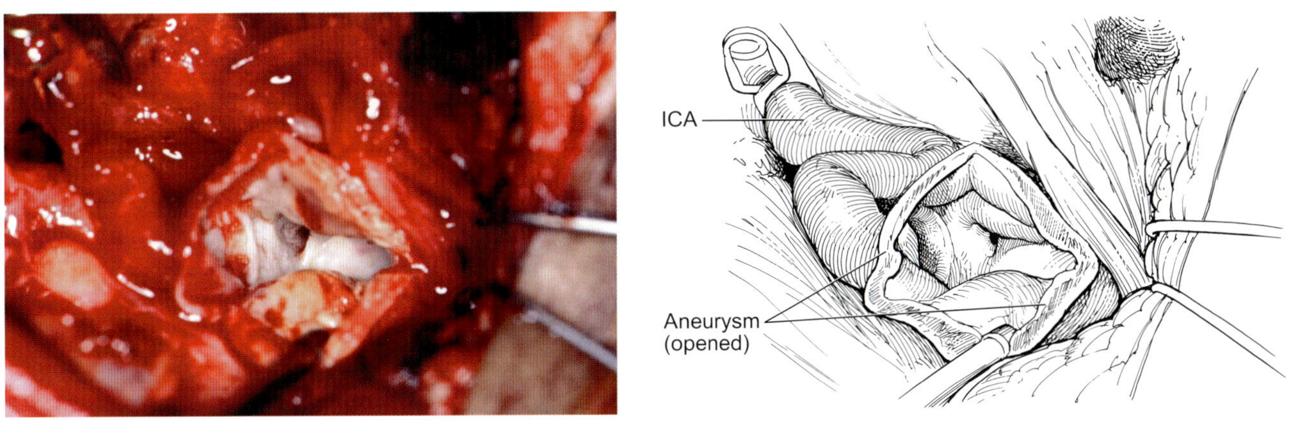

Fig. 10.1h The aneurysm is opened and the lumen is inspected.

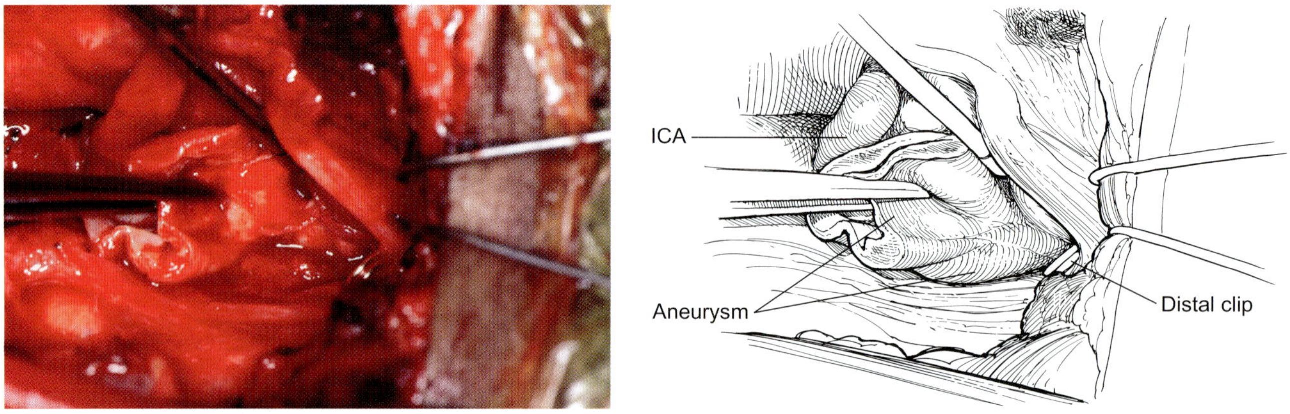

Fig. 10.1i The aneurysm dome is mobilized and cut from the proximal and distal ICA.

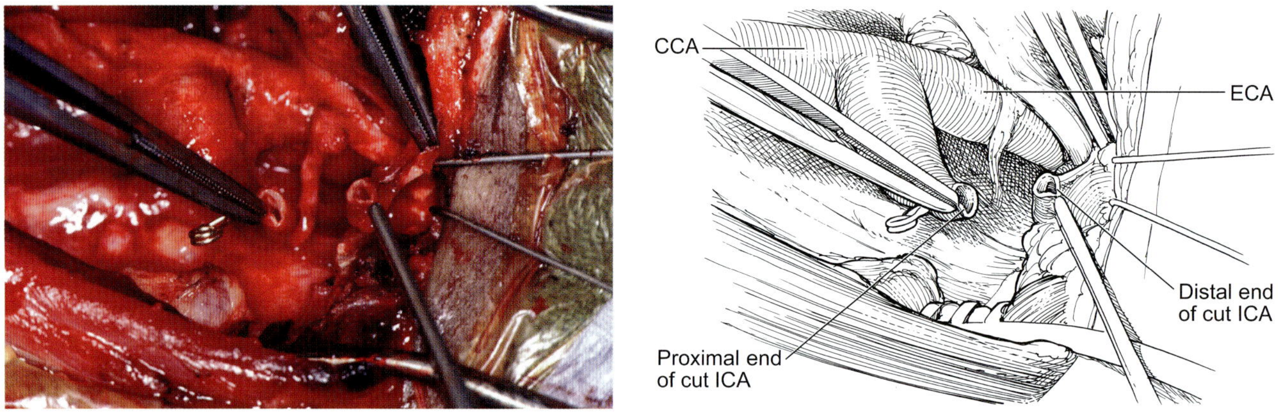

Fig. 10.1j The two cut ends of the ICA are mobilized to allow a tensionless anastomosis.

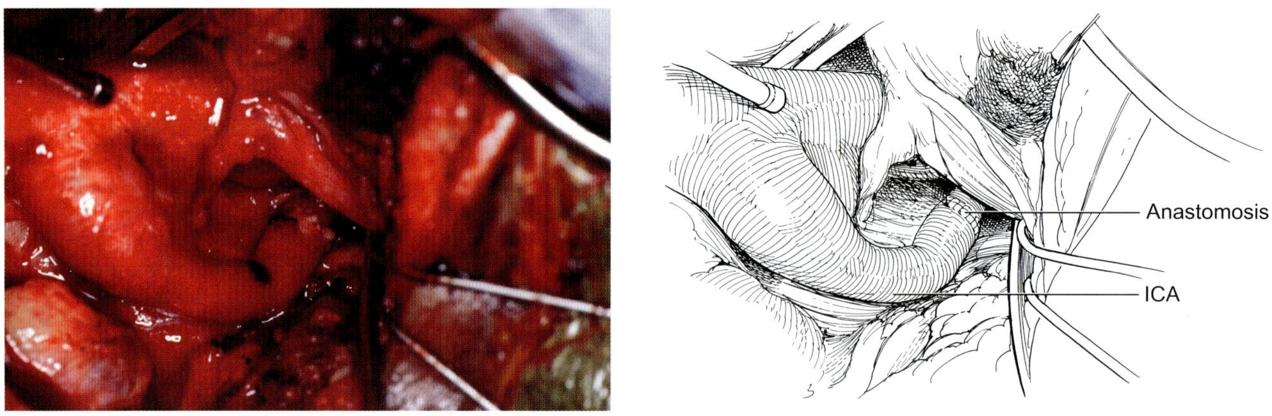

Fig. 10.1k A direct end-to-end anastomosis is performed between the cut ends.

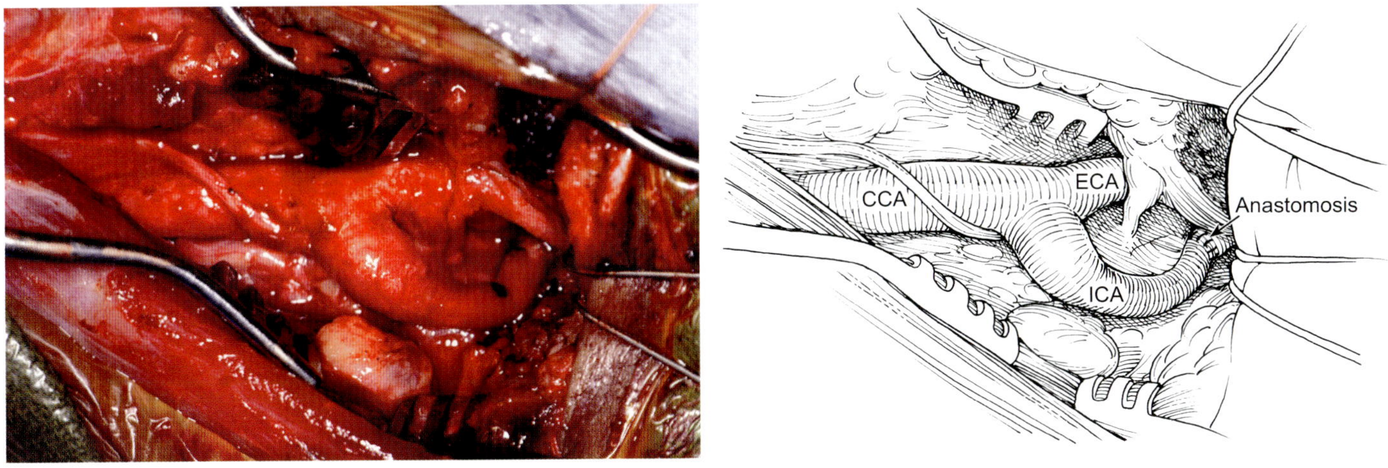

Fig. 10.1l The completed ICA reconstruction is shown.

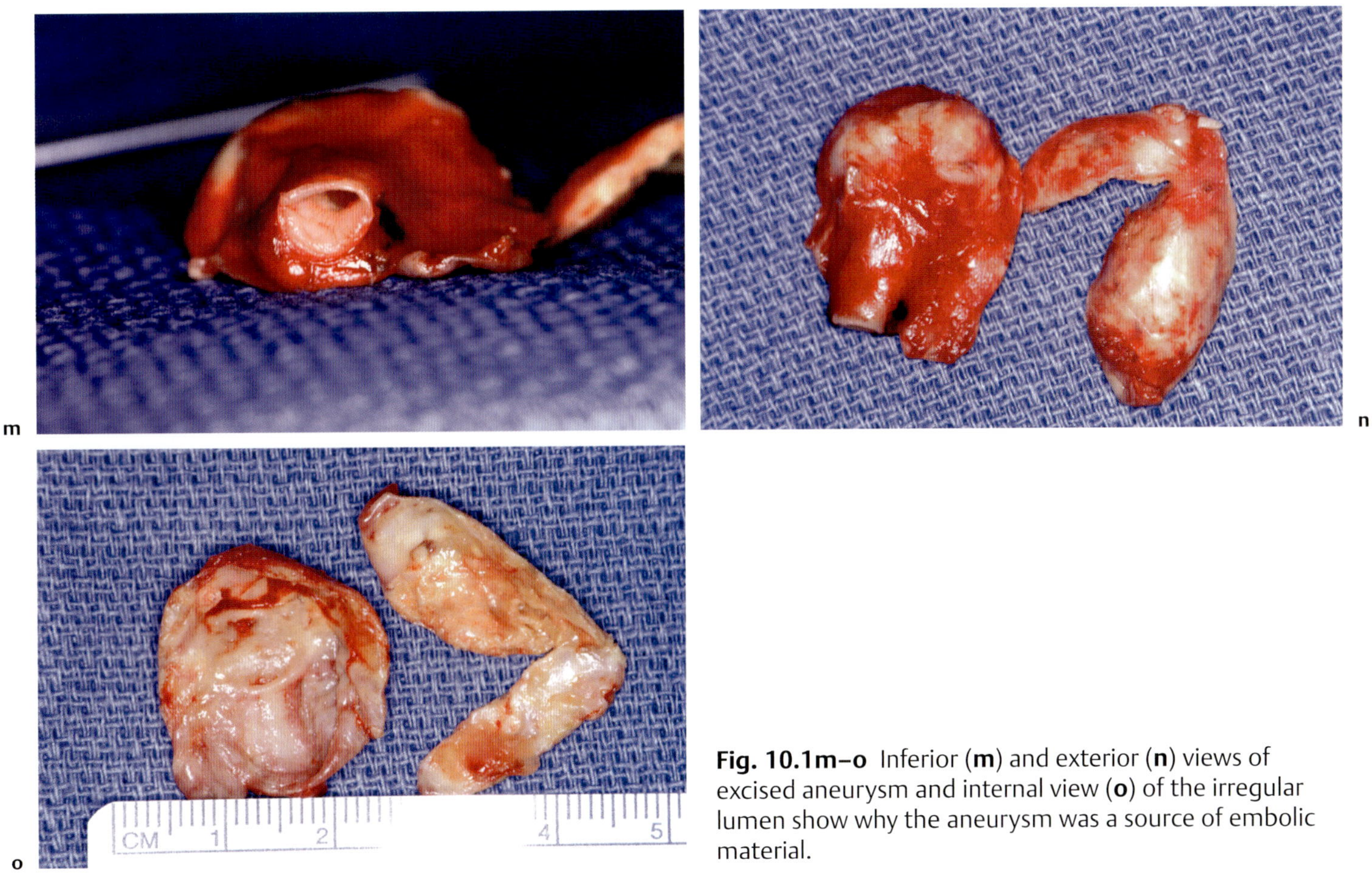

Fig. 10.1m–o Inferior (**m**) and exterior (**n**) views of excised aneurysm and internal view (**o**) of the irregular lumen show why the aneurysm was a source of embolic material.

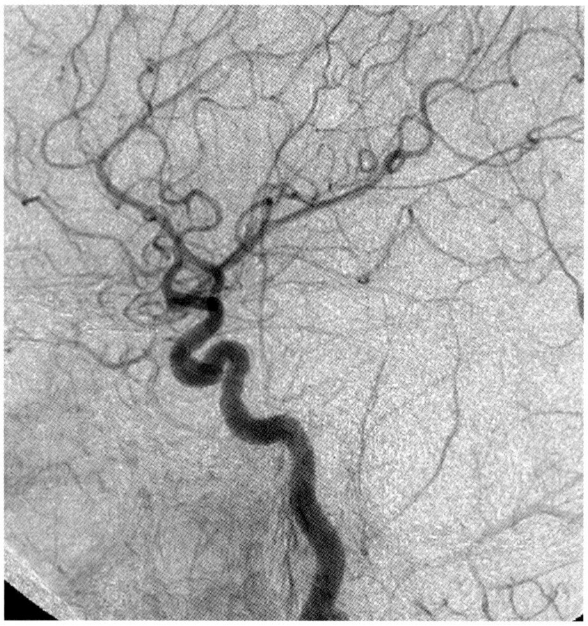

Fig. 10.1p Lateral angiographic view shows excision of the aneurysm and continued flow through the ICA.

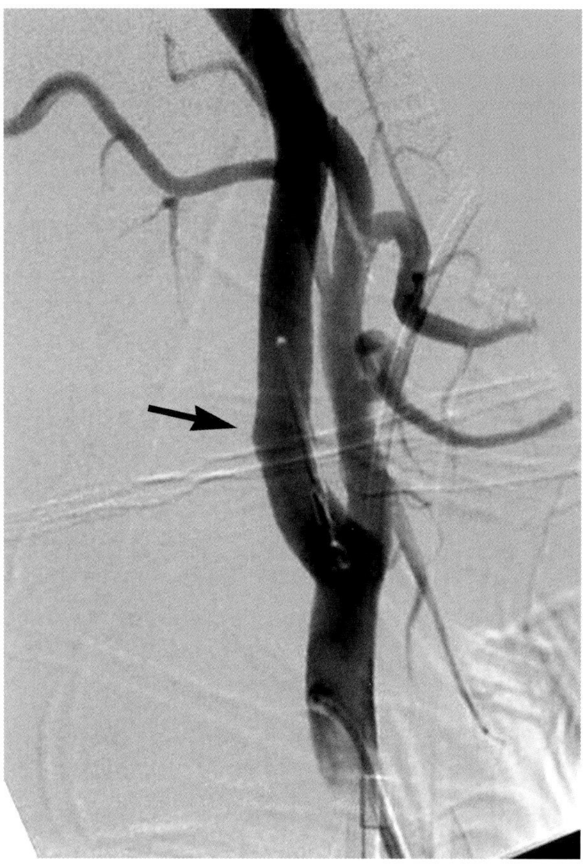

Fig. 10.1q Lateral angiographic view of the right carotid bifurcation shows the anastomosis (*arrow*) performed after the aneurysm was excised.

11 Subclavian Artery–to–CCA Bypass or Transposition

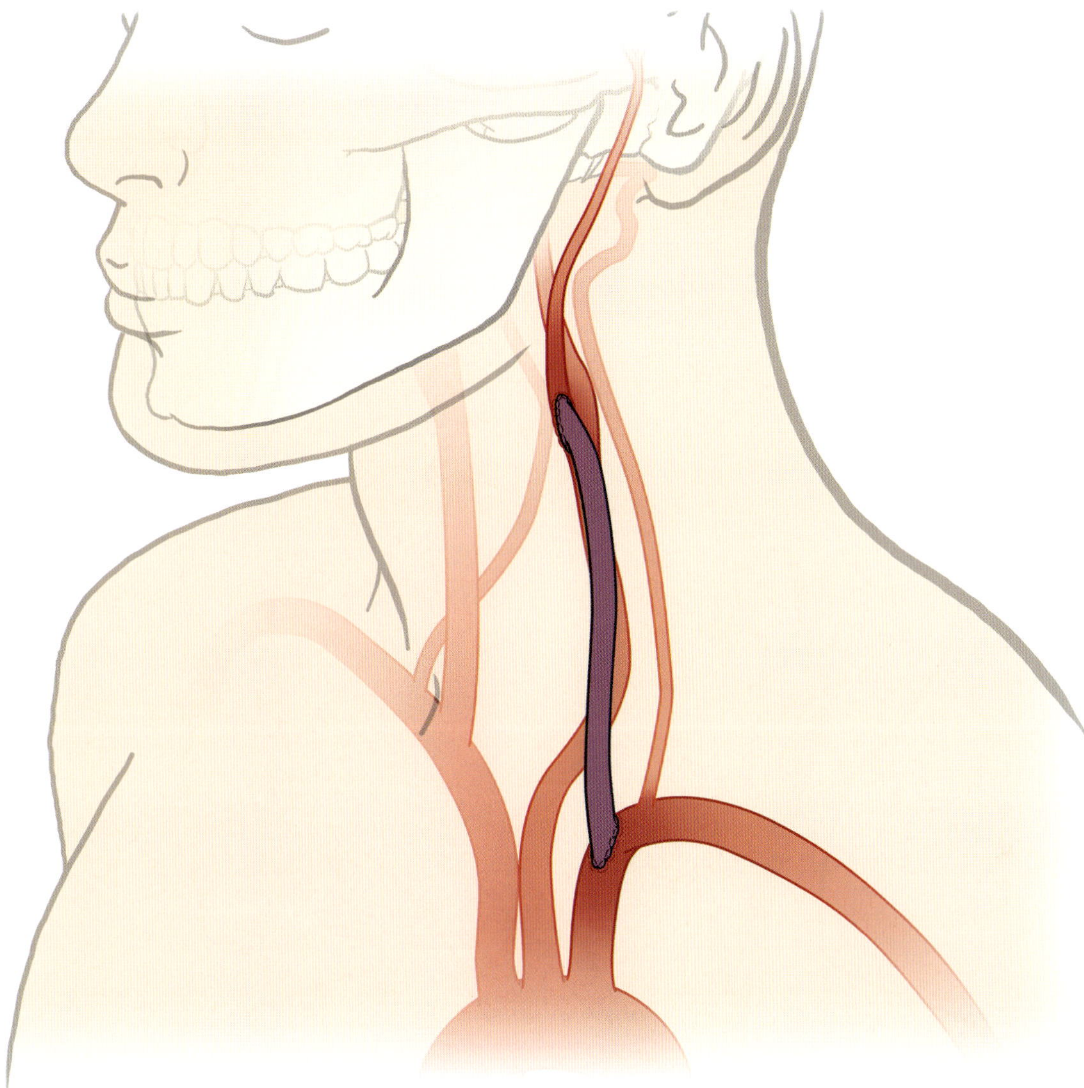

The subclavian artery, a large vessel located by the clavicle, is available as a donor site when needed. The subclavian artery is exposed through a transverse supraclavicular incision with bisection of at least part of the sternocleidomastoid muscle. The incision along the course of the CCA can be extended if the vessel must be exposed for any length or if a VA-to-CCA transposition will be performed.

On the left side, it is important to recognize the presence of the thoracic duct, whose integrity should be maintained. Once the duct and its branches have been identified, it can be cut after both ends are completely ligated. Ascertaining the anatomic location of the phrenic nerve and stellate ganglion can avoid injuries to these structures.

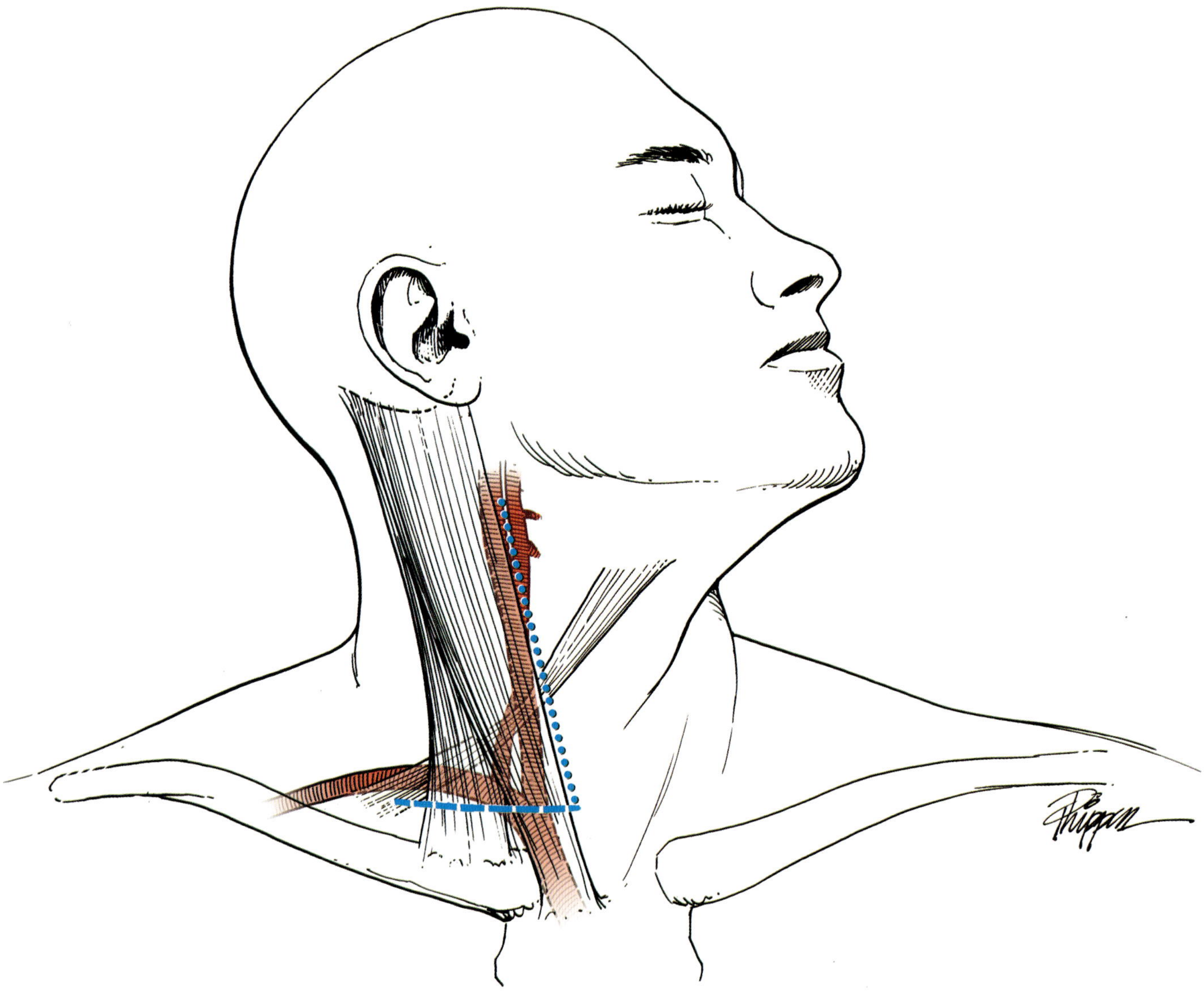

Fig. 11.0a The transverse supraclavicular incision (*dashed line*) is shown with a longitudinal extension (*dotted line*).

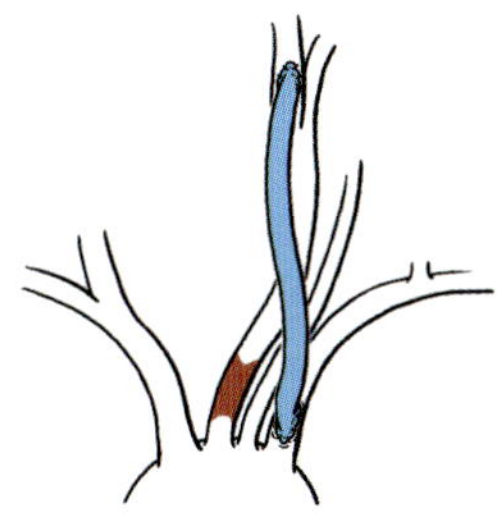

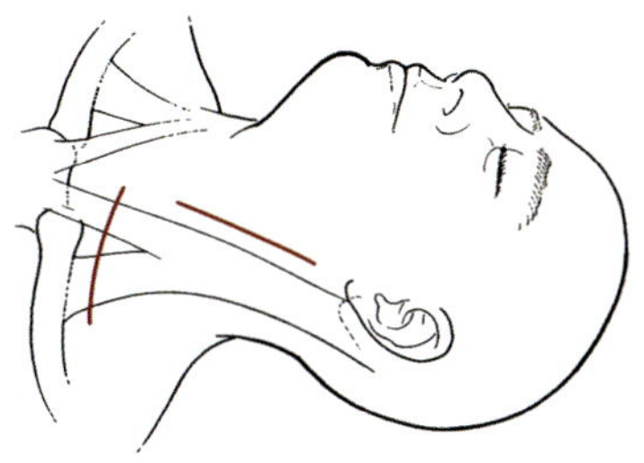

Case 11-1

Diagnosis: Radiation-induced occlusion of left CCA

Bypass: Subclavian artery-to-CCA bifurcation with saphenous vein graft

Approach: Left anterolateral cervical and left transverse supraclavicular

A 33-year-old man with a history of Hodgkin disease and left neck irradiation 18 years earlier complained of repeated episodes of tingling in his right hand.

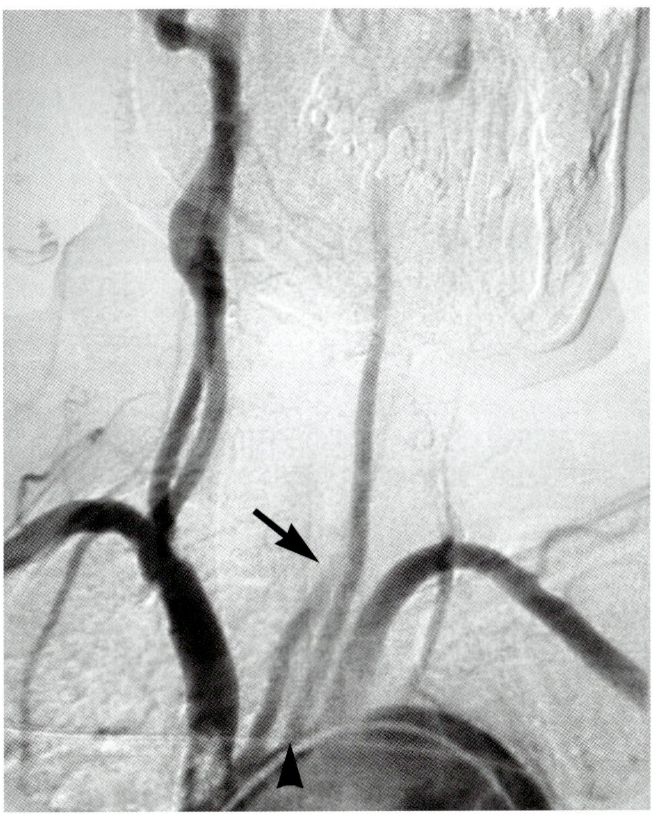

Fig. 11.1a Left anterior oblique aortic arch angiogram shows occlusion of the left CCA a few centimeters beyond its origin (*arrow*). The patient's left VA arises from his aortic arch (*arrowhead*), and it and his subclavian artery are widely patent.

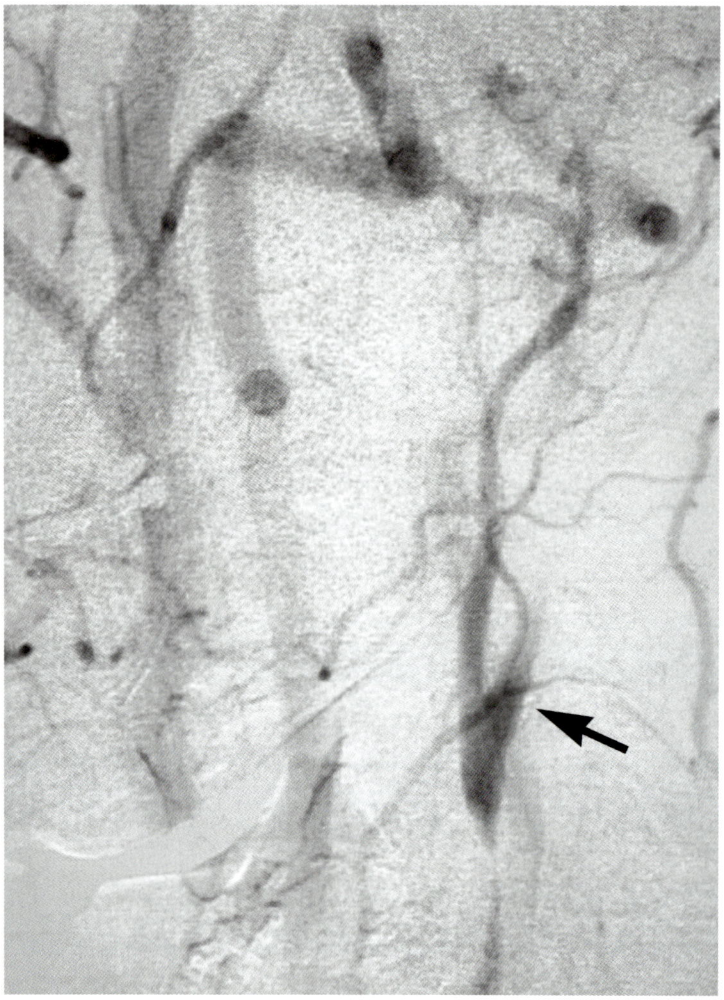

Fig. 11.1b Late-phase arch angiogram shows reconstitution of the carotid bifurcation (*arrow*) through ECA collaterals, primarily from muscular branches from the VA circulation.

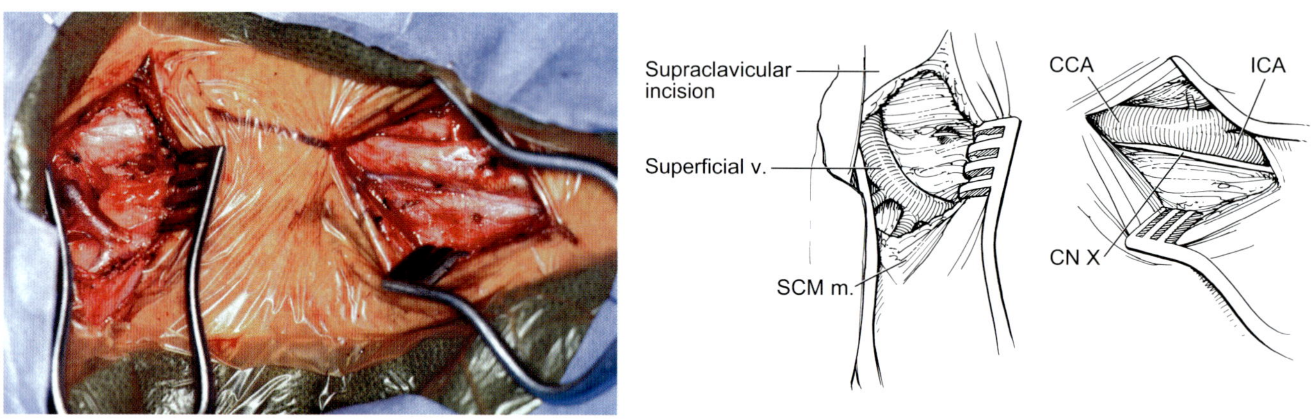

Fig. 11.1c A transverse supraclavicular incision is made and the SCM muscle is divided to provide access to the subclavian artery. An anterior cervical incision higher in the neck exposes the carotid bifurcation.

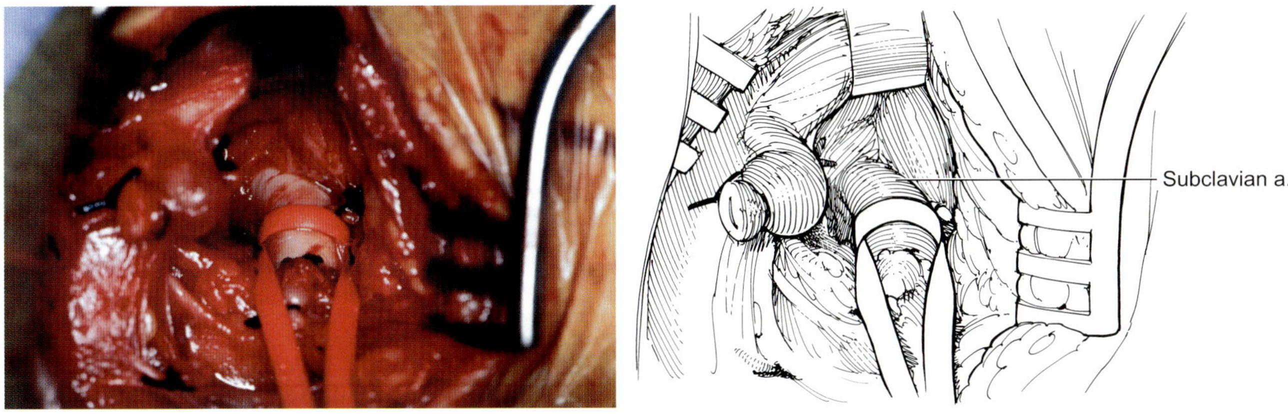

Fig. 11.1d As the transverse supraclavicular dissection proceeds downward, the subclavian artery is exposed as it arches beneath the left clavicle.

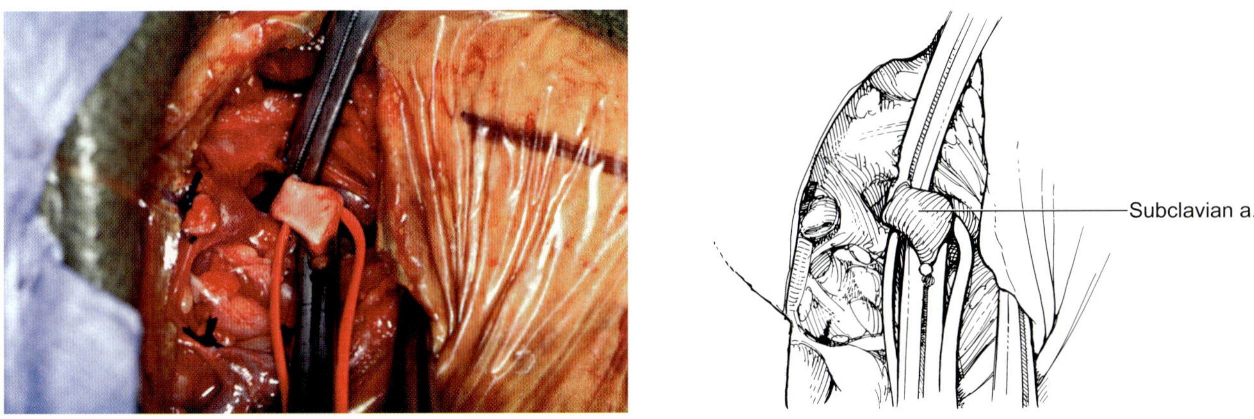

Fig. 11.1e A short segment of the subclavian artery is isolated between vascular clamps to provide a donor site for the proximal anastomosis. In this case, the lower anastomosis is the most difficult and therefore is performed first.

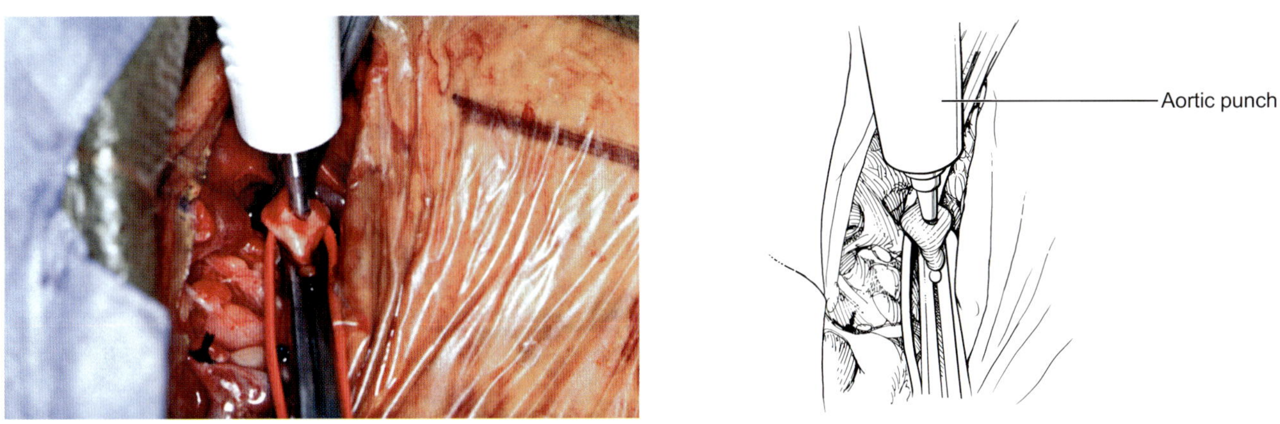

Fig. 11.1f An arteriotomy is made with a no. 11 blade and enlarged with a 4-mm aortic punch.

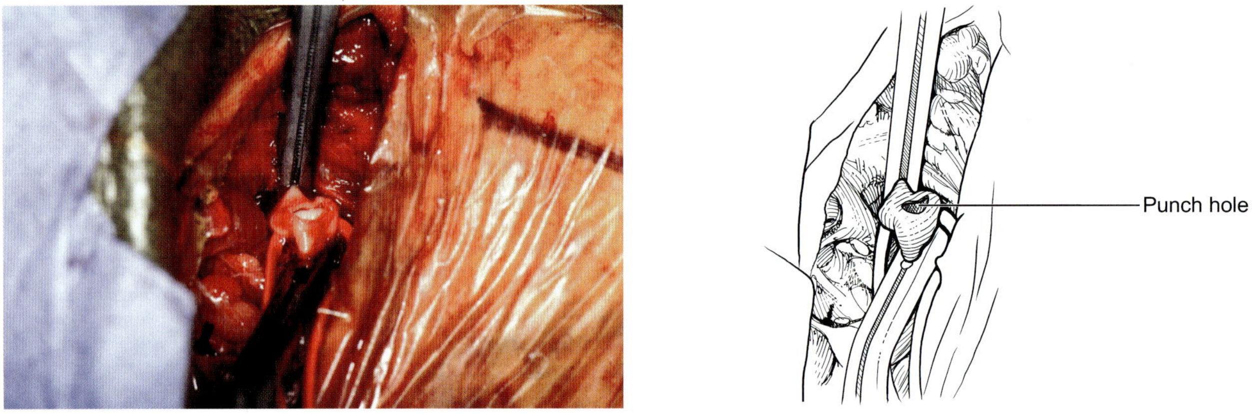

Fig. 11.1g The punch hole for the proximal anastomosis is inspected for debris and atheroma.

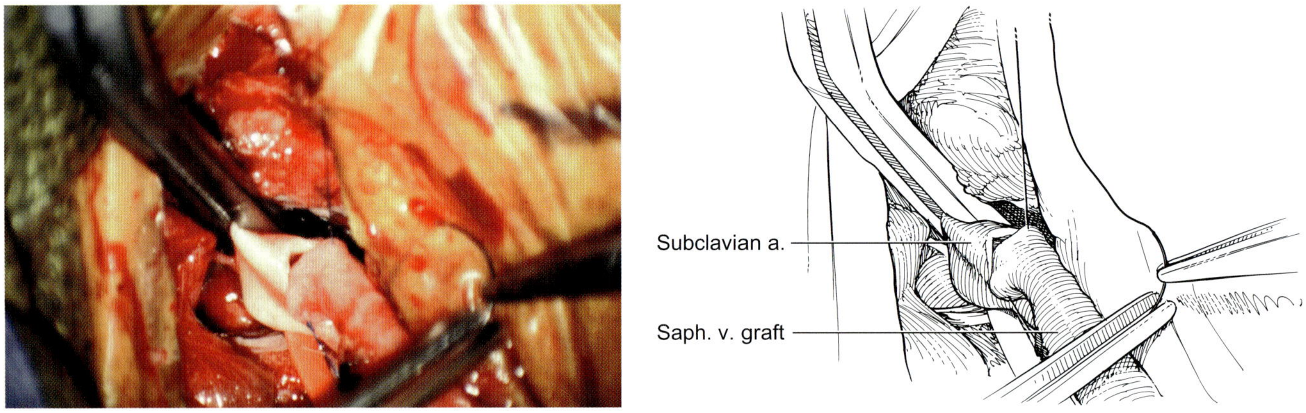

Fig. 11.1h The saphenous vein graft is tacked to the arteriotomy site at two points with 7–0 Prolene suture (Ethicon, Somerville, NJ) in preparation for the anastomosis.

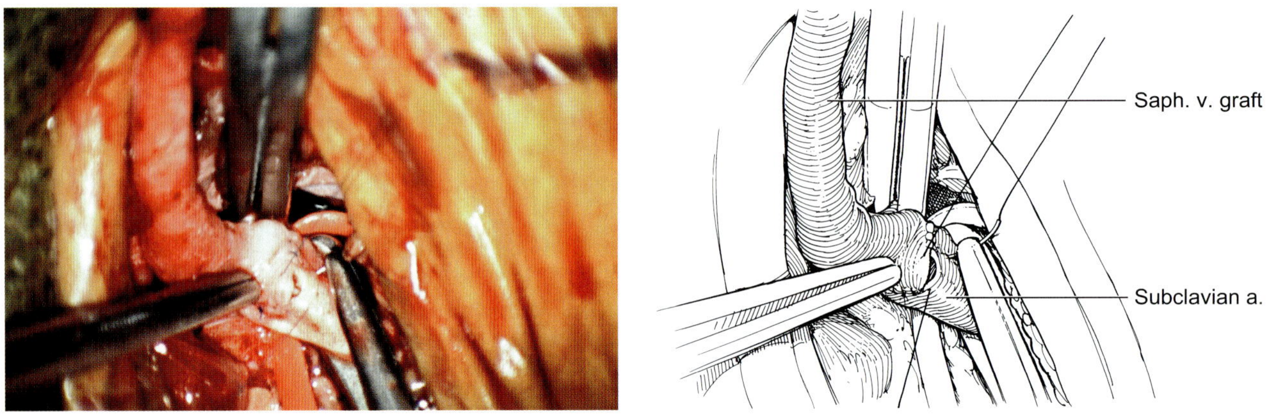

Fig. 11.1i After the back wall is sewn, the front wall of the proximal anastomosis is completed.

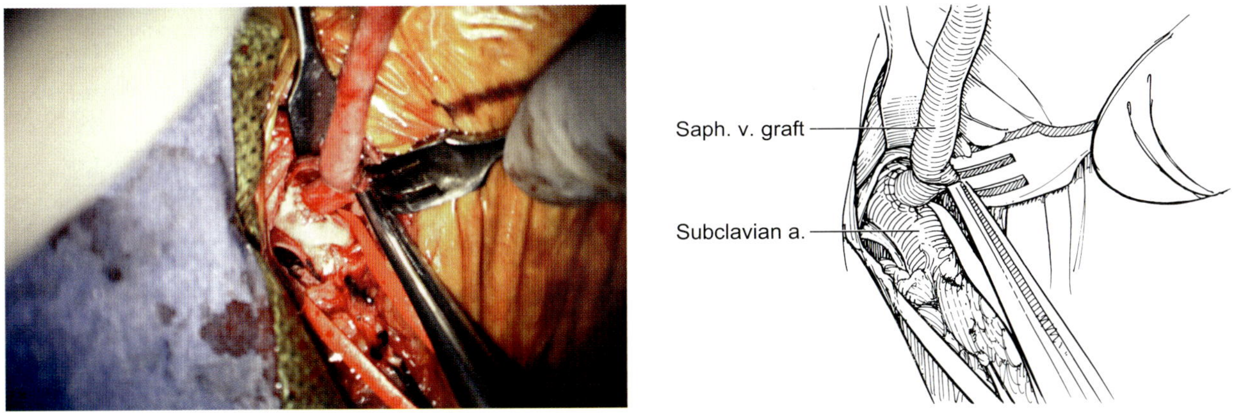

Fig. 11.1j The clamps are removed and the graft is allowed to fill. The anastomosis is inspected for hemostasis.

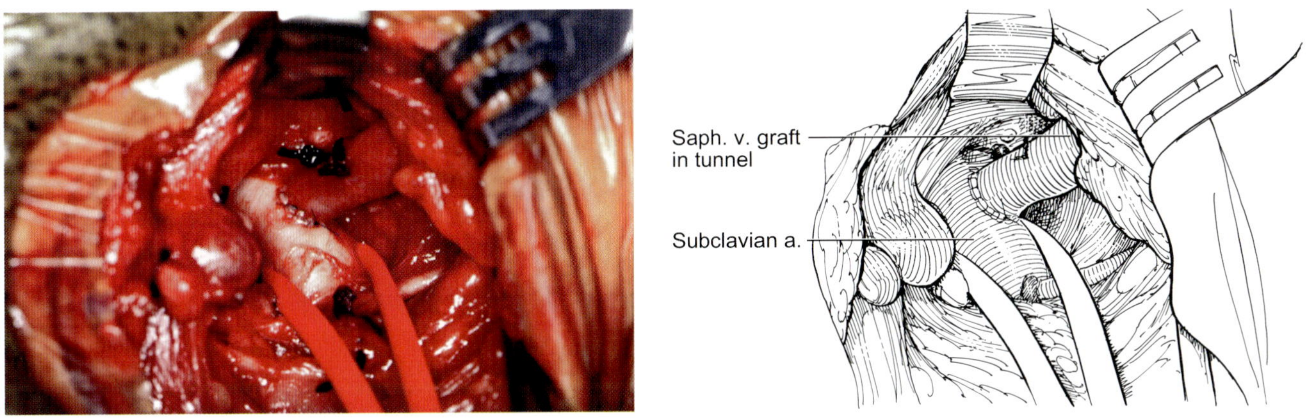

Fig. 11.1k The saphenous vein graft is tunneled subcutaneously to the incision over the carotid bifurcation. The graft must not be stretched, twisted, or kinked.

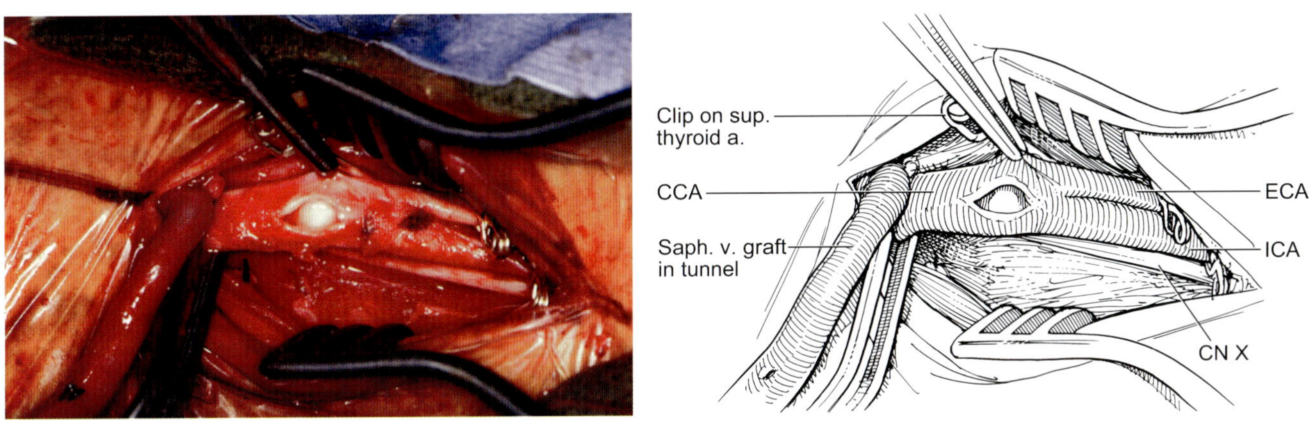

Fig. 11.1l At the level of the carotid bifurcation, a wide arteriotomy is made and then enlarged with an aortic punch. Temporary aneurysm clips occlude the superior thyroid artery, ICA, and ECA. The vein graft exits from the lower margin of the incision.

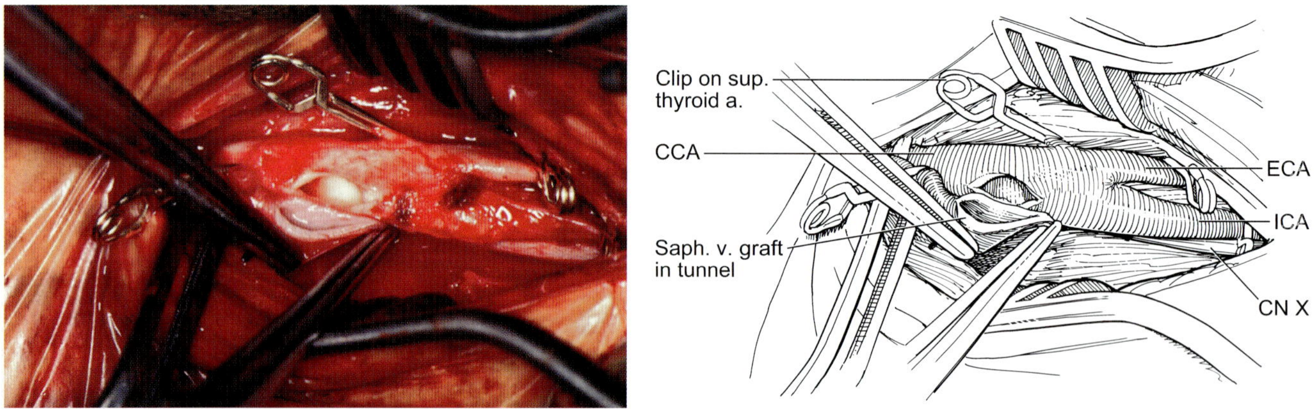

Fig. 11.1m The vein is shortened and trimmed to create a fishmouth opening to maximize the size of the anastomosis.

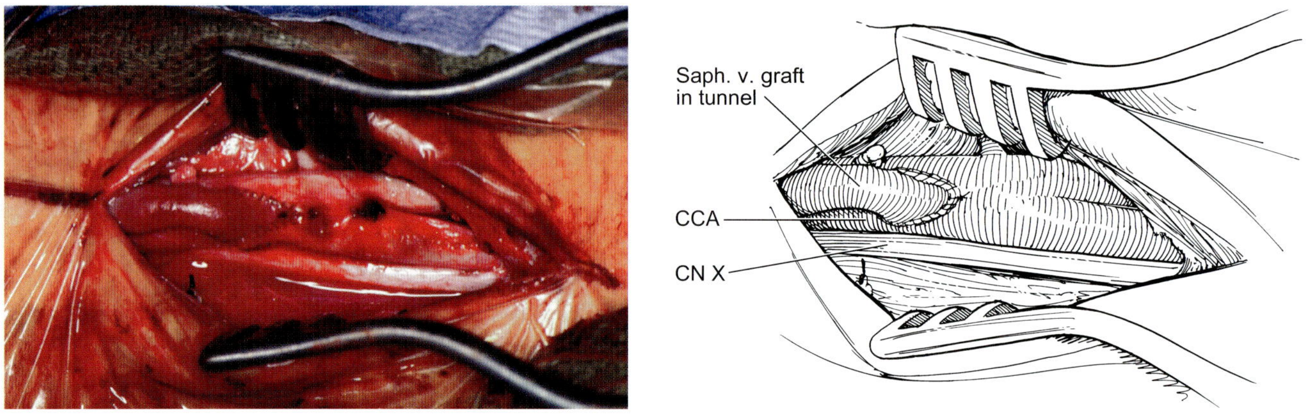

Fig. 11.1n A running 7–0 Prolene (Ethicon, Somerville, NJ) suture completes the anastomosis, which is then checked for hemostasis.

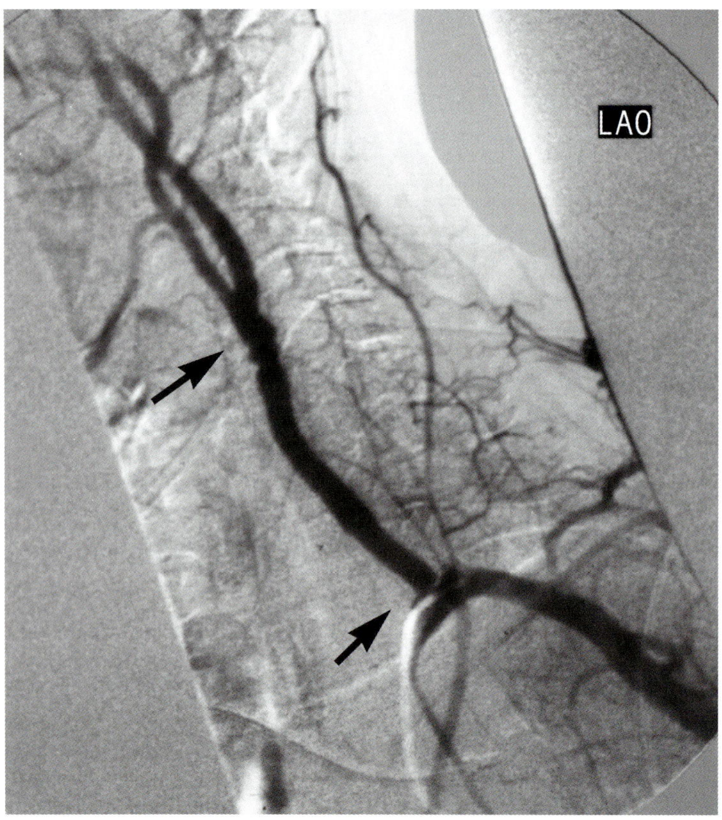

Fig. 11.1o The day after surgery, a selective subclavian angiogram in left anterior oblique projection shows the widely patent saphenous vein graft (*arrows*) from the subclavian artery to the carotid bifurcation rapidly filling the branches of the ECA and ICA.

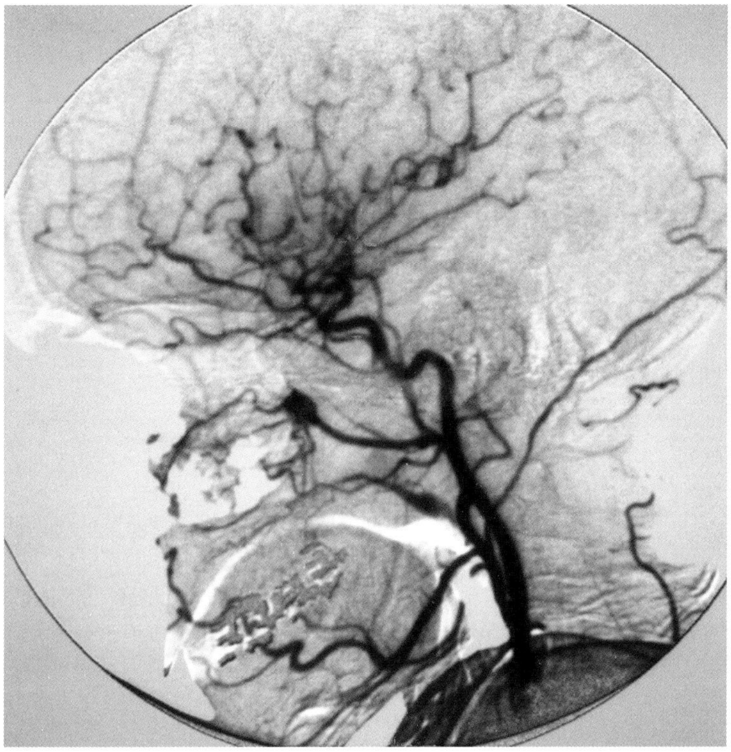

Fig. 11.1p Lateral left subclavian artery angiogram of the same injection shows the distal ICA with filling of the branches of the ACA and MCA. The patient tolerated the procedure without difficulty and was discharged on the fourth postoperative day.

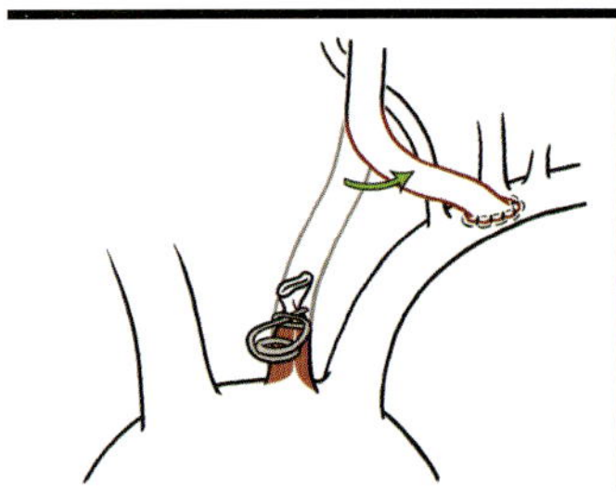

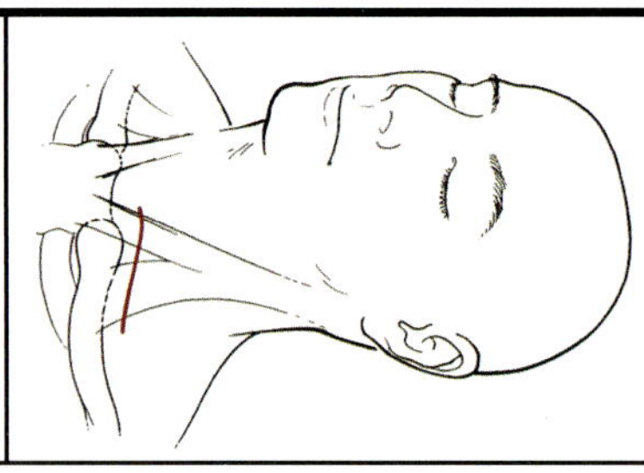

Case 11-2

Diagnosis: Severe stenosis at origin of left CCA

Bypass: CCA–to–subclavian artery transposition

Approach: Left transverse supraclavicular

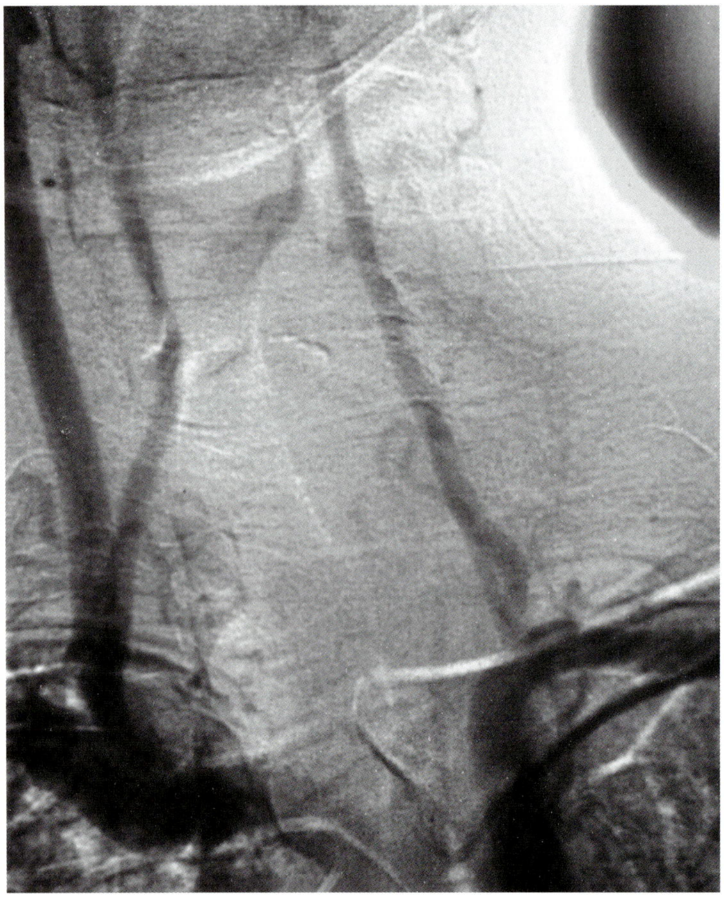

Fig. 11.2a Left anterior oblique arch angiogram of a 45-year-old man with repeated episodes of weakness and sensory changes on his right side is notable for the absence of the left CCA.

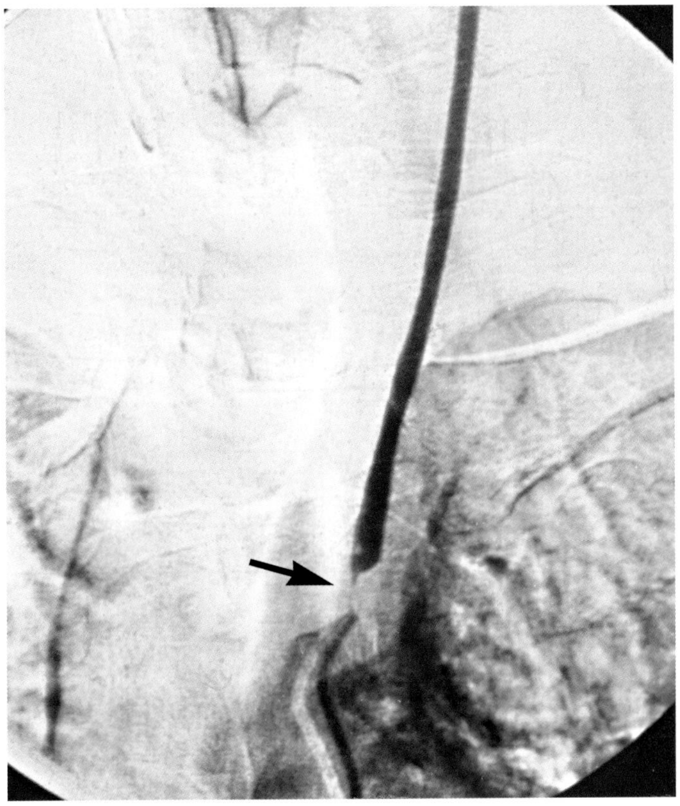

Fig. 11.2b Selective injection of the left CCA shows a short segment of severe stenosis (*arrow*) at the origin of the vessel.

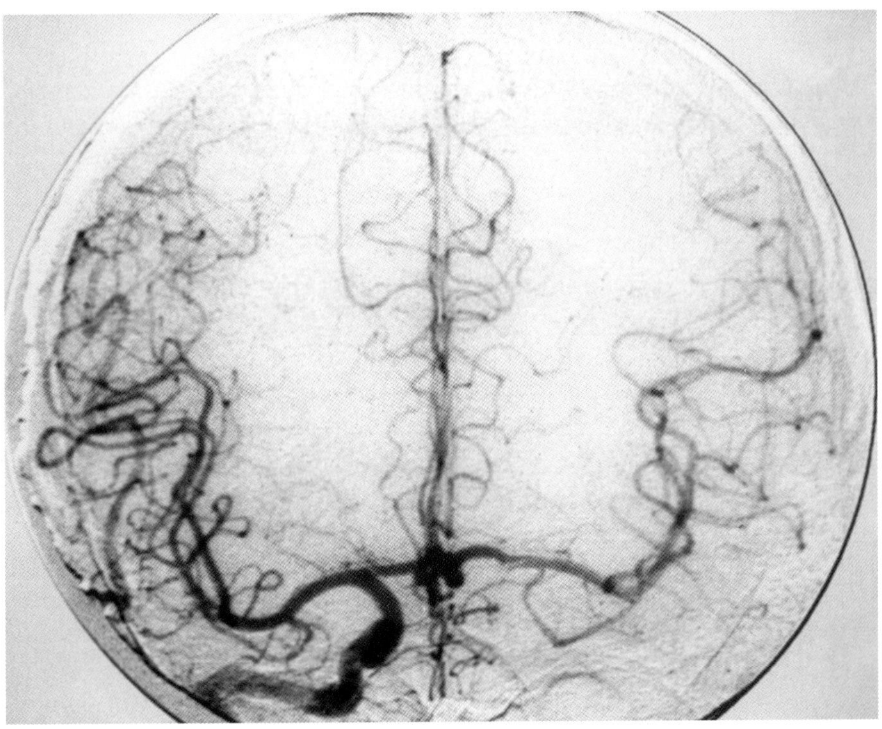

Fig. 11.2c Right anteroposterior CCA angiogram shows cross filling of the left ACA and MCA through the ACoA complex.

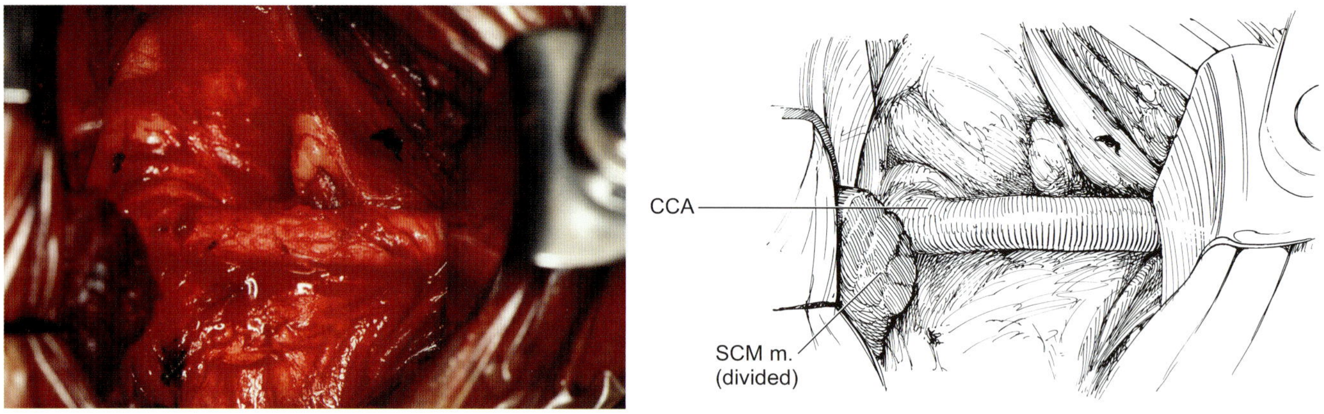

Fig. 11.2d A transverse supraclavicular incision with division of the SCM muscle is used to expose the lower portion of the CCA. Exposure is aided by the use of self-retaining anterior cervical diskectomy retractors. The ability to change blade length is particularly useful because the depth at which the surgeon works varies considerably.

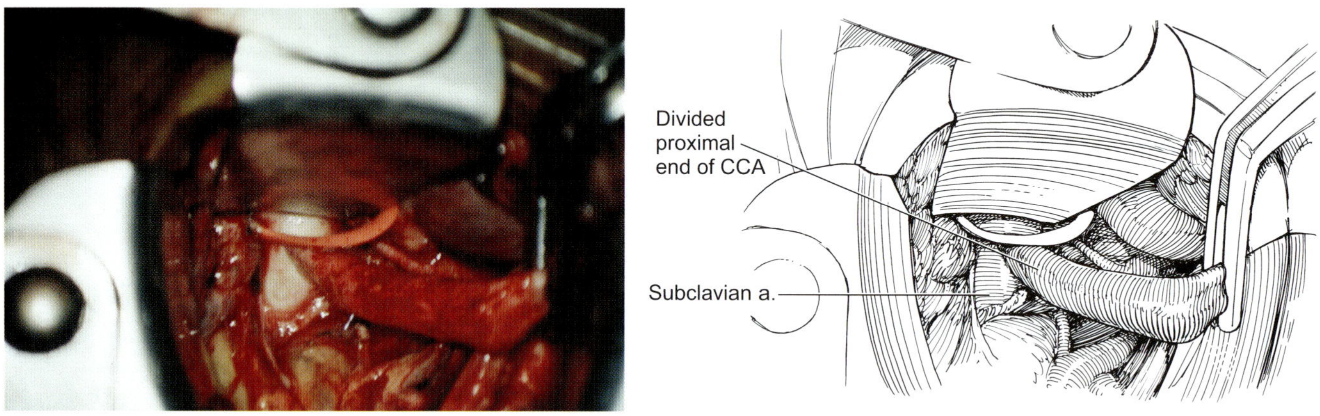

Fig. 11.2e The left subclavian artery, VA, and thyrocervical trunk are identified lateral and deep to the CCA. The CCA is mobilized and divided as proximally as possible to maximize the working length for transposition. The divided proximal end of the CCA is positioned over the subclavian artery at the site of the planned anastomosis. If additional length is needed, the CCA is dissected and mobilized distally.

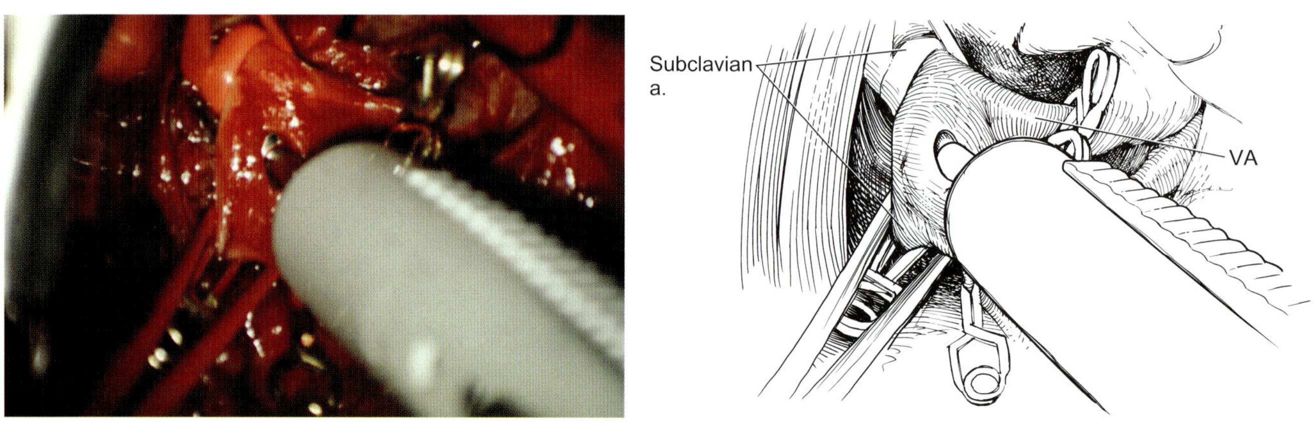

Fig. 11.2f A vascular loop is used to elevate a segment of subclavian artery. Its branches are occluded with temporary aneurysm clips. An arteriotomy is widened with a 5-mm aortic punch.

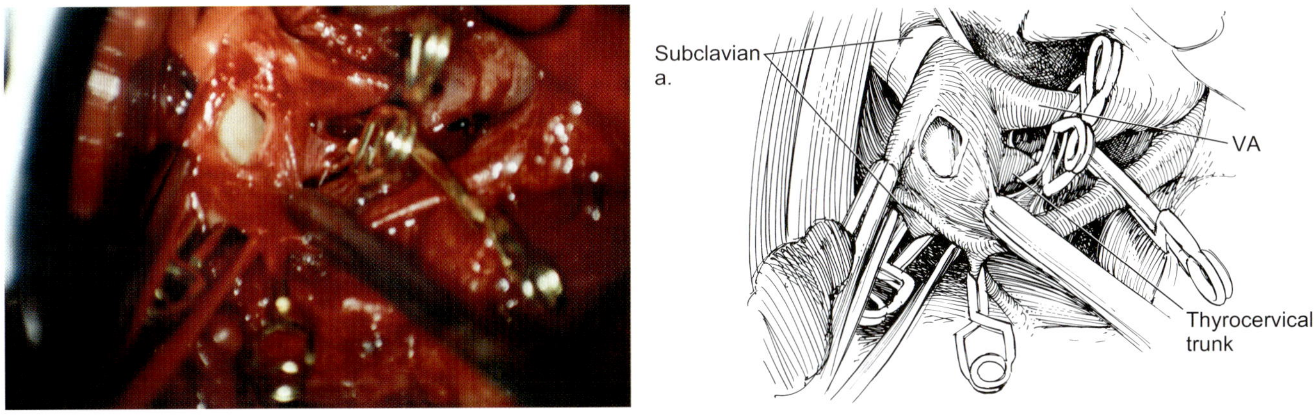

Fig. 11.2g The arteriotomy site is inspected. Note the smooth sides of the arteriotomy created with the aortic punch.

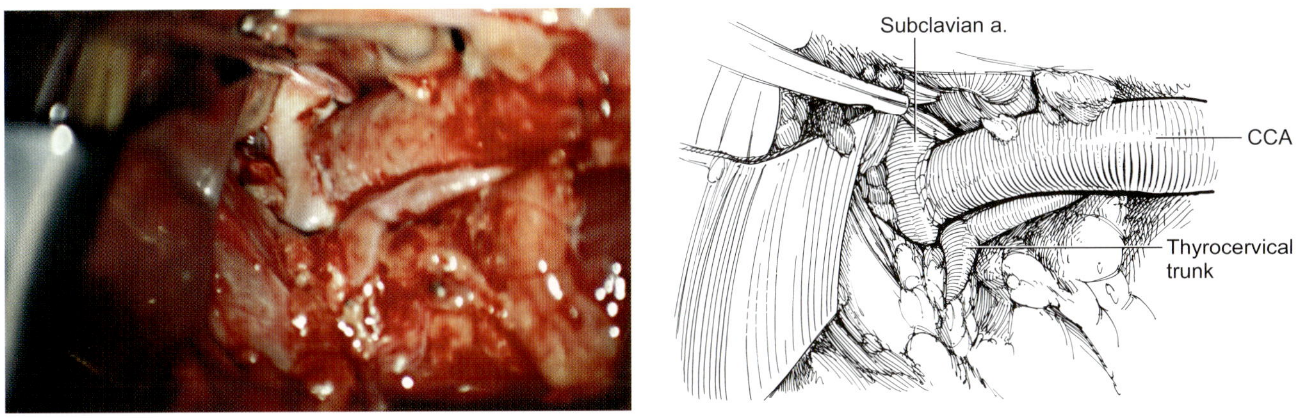

Fig. 11.2h A simple running 6–0 nylon suture is used to complete the anastomosis, which is inspected for hemostasis after all temporary clips are removed.

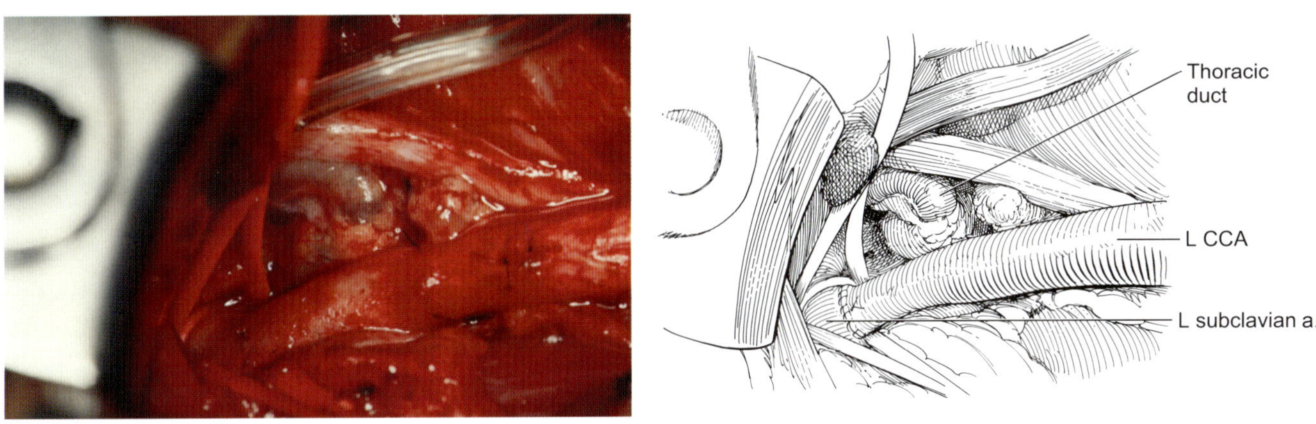

Fig. 11.2i The completed anastomosis is shown. The transposed CCA arises from the subclavian artery and is lateral to the thoracic duct and CN X.

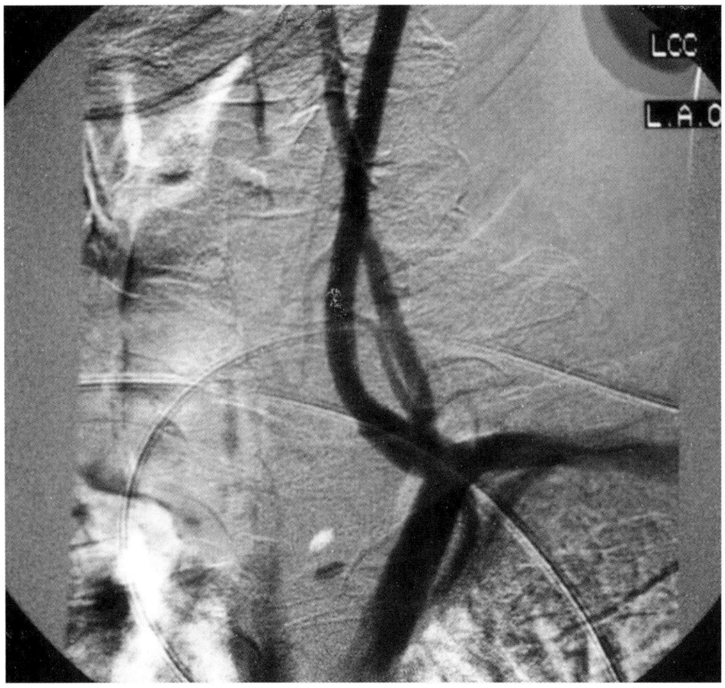

Fig. 11.2j Postoperative anterior oblique projection of a left subclavian artery angiogram shows the left CCA arising smoothly from the subclavian artery. The patient tolerated the procedure well and returned to work within 3 weeks.

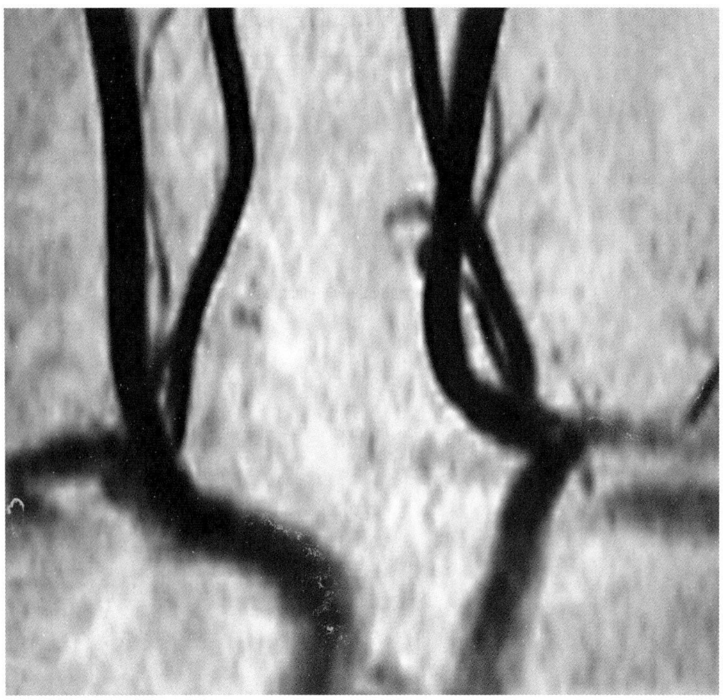

Fig. 11.2k MR angiogram obtained 3 years after surgery confirms excellent continued patency of the transposition. The patient remains asymptomatic.

12 STA-to-PCA and STA-to-SCA Bypass

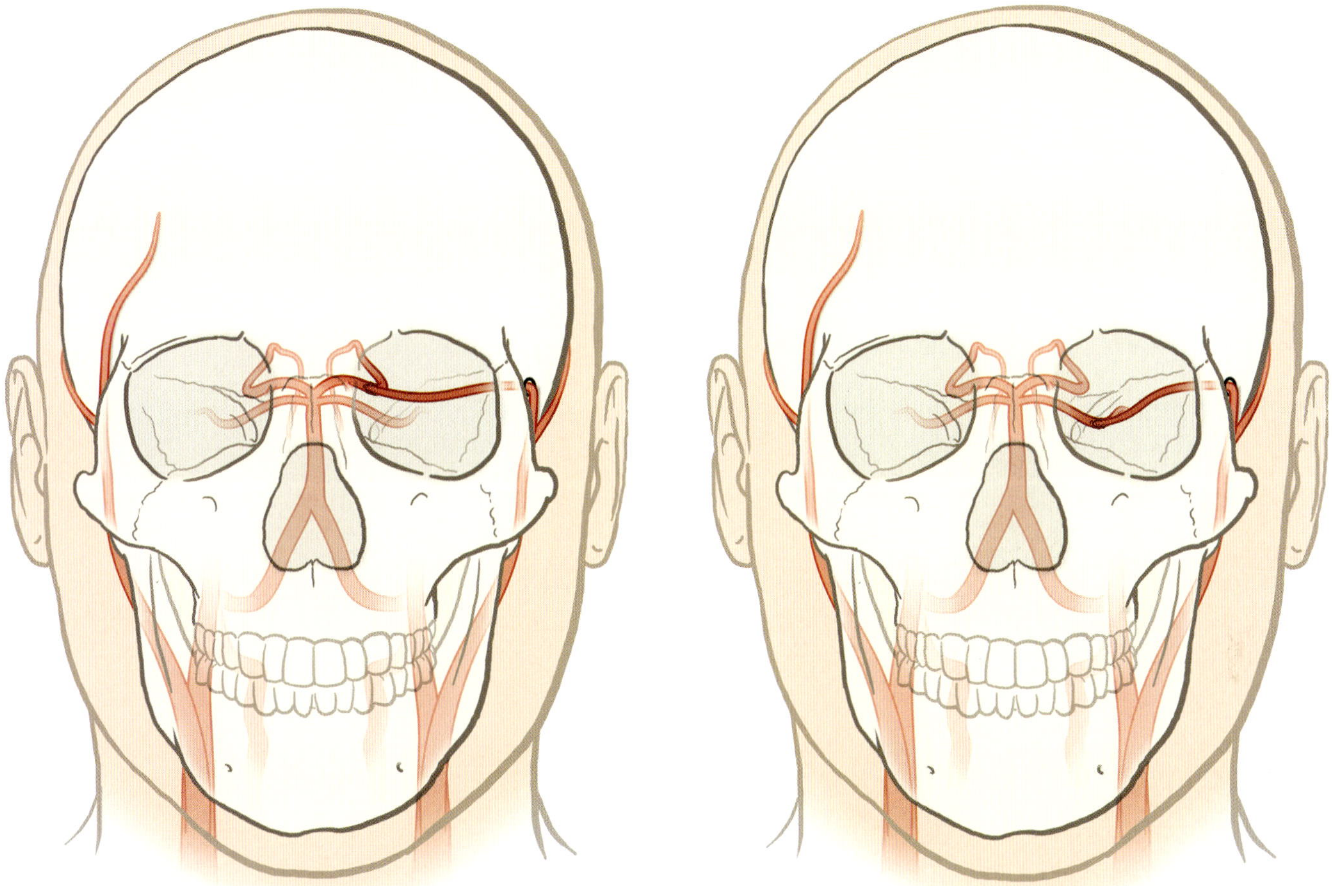

The recipient vessels for revascularization of the distal BA territory are the SCA and PCA. In the presence of normal anatomy, a bypass to either vessel perfuses the top of the BA and both SCAs and PCAs.

The STA is isolated in the same fashion as described in Section 2. An orbitozygomatic craniotomy is performed. This approach allows anterior mobilization of the temporalis muscle, creating more room for performing the anastomosis. The craniotomy needs to be flush with the floor of the middle fossa.

The SCA lies just at or below the tentorial edge. It is often advantageous to cut the edge of the tentorium to improve access to this artery. Care must be taken to identify and protect CN IV where it lies below the tentorial edge.

A 10-mm segment of the SCA without perforating vessels is isolated. There must be room for temporary clips on either side. A dam is placed under the vessel. A small piece of Gelfoam (Pfizer, New York, NY) also can be placed underneath the dam to elevate the vessel for easier access. The STA must be long enough that it can be swung back and forth as the anastomosis is performed. There must be enough redundancy of the STA that it can lie on floor of the middle fossa without tension and can accommodate the temporal lobe as the lobe assumes its normal position.

The STA-to-PCA bypass is performed in similar fashion, except that the tentorium does not need to be divided and the temporal lobe needs more mobilization.

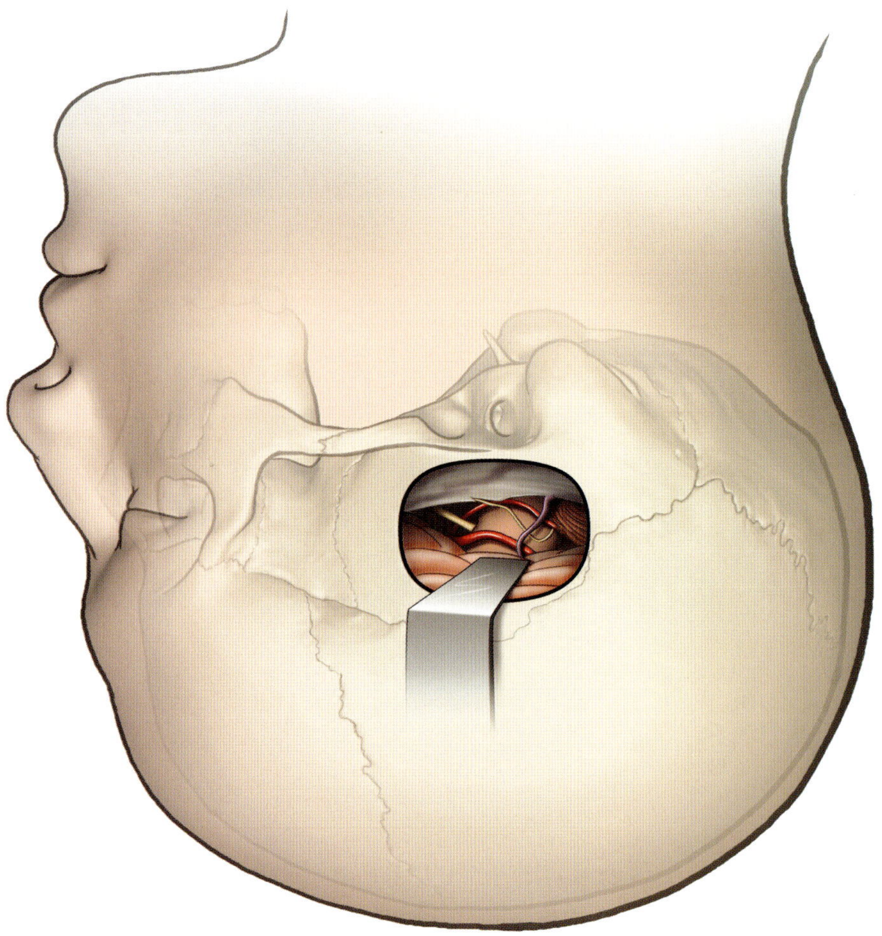

Fig. 12.0a Schematic representation shows the flat exposure needed to access the PCA and SCA.

Anatomy of the STA-to-PCA Bypass

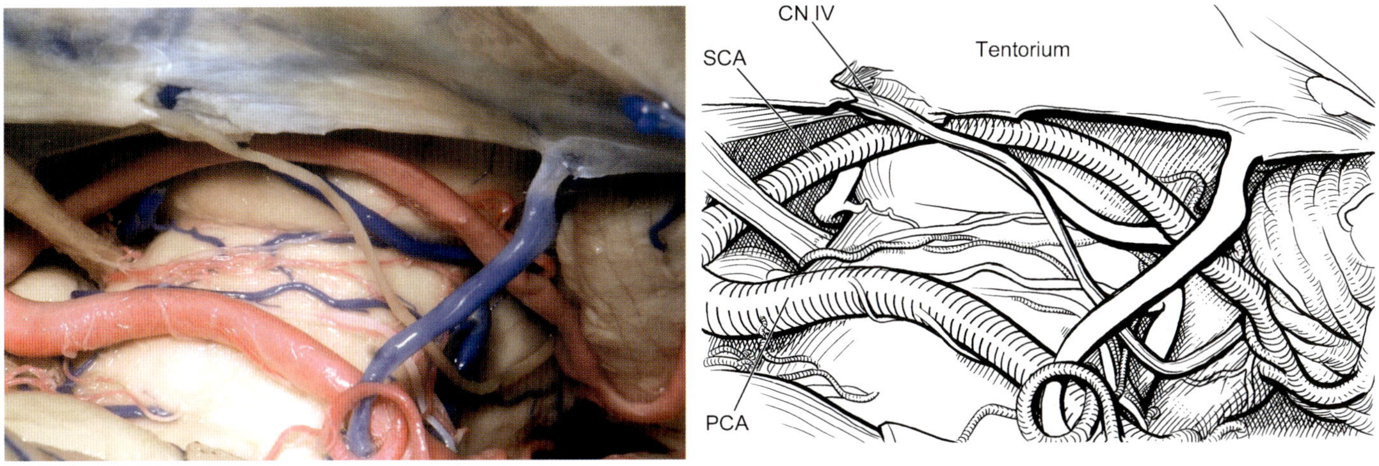

Fig. 12.0b Both the PCA and SCA are visible at the edge of the tentorium. CN IV has been exposed. (Photograph used with permission from *Journal of Neurosurgery*.)

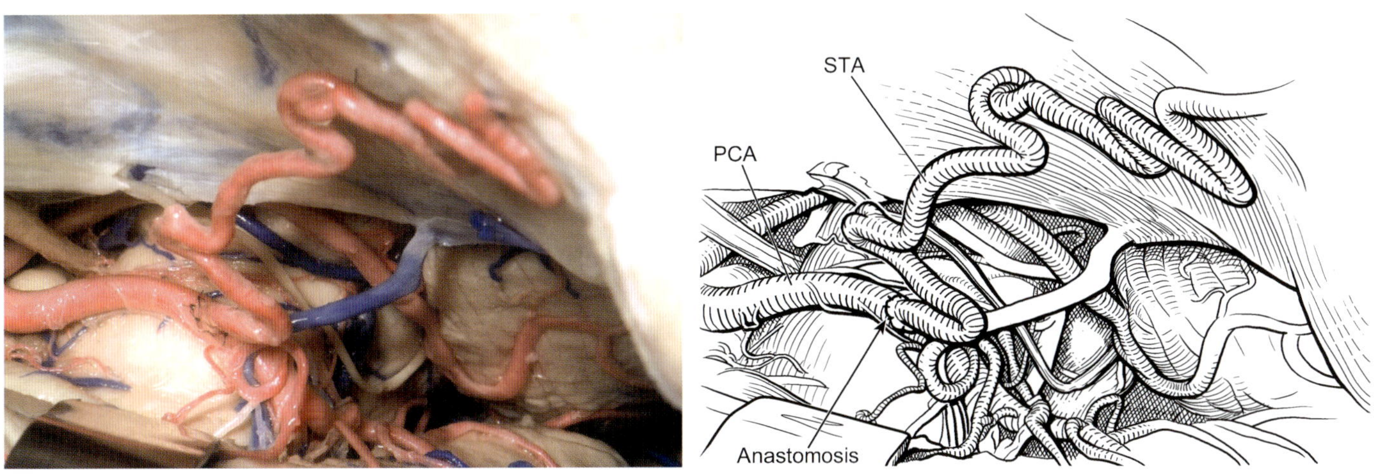

Fig. 12.0c A bypass has been performed between the STA and PCA. (Photograph used with permission from *Journal of Neurosurgery*.)

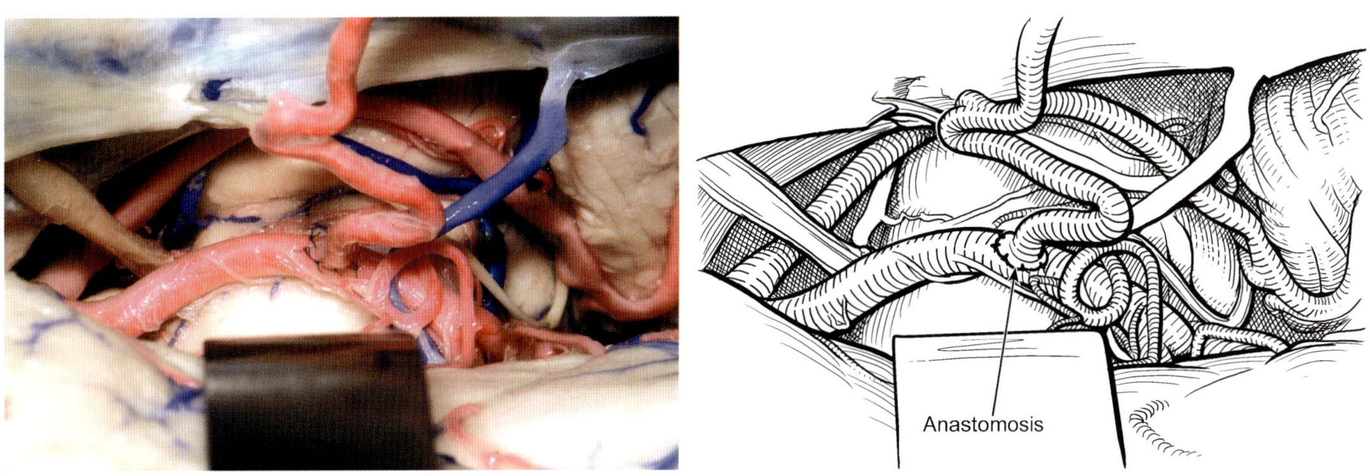

Fig. 12.0d Higher magnification view of an STA-to-PCA anastomosis. (Photograph used with permission from *Journal of Neurosurgery*.)

Anatomy of the STA-to-SCA Bypass

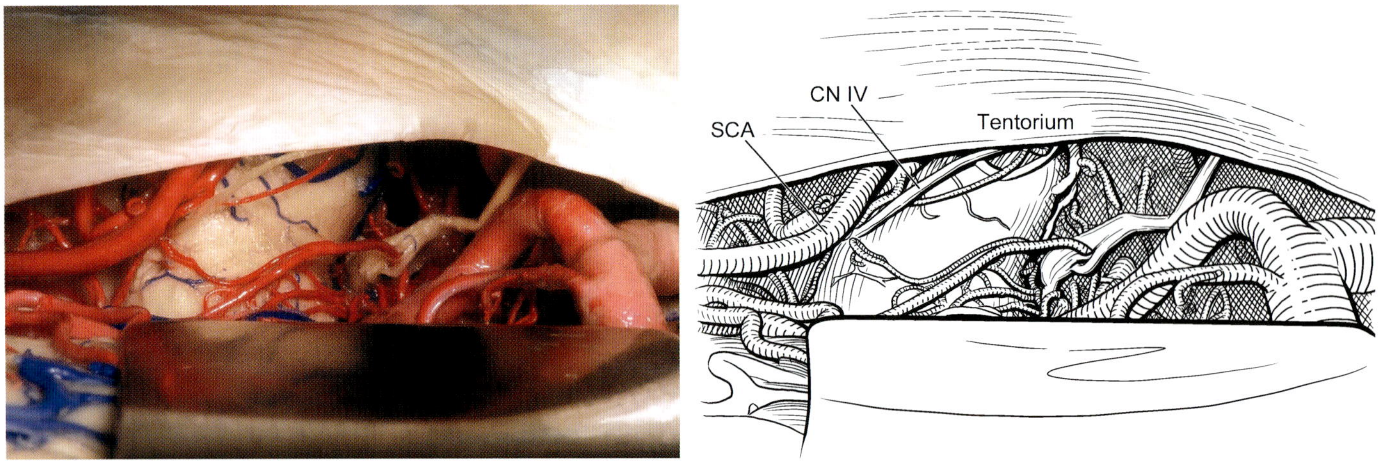

Fig. 12.0e On the left side, the edge of the tentorium is visualized along with the SCA as it tucks underneath the tentorium. CN IV is visible. (Photograph used with permission from *Journal of Neurosurgery*.)

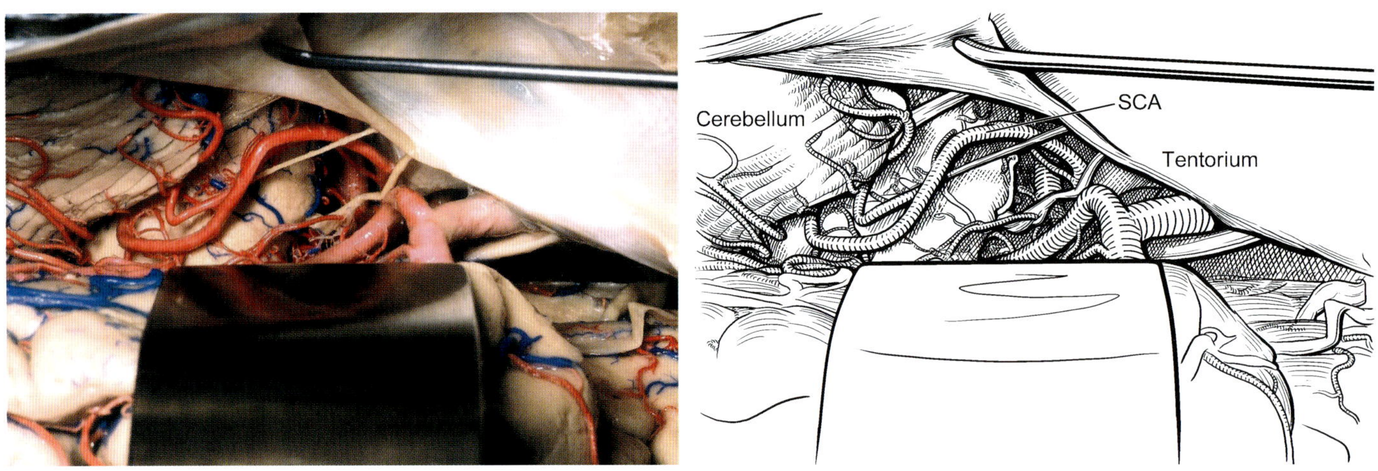

Fig. 12.0f The tentorial edge has been retracted, exposing the full course of the SCA in the ambient cistern. (Photograph used with permission from *Journal of Neurosurgery*.)

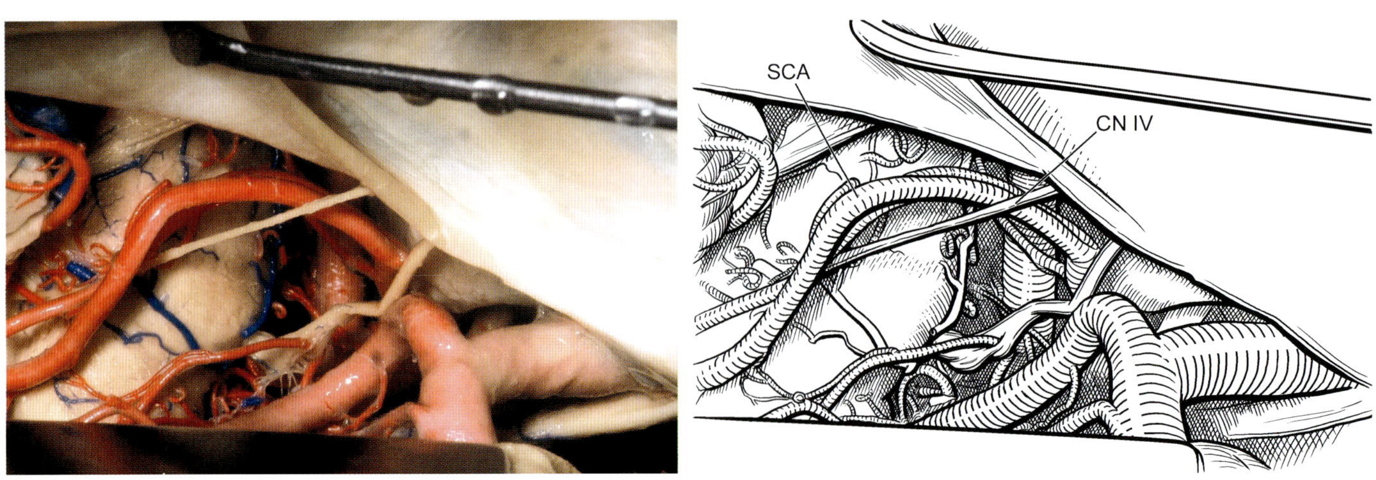

Fig. 12.0g High power view of CN IV and the SCA. (Photograph used with permission from *Journal of Neurosurgery*.)

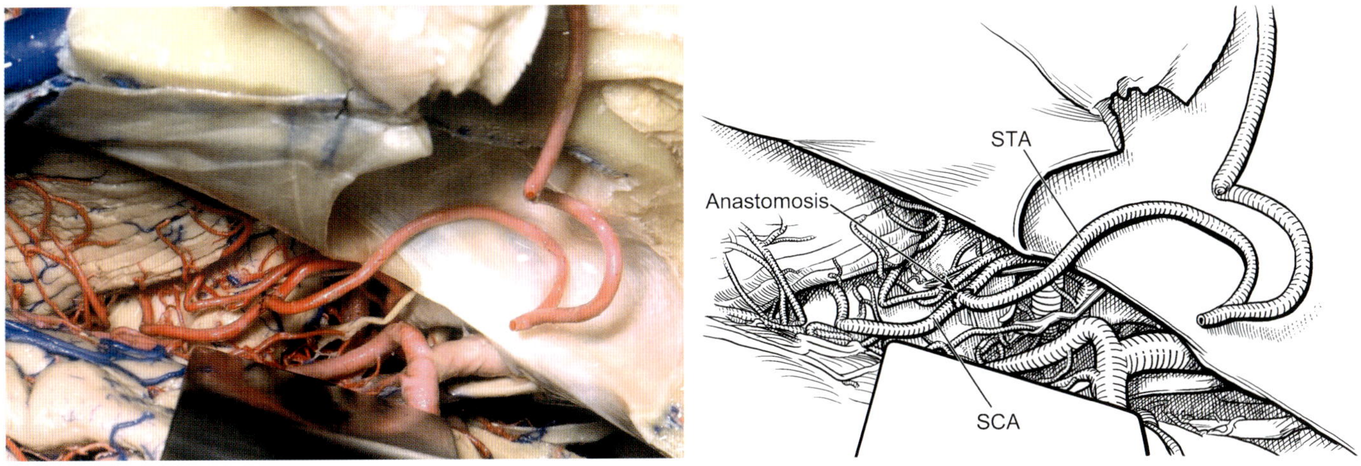

Fig. 12.0h A bypass has been performed between the STA and the SCA. (Photograph used with permission from *Journal of Neurosurgery*.)

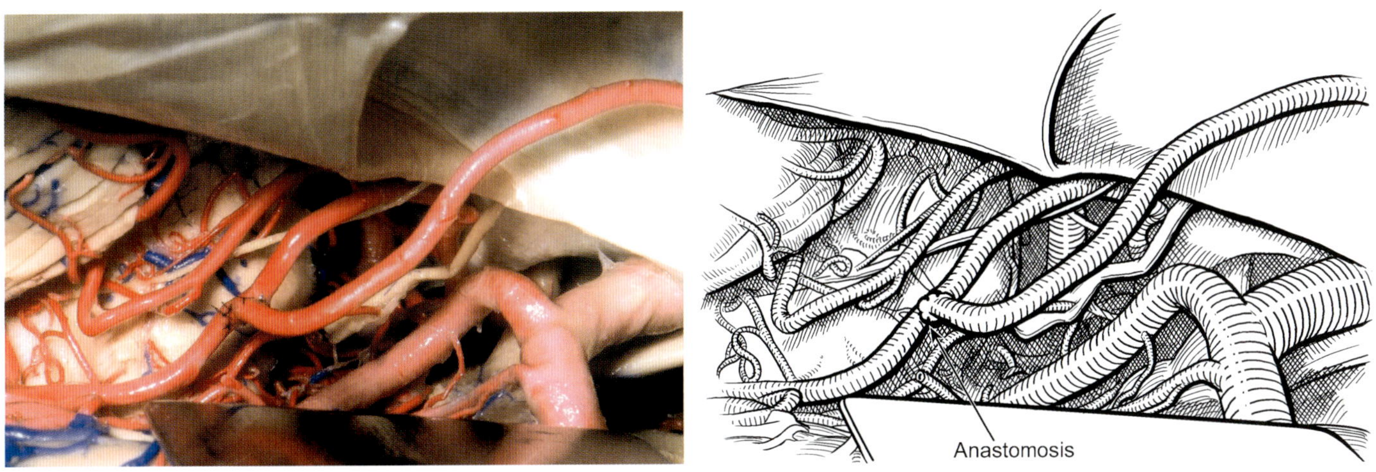

Fig. 12.0i High power view of the left STA-to-SCA bypass. (Photograph used with permission from *Journal of Neurosurgery*.)

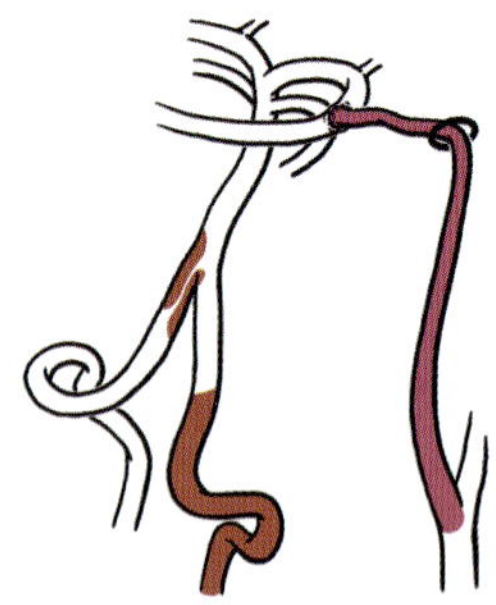

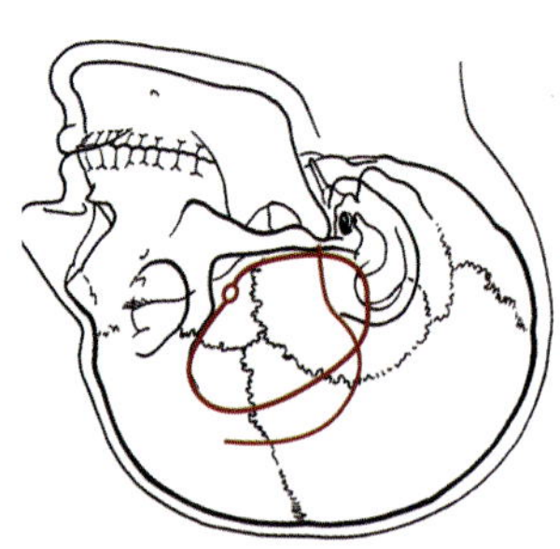

Case 12-1

Diagnosis: Complete occlusion of the right VA and severe stenosis of left VA with vestigial PCoAs

Bypass: STA-to-PCA

Approach: Right pterional with low temporal exposure

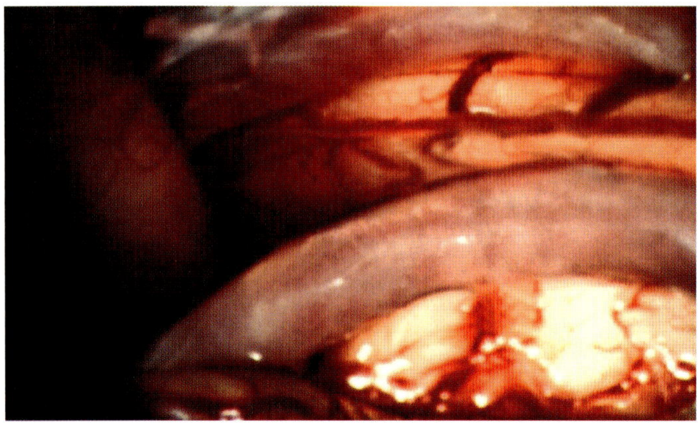

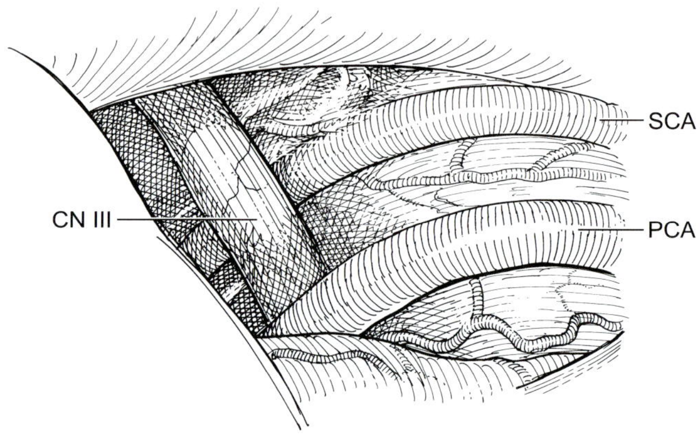

Fig. 12.1a The PCA and SCA are exposed in the ambient cistern.

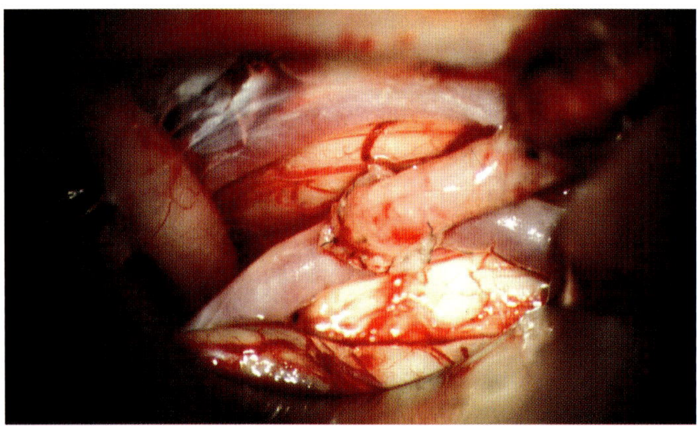

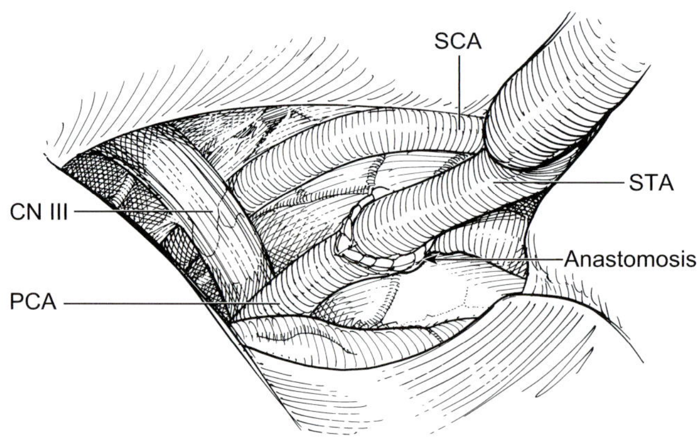

Fig. 12.1b An STA-to-PCA bypass has been performed.

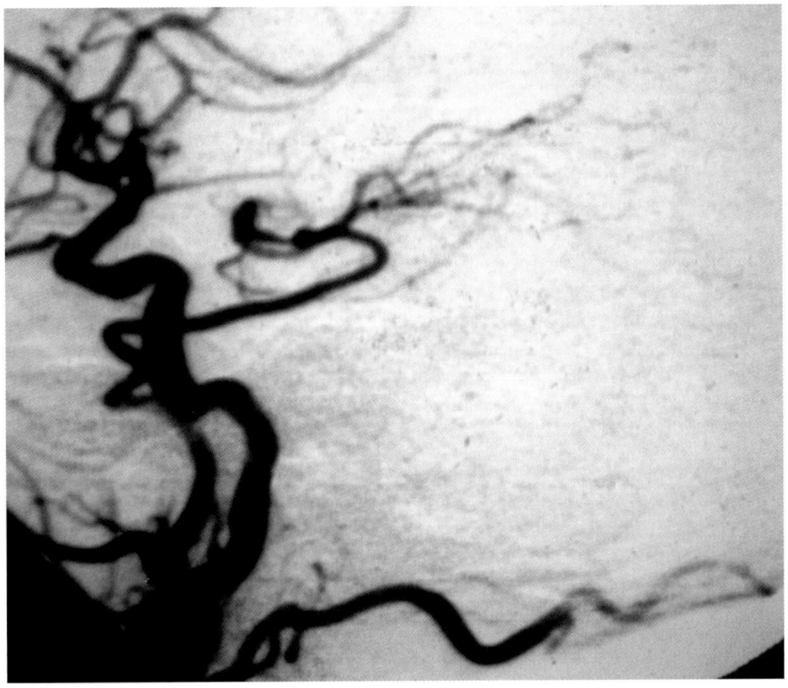

c

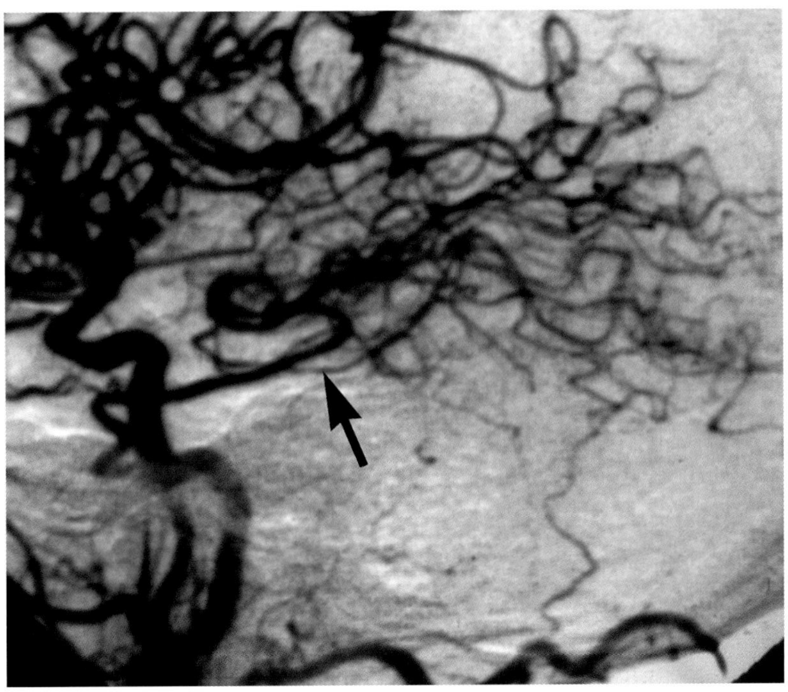

d

Fig. 12.1c, d Postoperative early and late lateral angiograms confirm patency of the STA-to-PCA bypass and excellent filling of the PCA (*arrow*) and upper BA territory.

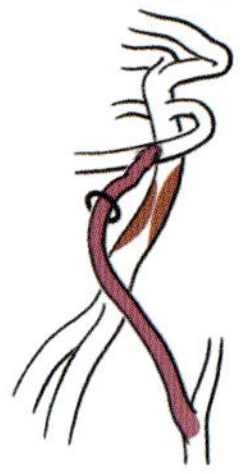

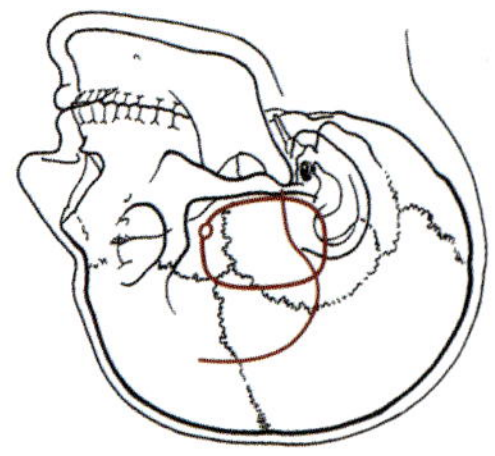

Case 12-2

Diagnosis: Symptomatic stenosis of mid-BA

Bypass: STA-to-SCA

Approach: Right subtemporal

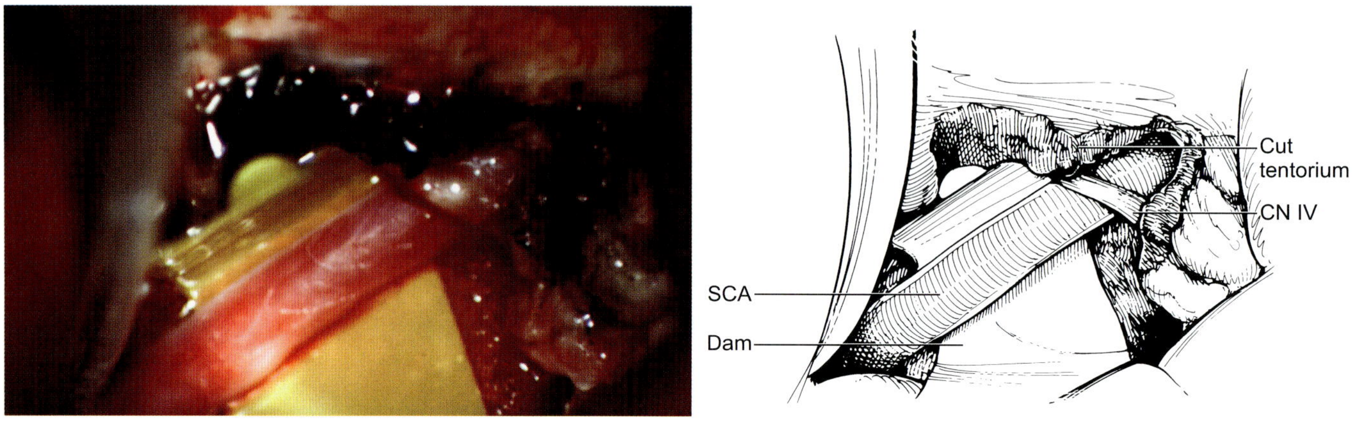

Fig. 12.2a The SCA is exposed via a right subtemporal approach. The edge of the tentorium is cut and coagulated, and a small latex dam is placed beneath the artery to improve visualization.

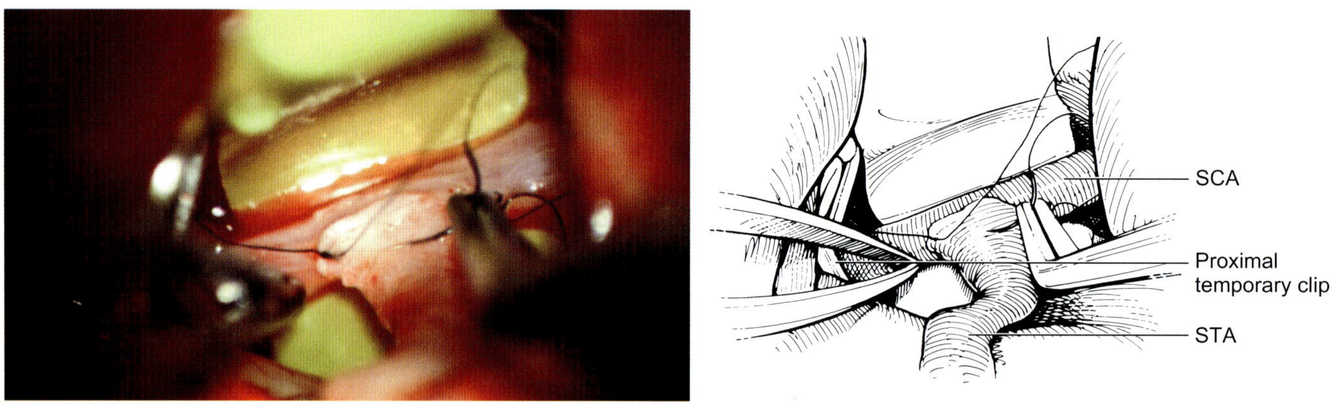

Fig. 12.2b A short segment of the SCA is isolated between temporary aneurysm clips. The distal end of the STA is tacked to the SCA at two points in preparation for the end-to-side anastomosis.

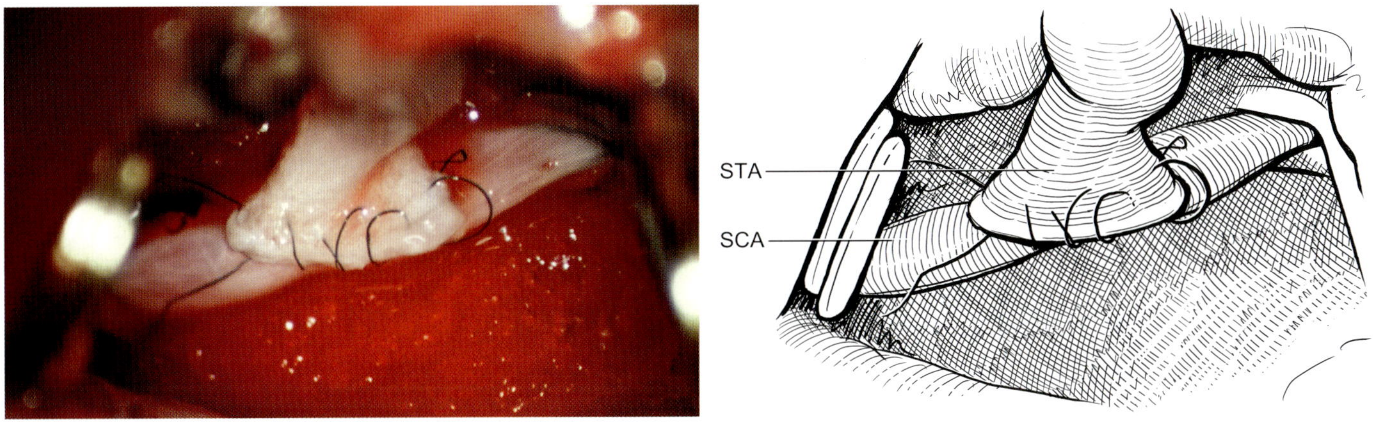

Fig. 12.2c A loose running 10–0 suture is placed along one wall. Waiting to tighten the sutures until they have all been placed helps the surgeon to visualize the vessel walls for these deep anastomoses, ensures uniform suture tension, and improves hemostasis.

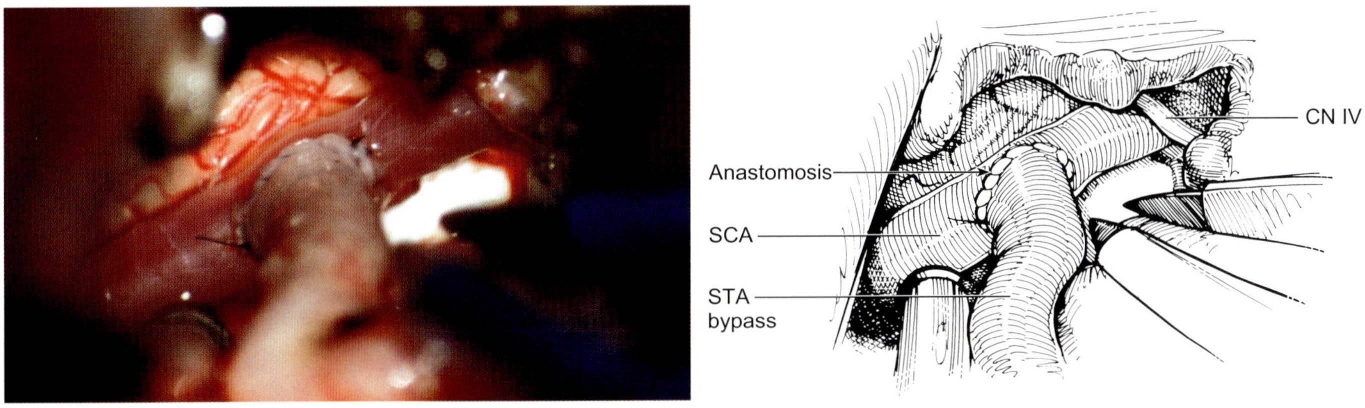

Fig. 12.2d The anastomosis is completed and inspected for hemostasis.

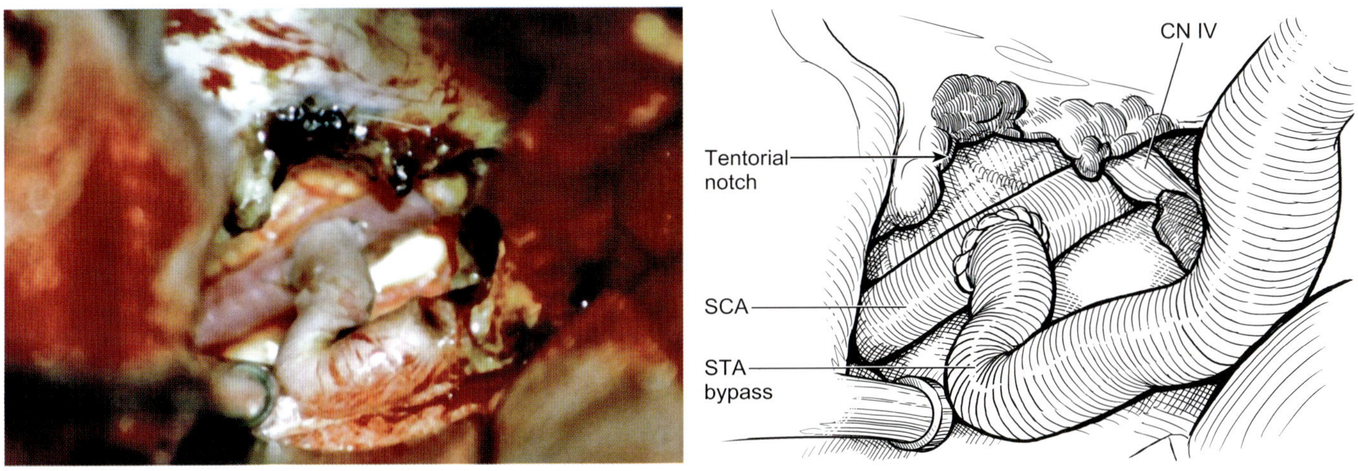

Fig. 12.2e Low power view shows the completed bypass. The STA must be sufficiently slack that the graft is not stretched when the temporal lobe returns to its normal position after the retractor is removed.

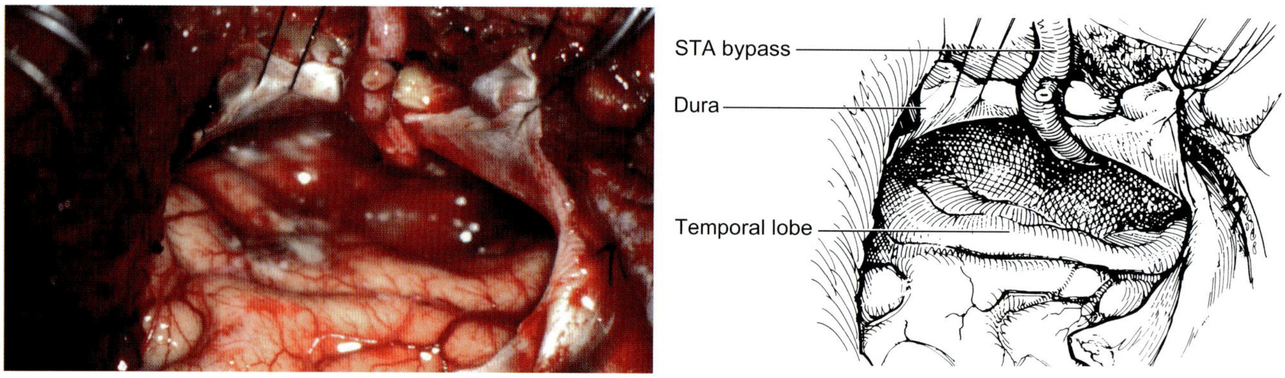

Fig. 12.2f Overview of the operative field shows the STA coursing over the floor of the middle fossa. Drilling the lateral wall of the middle fossa flat in relation to the floor maximizes subtemporal exposure while minimizing the need for retraction.

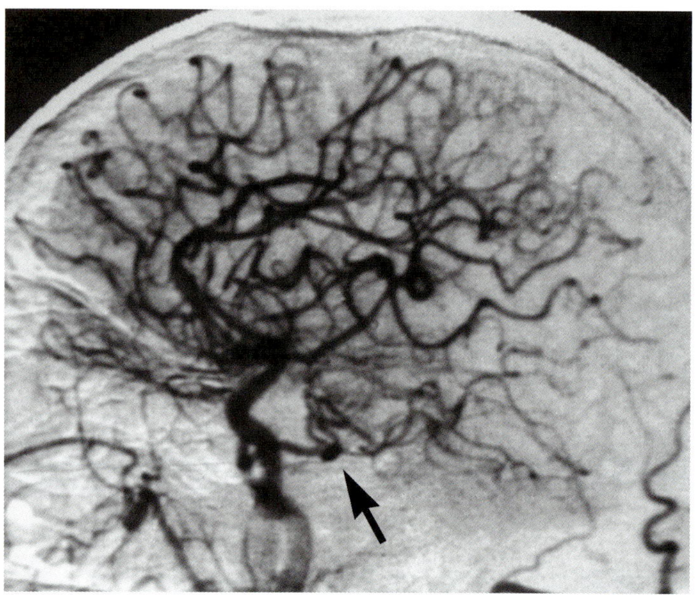

Fig. 12.2g Postoperative lateral angiogram of the right CCA demonstrates rapid filling of the SCAs and right PCA through the patent bypass (*arrow*).

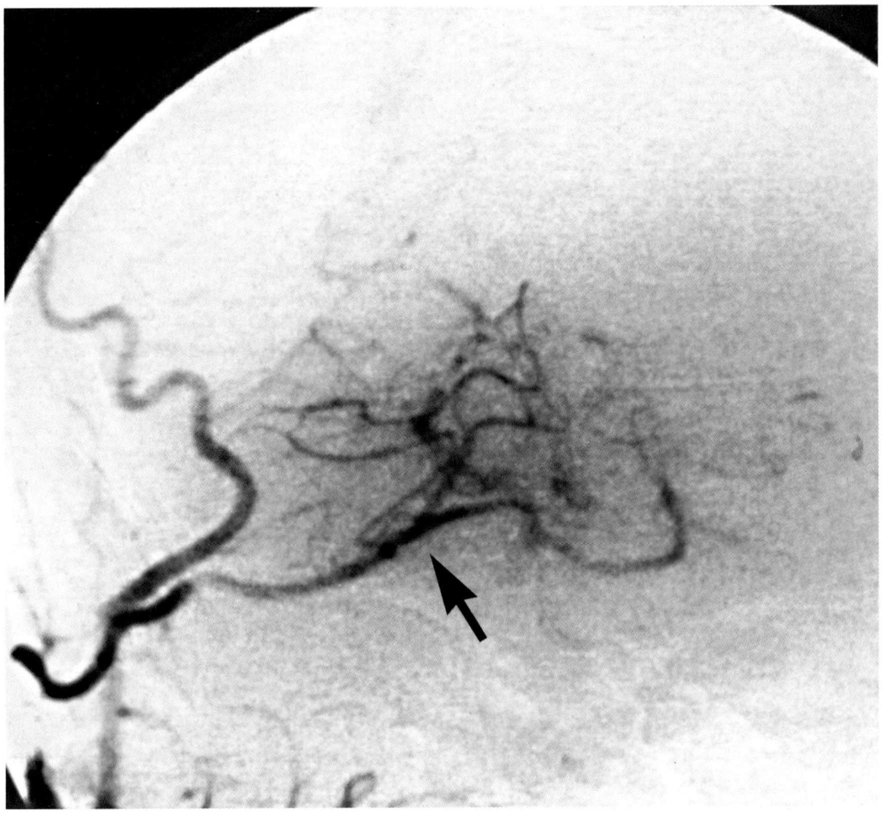

Fig. 12.2h Magnified postoperative selective angiogram of the right ECA shows the STA-to-SCA bypass (*arrow*).

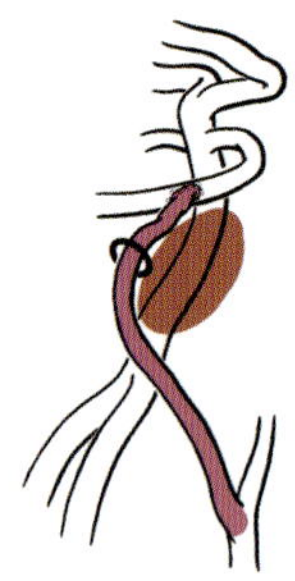

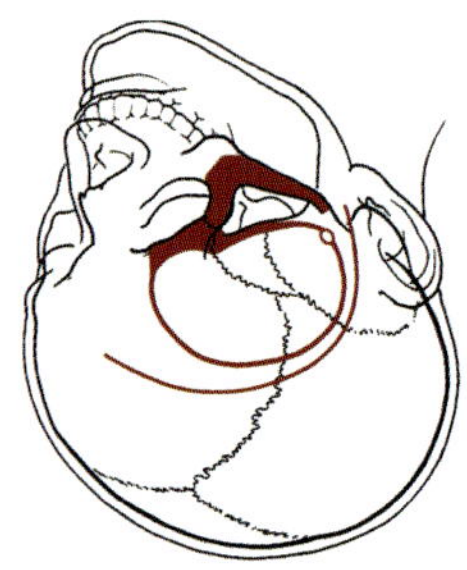

Case 12-3

Diagnosis: Complex BA aneurysm

Bypass: Right STA-to-SCA

Approach: Right orbitozygomatic

Video

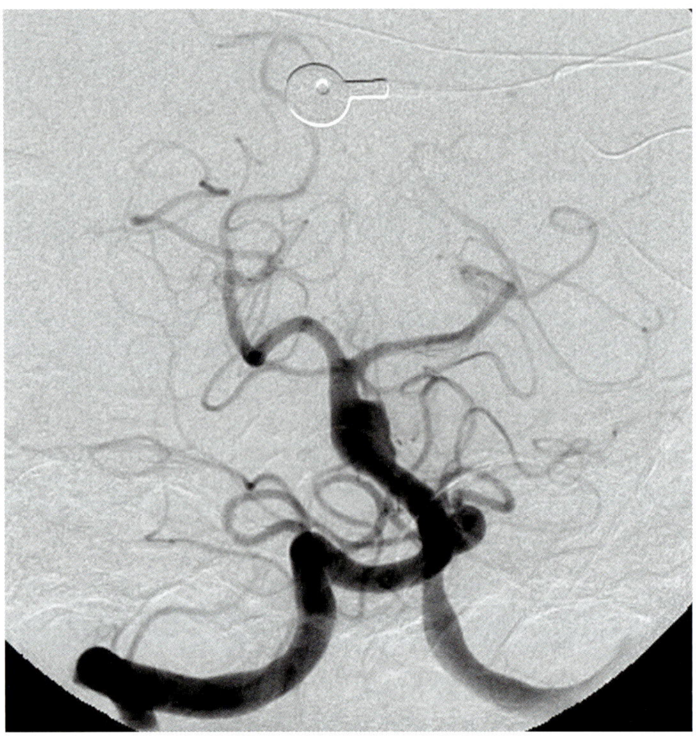

Fig. 12.3a A 50-year-old man with headaches underwent angiography, which showed a dissecting BA aneurysm.

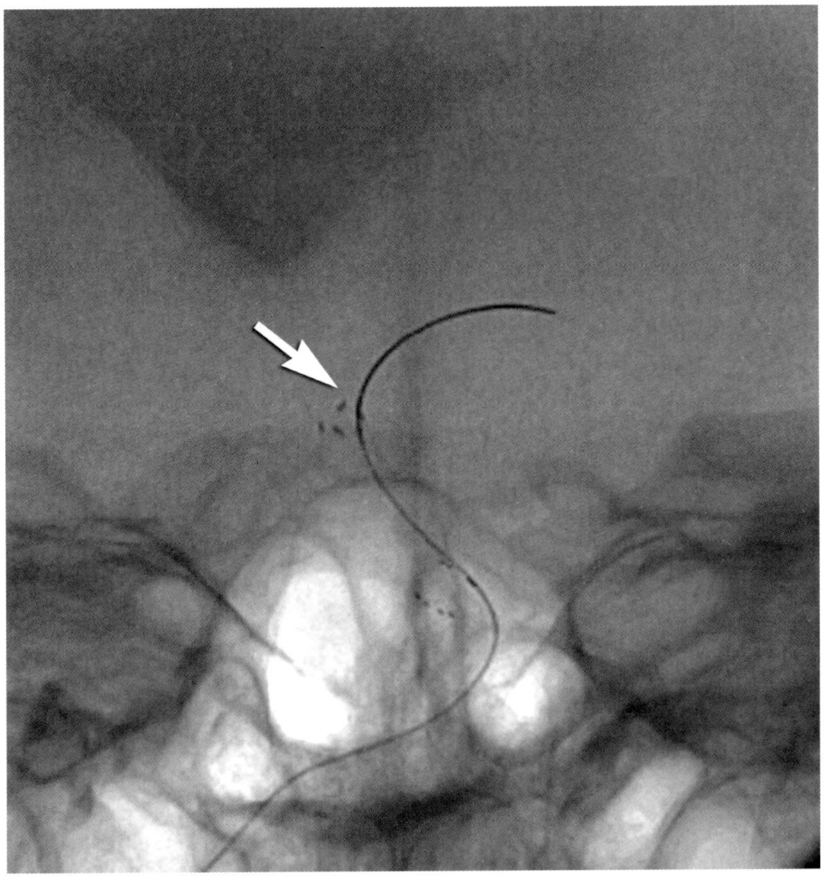

Fig. 12.3b A stent (*arrow*) is placed in the aneurysm.

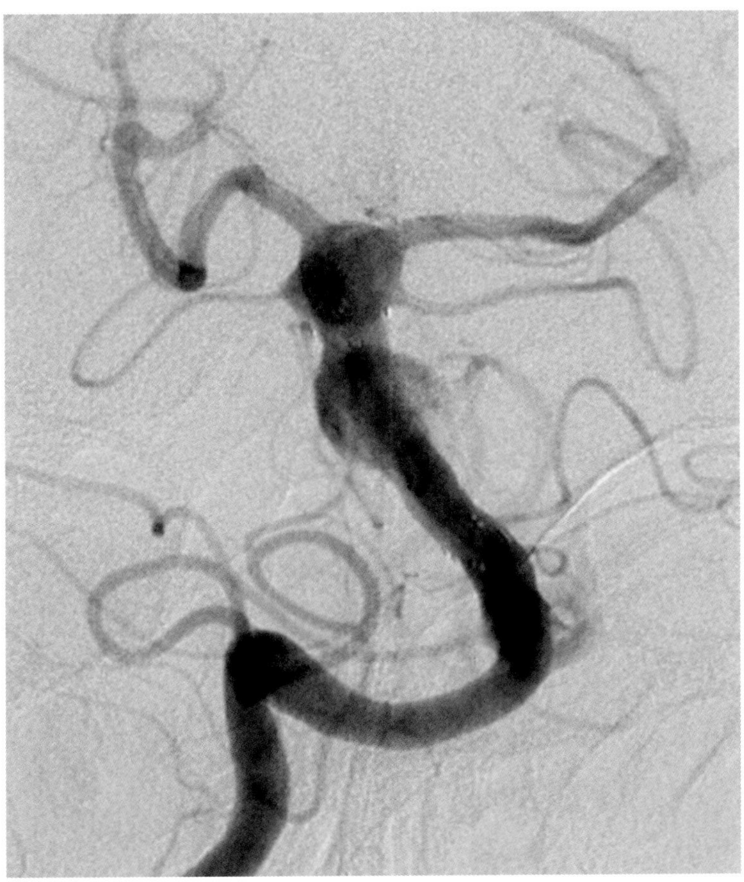

Fig. 12.3c Thirteen months after the stent was placed, further enlargement of the aneurysm was observed.

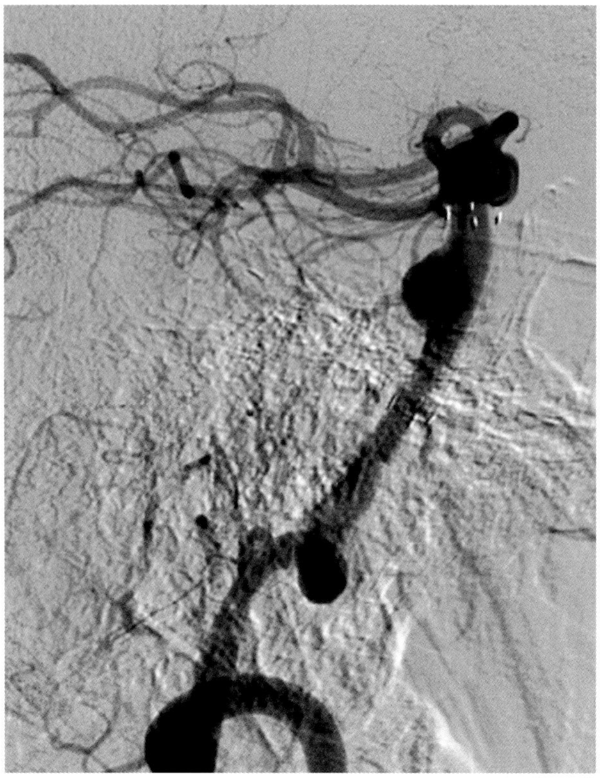

Fig. 12.3d Angiogram shows progressive enlargement of the original aneurysm through the stent as well as enlargement distal to the end of the stent.

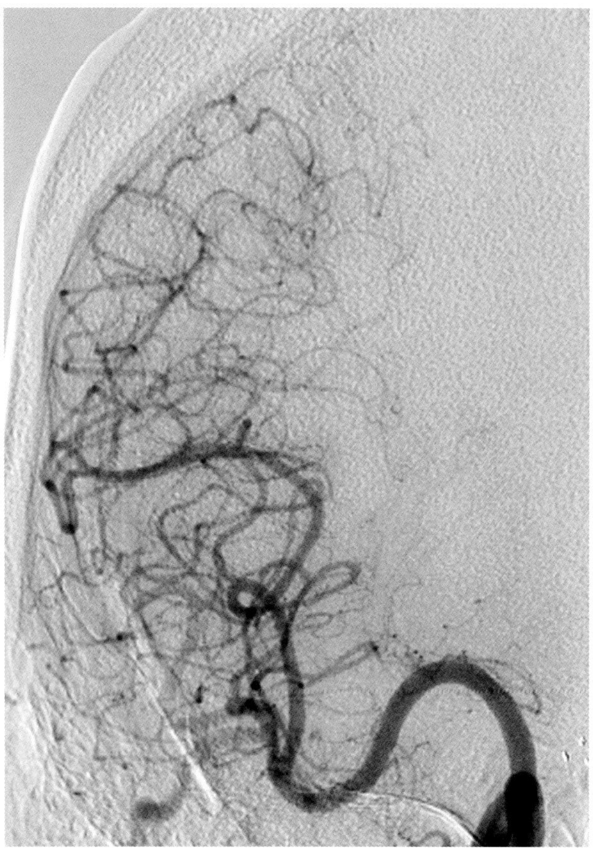

e

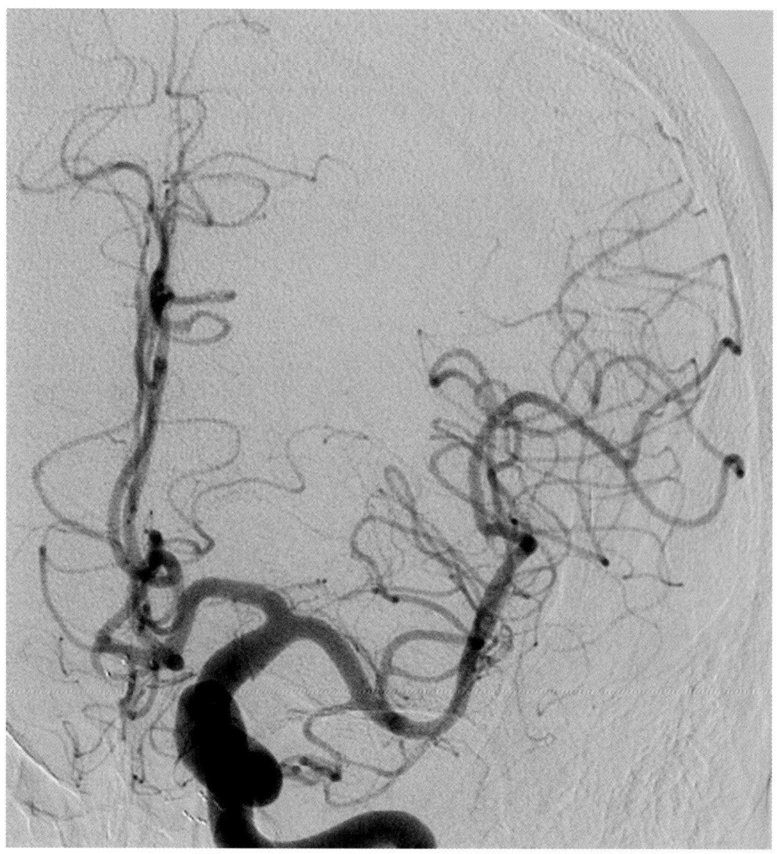

f

Fig. 12.3e, f The patient underwent an Alcock test, but no PCoA was identified.

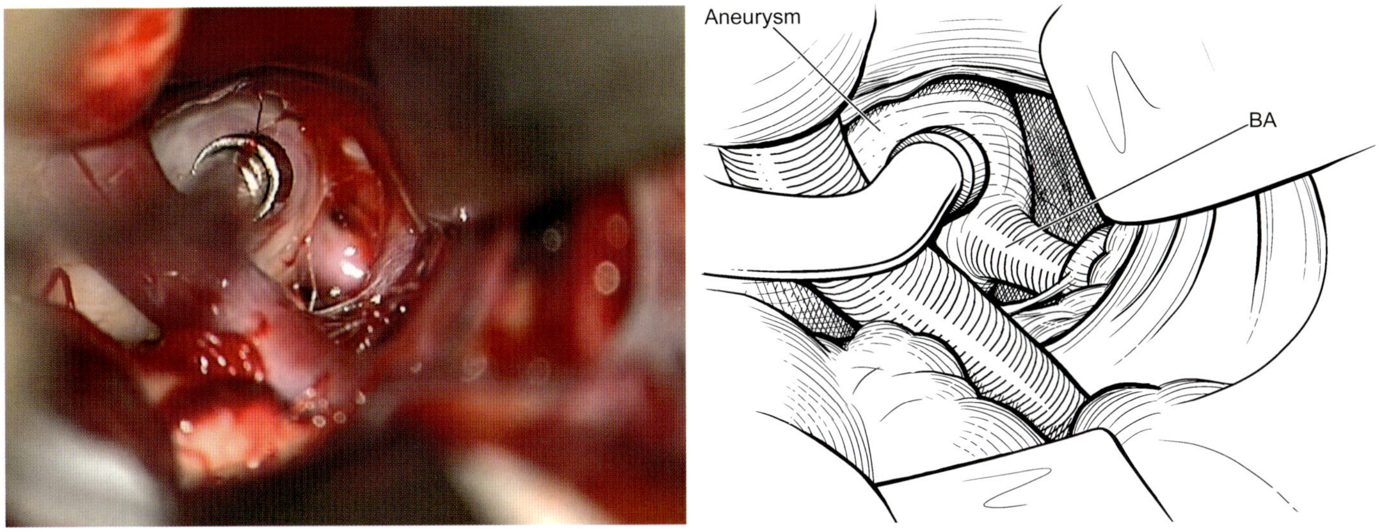

Fig. 12.3g Through a right orbitozygomatic approach, the distal BA aneurysm is visible.

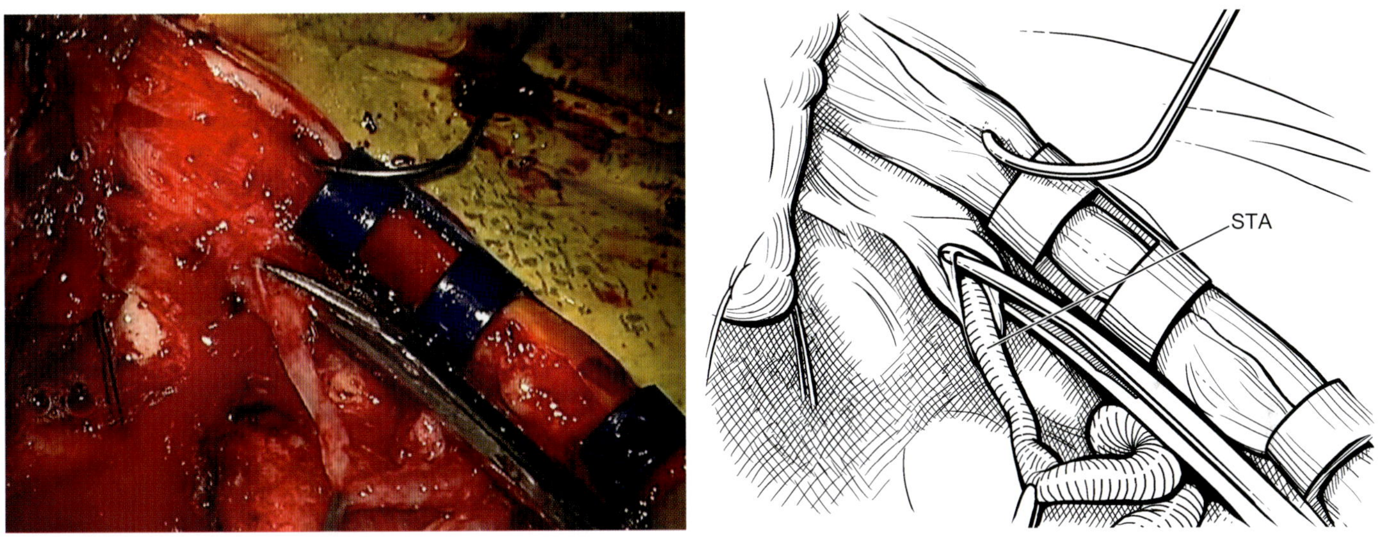

Fig. 12.3h The STA is freed and prepared for anastomosis.

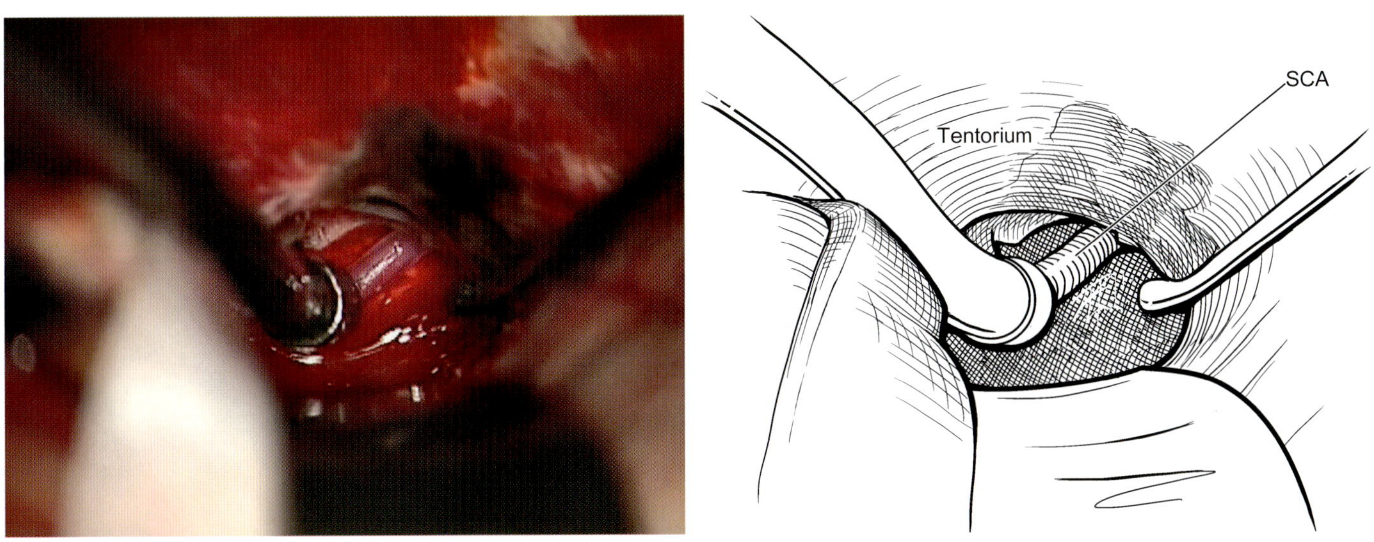

Fig. 12.3i The SCA is exposed through the incision in the tentorium.

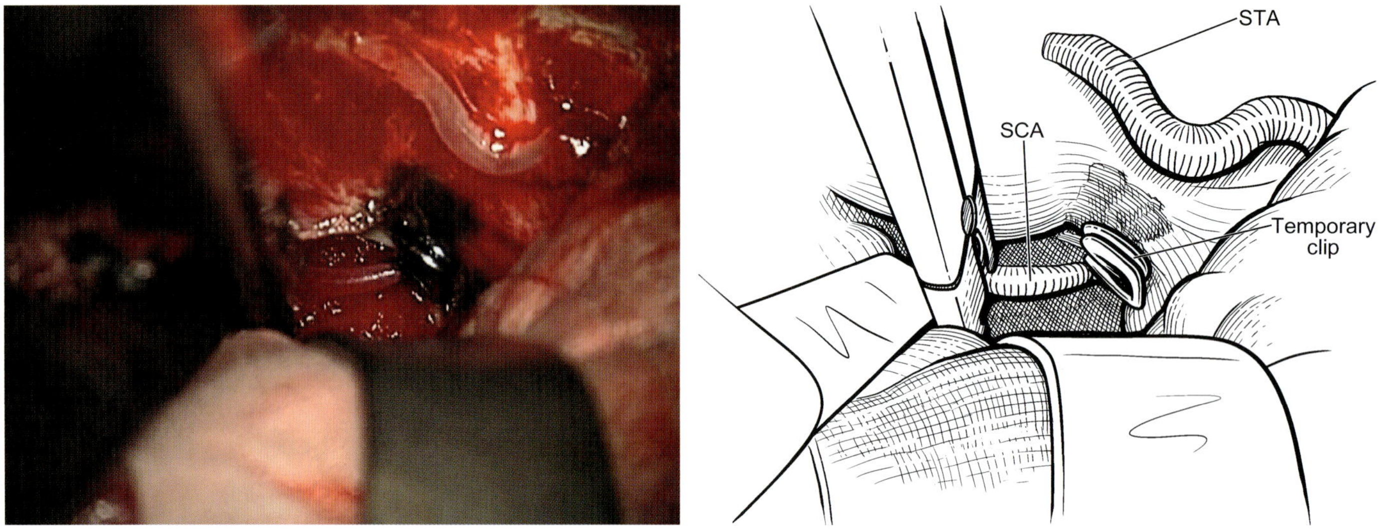

Fig. 12.3j Temporary clips are placed on the SCA.

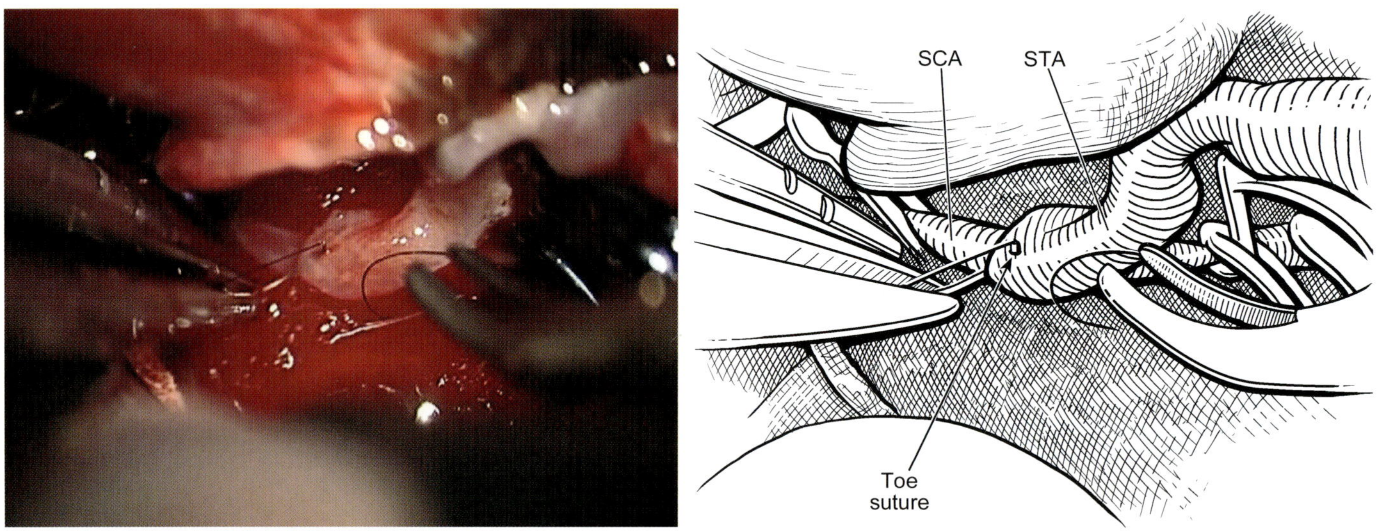

Fig. 12.3k After the SCA arteriotomy is made, the cut end of the STA is tacked to the SCA with heel and toe sutures.

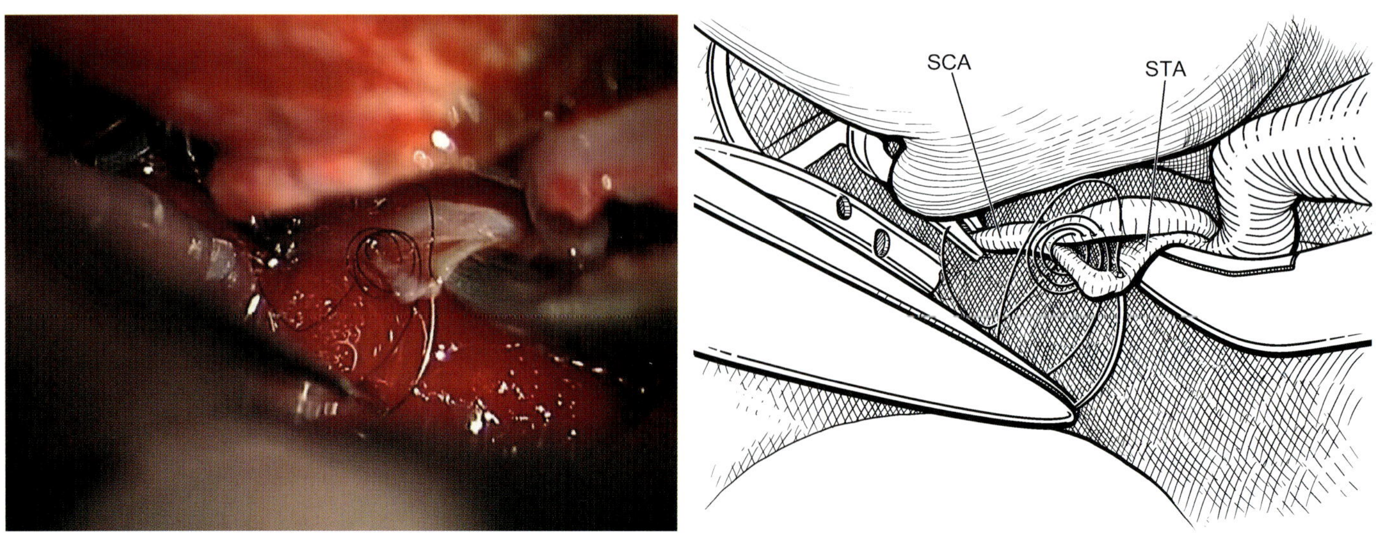

Fig. 12.3l Continuous running sutures are placed loosely in the back wall of the anastomosis.

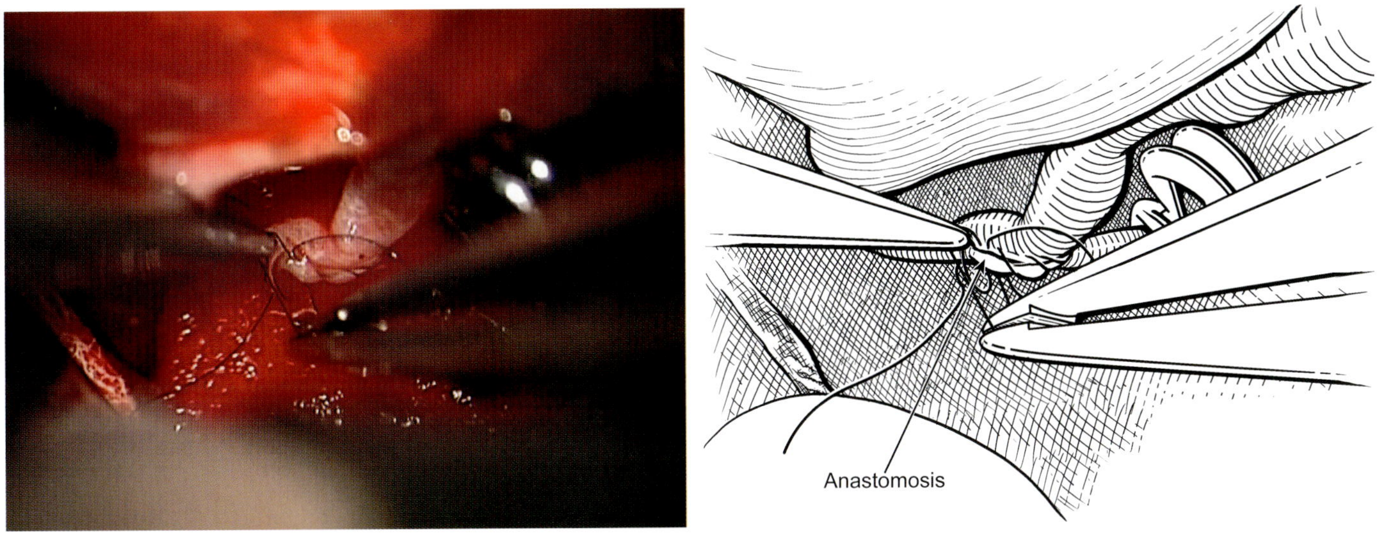

Fig. 12.3m The sutures are tightened.

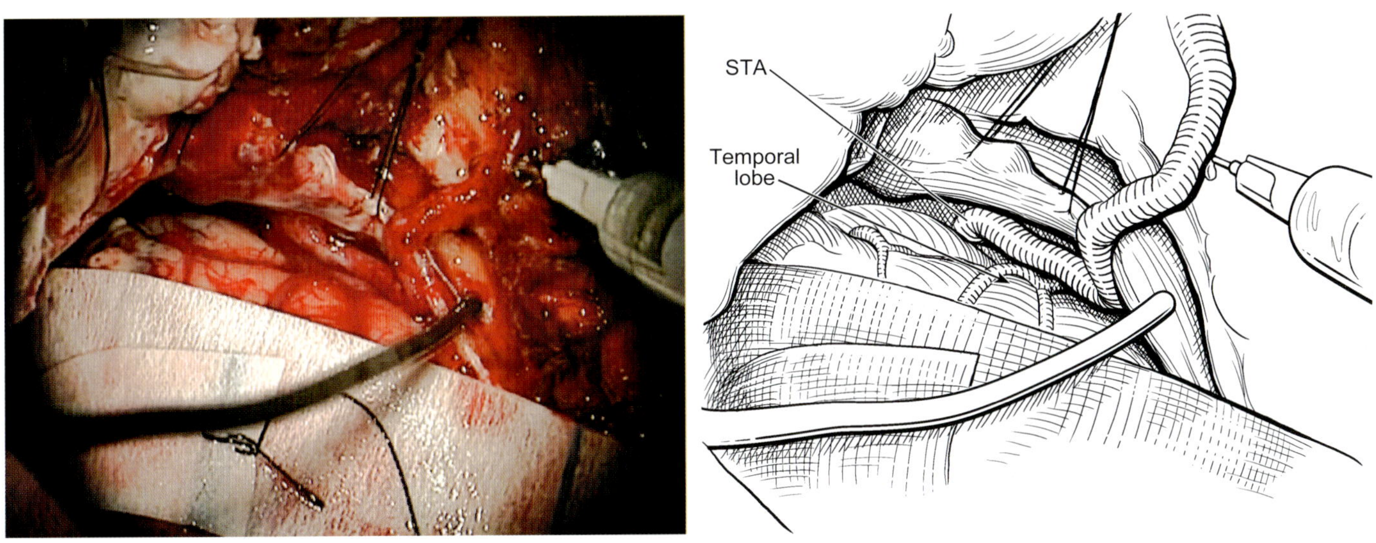

Fig. 12.3n Overview of the exposure shows the STA as it lies below the temporal lobe on its way to the anastomotic site.

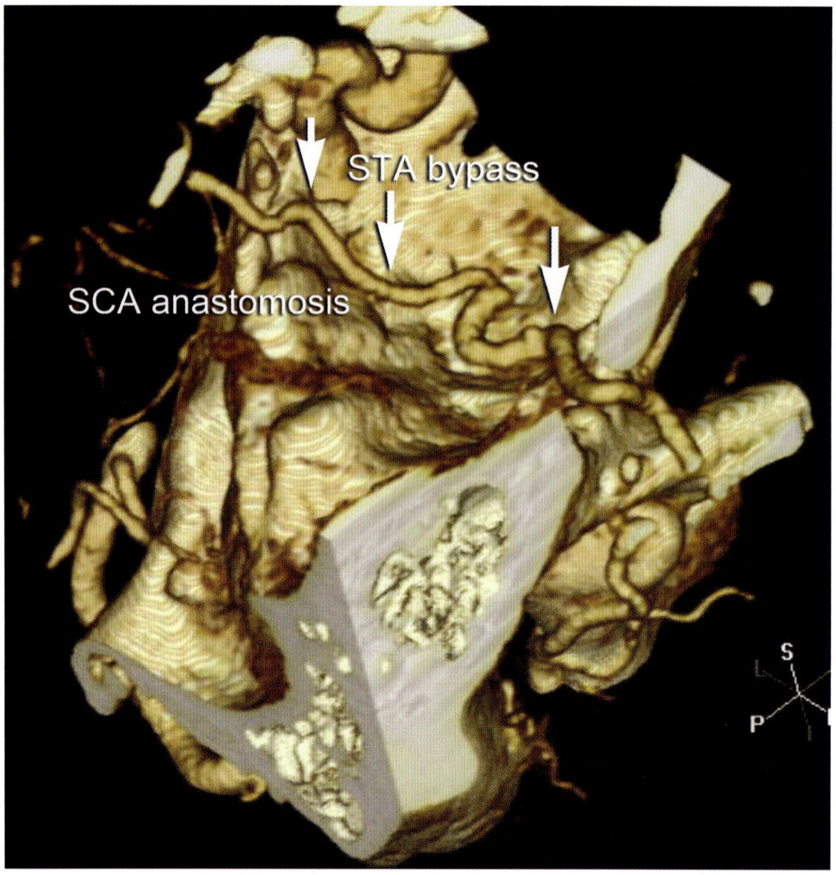

Fig. 12.3o Three-dimensional reconstruction shows the STA-to-SCA bypass (*arrows*).

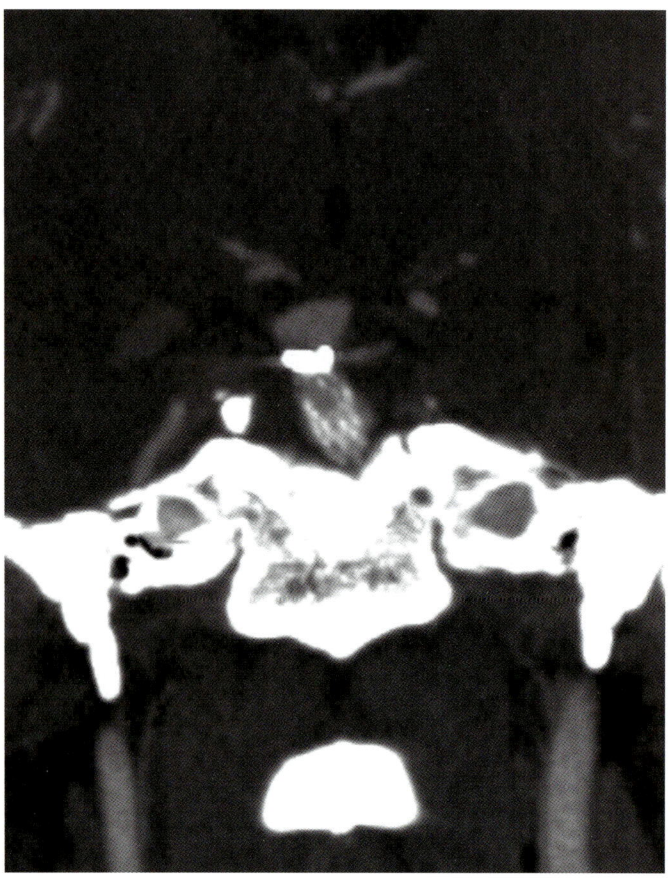

Fig. 12.3p CT angiogram shows the clips above the stent and below the SCA.

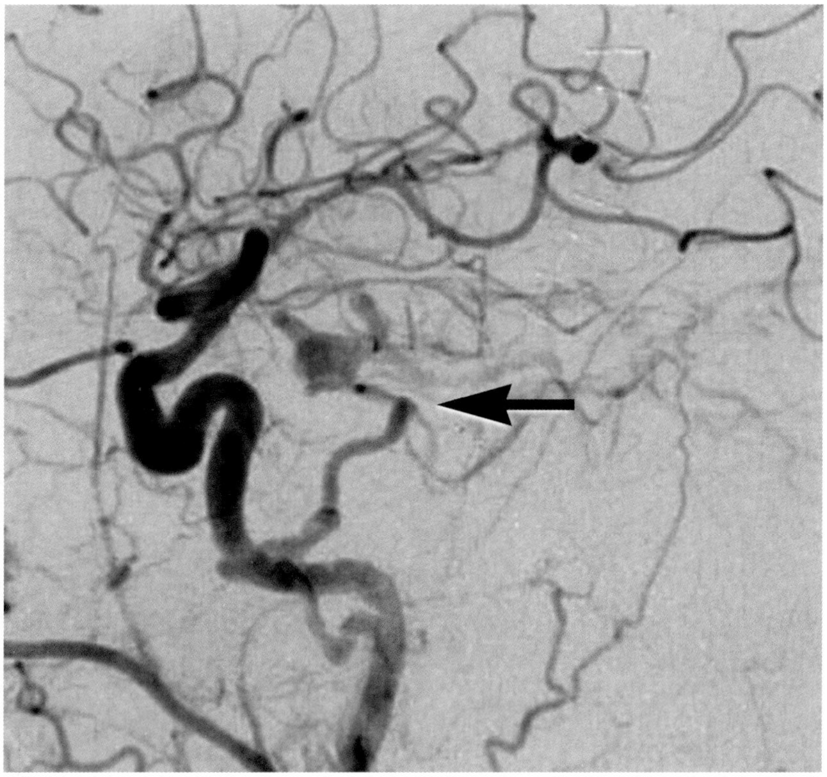

Fig. 12.3q Lateral right CCA injection demonstrates the STA-to-SCA bypass (*arrow*).

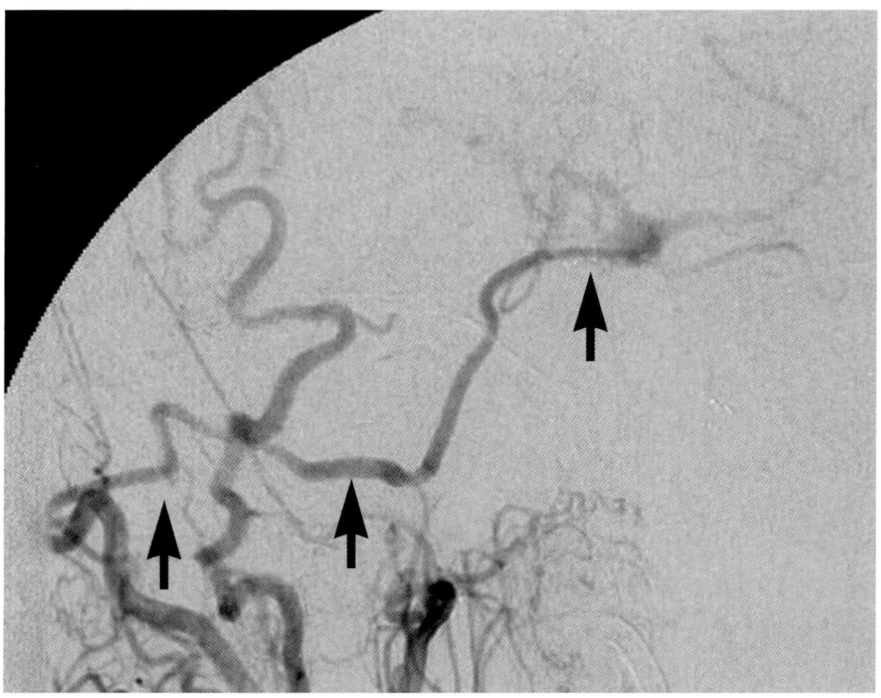

Fig. 12.3r Close-up anteroposterior angiographic view shows the STA-to-SCA bypass (*arrows*).

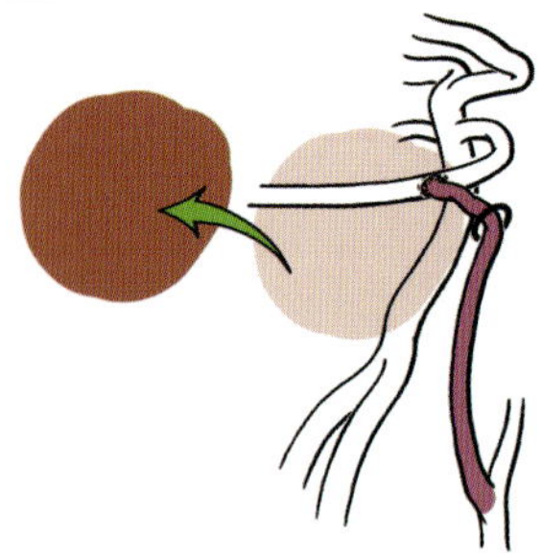

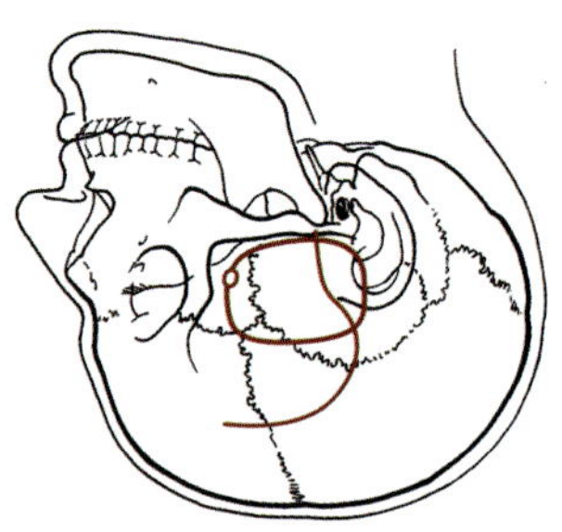

Case 12-4

Diagnosis: Giant serpentine BA trunk aneurysm

Bypass: STA-to-SCA

Approach: Staged right subtemporal, endovascular occlusion of BA and right retrolabyrinthine with aneurysmorrhaphy

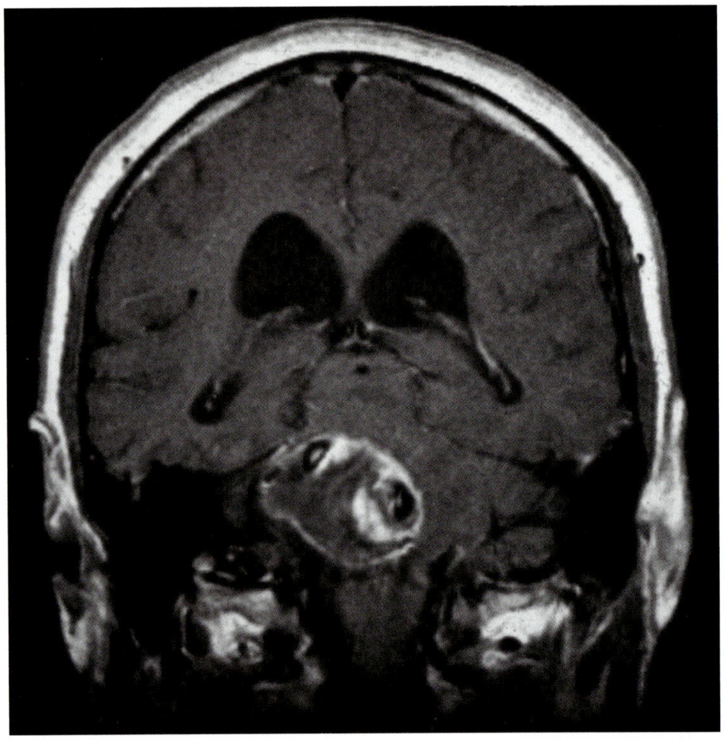

a

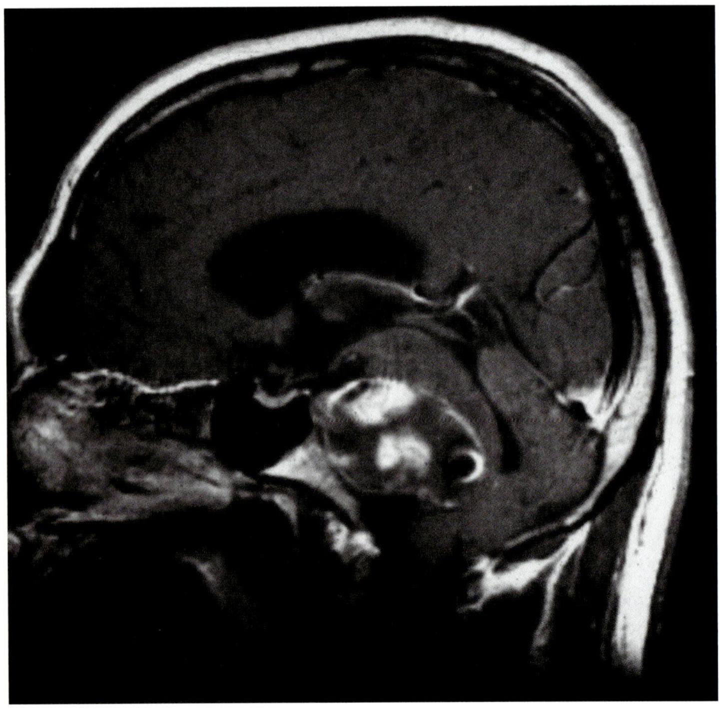

b

Fig. 12.4a, b Coronal and sagittal T1-weighted MR images of a 45-year-old man with rapidly progressive symptoms of brainstem compression show a giant BA aneurysm with flow voids.

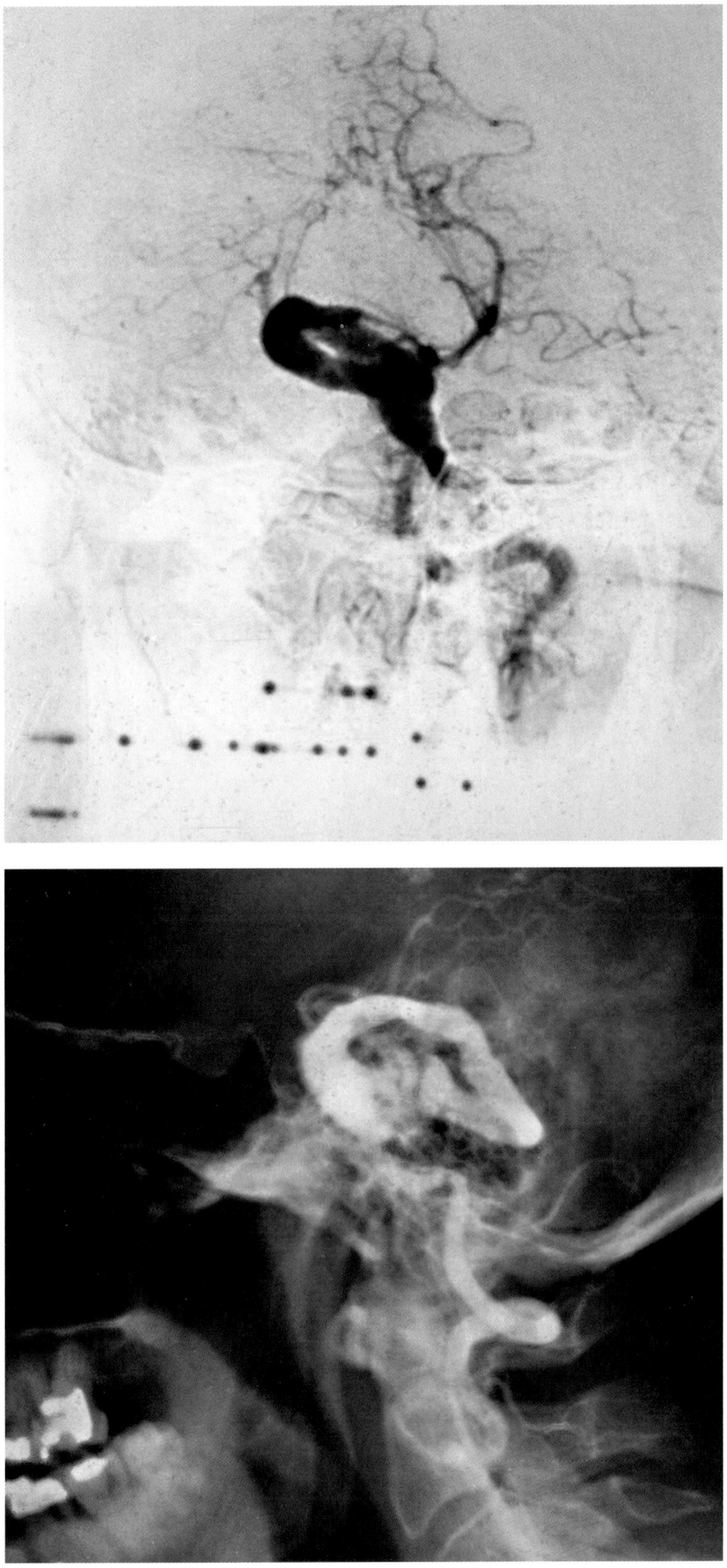

c

d

Fig. 12.4c, d Subtracted anteroposterior and unsubtracted lateral VA angiograms show the complex channel through the aneurysm that ultimately fills the circulation of the upper brainstem and distal PCA.

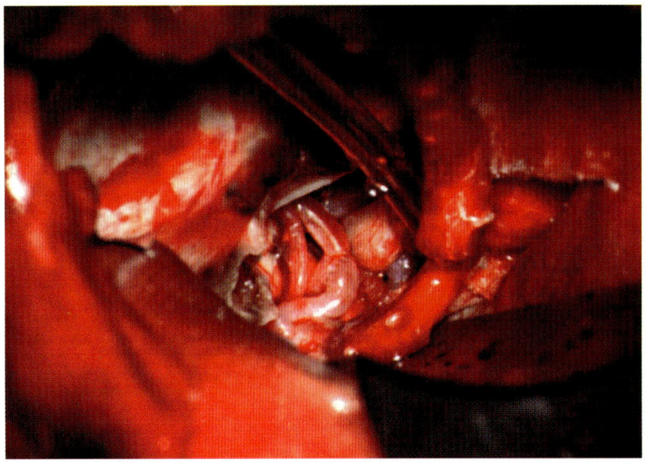

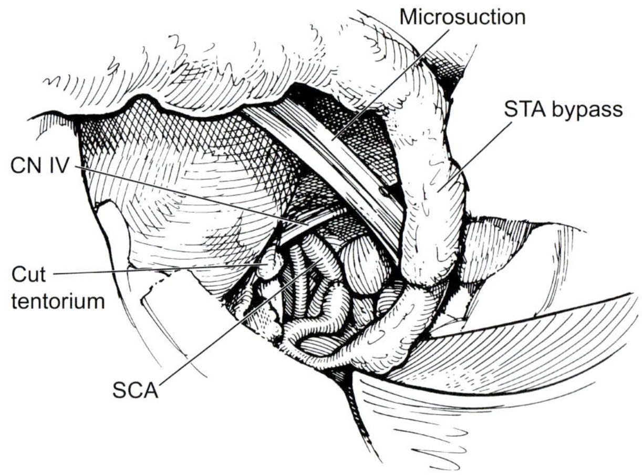

Fig. 12.4e The STA-to-SCA bypass is exposed via the subtemporal approach. The STA is long enough that the bypass will not kink when the temporal lobe reassumes its normal position.

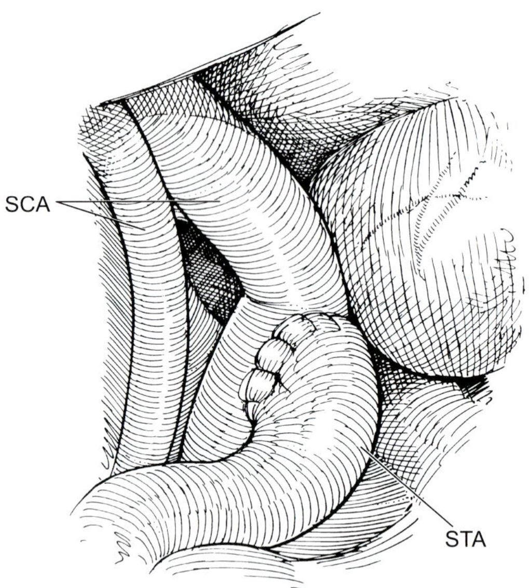

Fig. 12.4f High magnification view of the STA-to-SCA anastomosis.

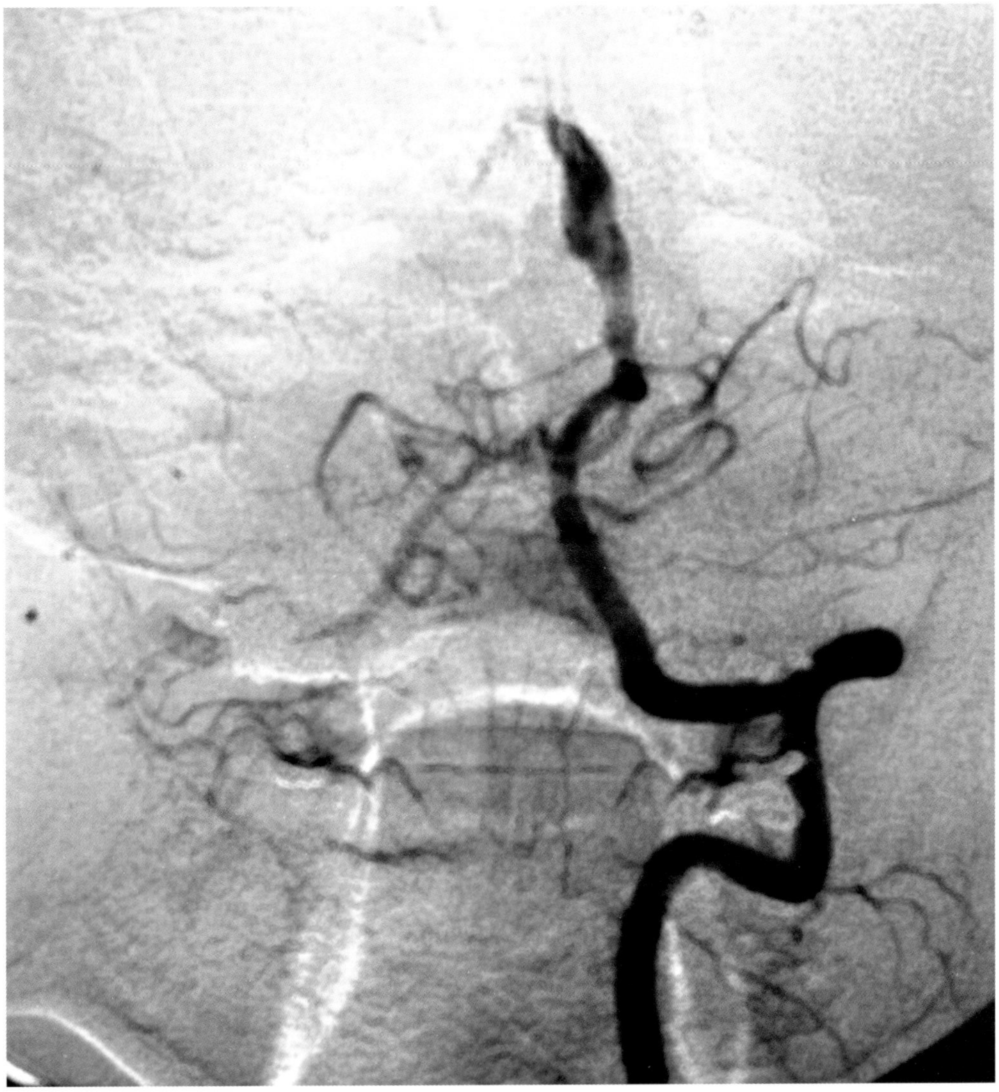

Fig. 12.4g Anteroposterior left VA angiographic injection shows that most of the serpiginous channel in the aneurysm has occluded and no longer fills the upper brainstem territory.

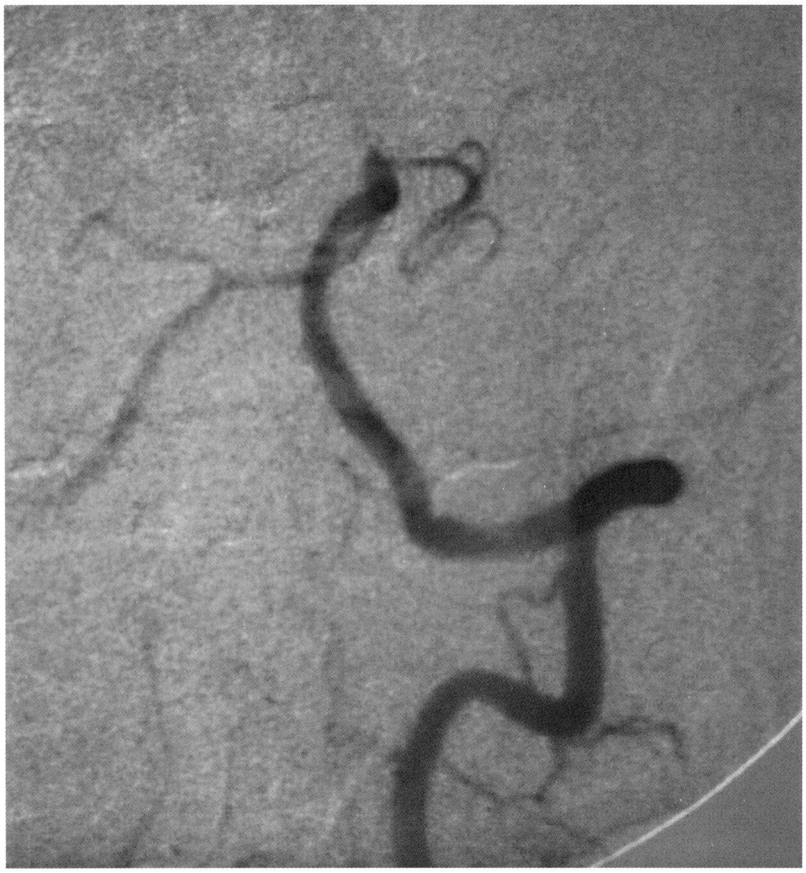

Fig. 12.4h Final VA angiogram of the endovascular occlusion of the stump of the serpentine channel demonstrates no further filling of the BA above the AICA.

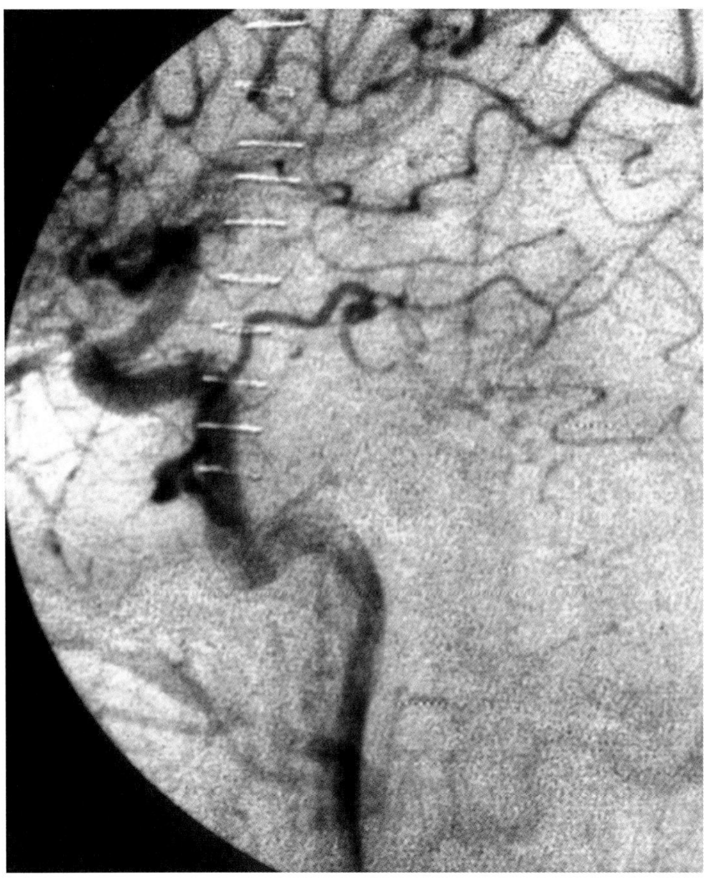

Fig. 12.4i Lateral left CCA angiogram confirms patency of the bypass.

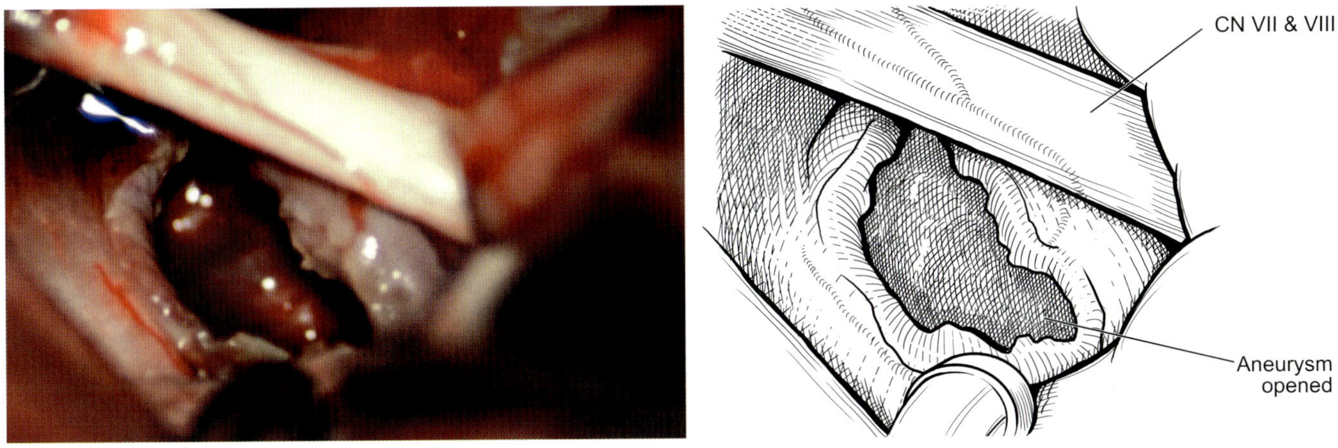

Fig. 12.4j Two weeks after bypass operation, the patient underwent debulking of the aneurysm through a right retrolabyrinthine approach. Intraoperative photograph shows the opening into the aneurysm below the CN VII and VIII complex.

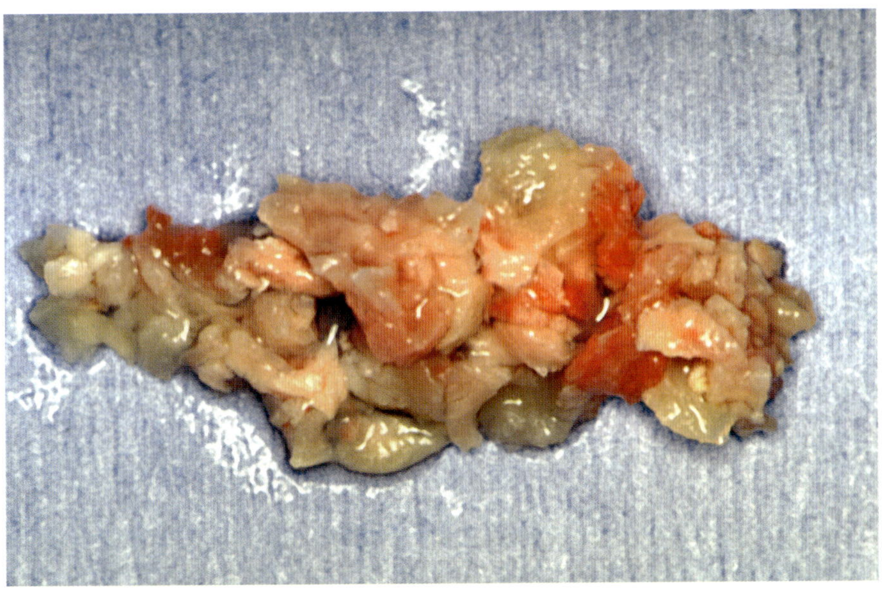

Fig. 12.4k Within the aneurysm, the chronic thrombus was highly organized. The patient has done well for more than 12 years.

13 OA Bypass

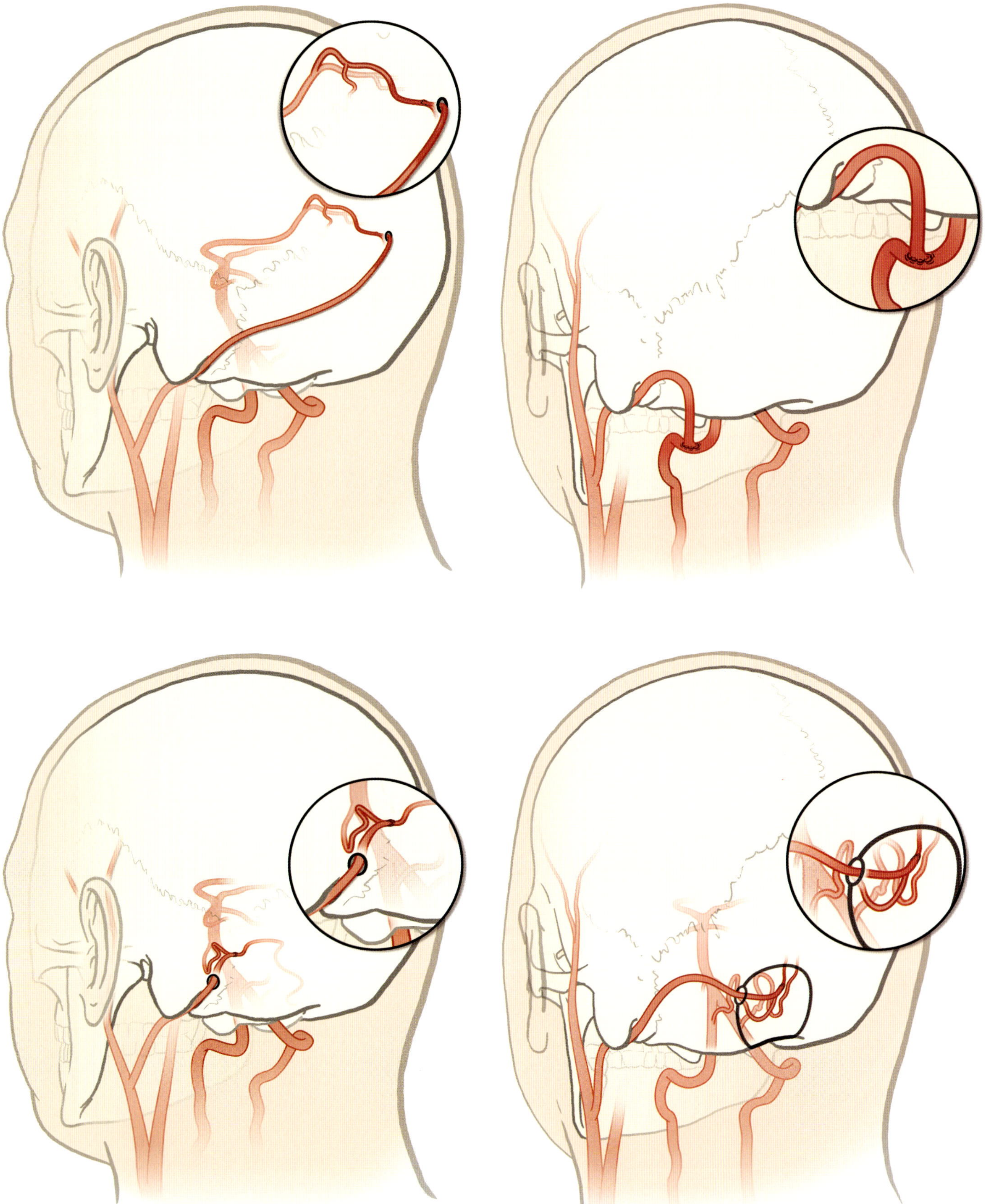

OA Bypass

The most common indication for an OA-to-PCA bypass is treatment of aneurysms involving the P2 or P3 segments. These aneurysms are often large and fusiform. The bypass only needs to support the cortical blood supply of the distal PCA. The important posterior medial and posterior lateral choroidal arteries and the direct PCA perforating vessels to the brainstem usually arise proximal to the aneurysm.

The OA–to–cortical PCA bypass is performed by making an incision directly over the OA and dissecting the artery free. Over the occipital lobe, the OA is above the neck muscles and relatively superficial. Very little inferior exposure of the OA is necessary for this bypass. The incision proceeds superiorly over the ipsilateral occipital cortex, which is exposed via an occipital craniotomy. If the patient is placed in the prone position, a lumbar drain may be useful to prevent the occipital lobe from swelling. A cortical (P4) branch of the PCA is dissected over the convexity at the edge of the occipital lobe. These branches are very small, usually less than 0.5 mm in diameter. Because the vessel is small, the anastomosis is performed in the usual manner with 11–0 suture.

The OA-to-VA bypass is used to increase blood flow to the posterior circulation.

The OA-to-AICA bypass is used to replace blood flow to the AICA itself or to treat vertebrobasilar ischemia above the origin of both PICAs. In the latter case, the PICA, if available, is preferred over the AICA as a recipient vessel. The PICA is easier to access and, in most individuals, a better match in size to the OA than the AICA.

The patient is placed in the lateral or park bench position. A hockey stick incision is made and the OA is harvested as described. A retrosigmoid craniotomy is performed at the midpoint of the sigmoid sinus. The cerebellopontine angle is opened. A distal branch over the cerebellum is freed. The OA pedicle is tunneled into the segment of the AICA just distal to the origin of branches supplying the internal auditory meatus, and the anastomosis is performed.

The OA-to-PICA bypass is a workhorse bypass for revascularizing the posterior circulation of the lower brainstem. It provides good blood flow and hypertrophies with time.

The patient is placed in the park bench position. A hockey stick incision is made behind the ear. The OA is identified and a segment of it is dissected. A craniotomy is fashioned to include the foramen magnum at the midline. Doing so usually requires extending the typical far lateral opening slightly medially.

The dura is opened and the tonsils are separated, exposing the PICA at the midline in its most superficial location. The OA is anastomosed to the PICA.

The OA is the most posterior of the eight branches of the ECA. It is a robust artery that passes through the neck and underneath the SCM and splenius capitis muscles to feed the scalp.

The OA is harvested by locating the artery posterior and medial to the mastoid process. The artery's course is traced using a handheld Doppler probe. The artery can be dissected by incising directly over it or by raising a large flap and cutting the artery from underneath. In either case, the OA is much more difficult to free from the surrounding tissue than the STA. Blunt and sharp scissors are used to dissect the OA from the muscular tissue to which it is densely adherent. Frequent muscular branches must be coagulated and divided. Distally, the OA courses with the occipital nerve in a shared fascial sheath.

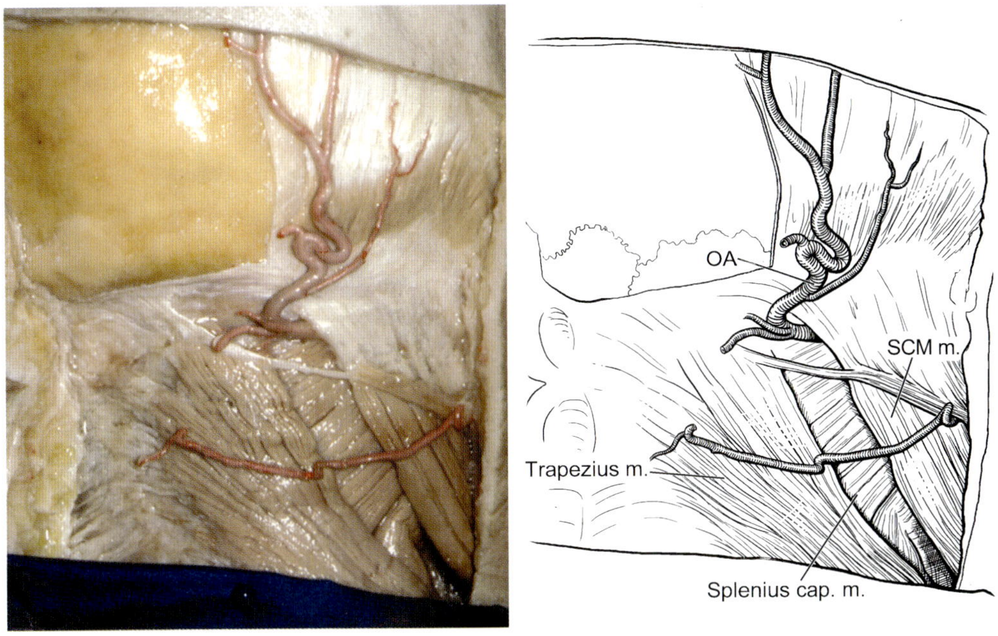

Fig. 13.0a The OA has been dissected out as it emerges from around the mastoid tip. (Photograph used with permission from *Journal of Neurosurgery*.)

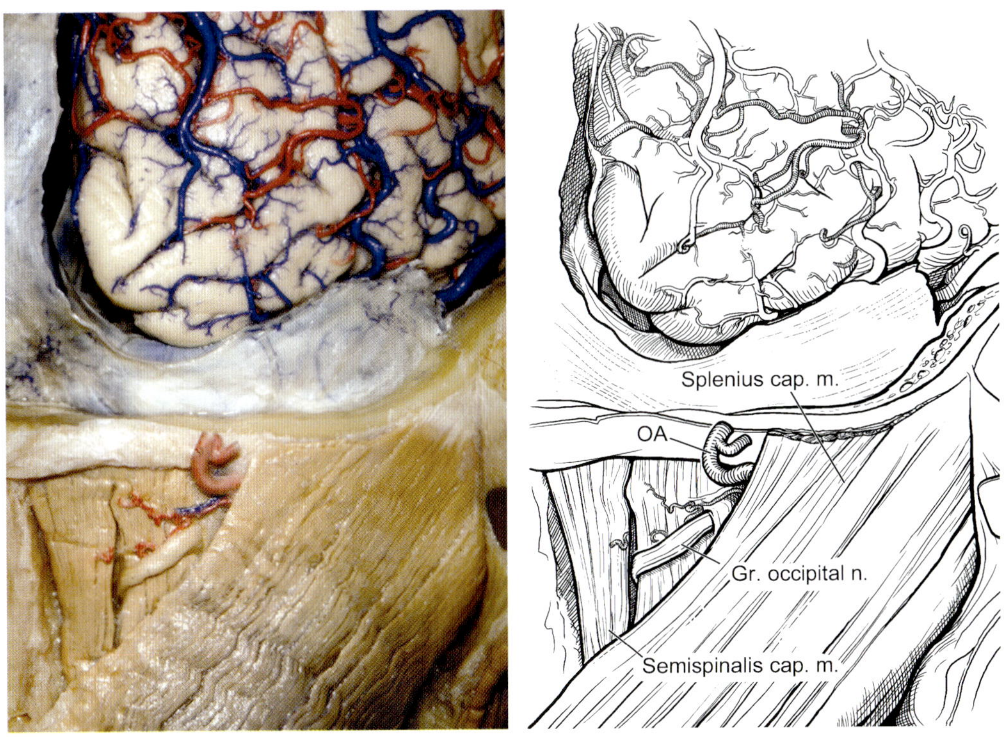

Fig. 13.0b The occipital lobe has been exposed. (Photograph used with permission from *Journal of Neurosurgery*.)

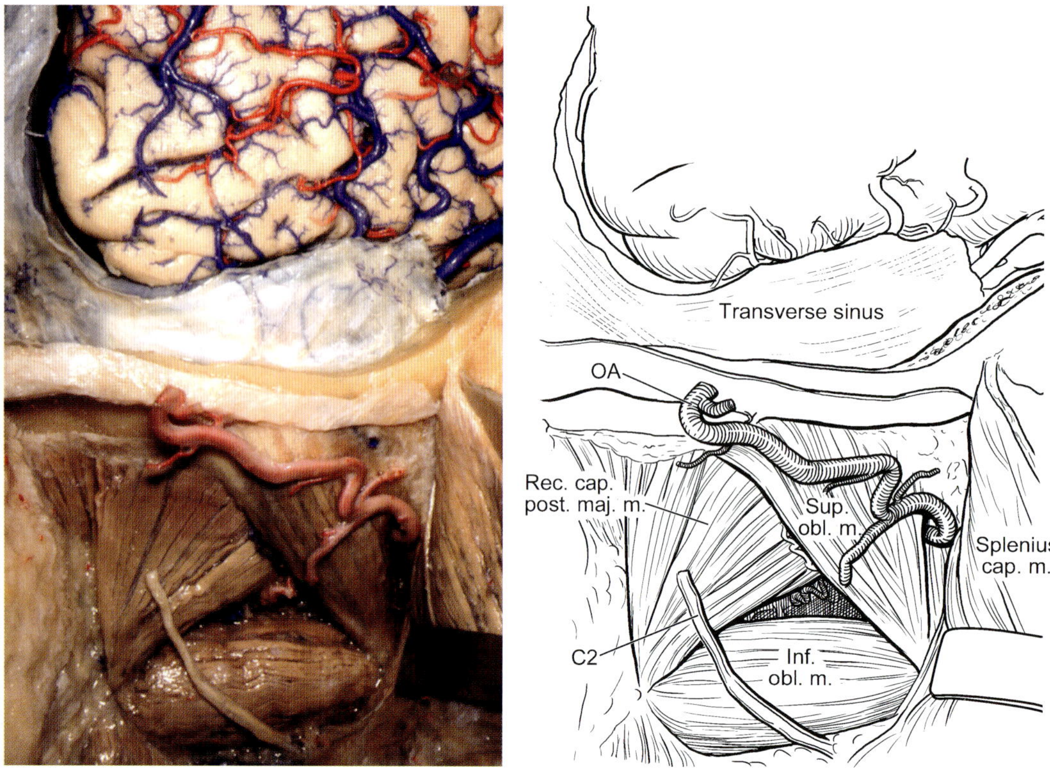

Fig. 13.0c Further dissection of the OA has been performed. (Photograph used with permission from *Journal of Neurosurgery*.)

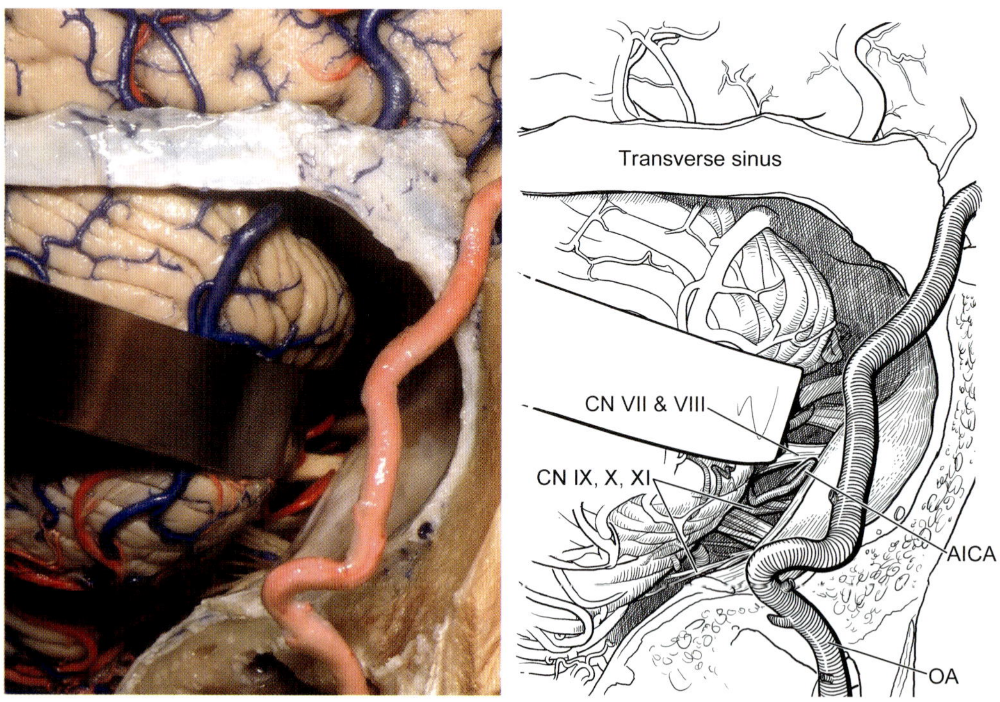

Fig. 13.0d The right posterior fossa and cerebellopontine angle are shown from a right retrosigmoid view. The right OA has been dissected free. (Photograph used with permission from *Journal of Neurosurgery*.)

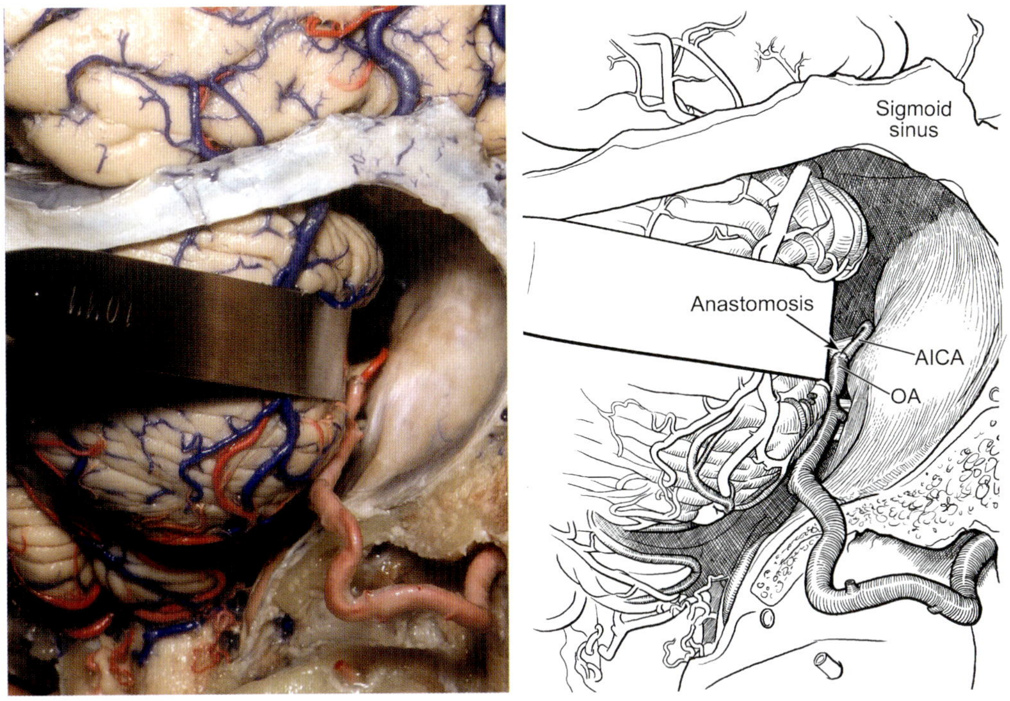

Fig. 13.0e The OA is introduced into the cerebellopontine angle to join the AICA distal to any branches that might contribute to the internal auditory canal. (Photograph used with permission from *Journal of Neurosurgery*.)

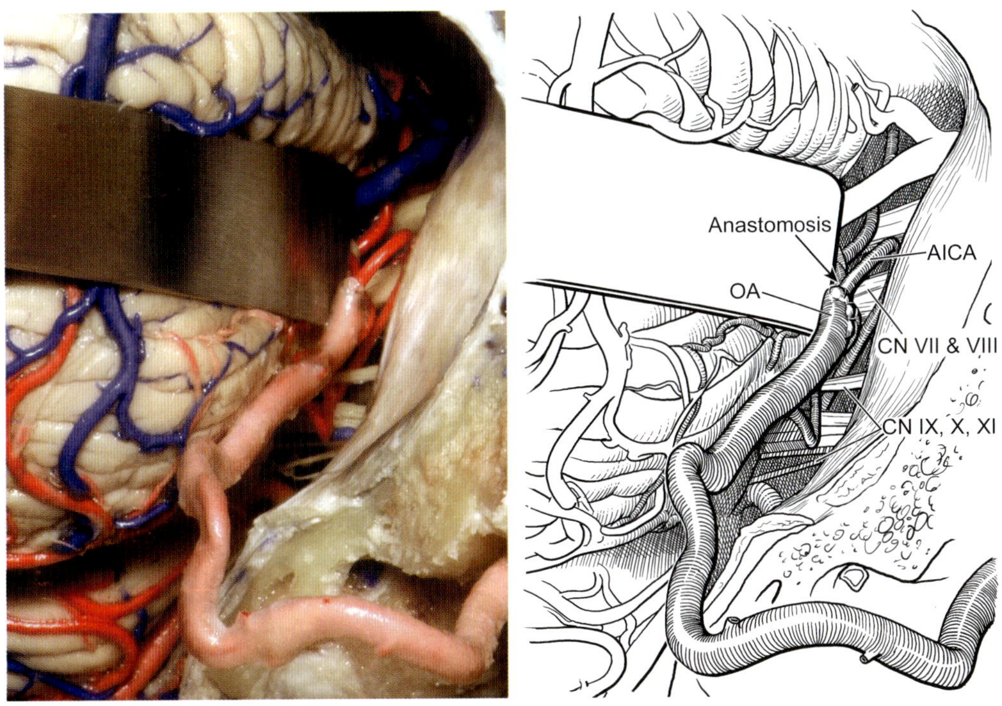

Fig. 13.0f Magnified view shows the lower cranial nerves. The bypass is sutured posterior to the nerves in the narrow corridor between the petrous bone and the cerebellar hemisphere. (Photograph used with permission from *Journal of Neurosurgery*.)

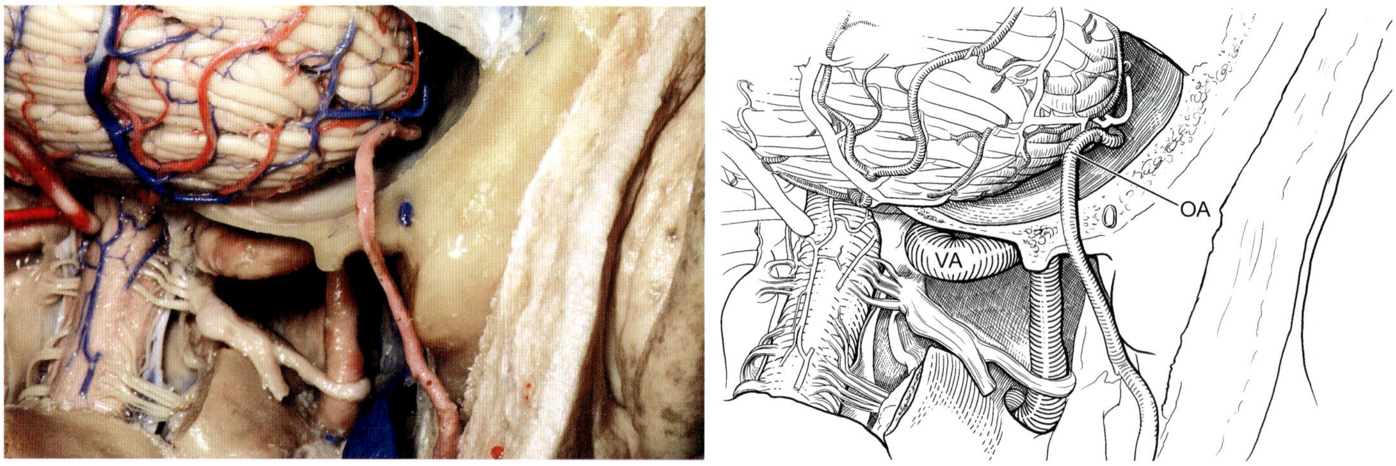

Fig. 13.0g An overview of the OA-to-AICA bypass. (Photograph used with permission from *Journal of Neurosurgery*.)

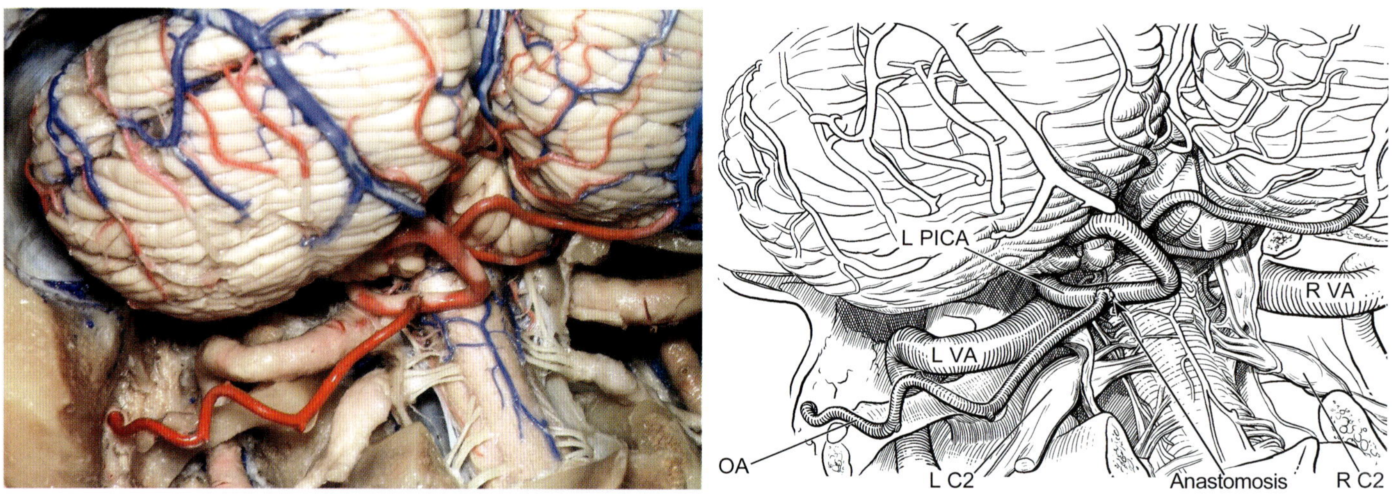

Fig. 13.0h OA-to-PICA bypass in a cadaver. (Photograph used with permission from *Journal of Neurosurgery*.)

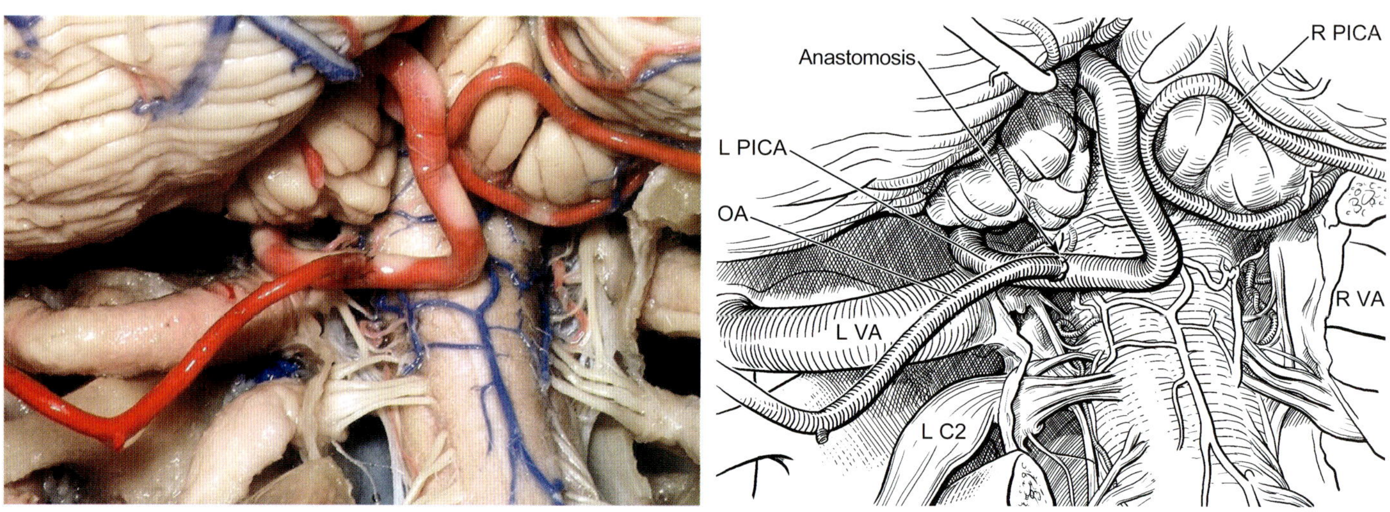

Fig. 13.0i High magnification view of the OA-to-PICA bypass. (Photograph used with permission from *Journal of Neurosurgery*.)

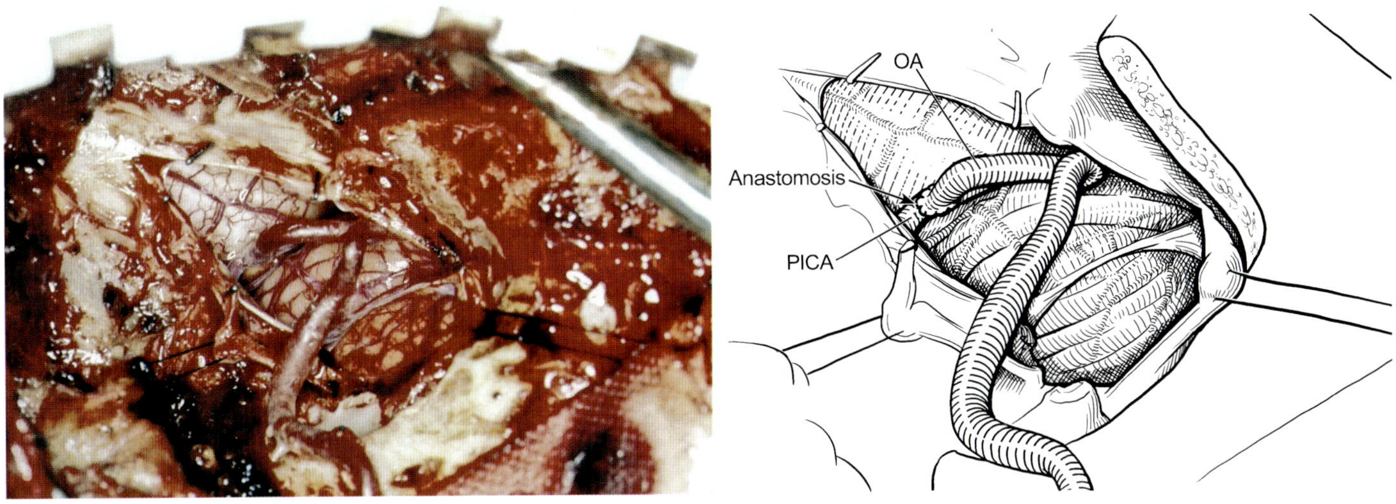

Fig. 13.0j Example of OA-to-PICA bypass.

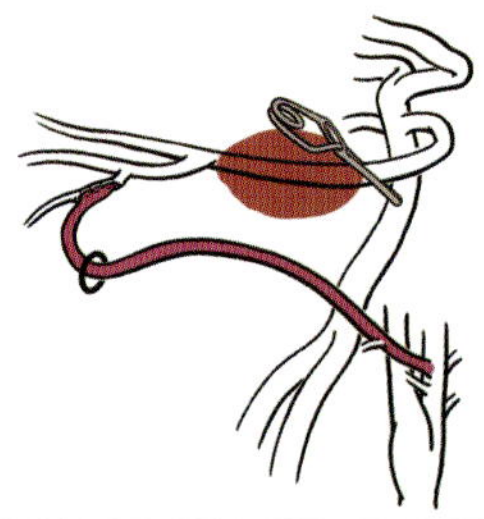

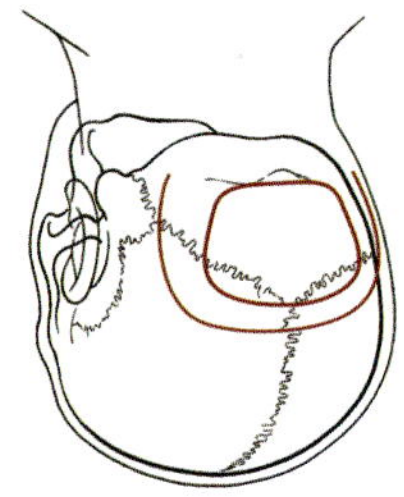

Case 13-1

Diagnosis: Giant fusiform left P2-P3 junction aneurysm

Bypass: OA-to-PCA

Approach: Bilateral occipital

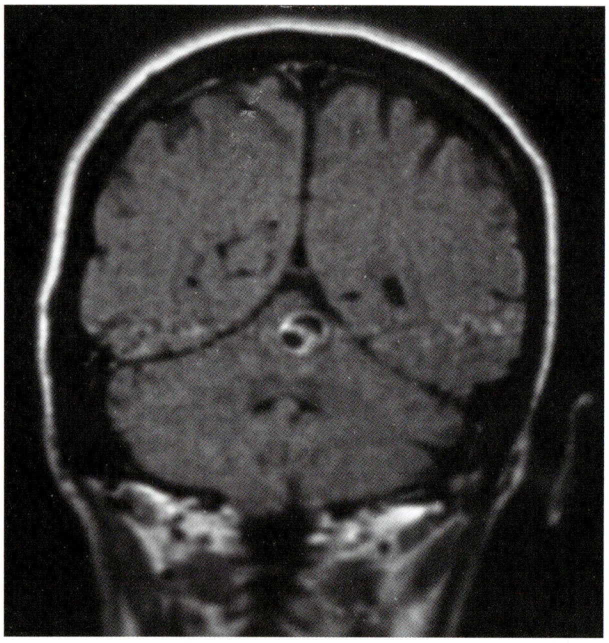

Fig. 13.1a Coronal T1-weighted MR image of a patient with headaches shows a distal PCA aneurysm.

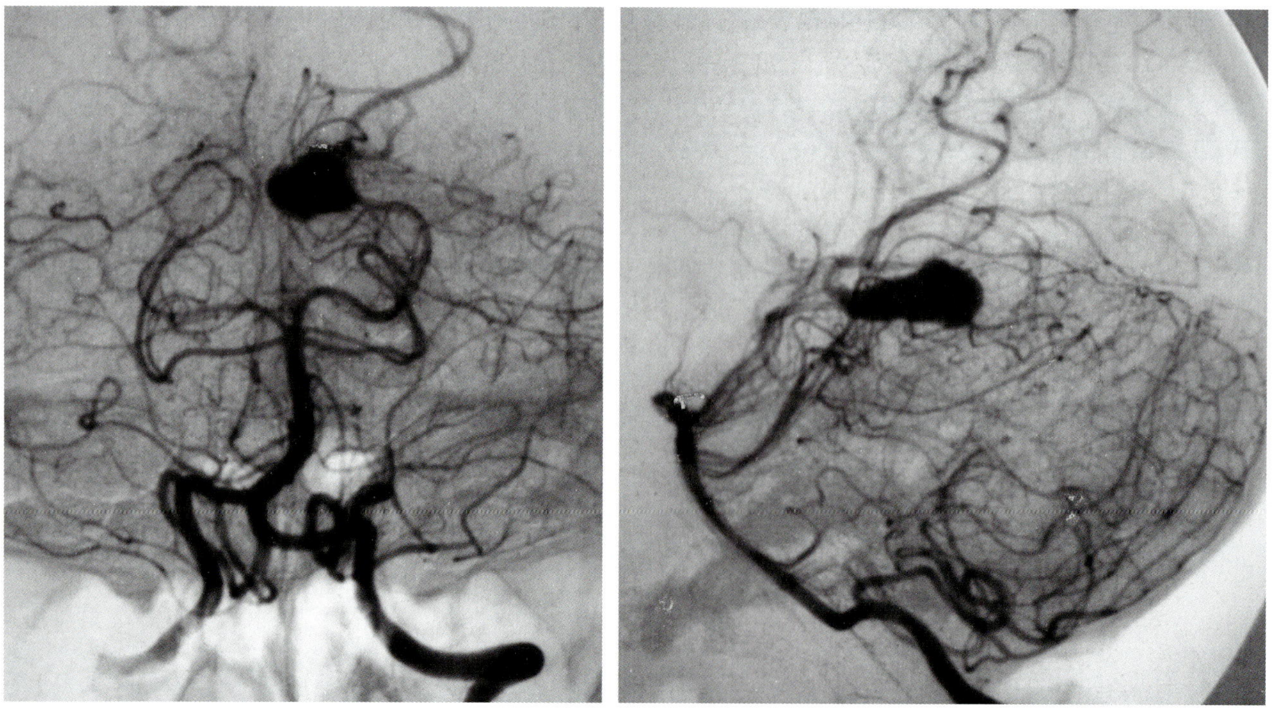

b

c

Fig. 13.1b, c Anteroposterior and lateral left VA angiograms show a giant fusiform aneurysm at the left P2-P3 junction.

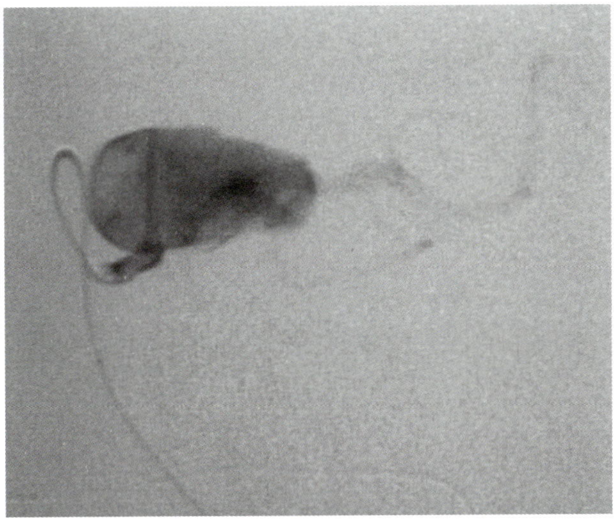

Fig. 13.1d Magnified superselective left PCA angiogram confirms the fusiform anatomy of the aneurysm.

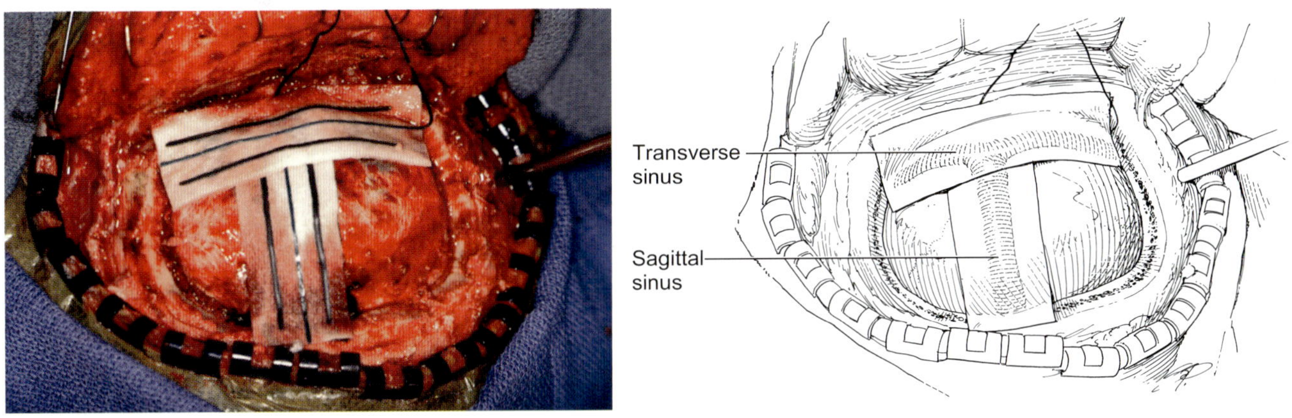

Fig. 13.1e A large U-shaped flap on the posterior fossa exposes the torcular, superior sagittal sinus, and transverse sinuses, which are all covered by Cottonoids (Codman, Raynham, MA).

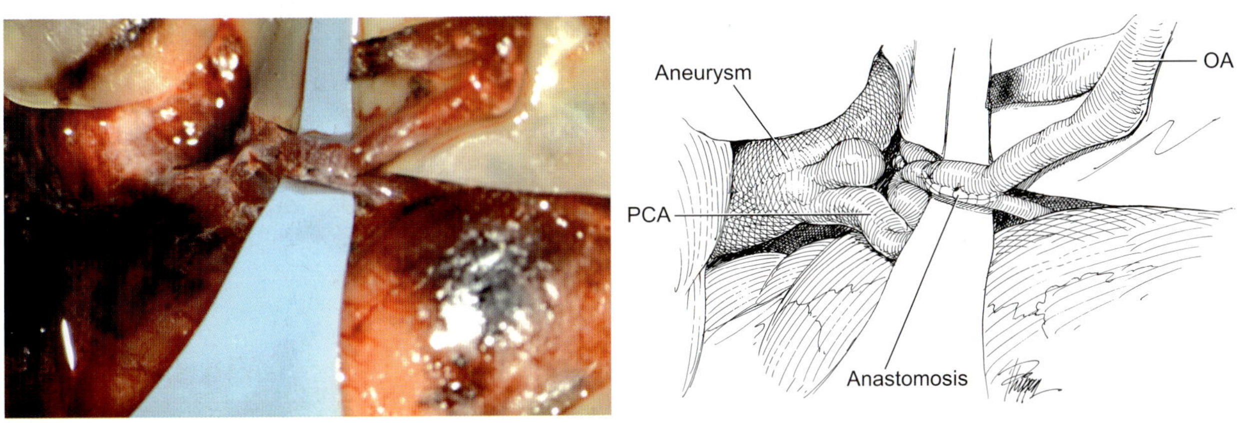

Fig. 13.1f A tiny cortical branch of the left PCA is isolated and an OA-to-PCA bypass is performed with 11–0 nylon sutures.

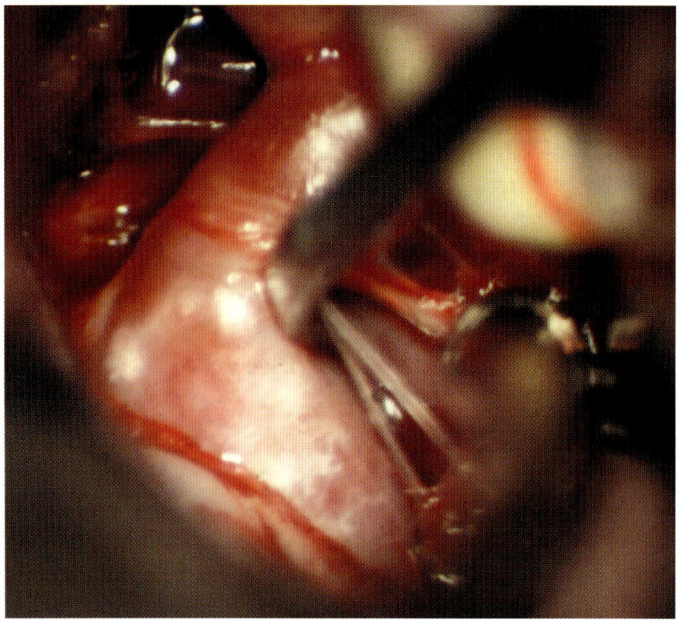

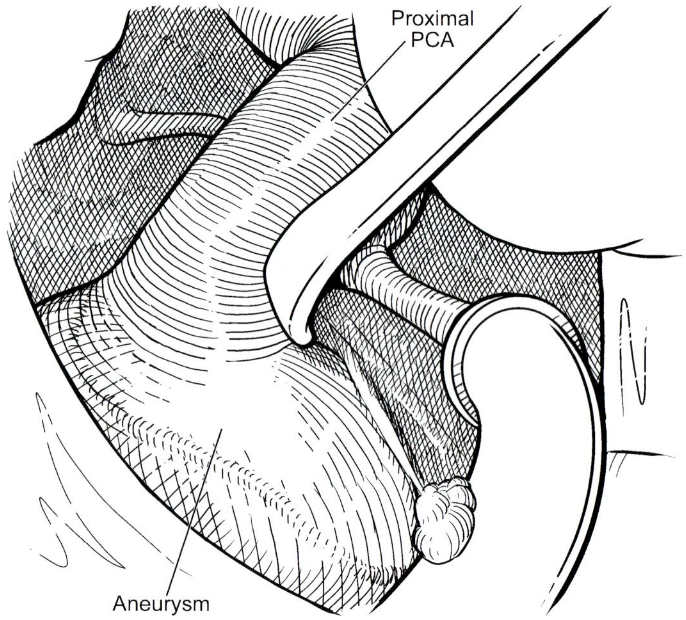

Fig. 13.1g The aneurysm is inspected and the PCA is clipped proximal to the aneurysm. Endovascular sacrifice of the parent vessel is also an option.

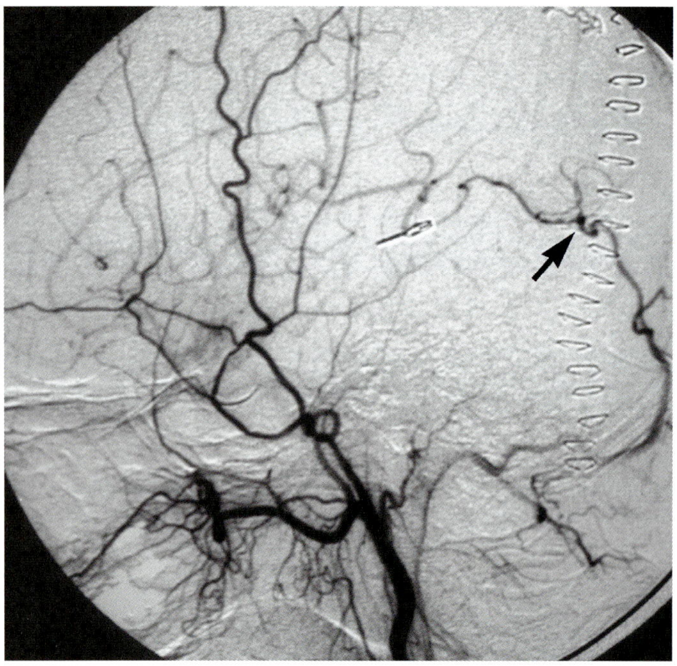

Fig. 13.1h Lateral left ECA angiogram shows the OA-to-PCA bypass (*arrow*) filling the distribution of the PCA.

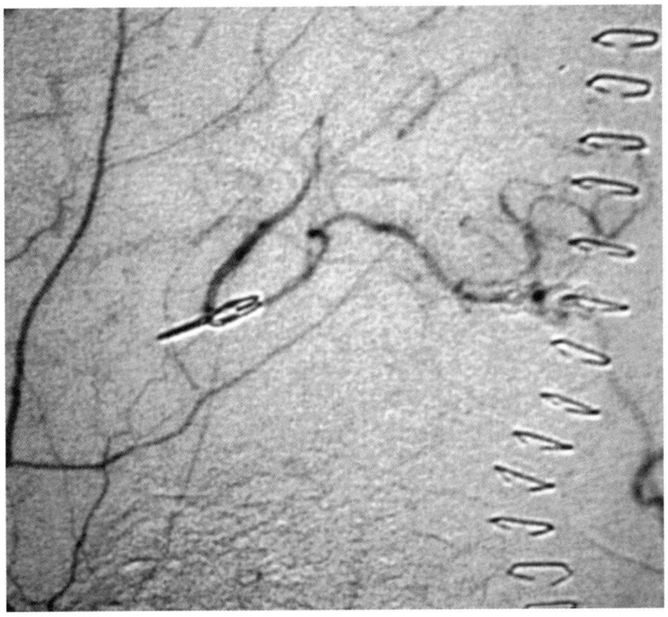

Fig. 13.1i Magnified angiographic view shows backfilling as far as the aneurysm clip.

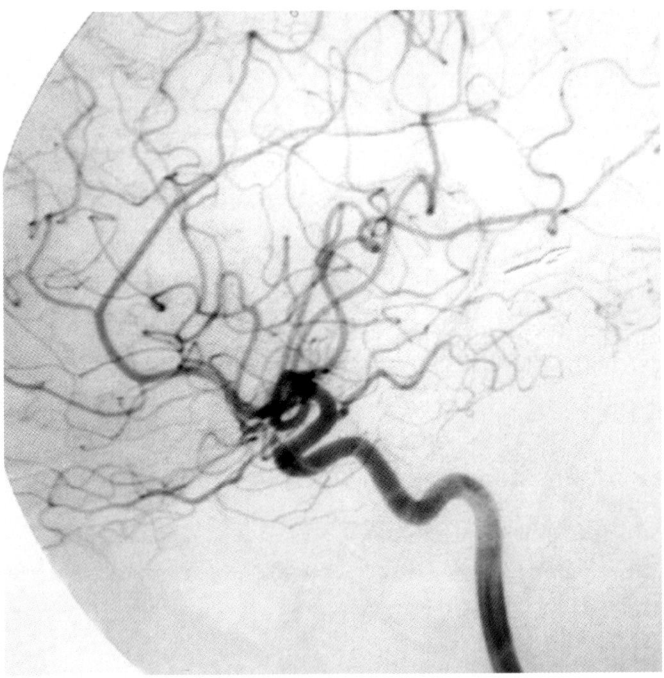

Fig. 13.1j Left ICA angiogram shows occlusion of the aneurysm and the clip on the PCA.

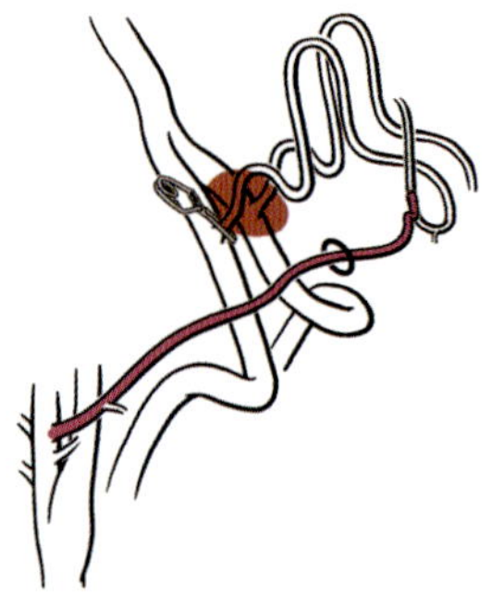

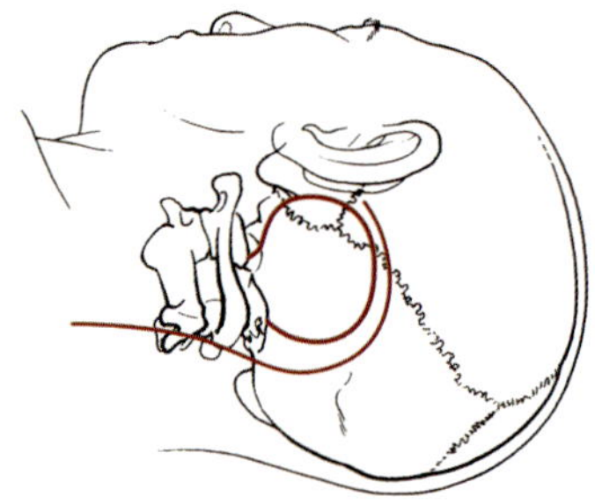

Case 13-2

Diagnosis: Complex, previously coiled left PICA aneurysm

Bypass: OA-to-PICA

Approach: Left far lateral

Video

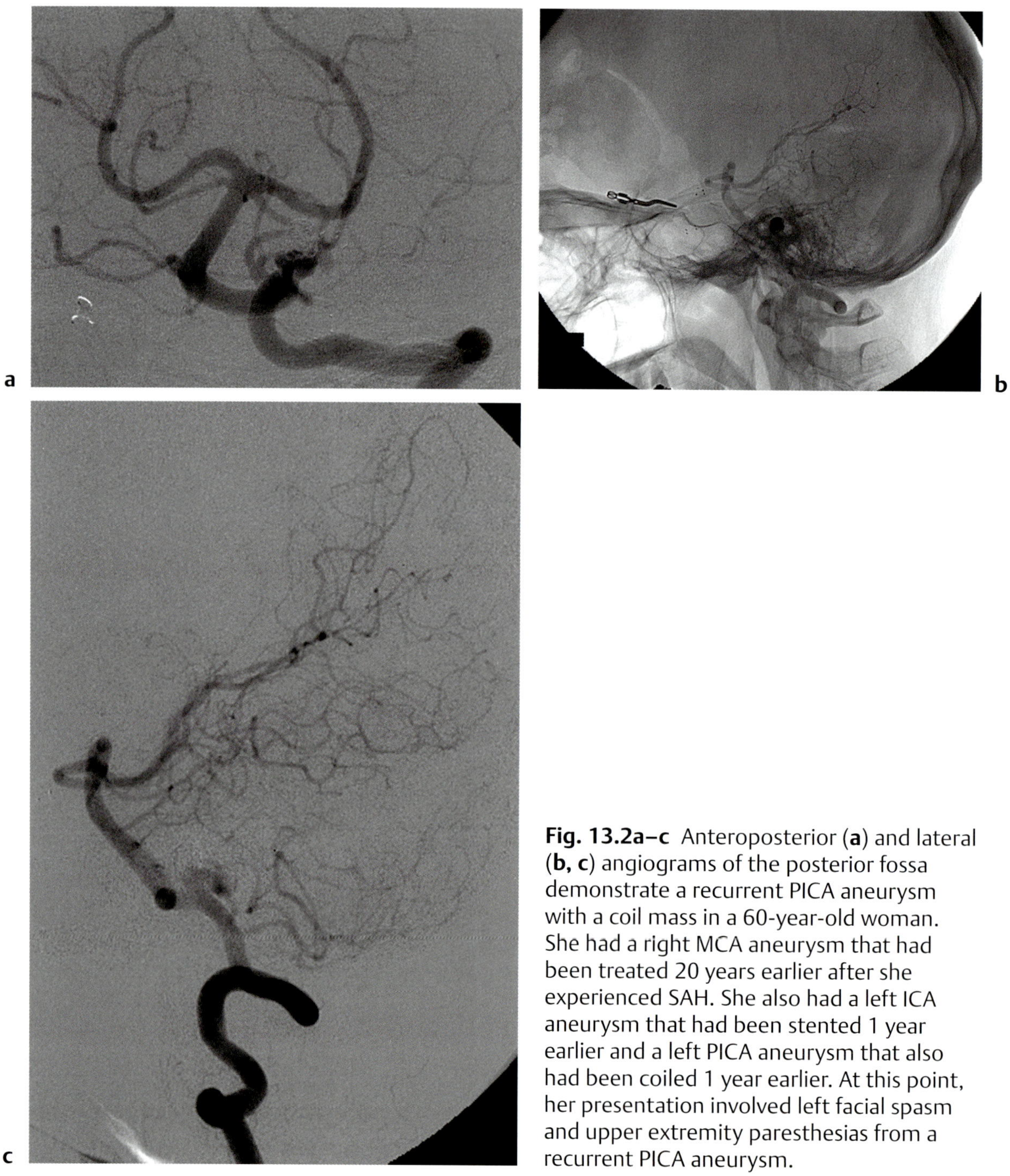

Fig. 13.2a–c Anteroposterior (**a**) and lateral (**b, c**) angiograms of the posterior fossa demonstrate a recurrent PICA aneurysm with a coil mass in a 60-year-old woman. She had a right MCA aneurysm that had been treated 20 years earlier after she experienced SAH. She also had a left ICA aneurysm that had been stented 1 year earlier and a left PICA aneurysm that also had been coiled 1 year earlier. At this point, her presentation involved left facial spasm and upper extremity paresthesias from a recurrent PICA aneurysm.

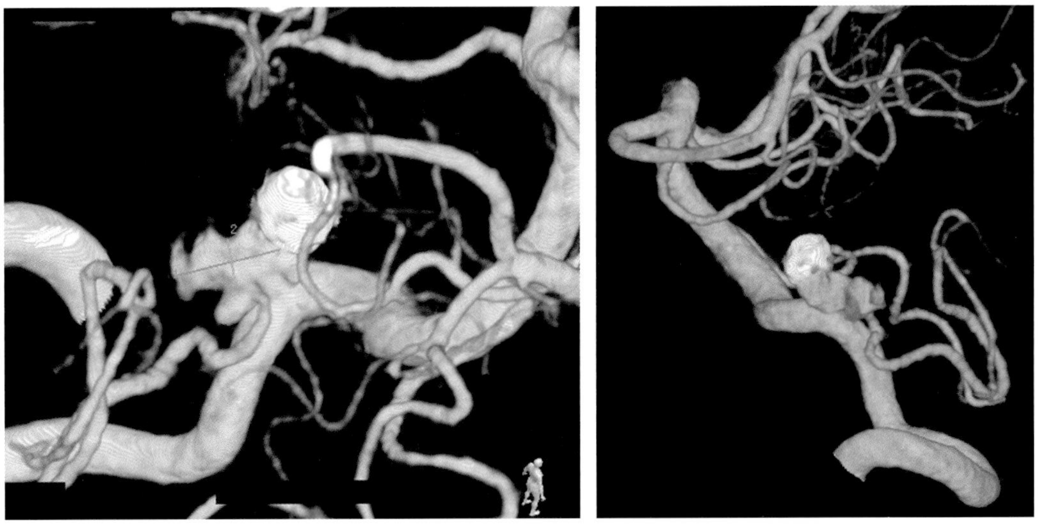

d e

Fig. 13.2d, e Three-dimensional CT reconstructions show the coil mass and the left PICA emerging from the base of the heavily calcified aneurysm.

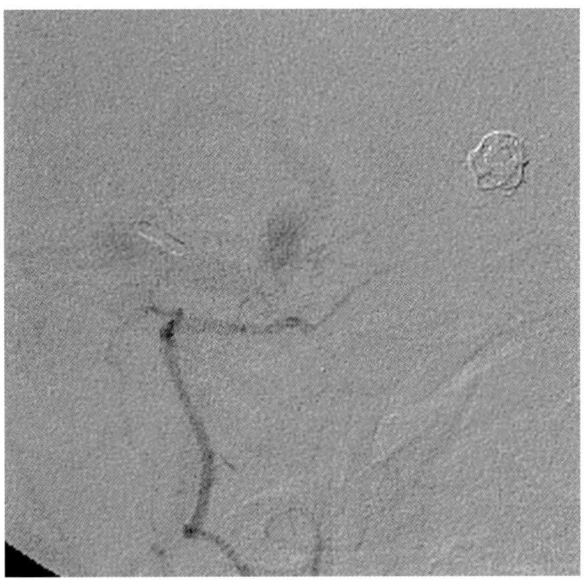

Fig. 13.2f Right lateral VA angiogram demonstrates that the right VA is vestigial and terminates in PICA.

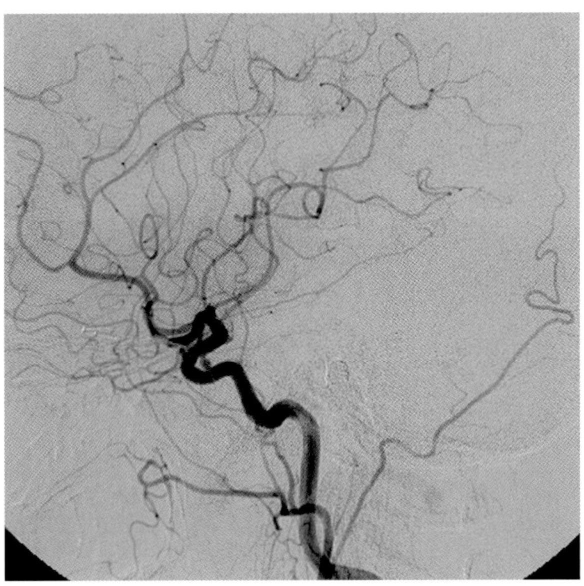

Fig. 13.2g Lateral CCA angiogram performed during an Alcock test shows no PCoA. The right injection also failed to reveal a PCA. Therefore, the left VA with the PICA aneurysm was the sole supply to the posterior fossa.

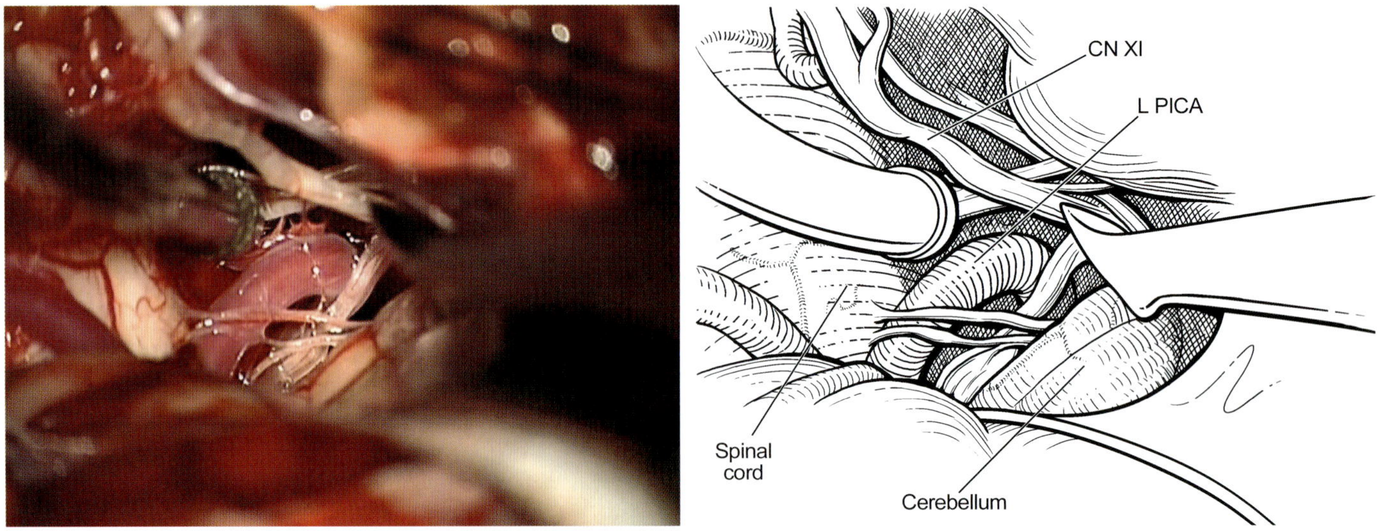

Fig. 13.2h Through a left far lateral approach, the left PICA is visible.

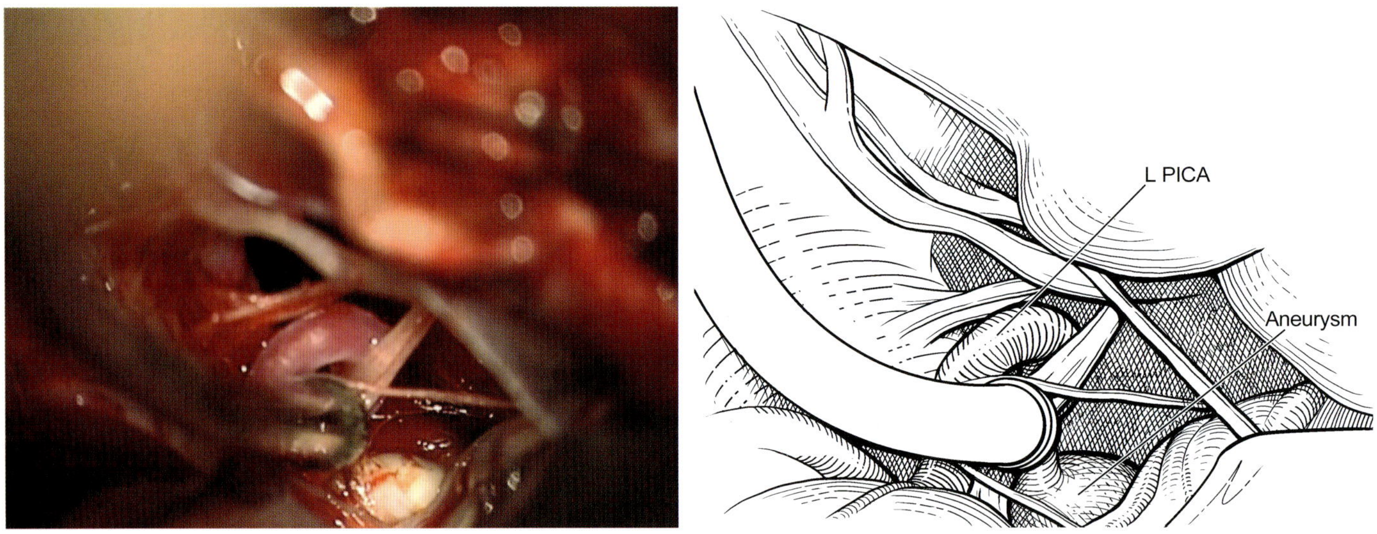

Fig. 13.2i After further dissection the calcified aneurysm is visible.

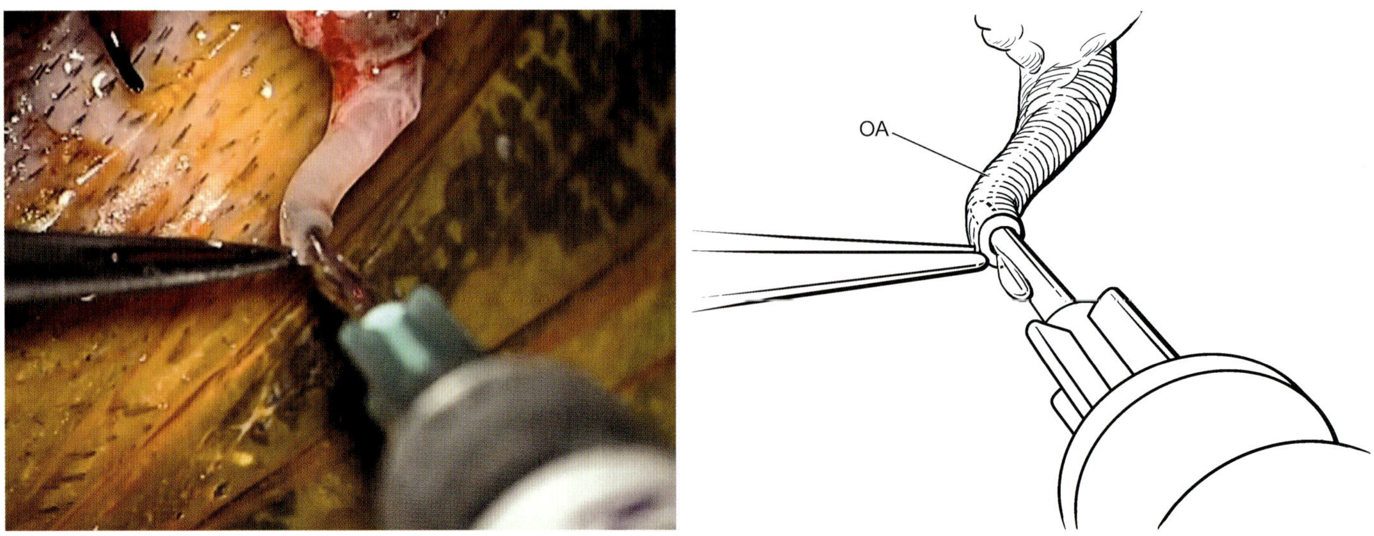

Fig. 13.2j The OA has been dissected from its bed in preparation for the bypass.

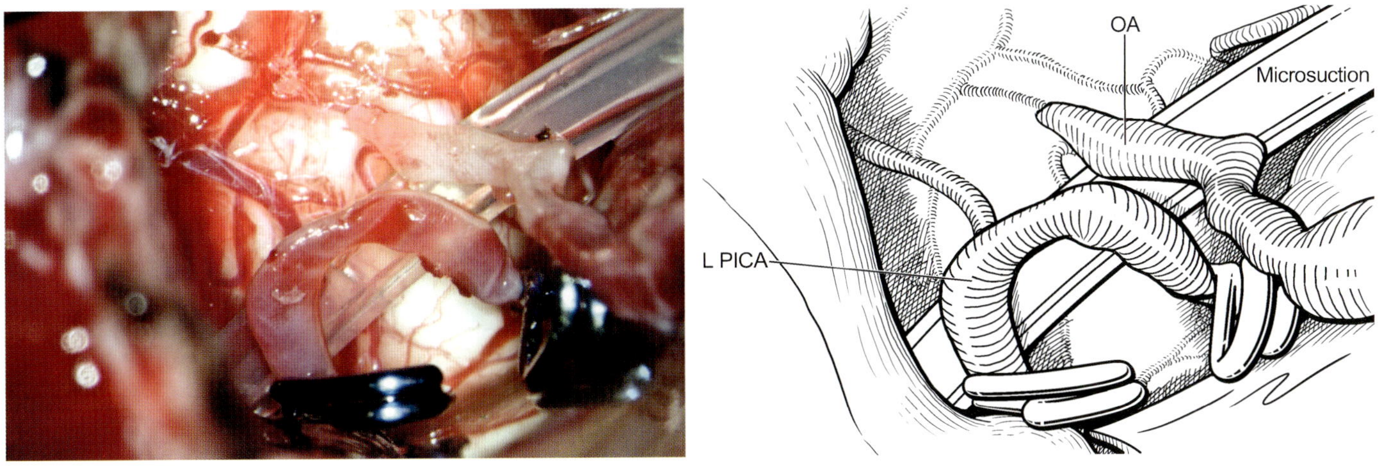

Fig. 13.2k Temporary clips are placed on the loop of the PICA distal to the aneurysm. A microsuction device is underneath the PICA and the obliquely cut OA has been placed in the surgical field.

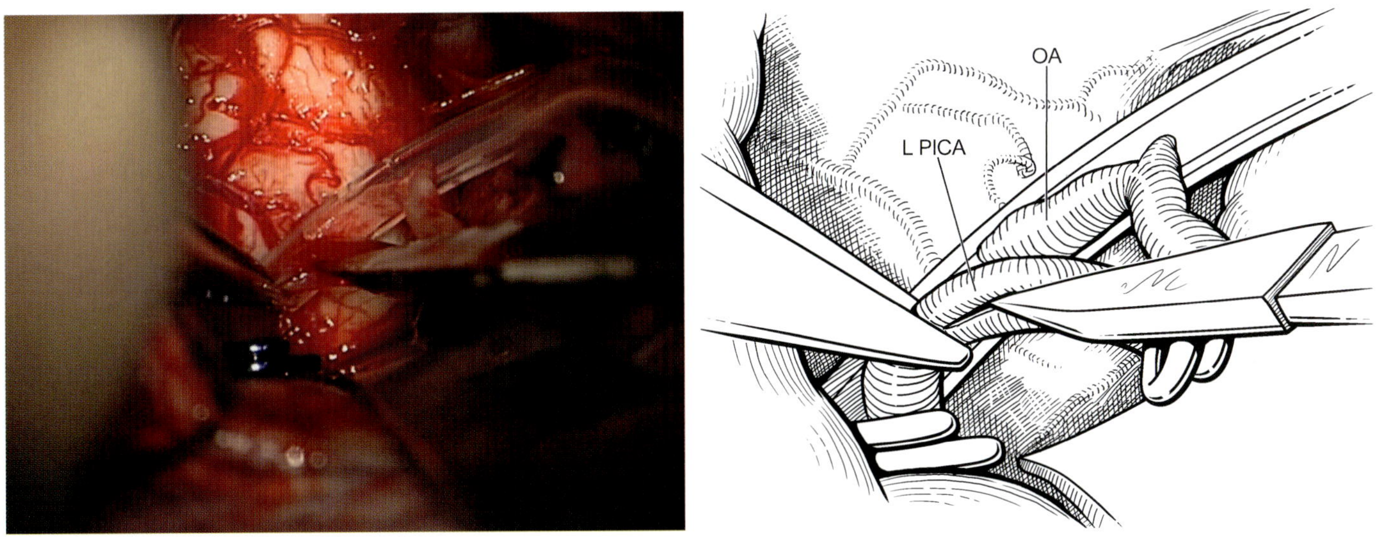

Fig. 13.2l The PICA is opened.

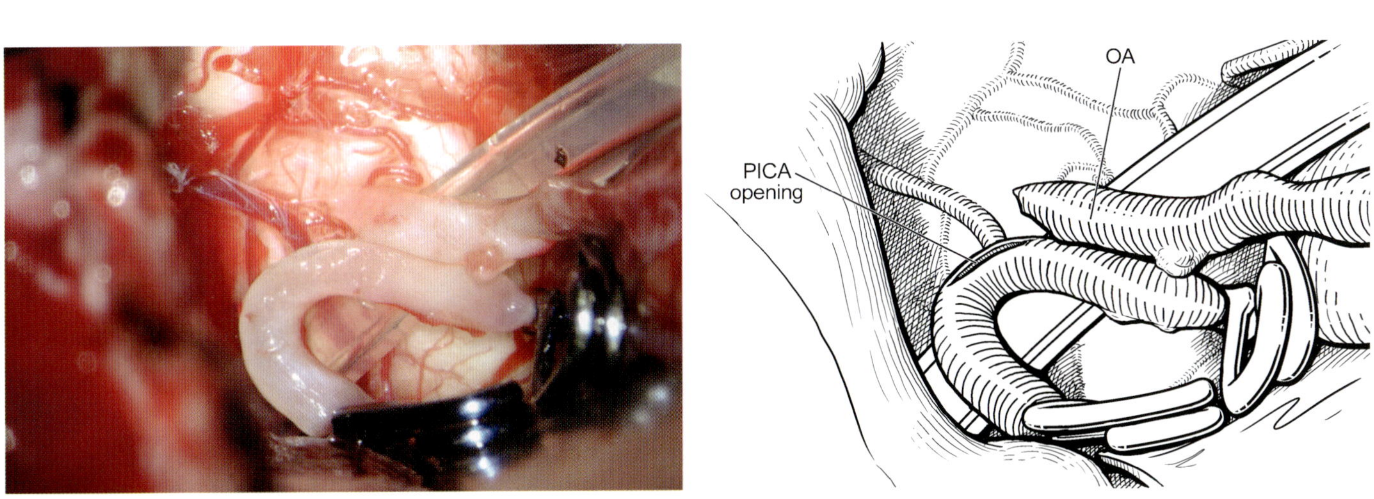

Fig. 13.2m The obliquely cut OA has been placed next to the PICA in preparation for the bypass.

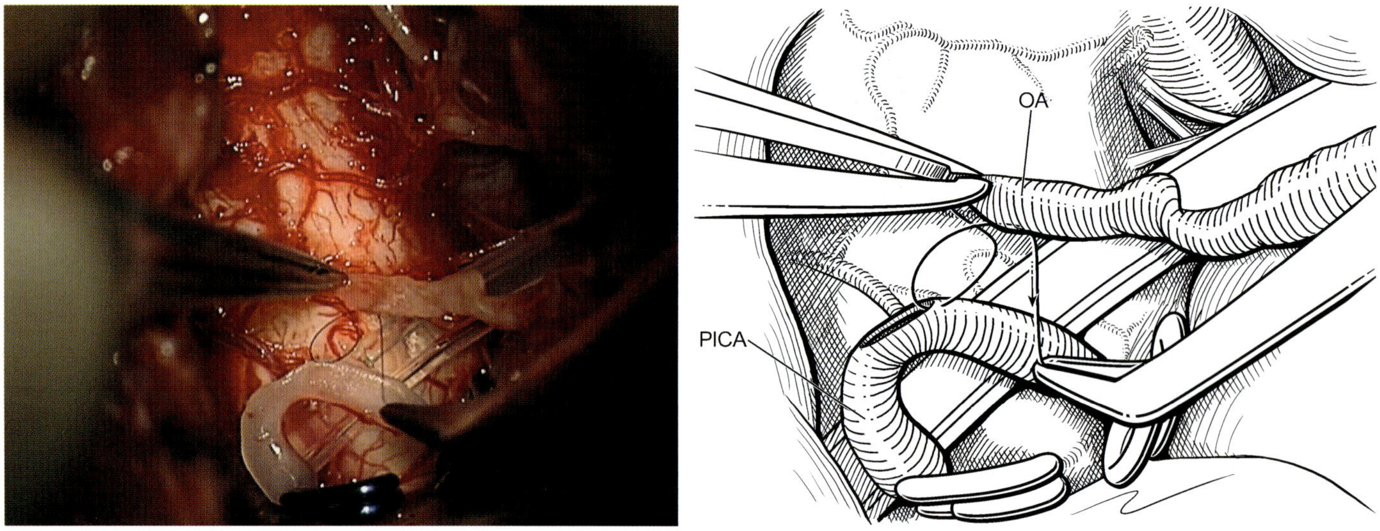

Fig. 13.2n The heel stitch is placed in the OA.

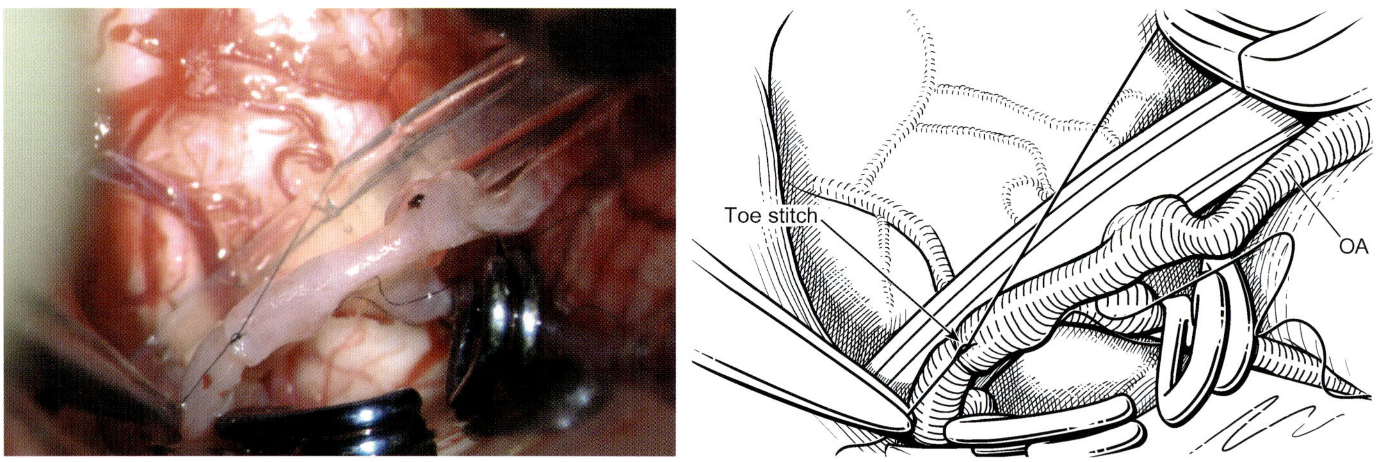

Fig. 13.2o The toe and heel stitches have been completed.

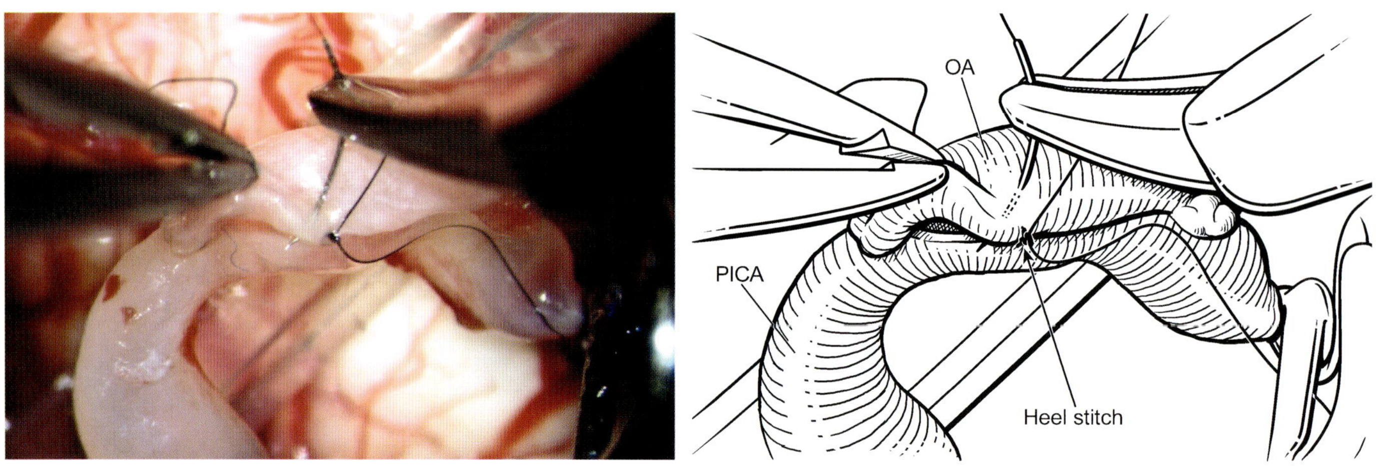

Fig. 13.2p A running stitch is performed.

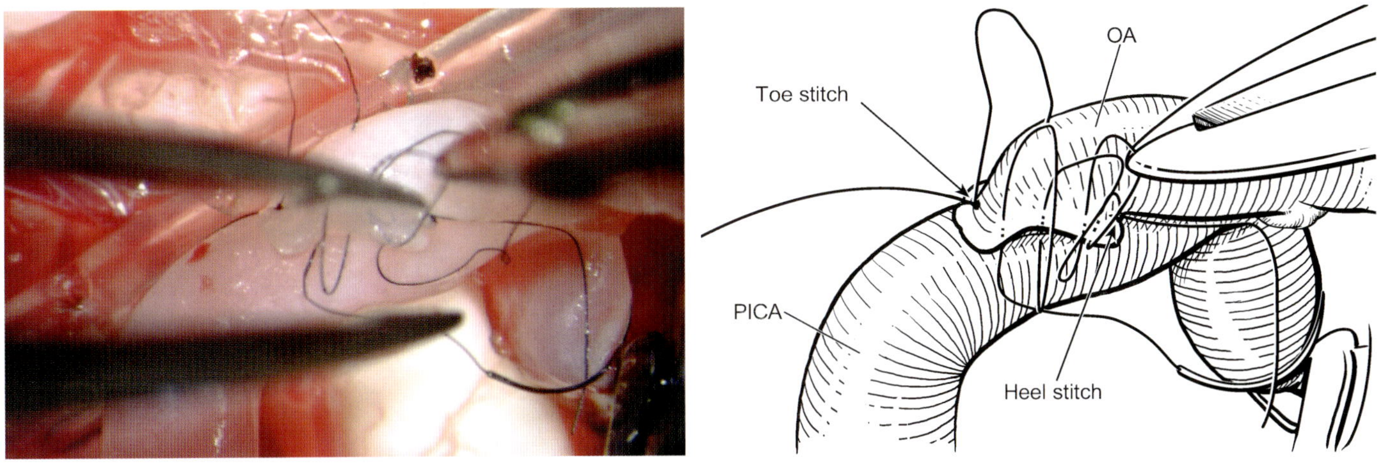

Fig. 13.2q The loops of the suture are straightened.

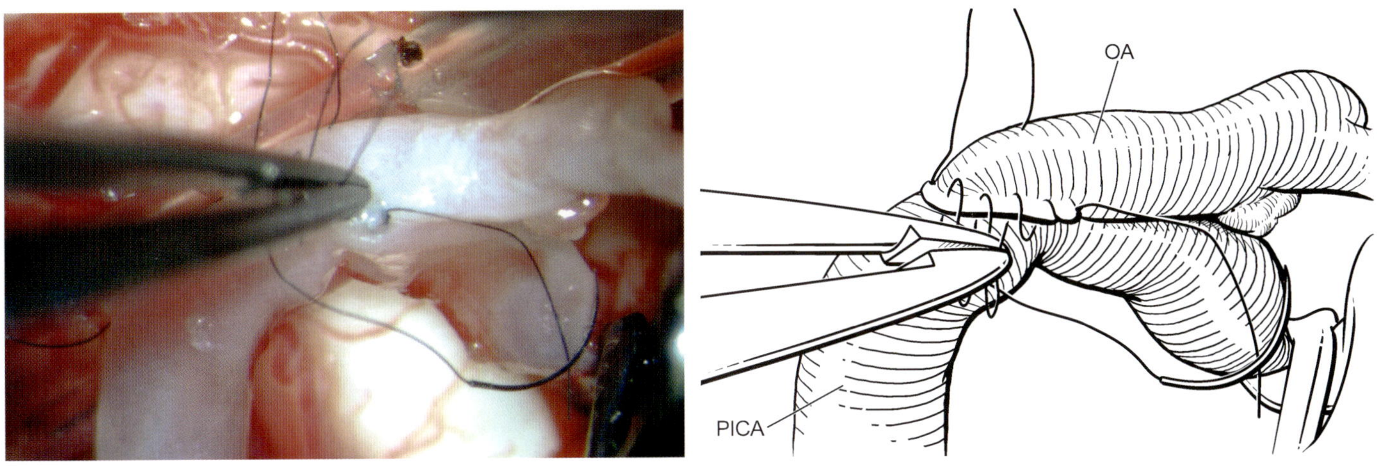

Fig. 13.2r The line of sutures is tightened.

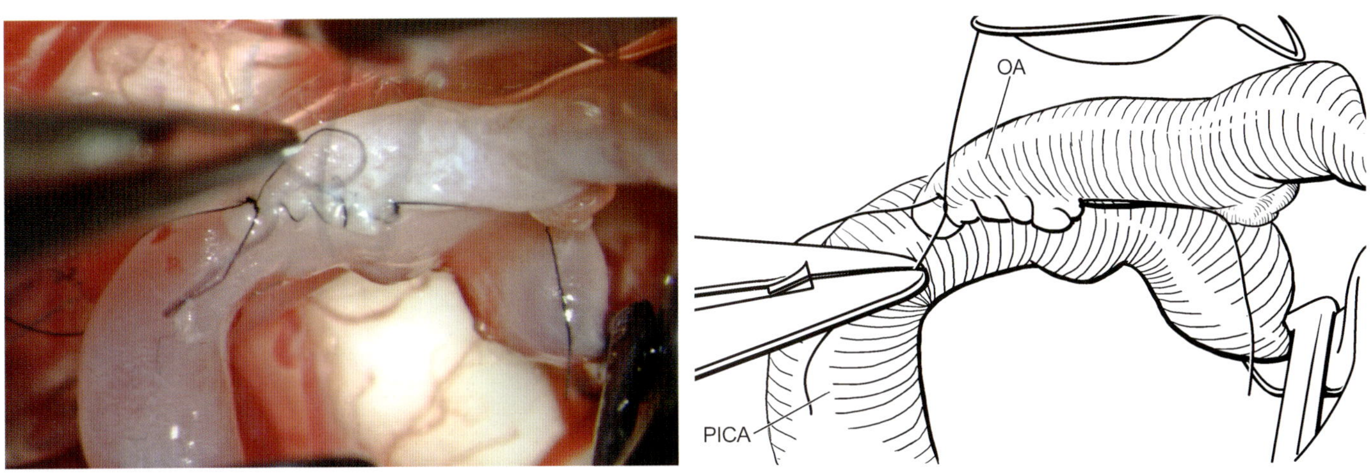

Fig. 13.2s One side of the anastomosis is completed and tied to the toe stitch.

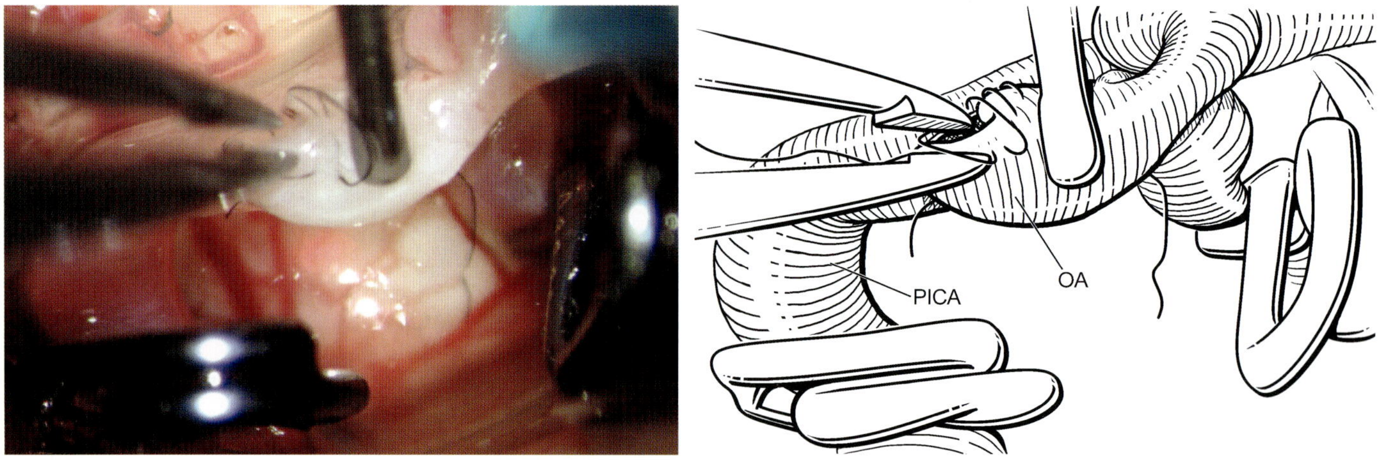

Fig. 13.2t The back wall of the anastomosis is performed.

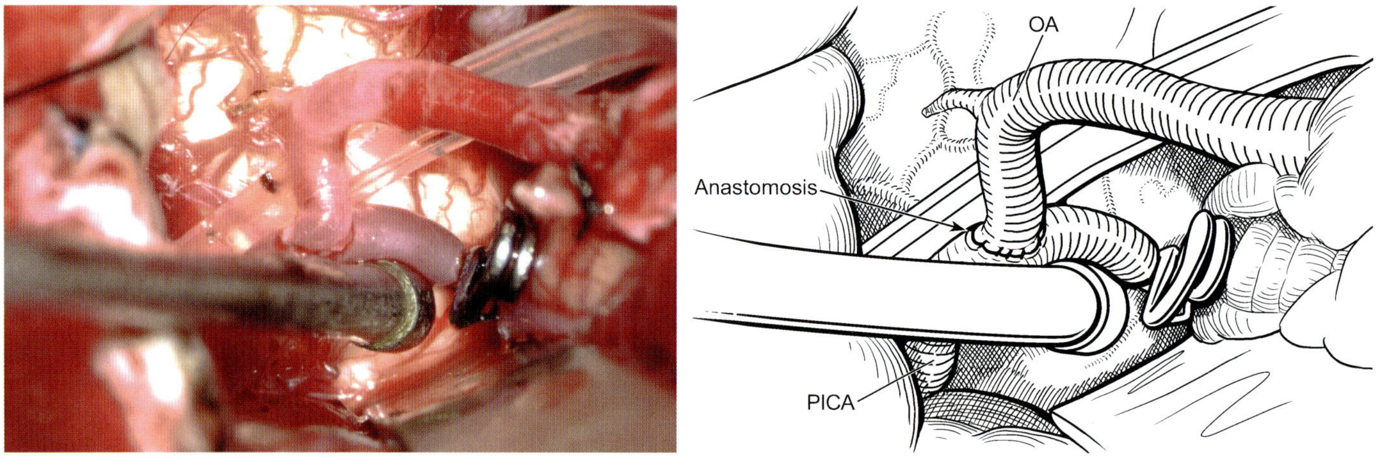

Fig. 13.2u The anastomosis is completed. Only one temporary clip remains in place.

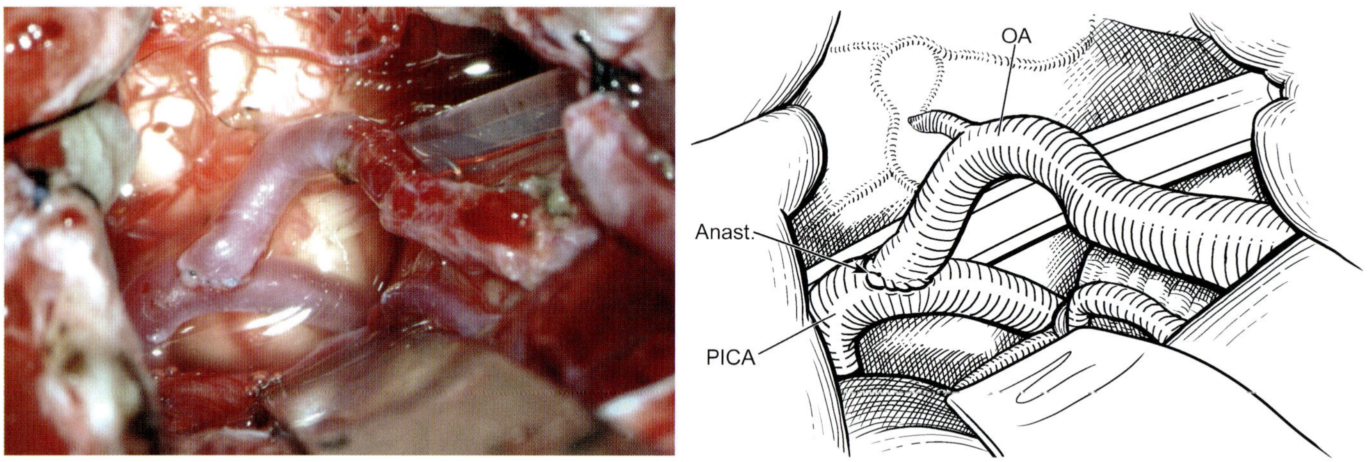

Fig. 13.2v The bypass is completed.

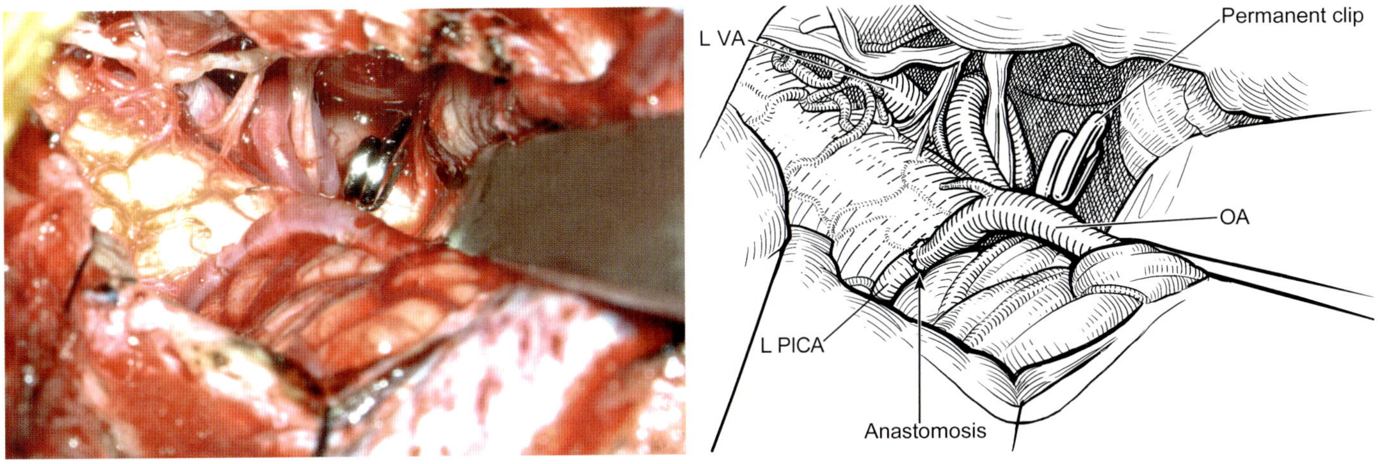

Fig. 13.2w A clip placed parallel to the VA occludes the aneurysm and the origin of the PICA.

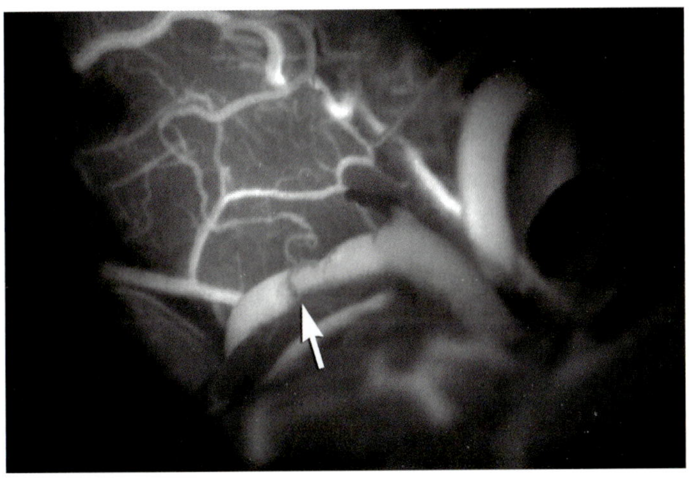

Fig. 13.2x ICG angiogram shows good patency of the OA bypass (*arrow*).

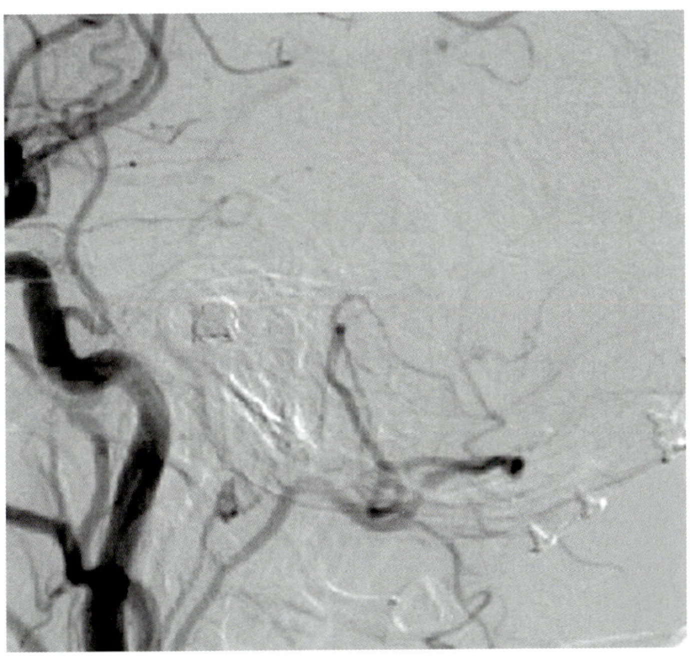

Fig. 13.2y CCA injection confirms good patency of the OA-to-PICA bypass.

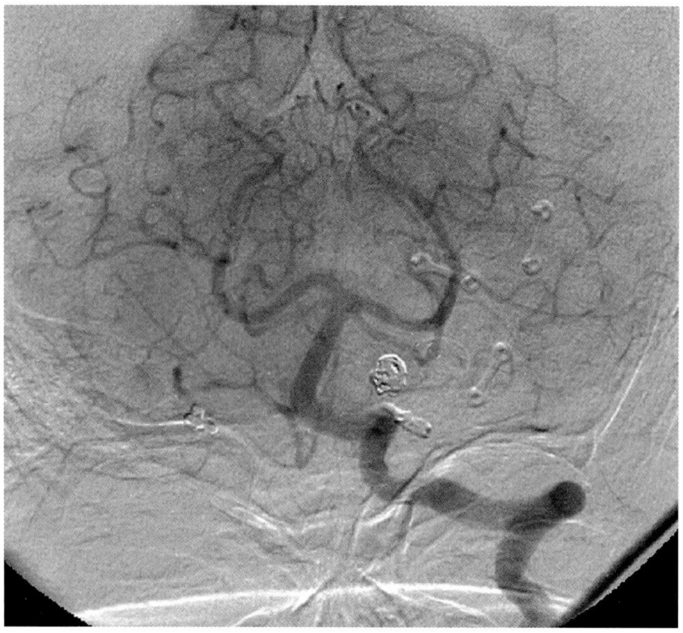

Fig. 13.2z Anteroposterior VA angiogram confirms patency of the VA and exclusion of the PICA aneurysm.

14 PICA-to-PICA Bypass

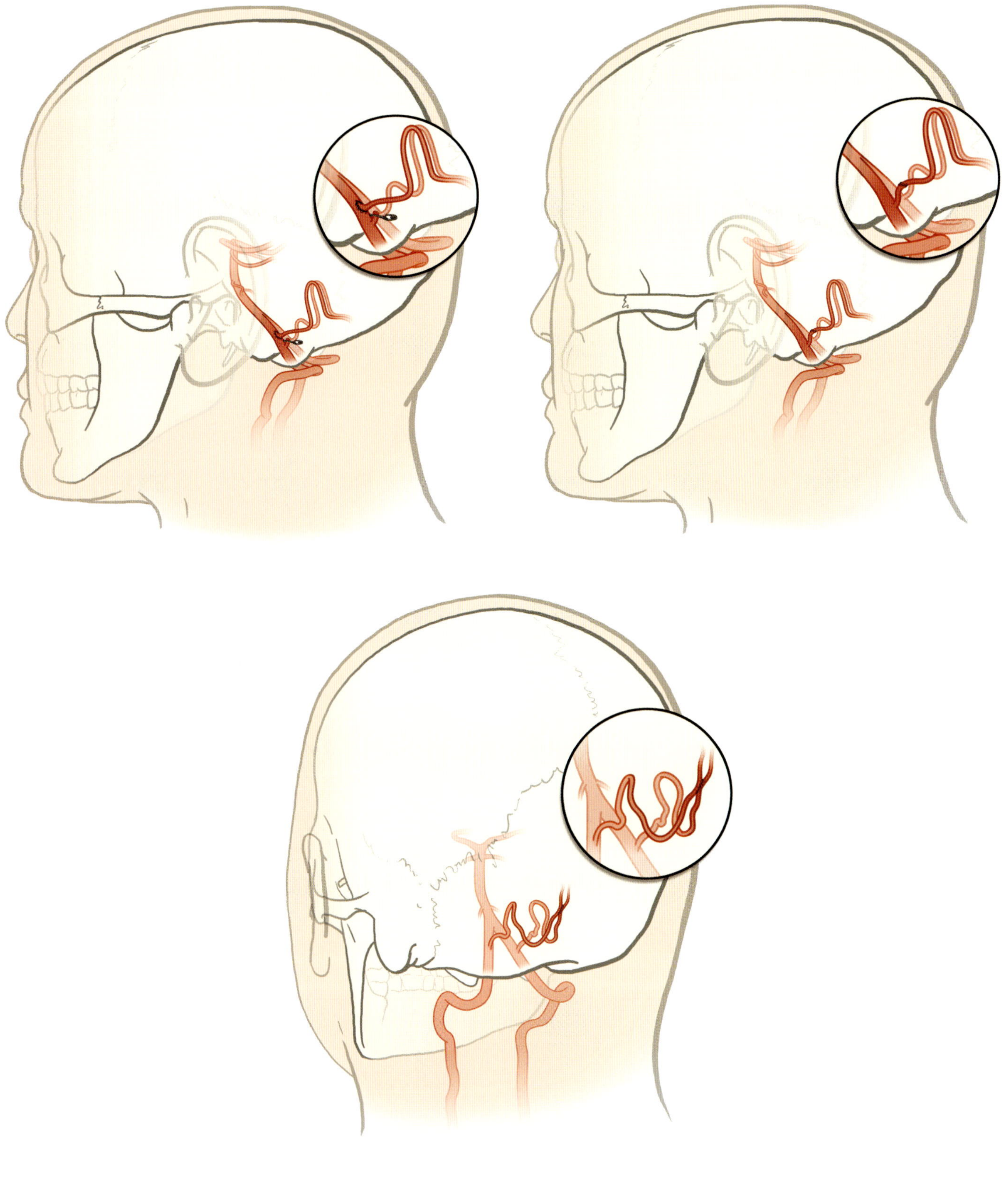

Several bypasses from the PICA can be performed using the PICA as a donor vessel. The most common PICA-to-PICA bypass takes advantage of the site where the two vascular loops lie closest to each other in the midline as the vessels course around the medial surface of the tonsil. When temporary clips are placed on the two PICAs, a slit opening can be made in each artery in a longitudinal fashion and the anastomosis can be performed. The back side of the anastomosis must be performed first. After the bypass is completed, usually with 10–0 or 11–0 suture, the clips are removed and the bypass's patency is checked with ICG angiography.

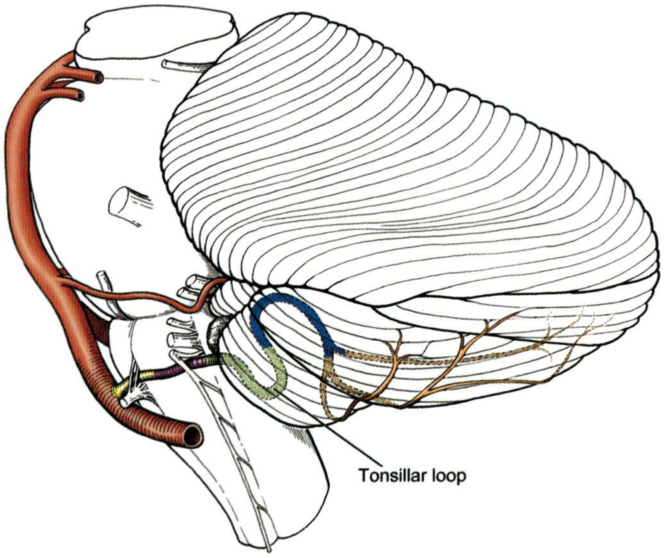

Fig. 14.0a Lateral schematic representation of a normal variant of the PICA. The tonsillar loop is the most common site of a PICA-to-PICA anastomosis.

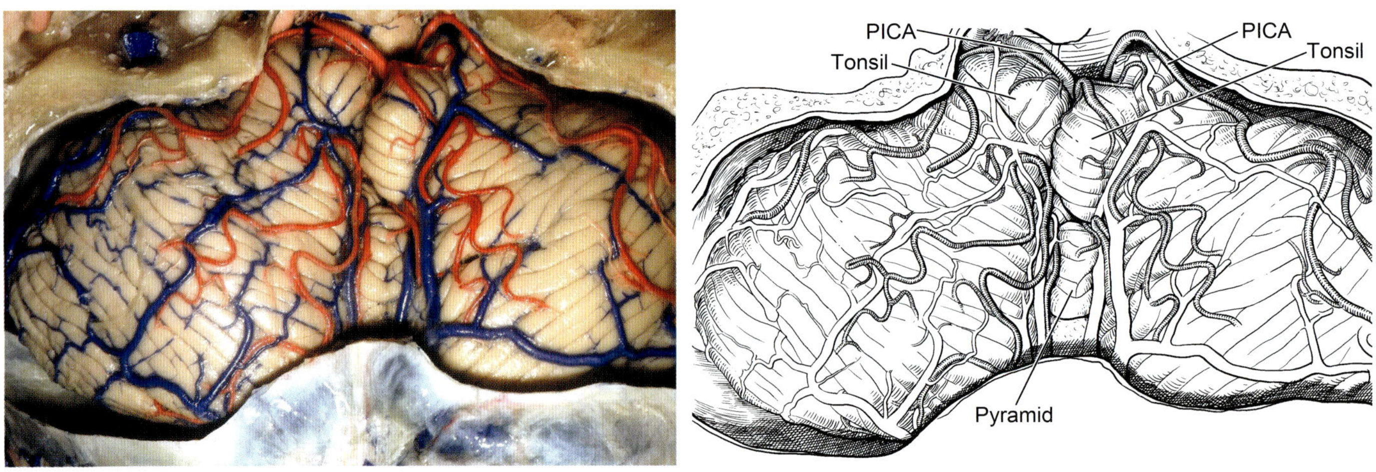

Fig. 14.0b A view of the cerebellar hemispheres, as seen from the surgeon's perspective, shows the cerebellar tonsils and their associated PICA segments. (Photograph used with permission from *Journal of Neurosurgery*.)

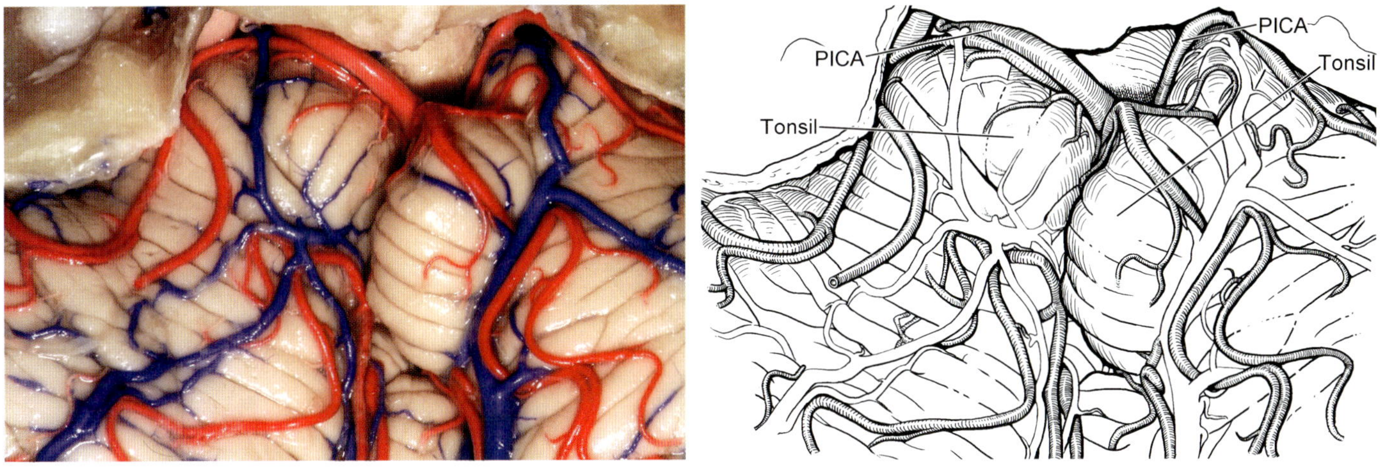

Fig. 14.0c High magnification view of the cerebellar tonsils and the branches of the PICA appropriate for anastomosis. (Photograph used with permission from *Journal of Neurosurgery*.)

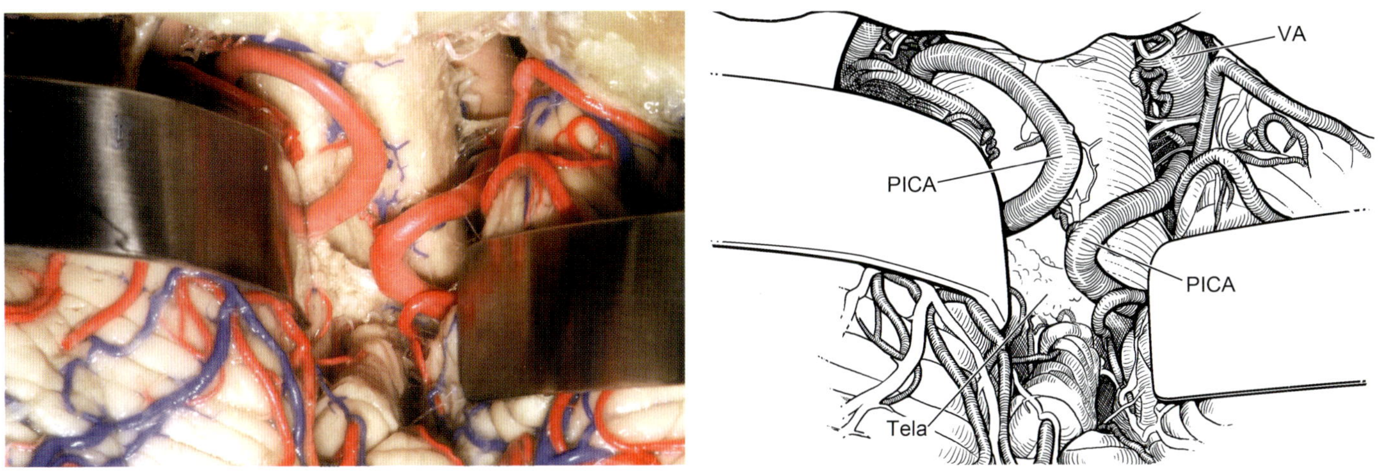

Fig. 14.0d The tonsils are retracted, demonstrating the two loops of the PICA. (Photograph used with permission from *Journal of Neurosurgery*.)

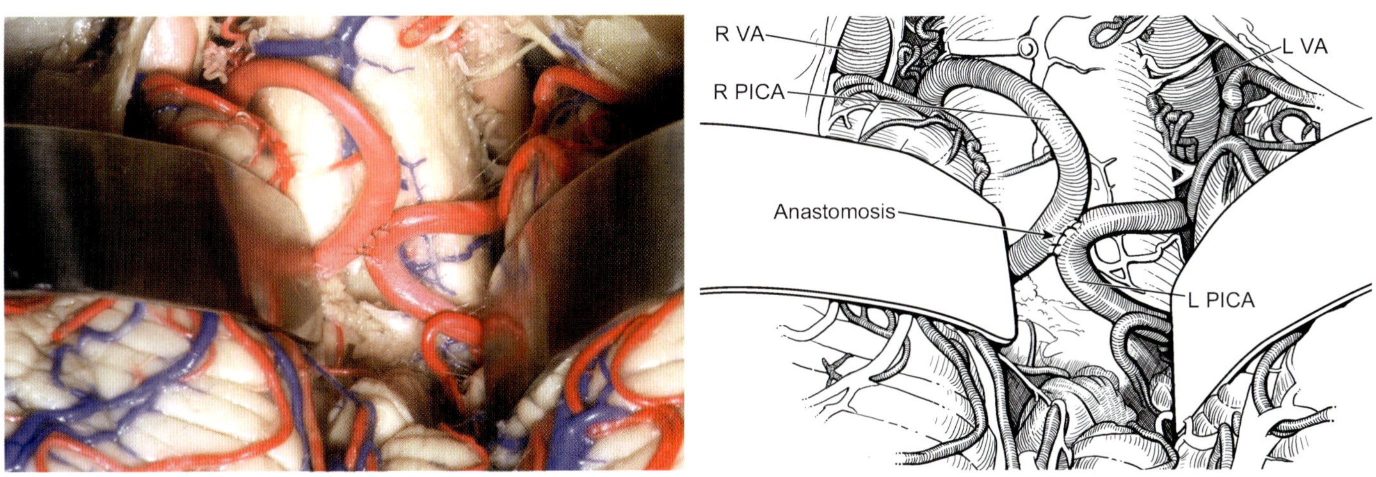

Fig. 14.0e A completed PICA-to-PICA bypass. (Photograph used with permission from *Journal of Neurosurgery*.)

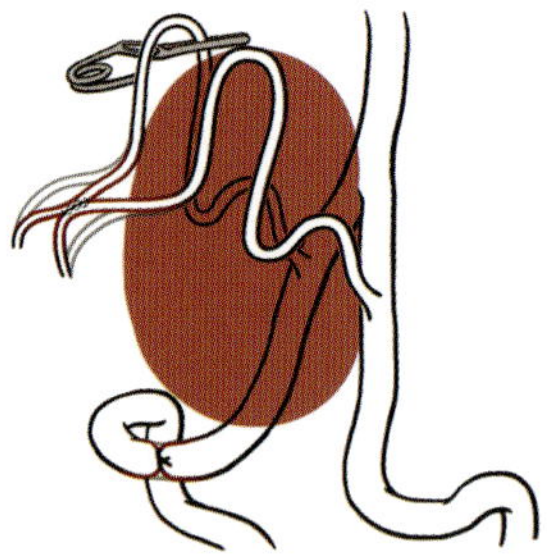

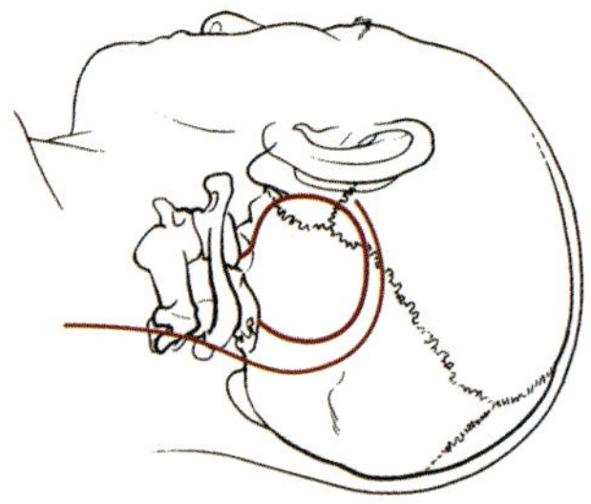

Case 14-1

Diagnosis: Giant left VA aneurysm

Bypass: PICA–to–contralateral PICA

Approach: Left far lateral

Video

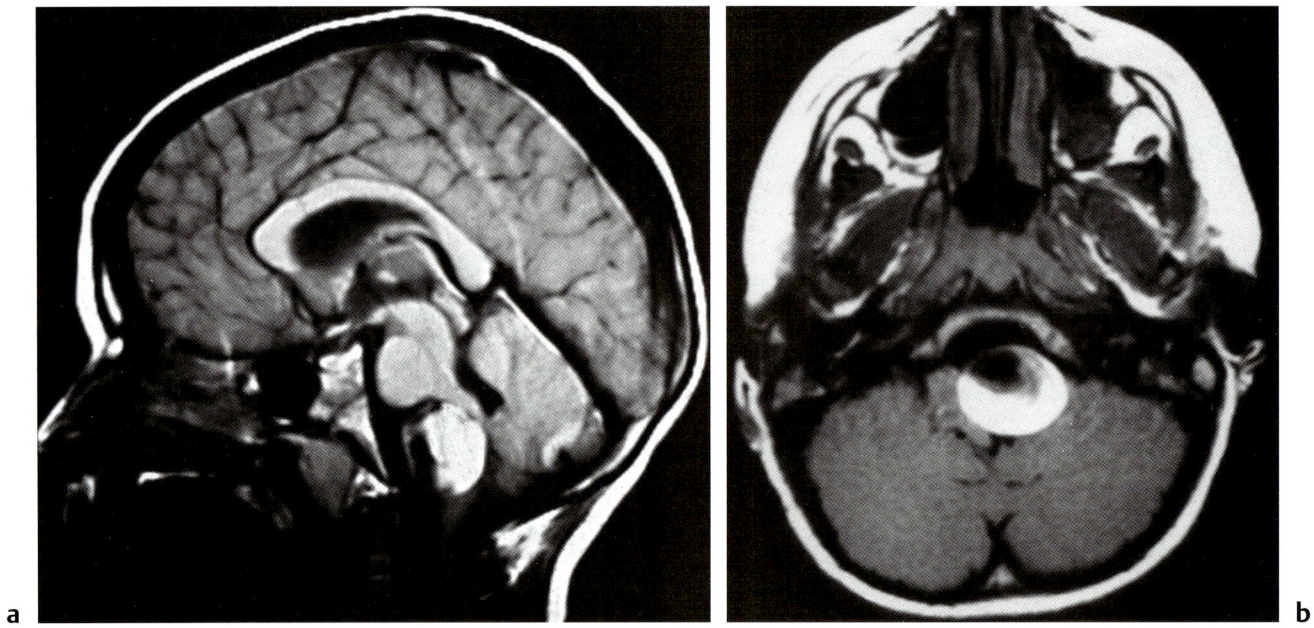

Fig. 14.1a, b Sagittal (**a**) and axial (**b**) MR images of the brain of a 5-year-old boy with acute SAH show a large aneurysm compressing the pontomedullary junction toward the left side. The bright T1-weighted signal suggests the presence of intraluminal thrombus.

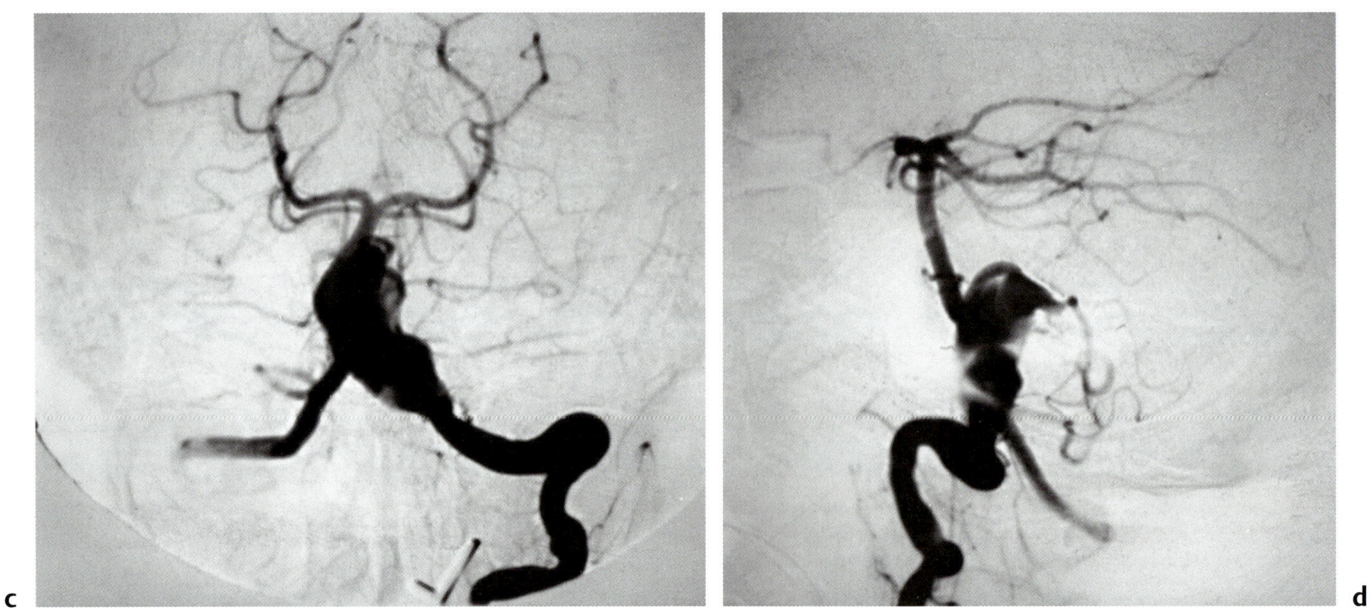

Fig. 14.1c, d Anteroposterior and oblique left VA angiograms show the aneurysm involving the left VA and PICA. (Used with permission from *Journal of Neurosurgery*.)

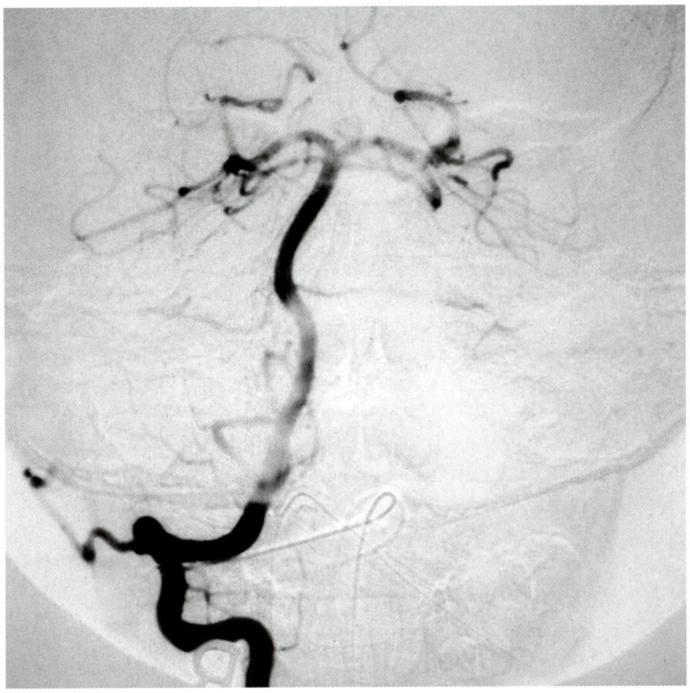

Fig. 14.1e The right VA angiographic injection does not show the aneurysm but does show a normal right VA, BA, and vertebrobasilar junction.

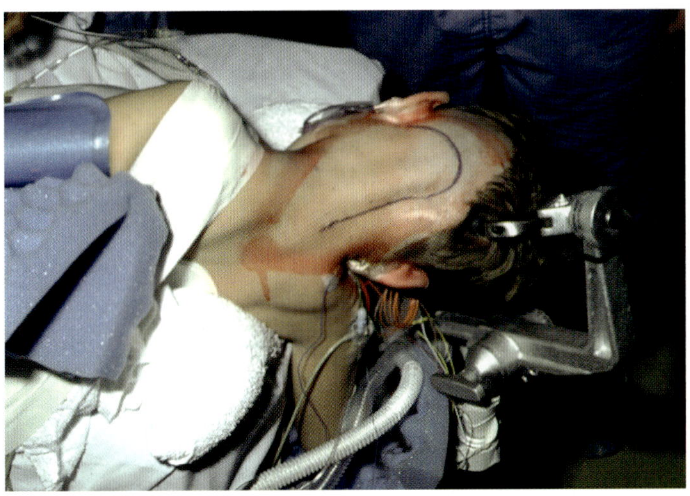

Fig. 14.1f The patient is placed in a park bench position and the hockey stick incision for the left far lateral approach is outlined on the skin.

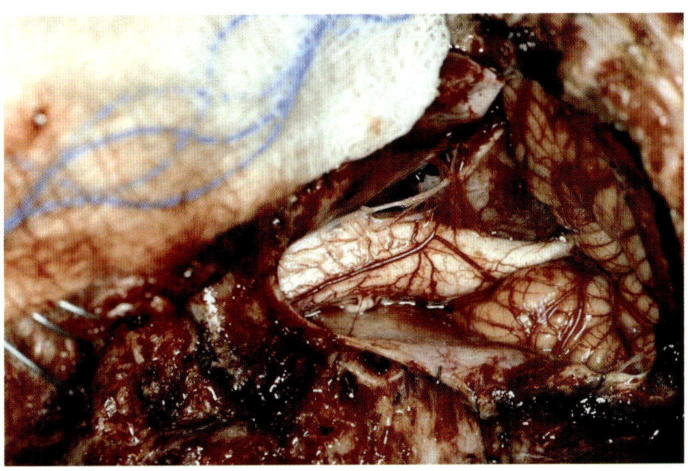

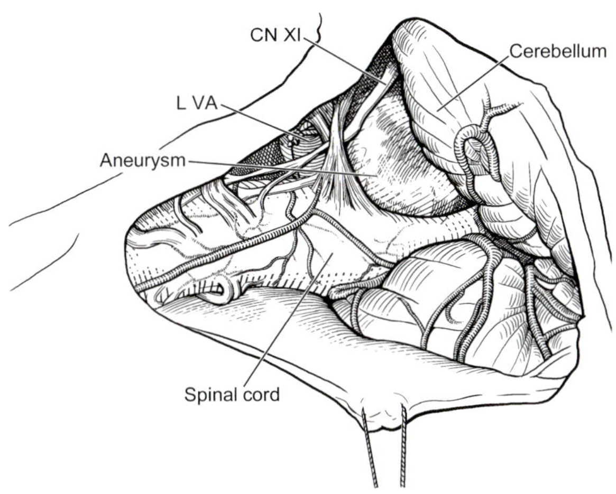

Fig. 14.1g The aneurysm is compressing the cervicomedullary junction.

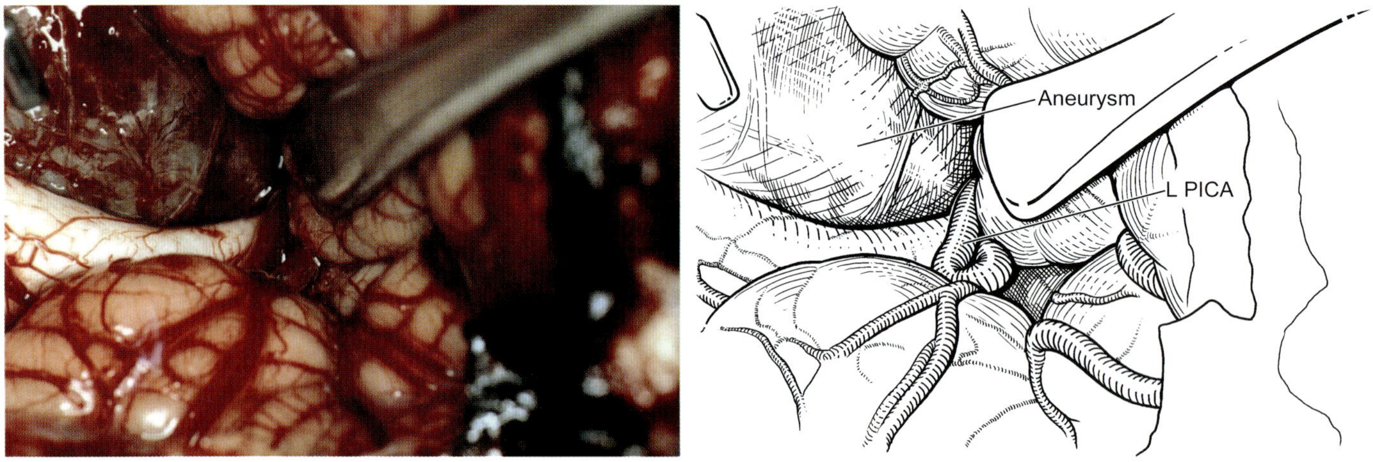

Fig. 14.1h High magnification view shows the PICA exiting the aneurysm. The working space near the origin of the PICA is severely restricted by the mass of the aneurysm.

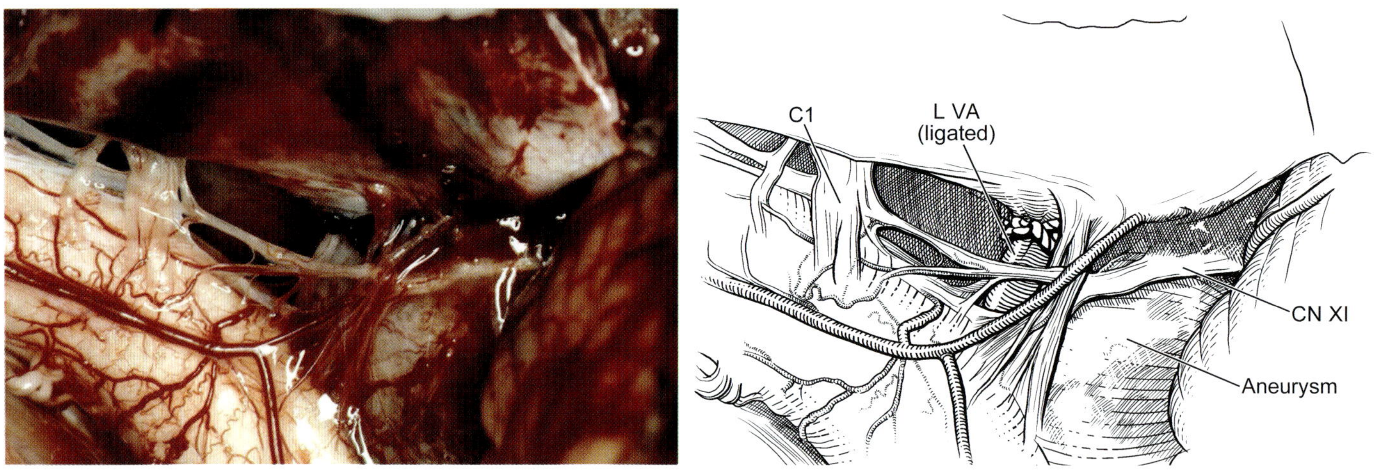

Fig. 14.1i The lower cranial nerves are splayed over the dome of the aneurysm. A ligature is placed on the left VA proximal to the aneurysm.

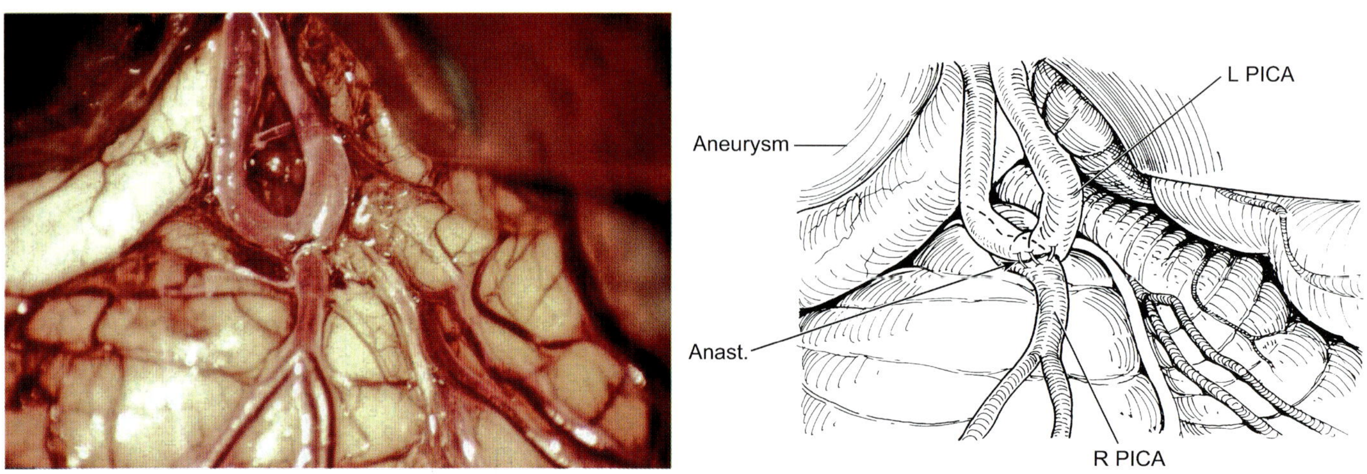

Fig. 14.1j A side-to-side anastomosis of the PICA loops is performed. (Used with permission from *Journal of Neurosurgery*.)

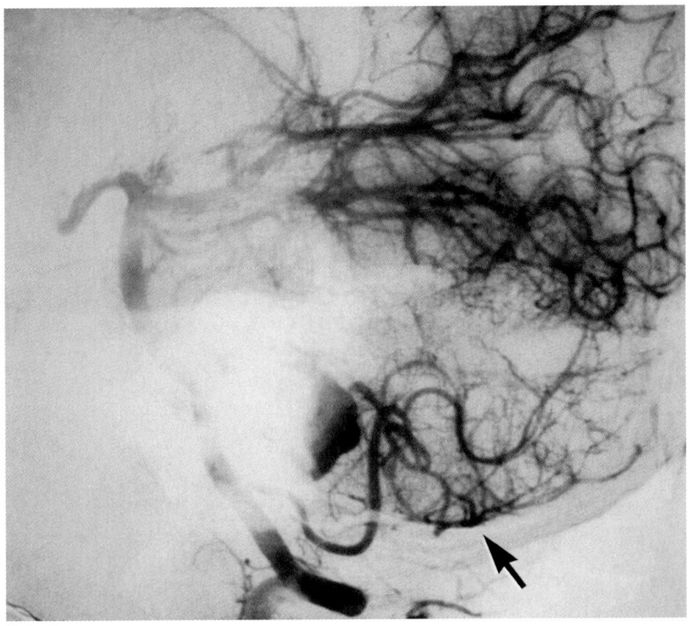

Fig. 14.1k Right VA angiographic injection shows filling of both PICA distributions *(arrow)*. The dome of the aneurysm is partially visible because of backfilling through the left PICA.

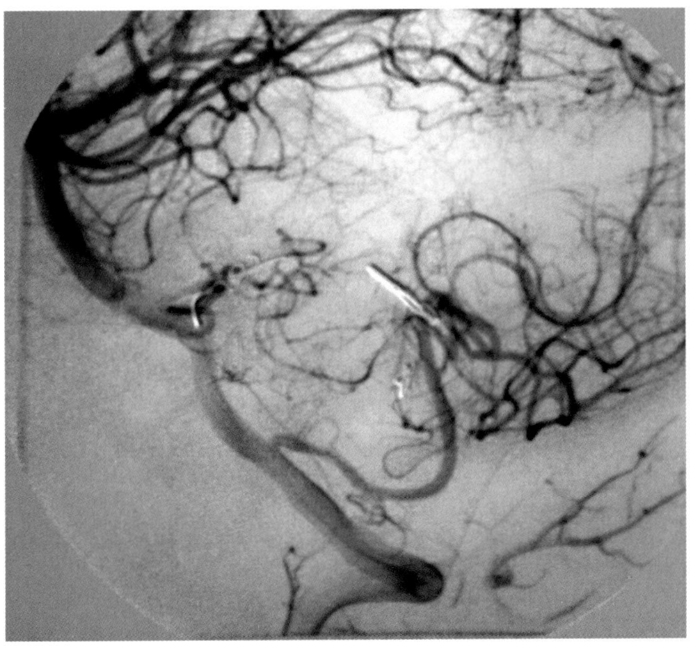

Fig. 14.1l Lateral right VA injection shows that permanent clipping of the left PICA at the aneurysm isolates the lesion distally. The distal left VA was coiled to obliterate residual filling from the contralateral VA. (Used with permission from *Journal of Neurosurgery*.)

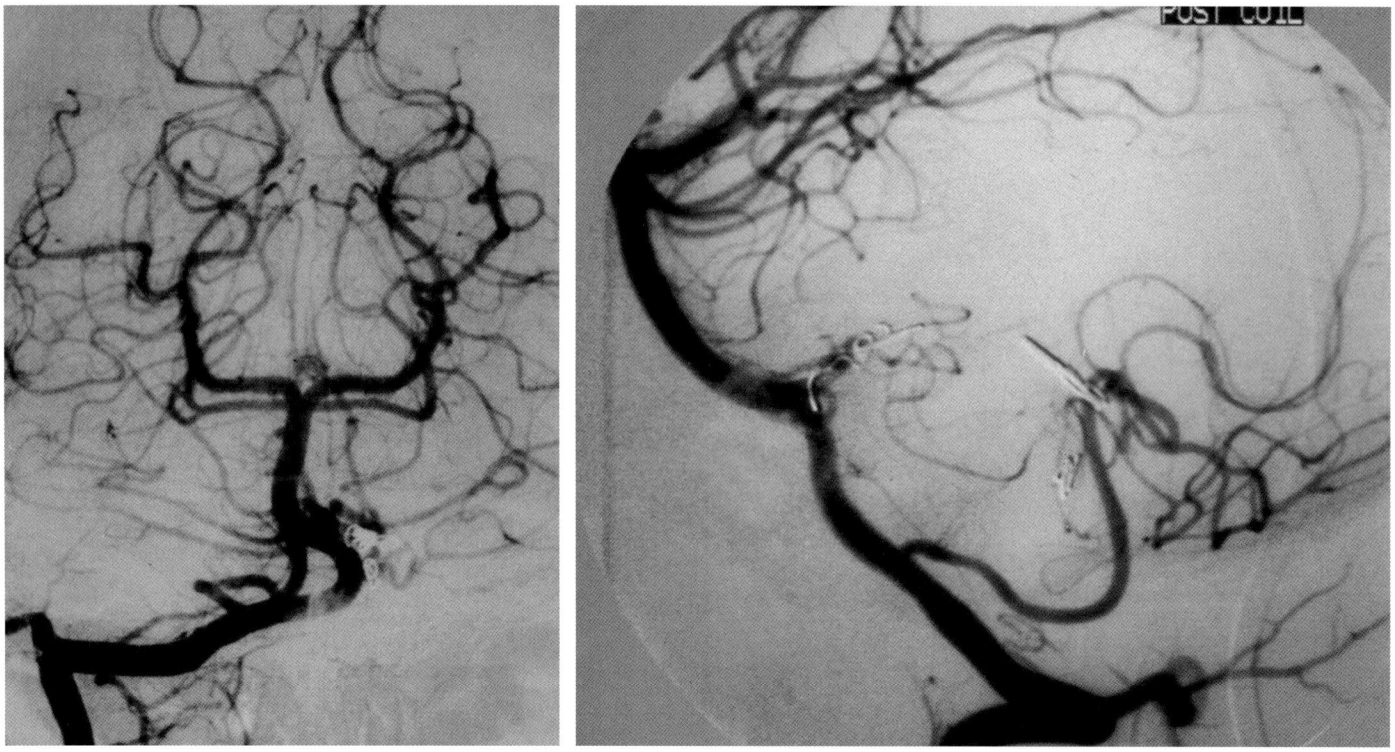

m n

Fig. 14.1m, n Anteroposterior and lateral right VA angiograms show the coils in the left distal aneurysm, the clip on the PICA distal to the aneurysm, and no further filling of the lumen of the aneurysm. (**Fig. 14.1n** used with permission from *Journal of Neurosurgery*.)

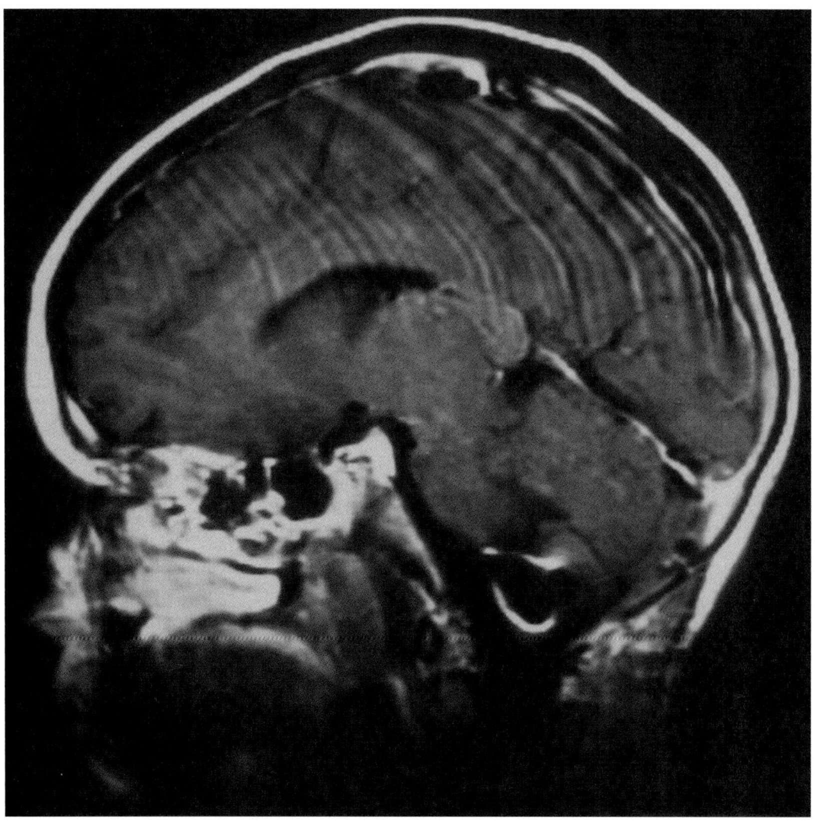

Fig. 14.1o Postoperative sagittal T1-weighted MR image shows improvement of the mass effect on the brainstem. Clip artifact is also visible. (Used with permission from *Journal of Neurosurgery*).

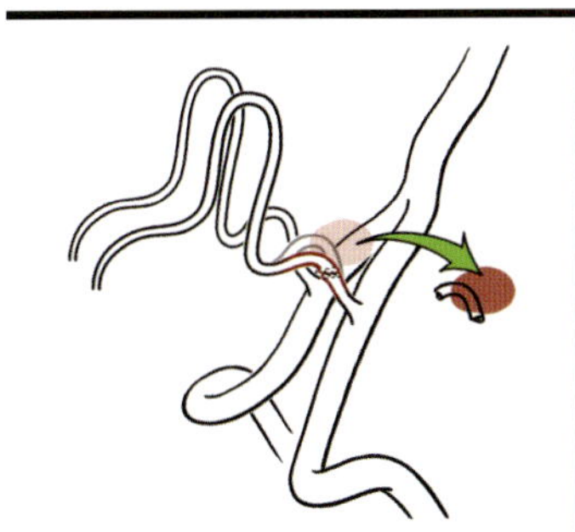

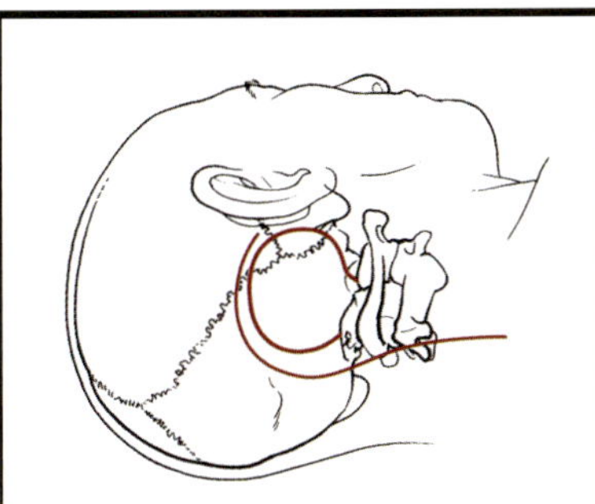

Case 14-2

Diagnosis: Right PICA aneurysm

Bypass: Direct PICA-to-PICA reanastomosis

Approach: Right far lateral

▶ Video

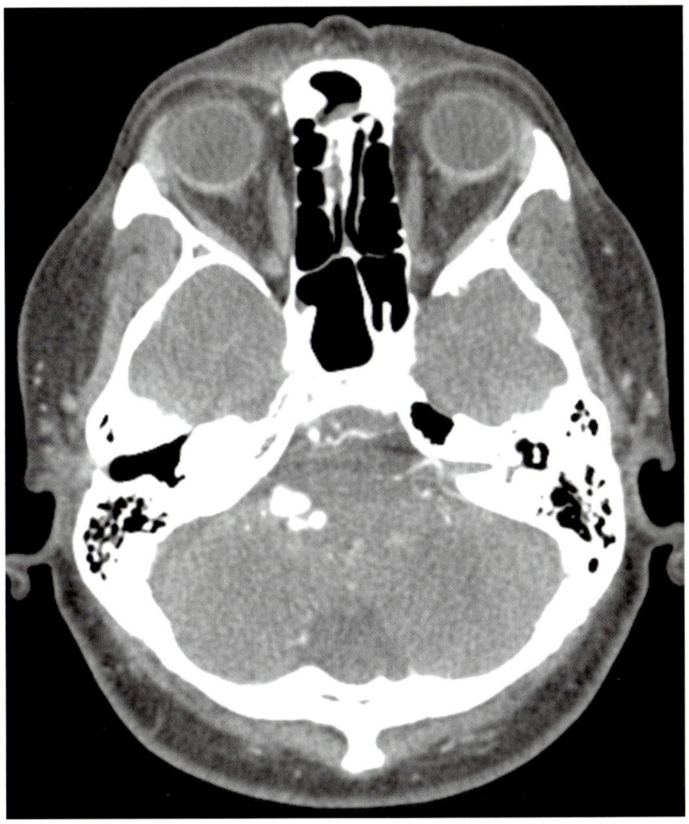

Fig. 14.2a CT scan shows a complex aneurysm in the region of the right PICA in a patient who presented with headache and dizziness.

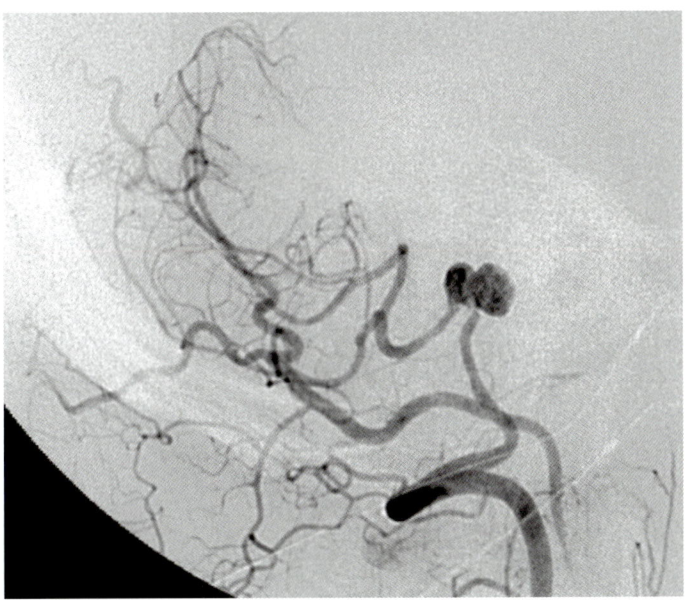

Fig. 14.2b Angiogram shows the complex dissecting PICA aneurysm.

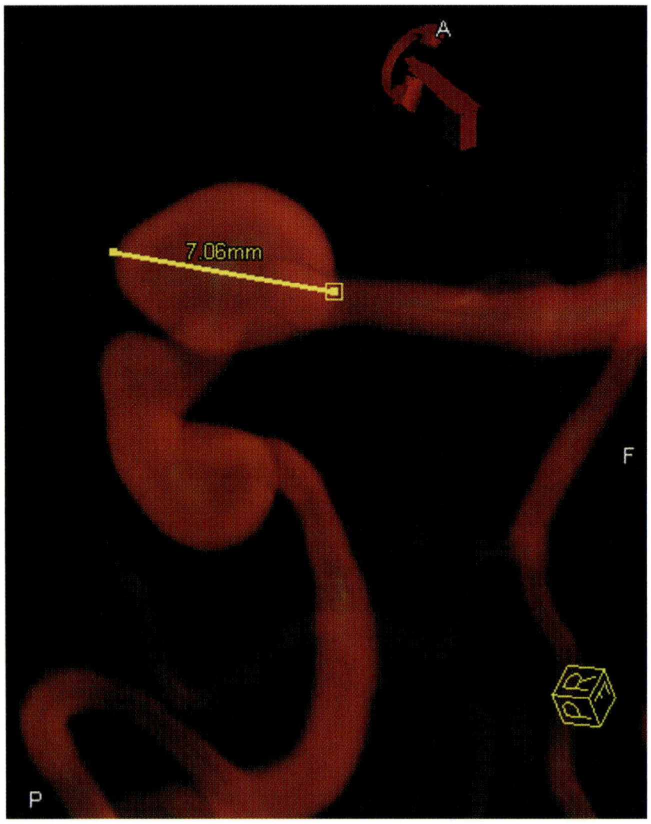

Fig. 14.2c Three-dimensional angiographic reconstruction shows the complex nature of the dissecting aneurysm.

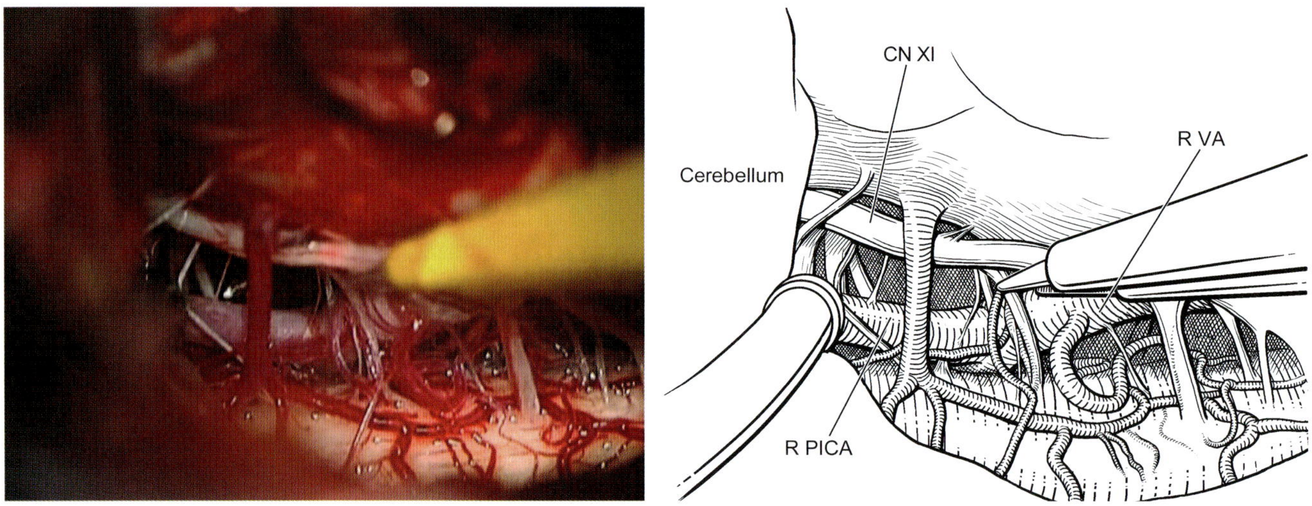

Fig. 14.2d The right VA and PICA are identified through a right far lateral approach.

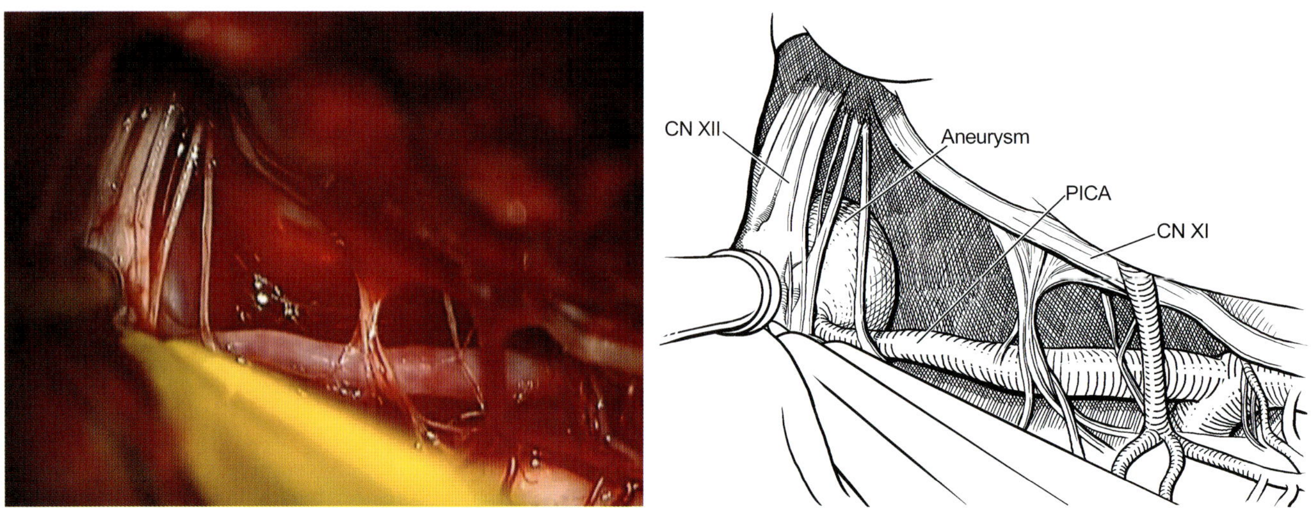

Fig. 14.2e The PICA is followed into the aneurysm.

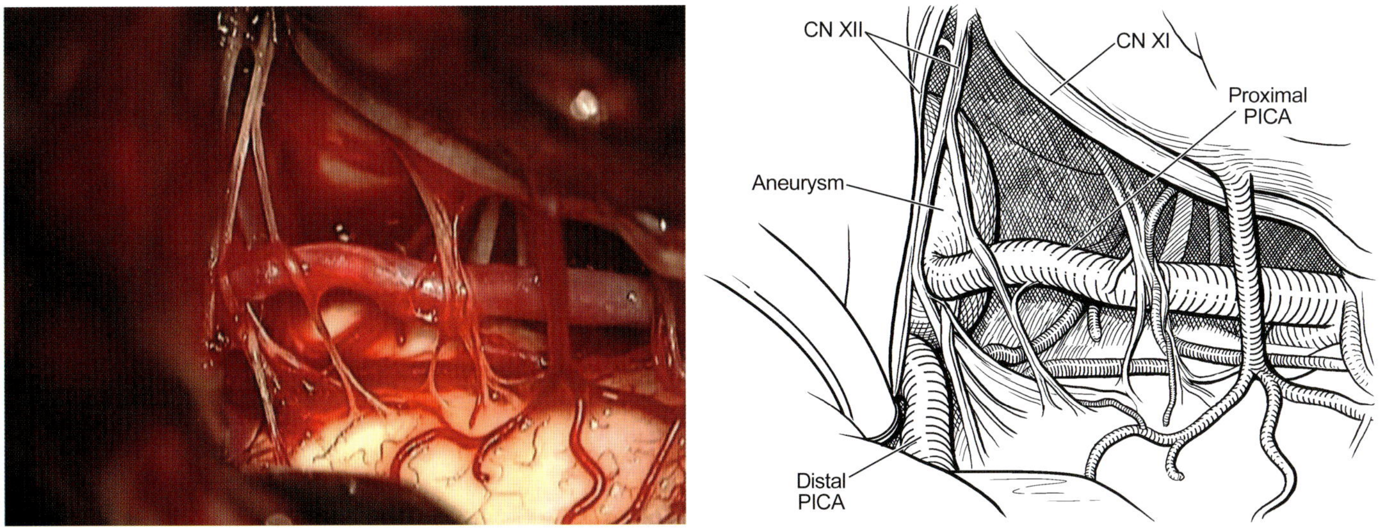

Fig. 14.2f Distal PICA is identified coursing between CN XII rootlets.

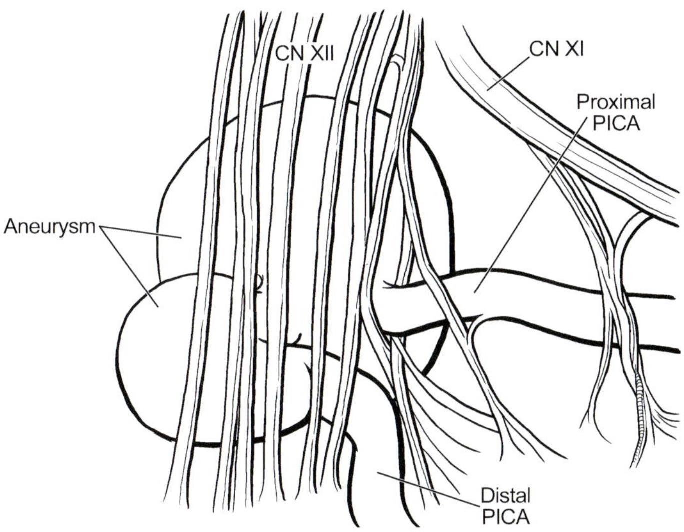

Fig. 14.2g Diagram illustrates the position of the complex aneurysm behind CN XII.

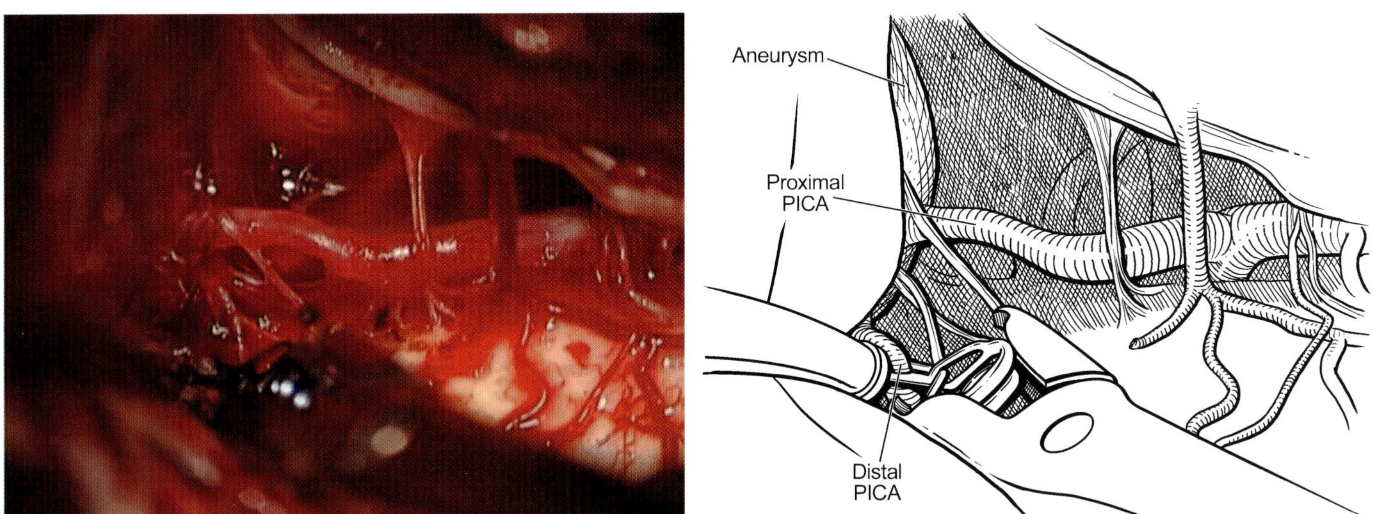

Fig. 14.2h A temporary clip is applied on the PICA outflow from the aneurysm.

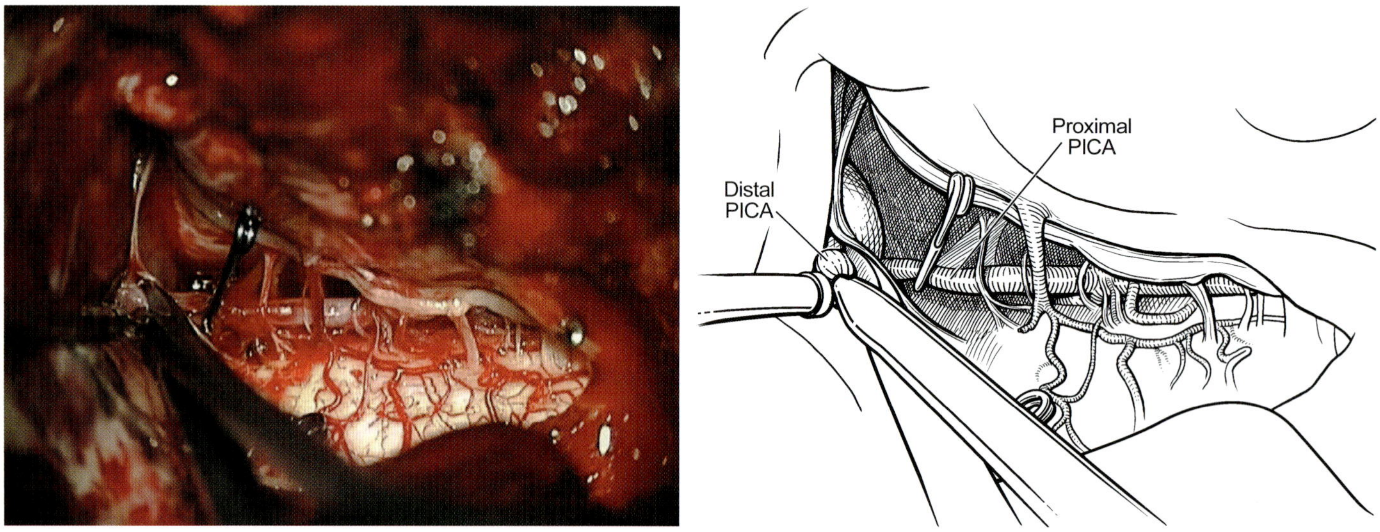

Fig. 14.2i After a clip is placed proximal to the aneurysm, the PICA is cut distal to the aneurysm.

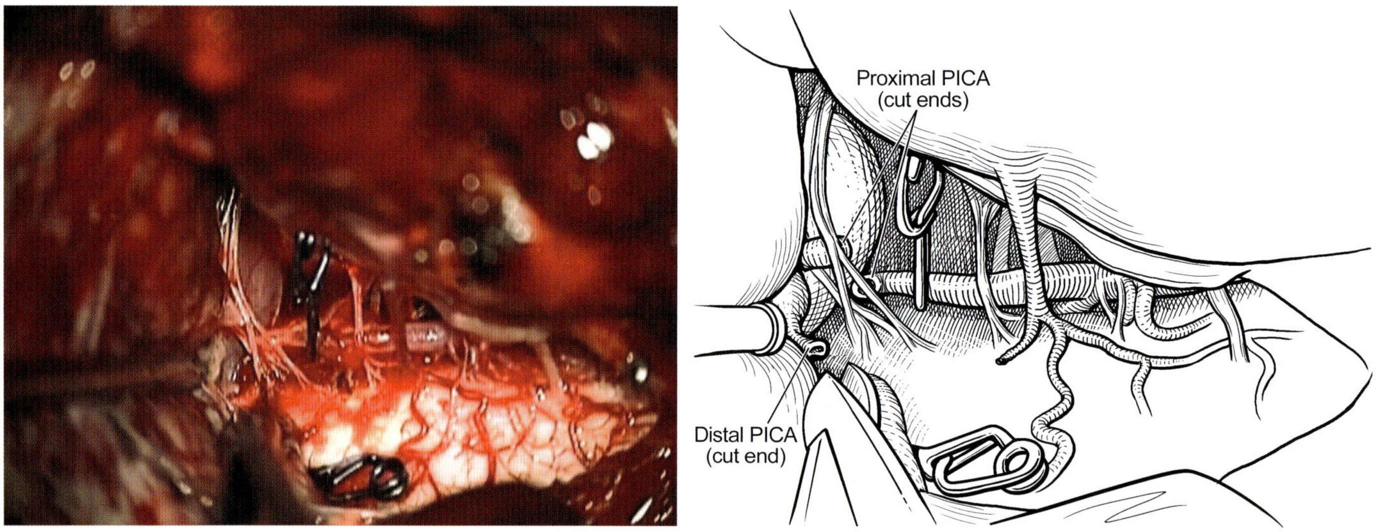

Fig. 14.2j The PICA is cut proximal to the aneurysm.

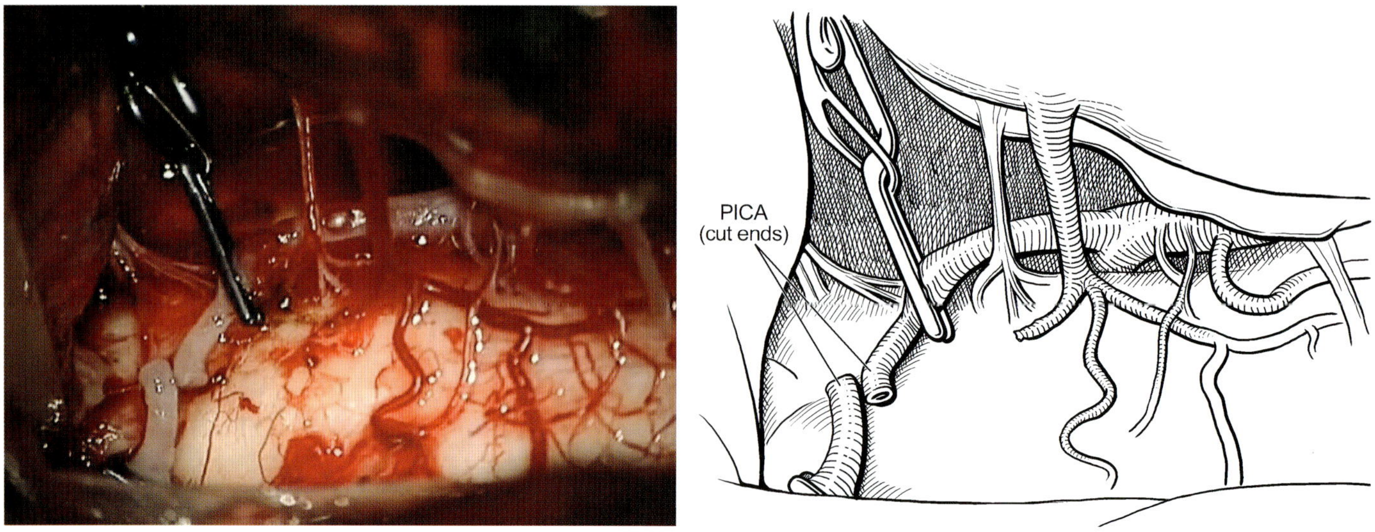

Fig. 14.2k The two cut ends of PICA are approximated.

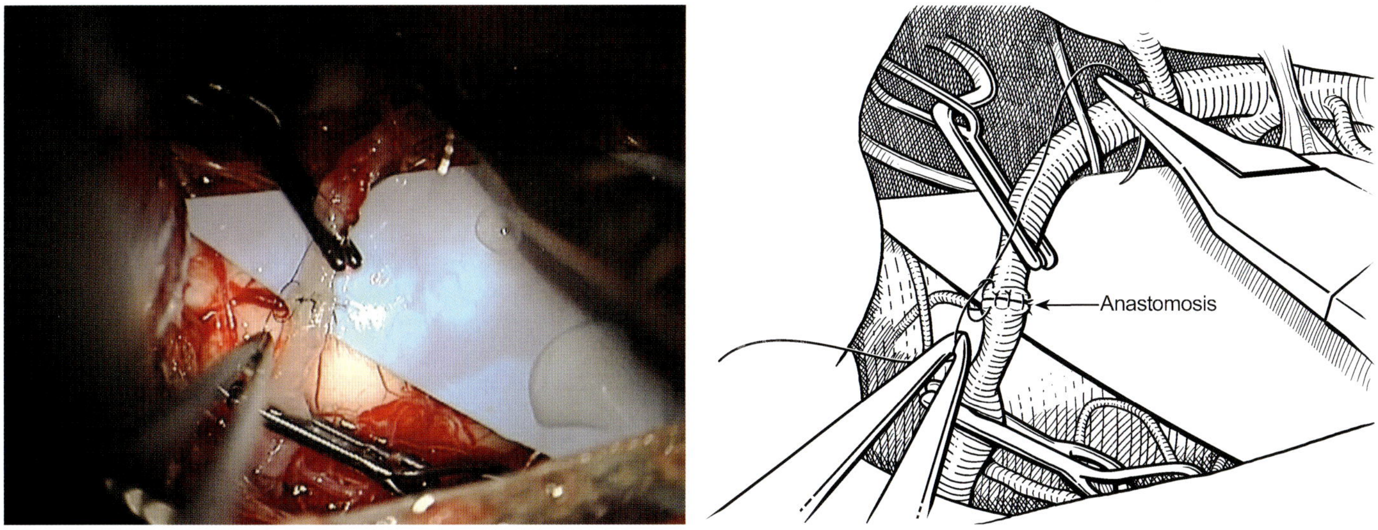

Fig. 14.2l The direct PICA-to-PICA reanastomosis is performed.

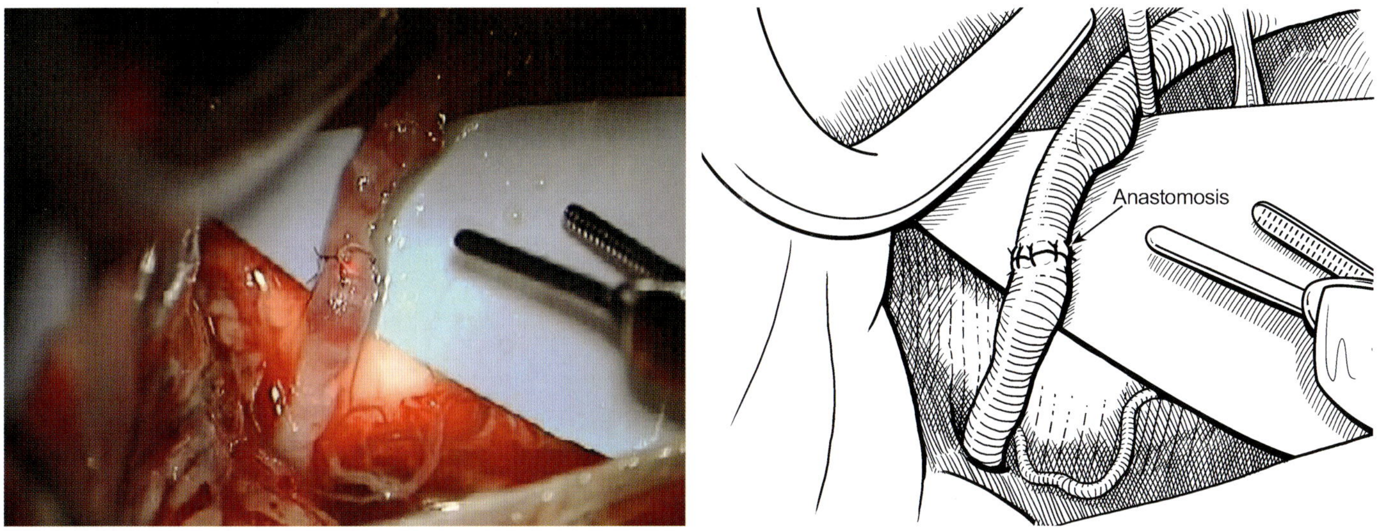

Fig. 14.2m The temporary clips are removed.

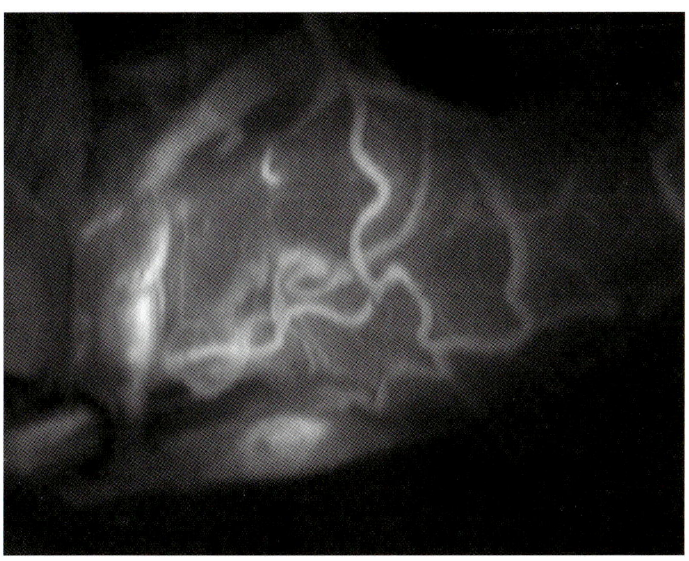

Fig. 14.2n Intraoperative ICG angiogram confirms patency of the PICA-to-PICA direct reanastomosis.

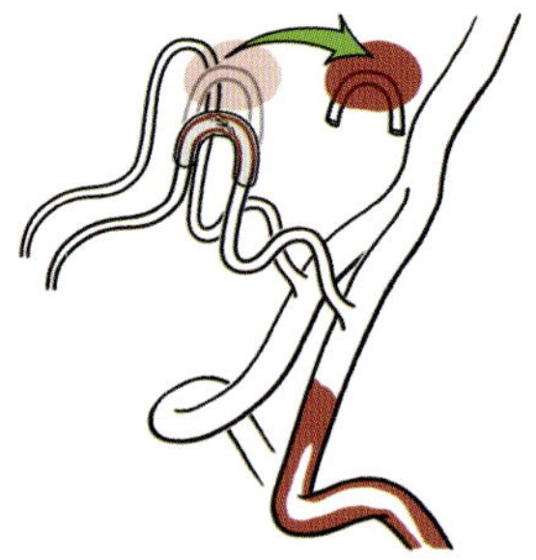

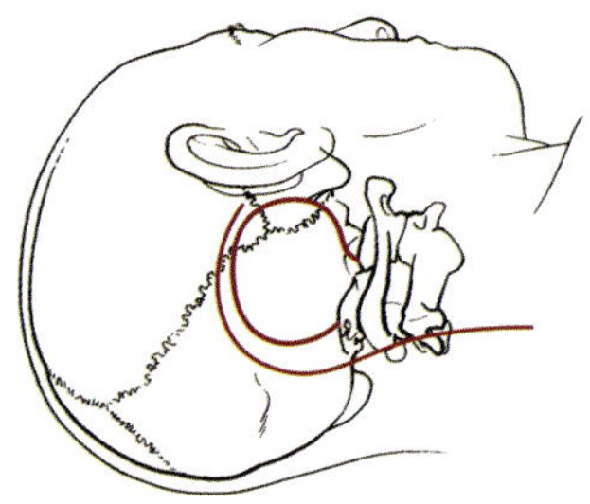

Case 14-3

Diagnosis: Complex right PICA aneurysm

Bypass: Direct end-to-end PICA-to-PICA

Approach: Right far lateral

Video

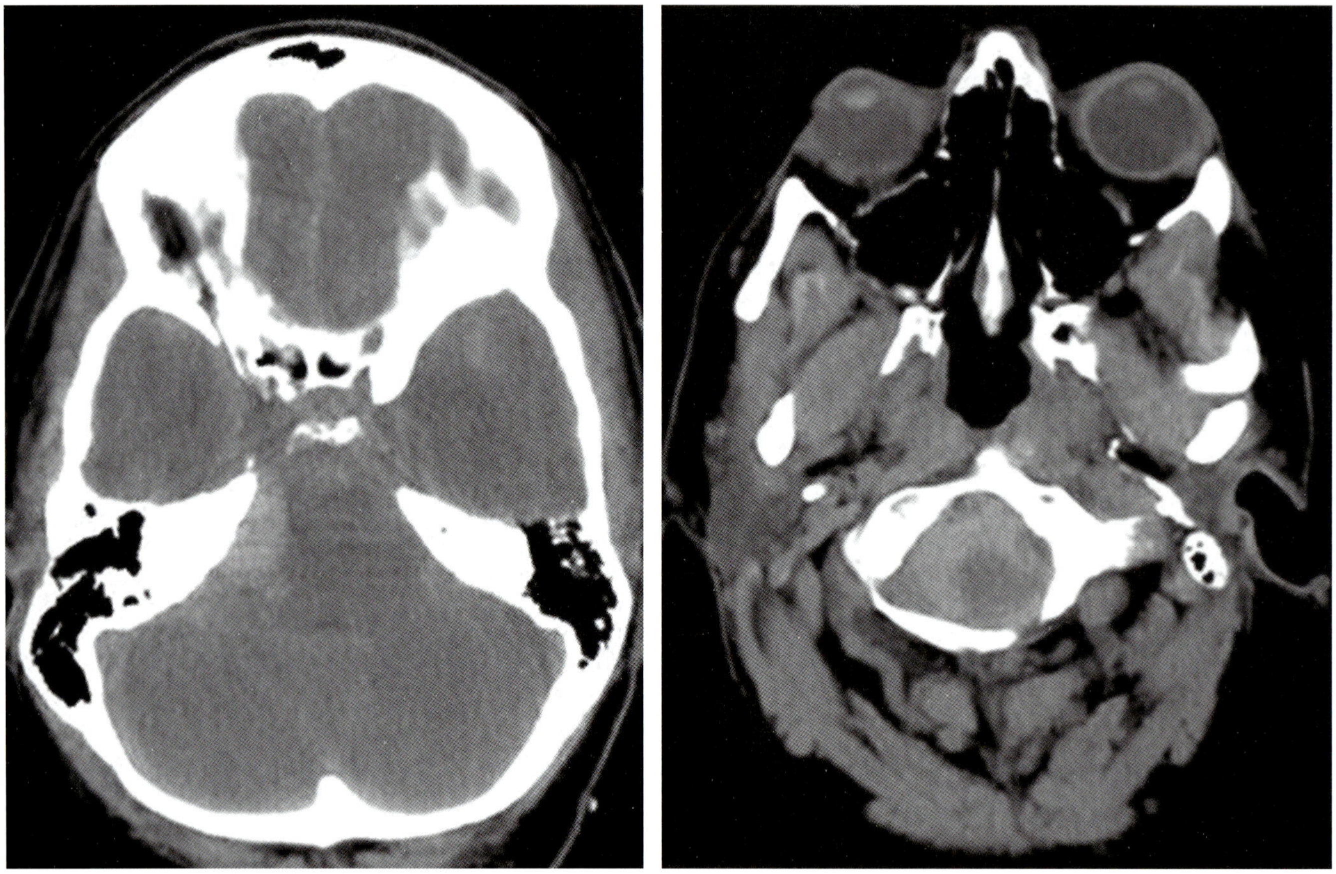

a b

Fig. 14.3a, b Axial CT scans of a 38-year-old woman show severe SAH.

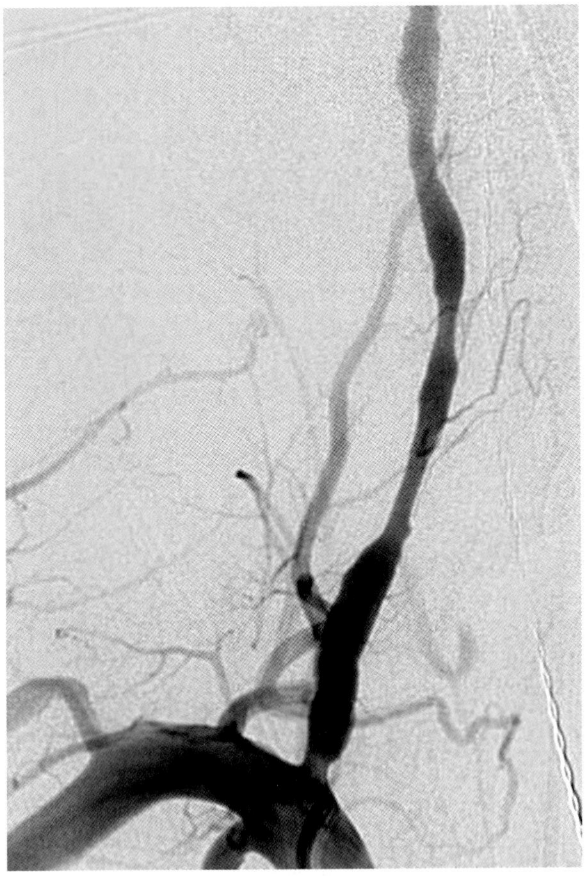

Fig. 14.3c Anteroposterior angiogram shows significant right VA disease associated with dissection of the VA, which was occluded at the skull base.

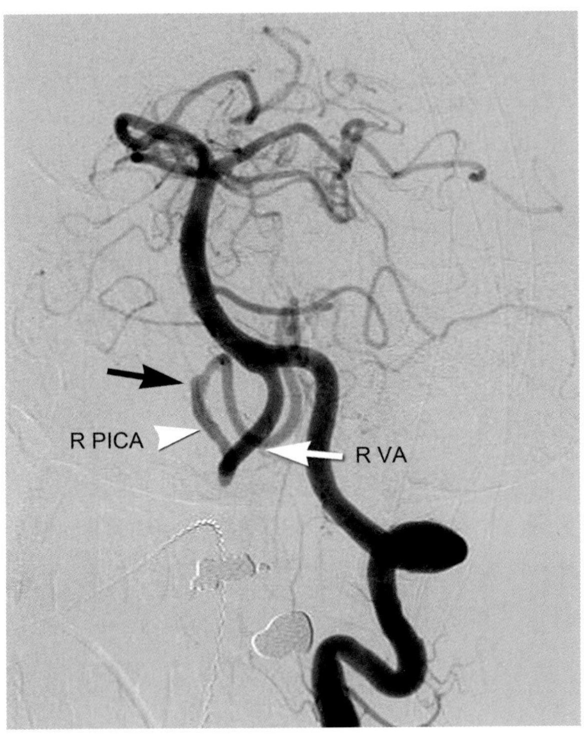

Fig. 14.3d The normal left VA feeds the right VA (*white arrow*) through retrograde flow to fill the right PICA *(white arrowhead)*. The dissecting aneurysm *(black arrow)* is seen on the cranial loop of the distal right PICA.

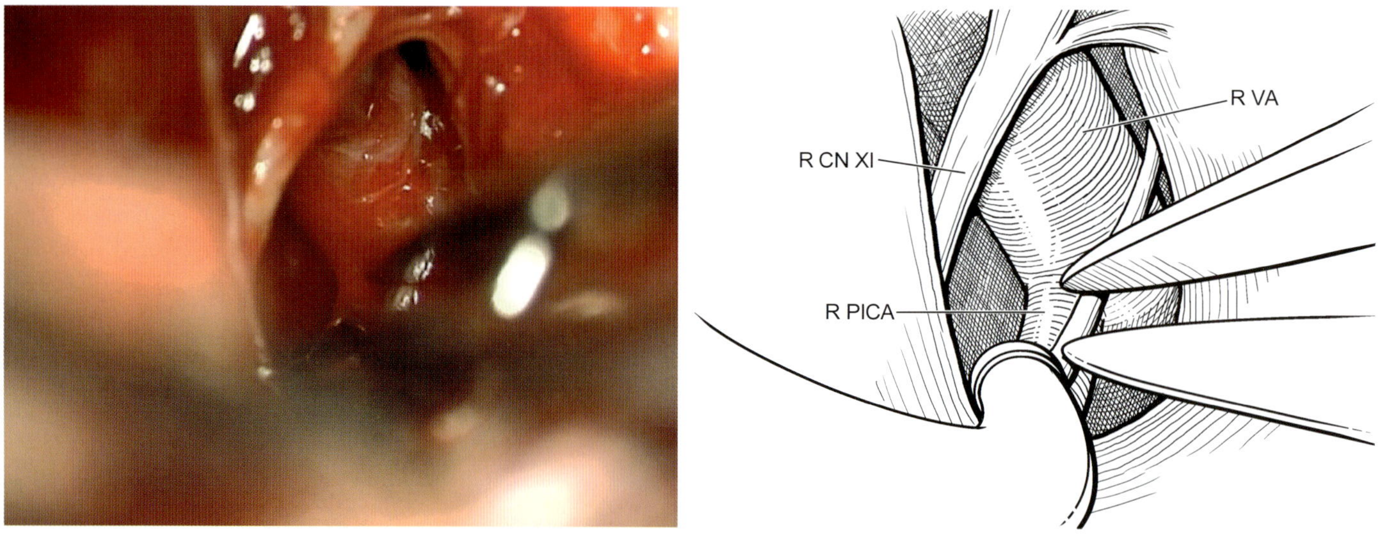

Fig. 14.3e Through a right far lateral approach, the VA is identified.

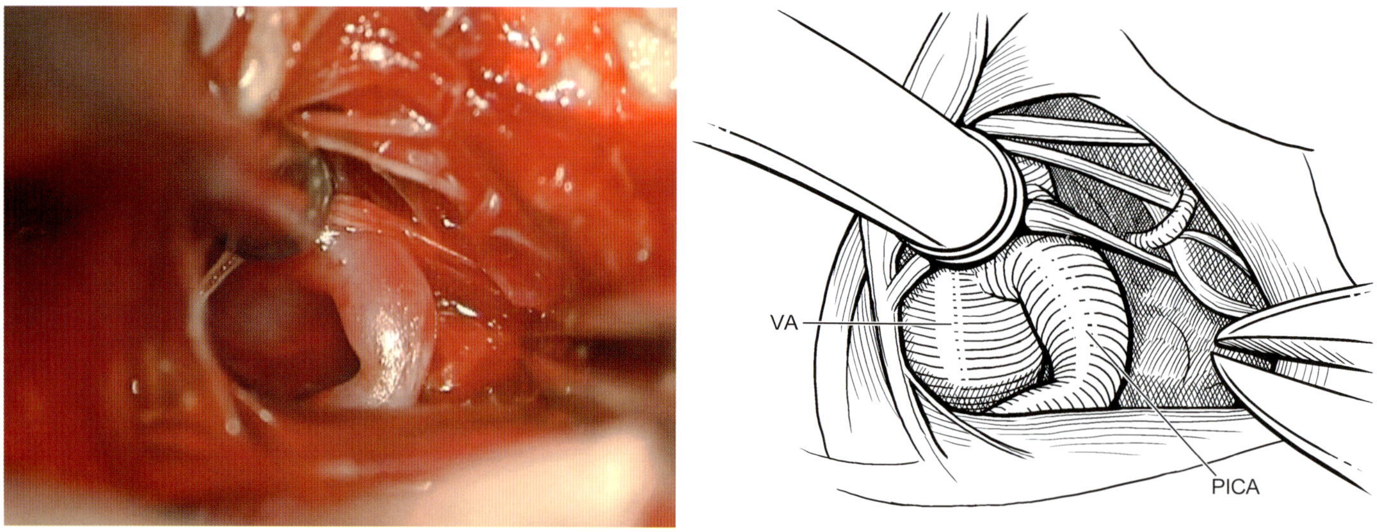

Fig. 14.3f The proximal portion of the PICA is exposed.

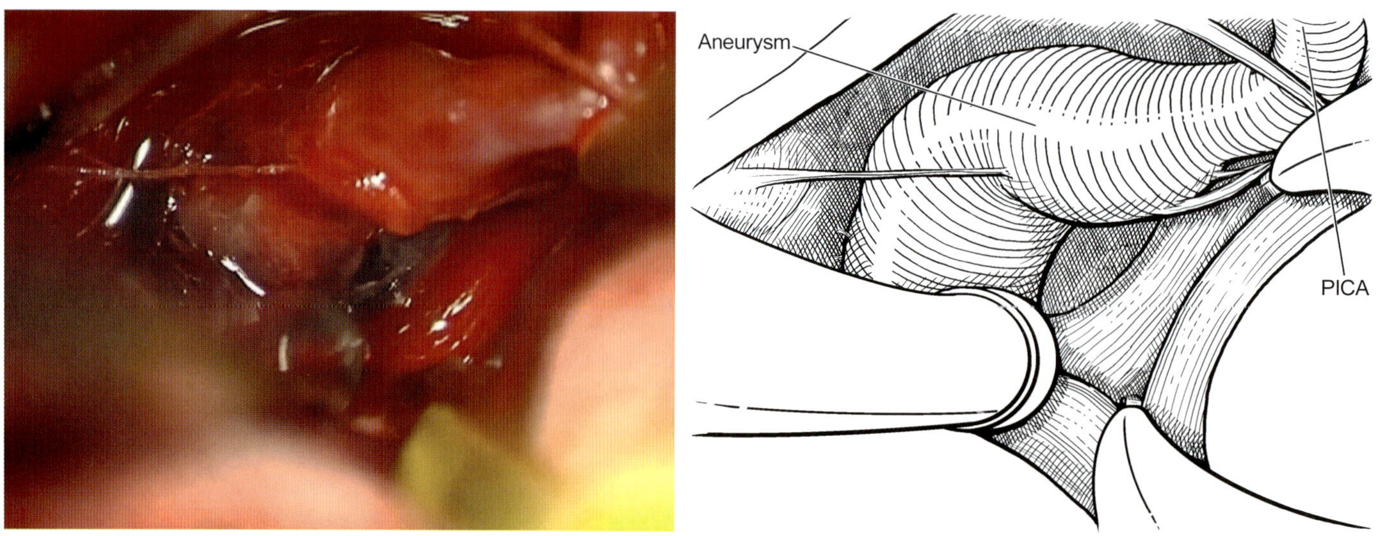

Fig. 14.3g The complex dissecting PICA aneurysm is identified.

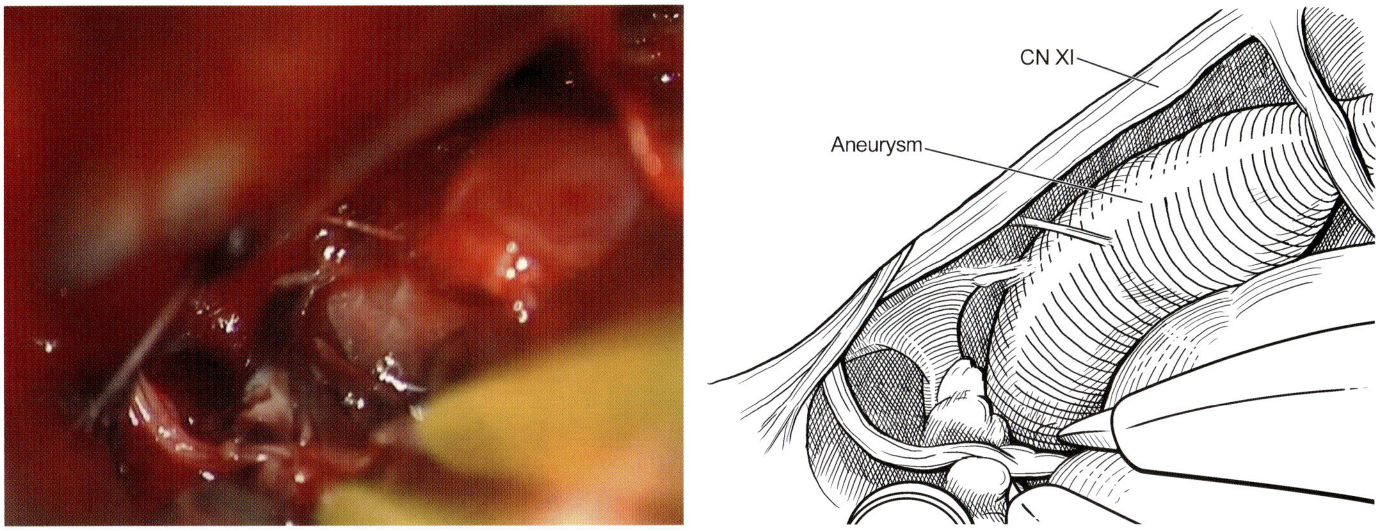

Fig. 14.3h The aneurysm is further exposed.

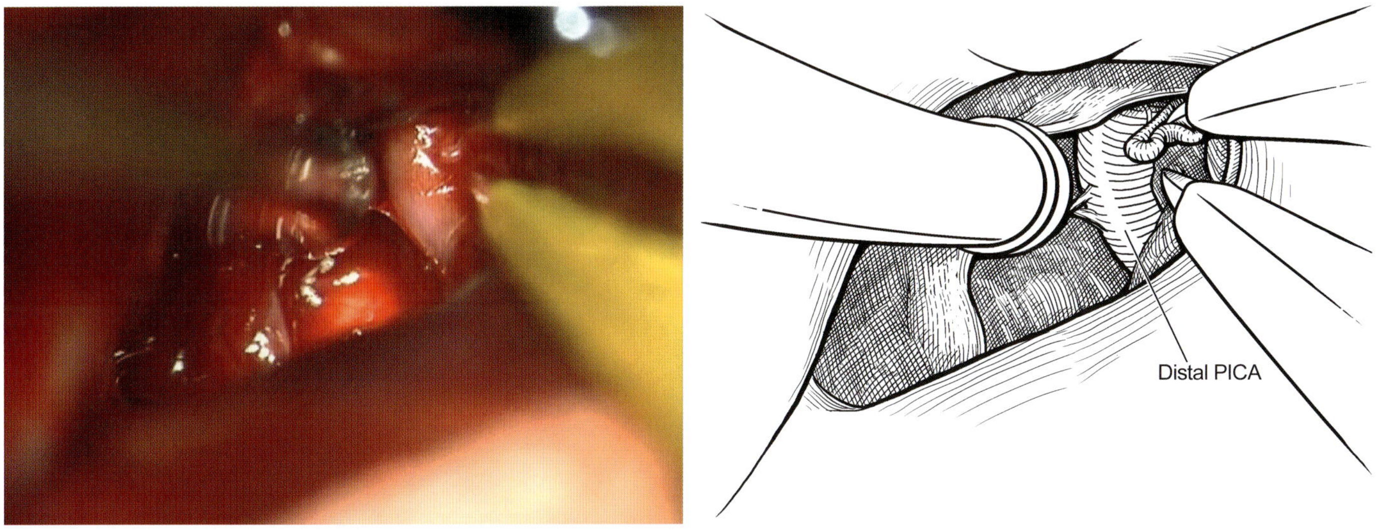

Fig. 14.3i The distal portion of the PICA is identified.

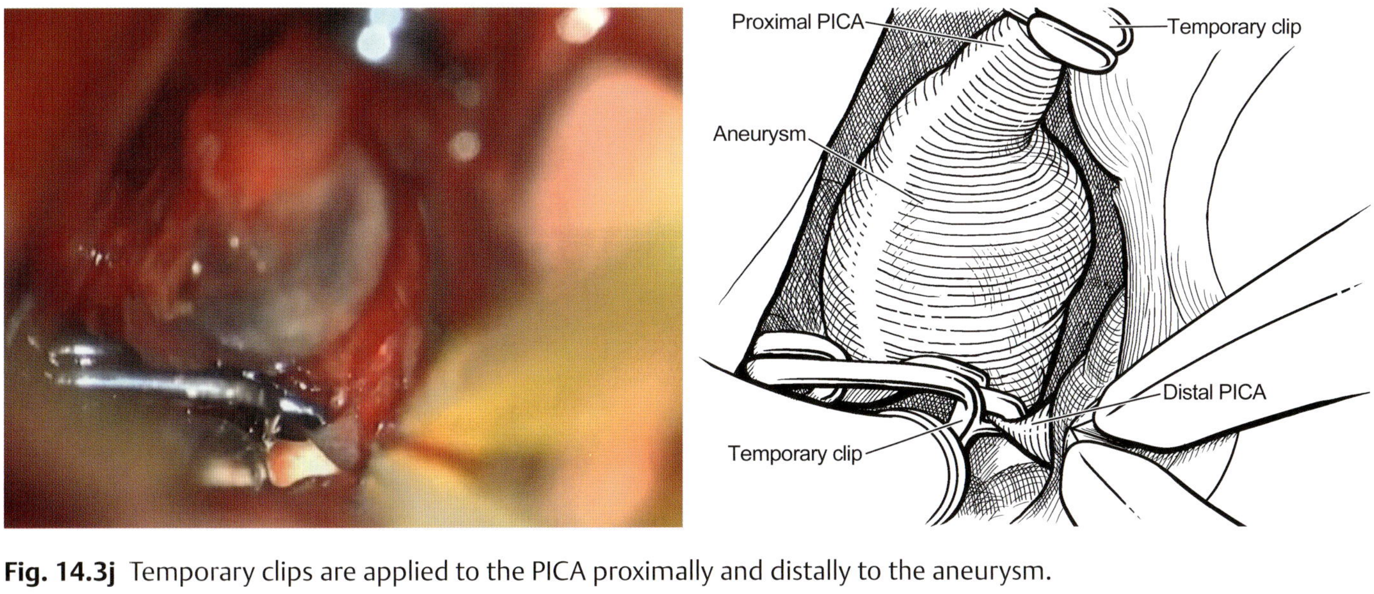

Fig. 14.3j Temporary clips are applied to the PICA proximally and distally to the aneurysm.

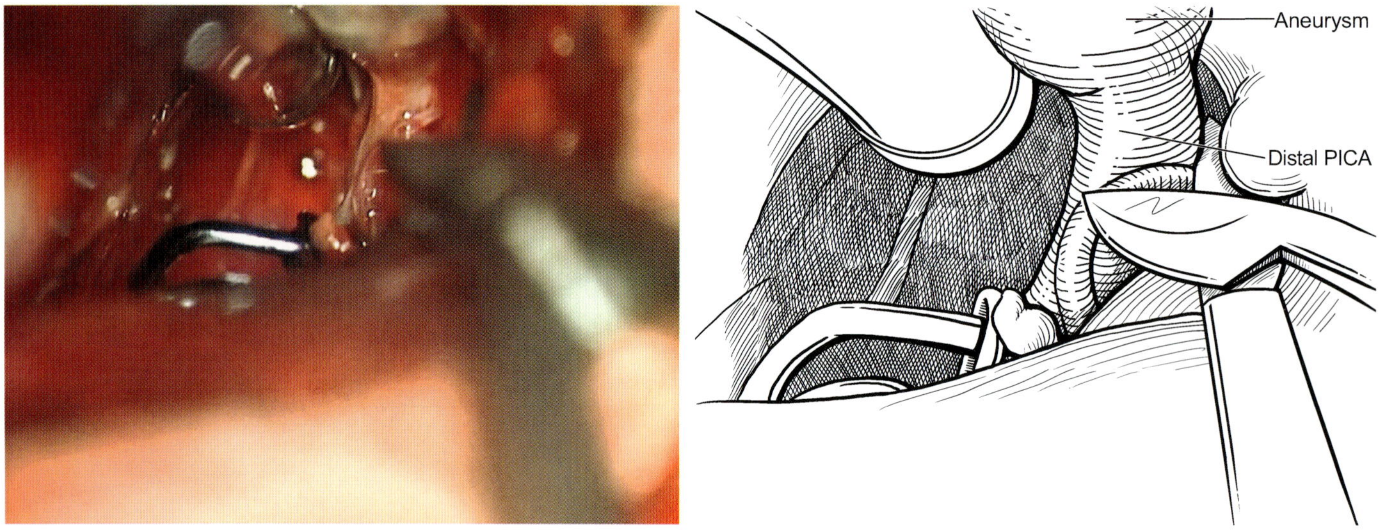

Fig. 14.3k The PICA is cut distal to the aneurysm.

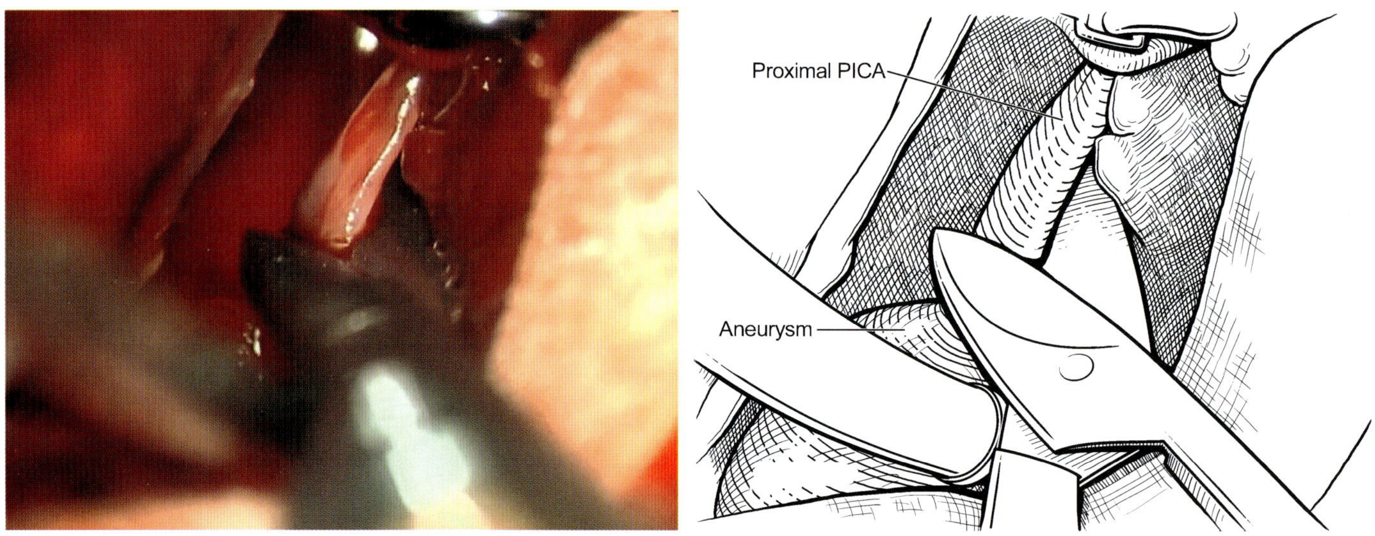

Fig. 14.3l The PICA is cut proximal to the aneurysm.

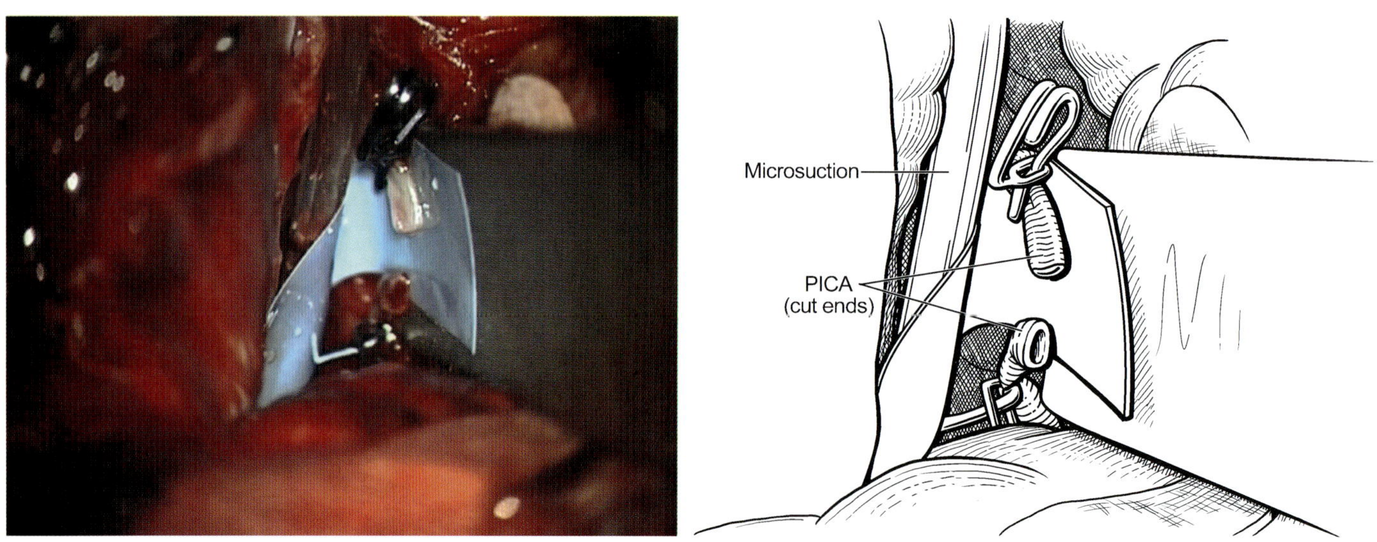

Fig. 14.3m The two cut ends of PICA are prepared for a direct end-to-end anastomosis.

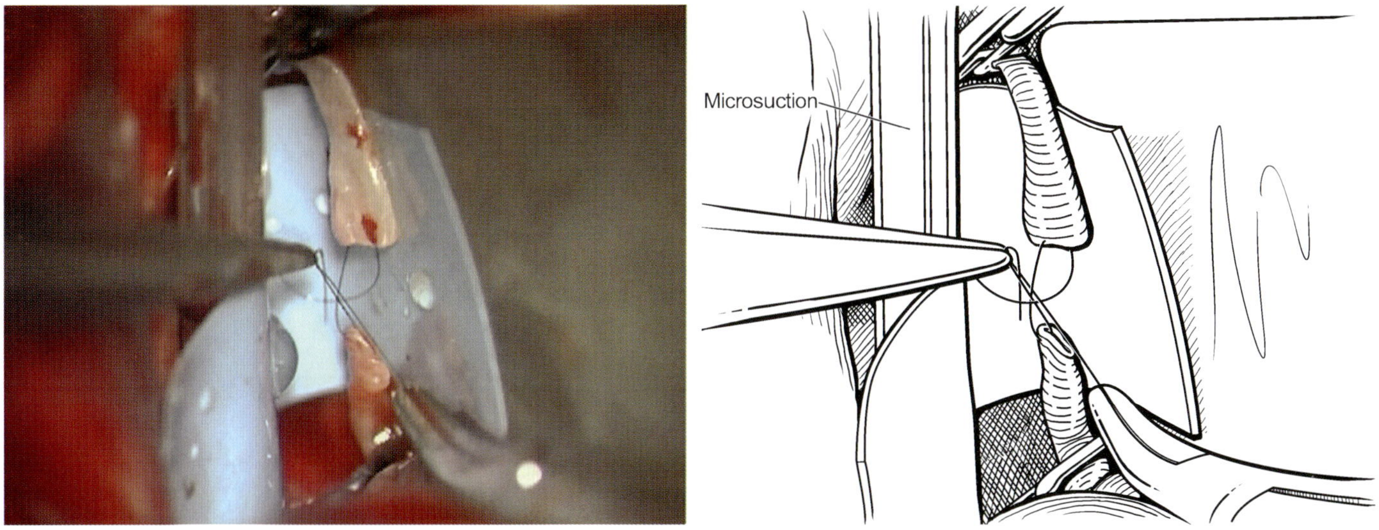

Fig. 14.3n The first stitch is placed.

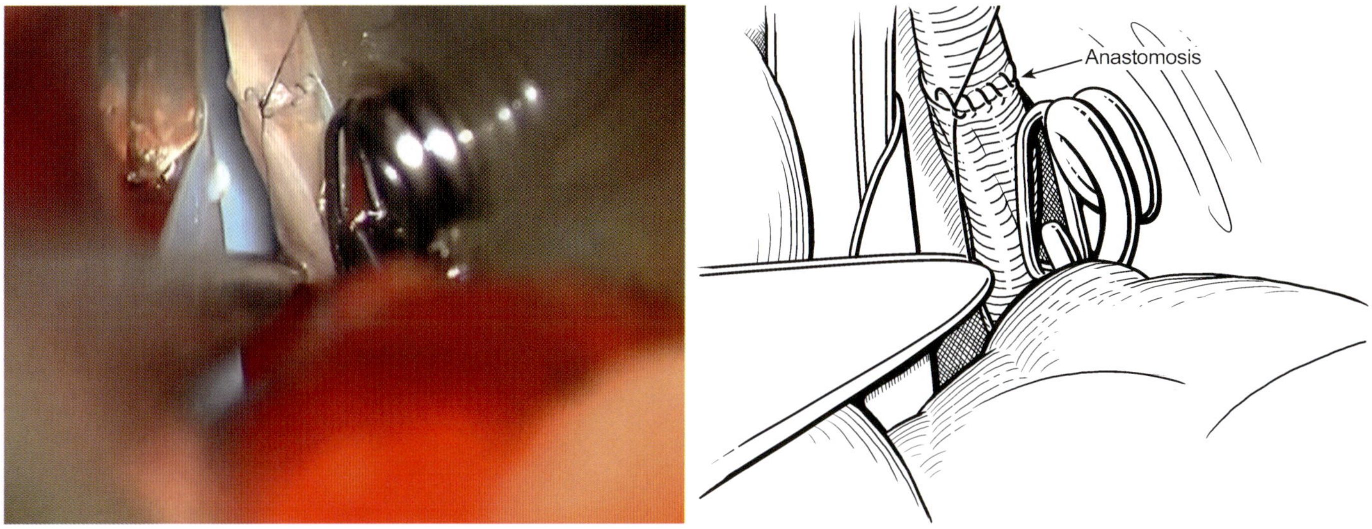

Fig. 14.3o The anastomosis is almost complete.

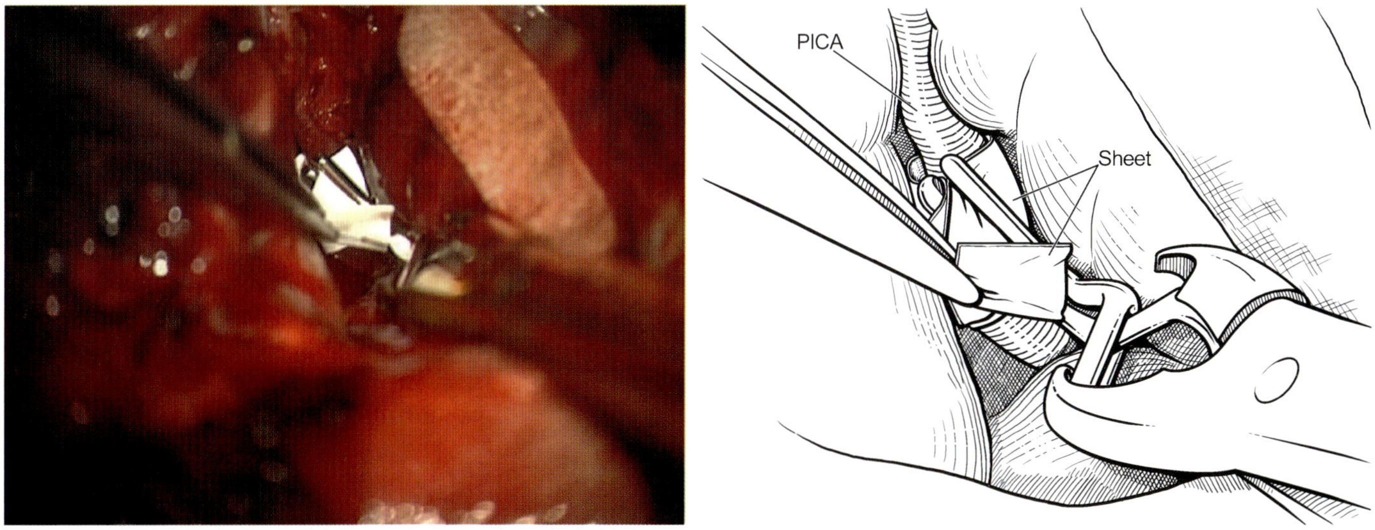

Fig. 14.3p A polytetrafluoroethylene sheet is placed around the anastomosis to prevent further dissection of the abnormal PICA.

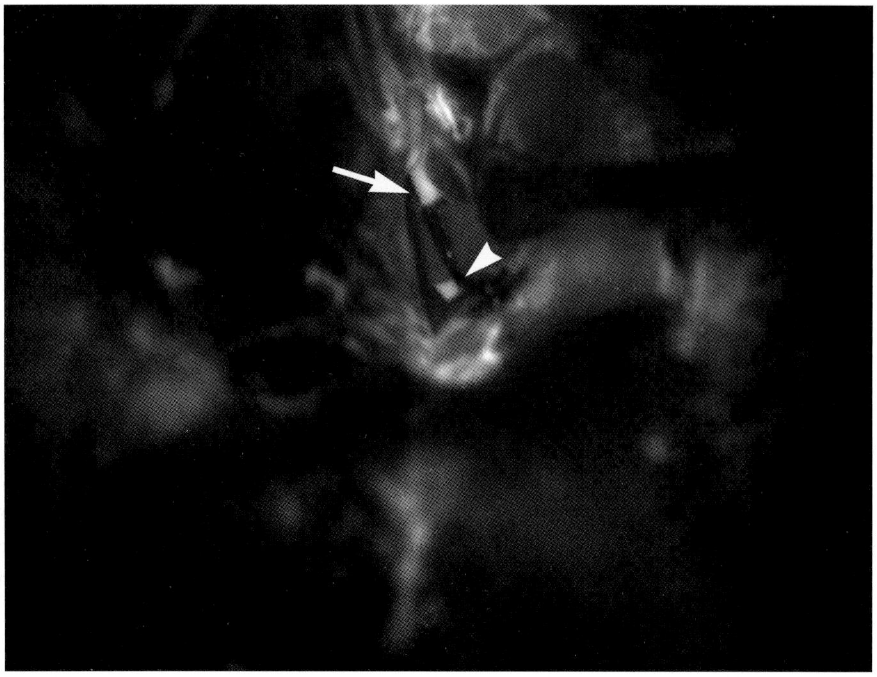

Fig. 14.3q ICG angiogram shows the patency of the bypass proximal (*arrow*) and distal *(arrowhead)* to the wrapping.

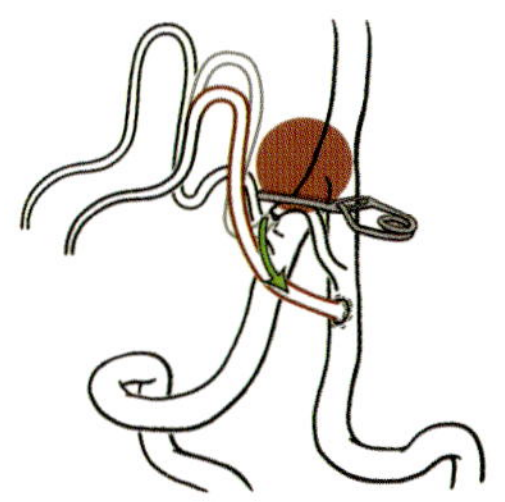

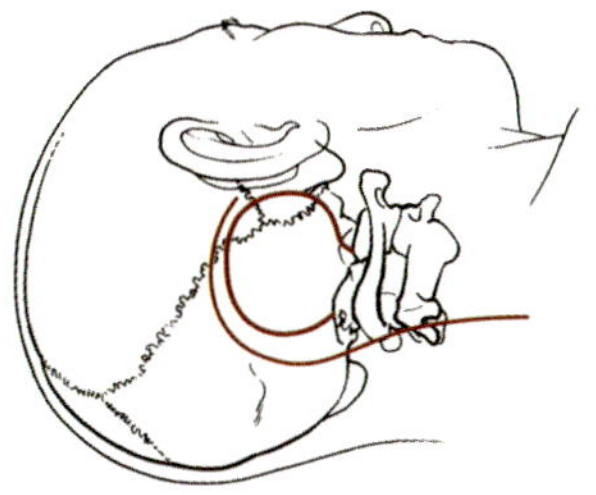

Case 14-4

Diagnosis: Previously coiled, large recurrent right PICA aneurysm

Bypass: PICA-to-VA direct reanastomosis

Approach: Right far lateral

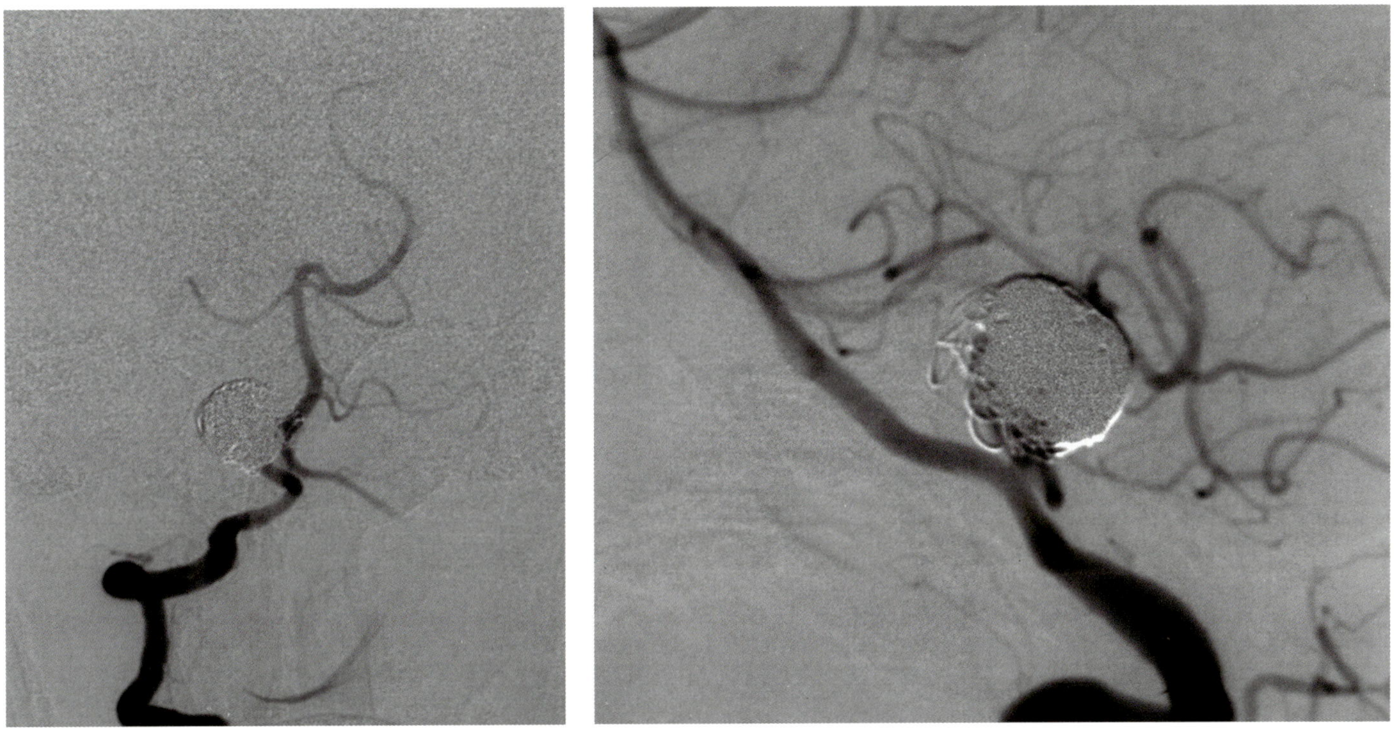

a b

Fig. 14.4a, b Anteroposterior and lateral VA angiograms show a successfully coiled PICA aneurysm.

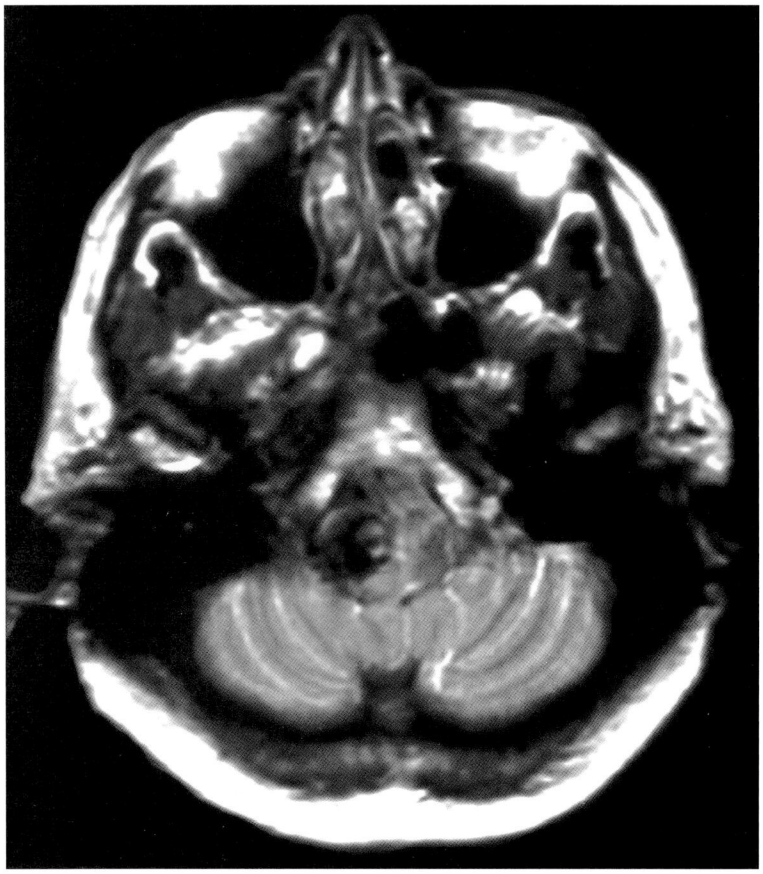

Fig. 14.4c CT scan shows the coiled aneurysm with some regrowth.

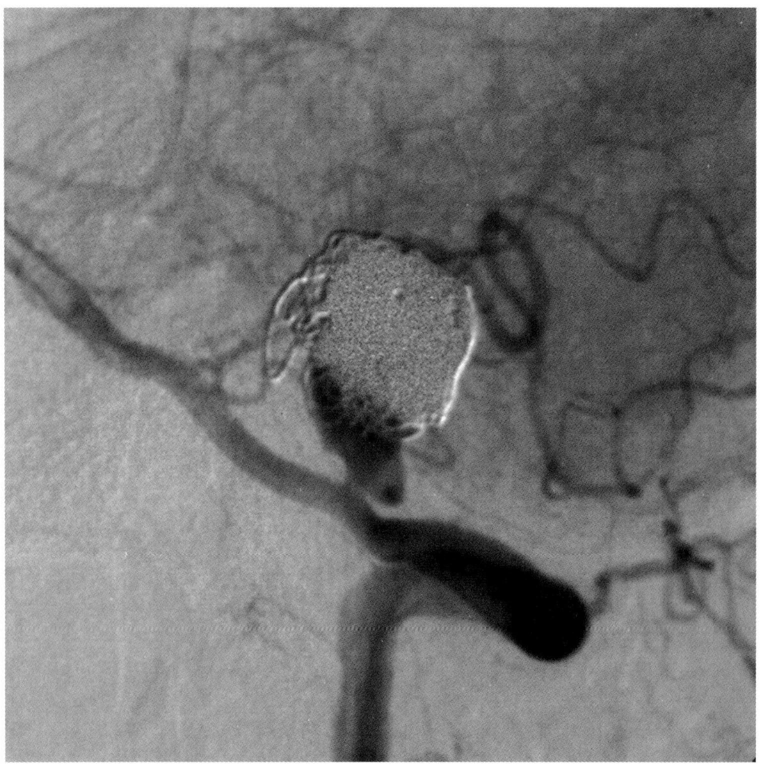

Fig. 14.4d Angiogram performed a year later showed regrowth at the base of the aneurysm. The patient had recurrent symptoms of brainstem compression.

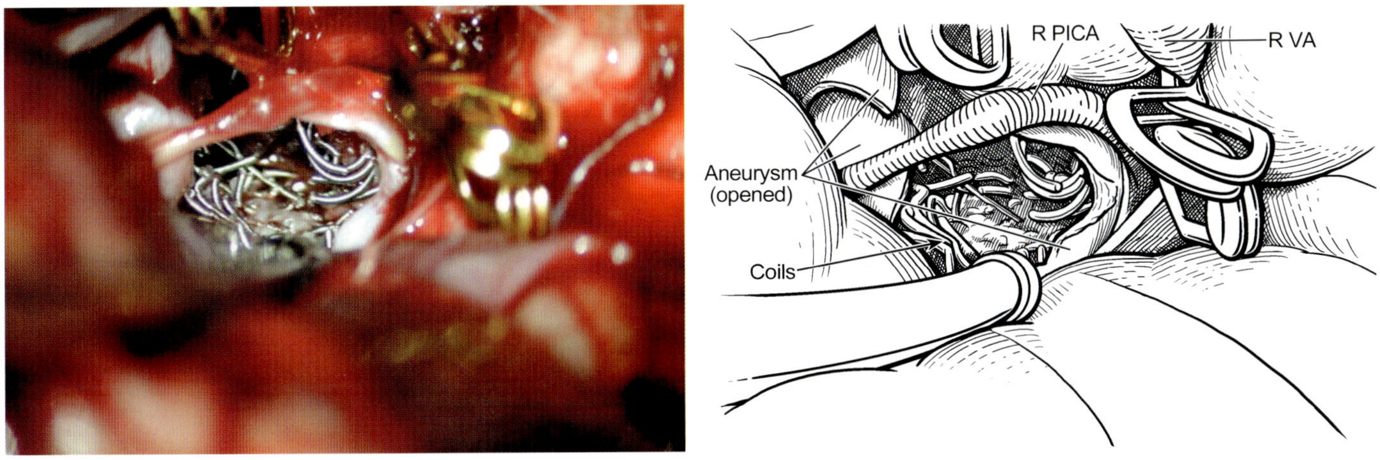

Fig. 14.4e Operative view shows the PICA and the opened aneurysm with the compacted coils. Temporary clips have been placed on the VA proximal and distal to the PICA.

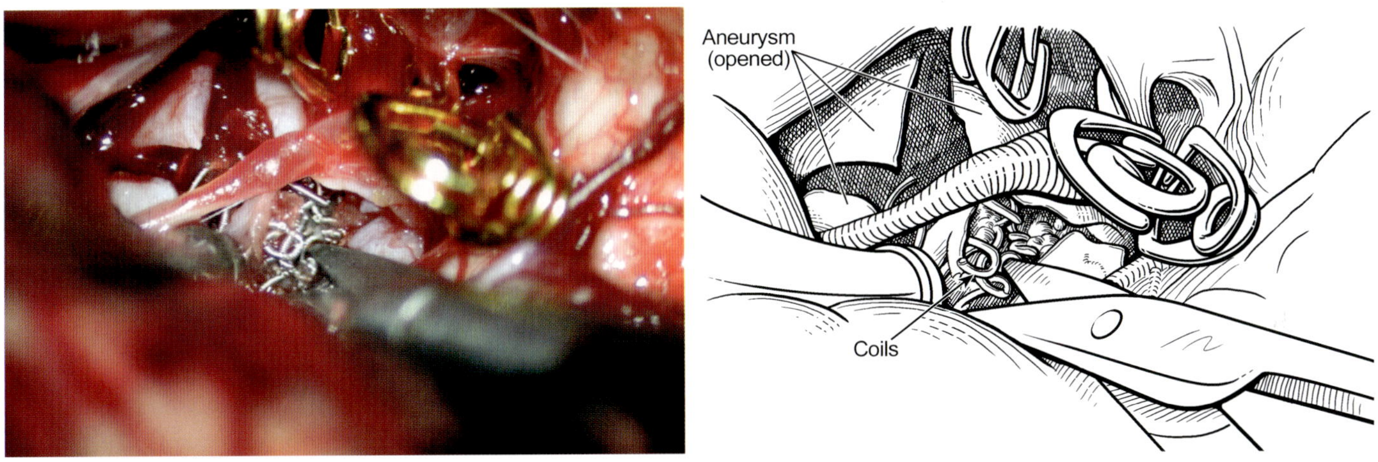

Fig. 14.4f The coils are cut with microscissors.

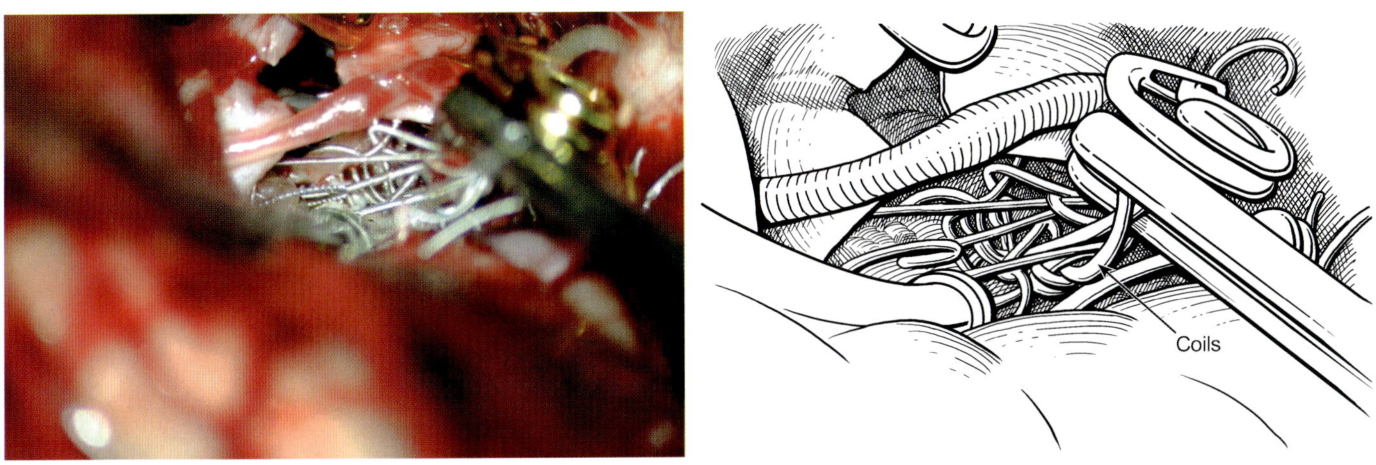

Fig. 14.4g Coils are removed to provide sufficient room for primary clipping.

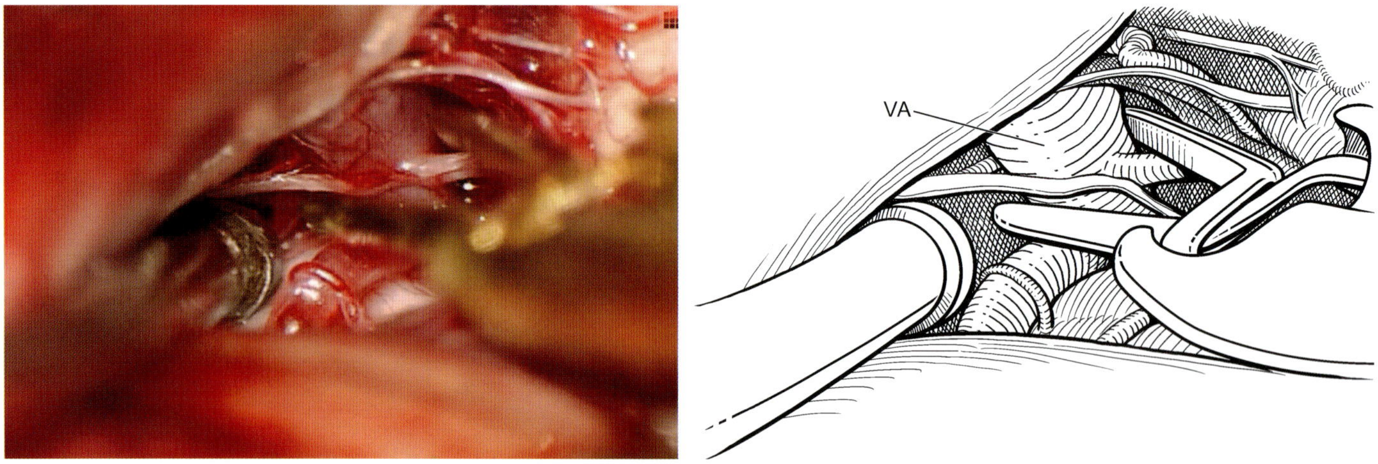

Fig. 14.4h A temporary clip is removed from the VA. At this point, there was significant hemorrhage from the base of the aneurysm because the permanent clip at its base had ruptured the neck of the aneurysm from the VA.

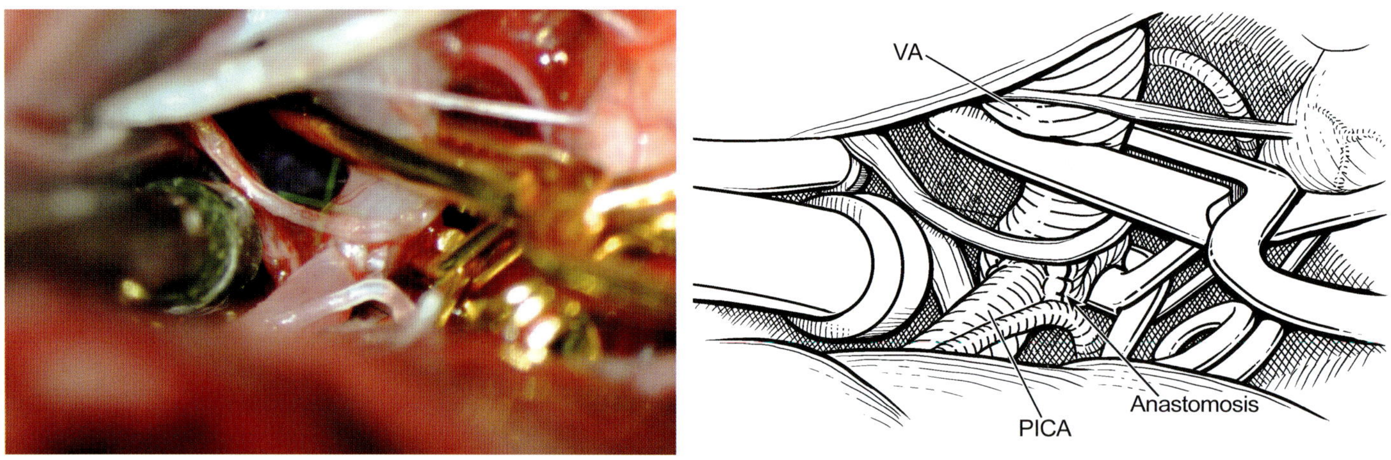

Fig. 14.4i The PICA has been removed distal to the aneurysm and reimplanted onto the VA.

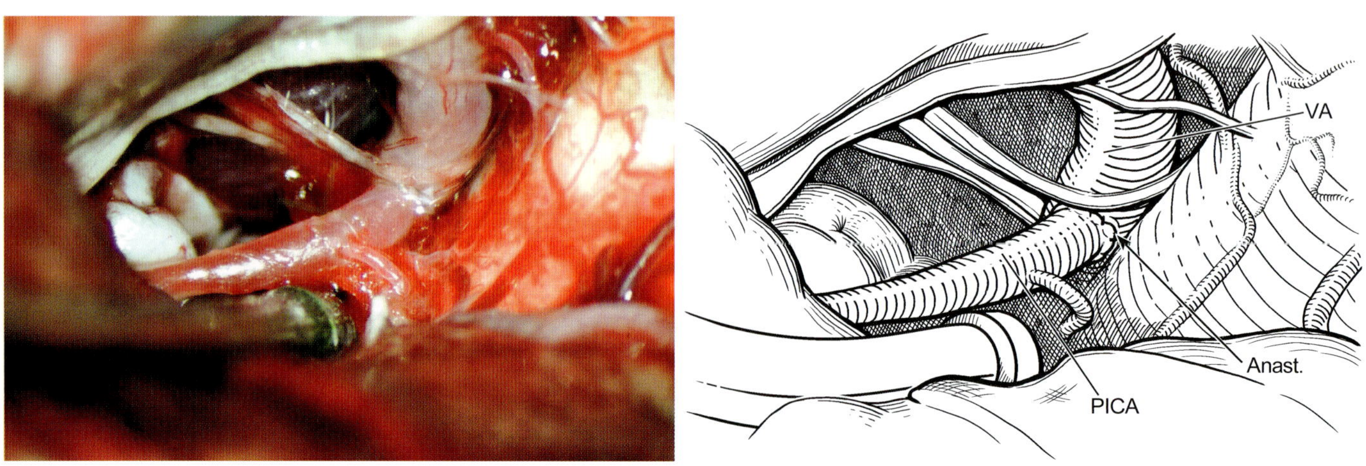

Fig. 14.4j Completed reimplantation of PICA to the VA.

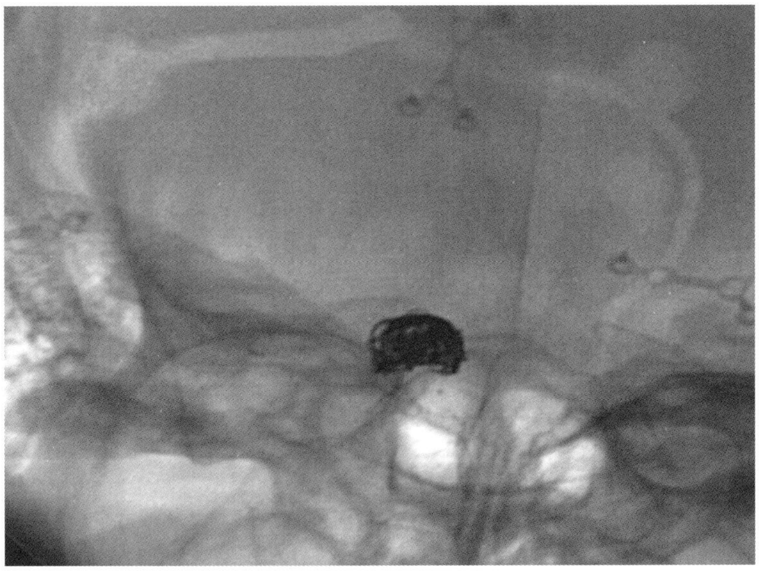

Fig. 14.4k Postoperative anteroposterior angiogram shows the residual coil mass.

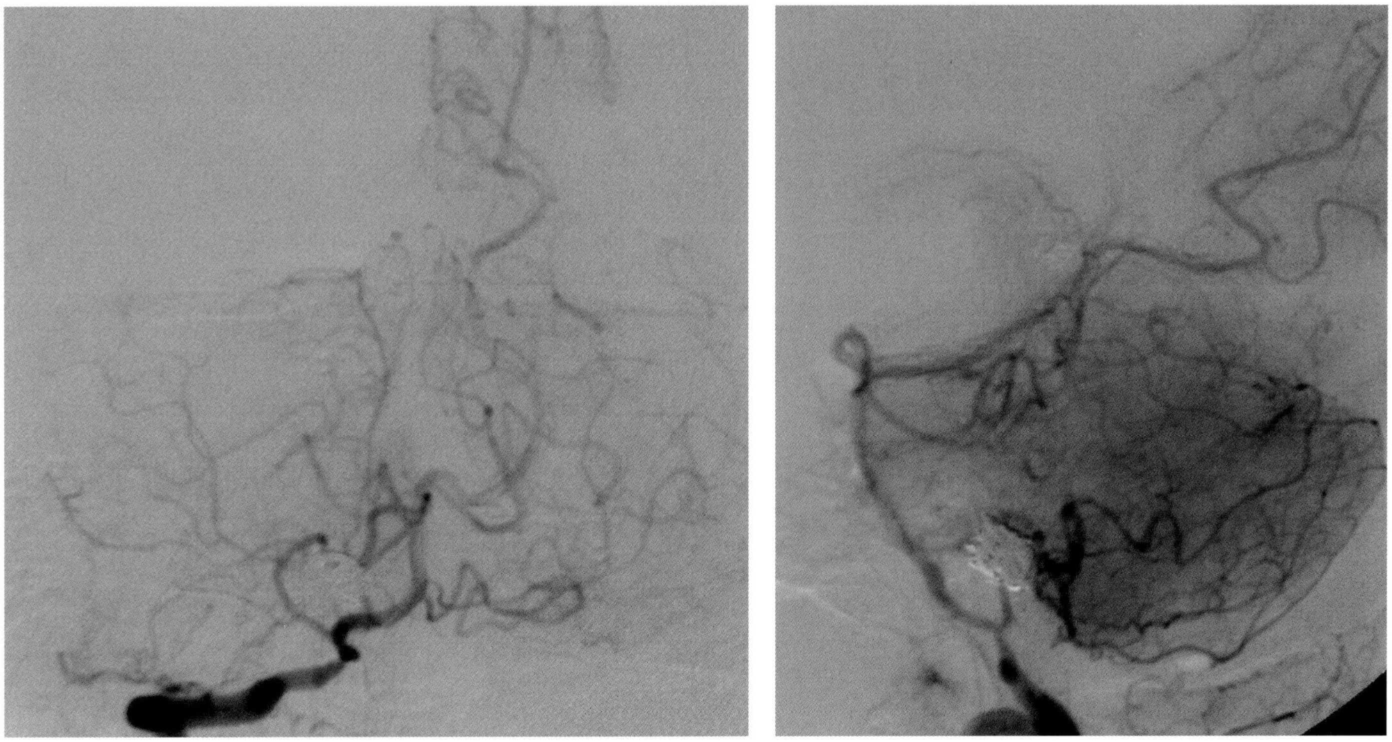

l m

Fig. 14.4l, m Anteroposterior and lateral angiographic views show excellent filling of the PICA reimplanted onto the VA.

15 FA-to-VA Bypass

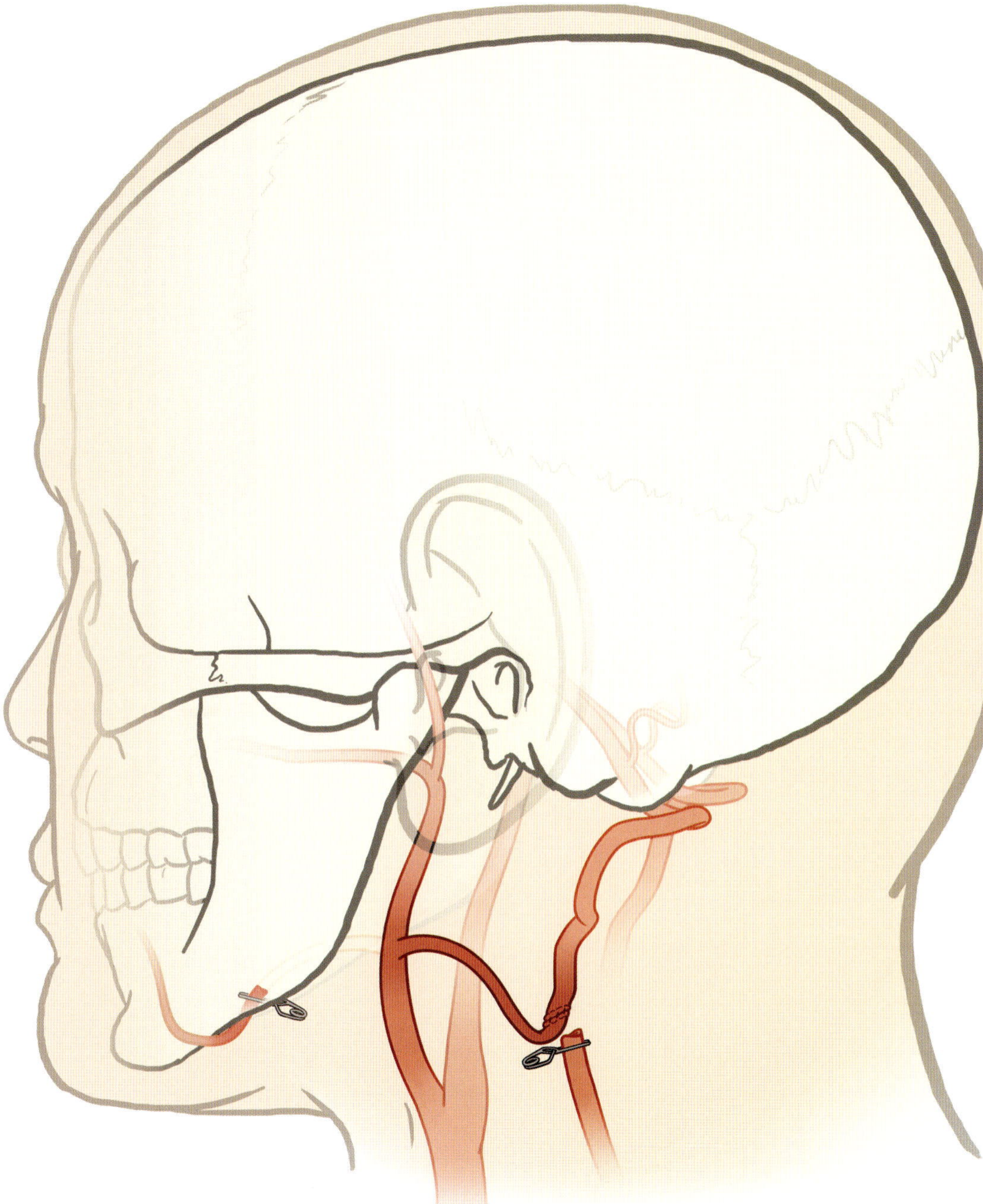

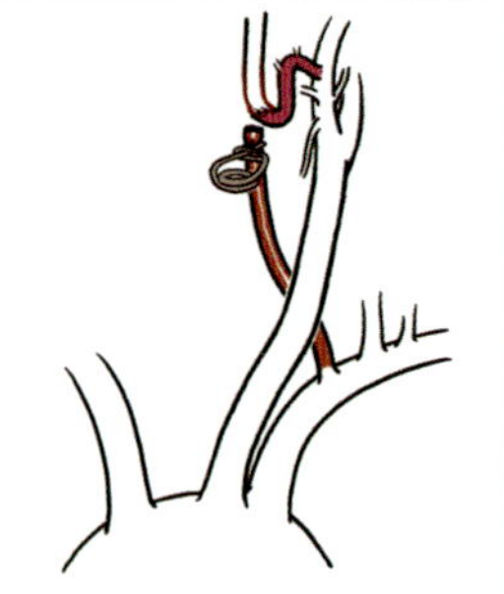

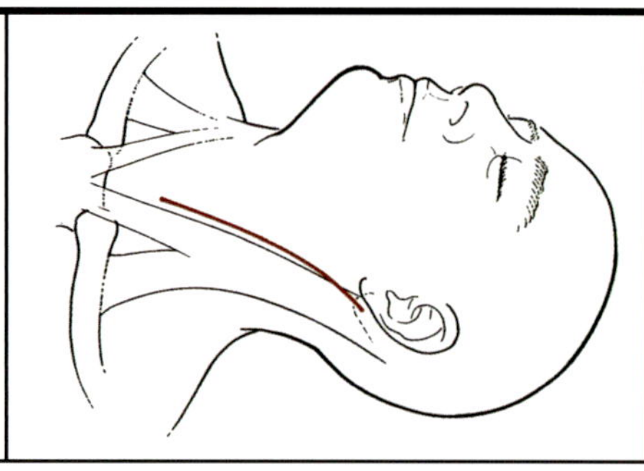

Case 15-1

Diagnosis: VA insufficiency

Bypass: FA-to-VA

Approach: Left anterior cervical

▶ Video

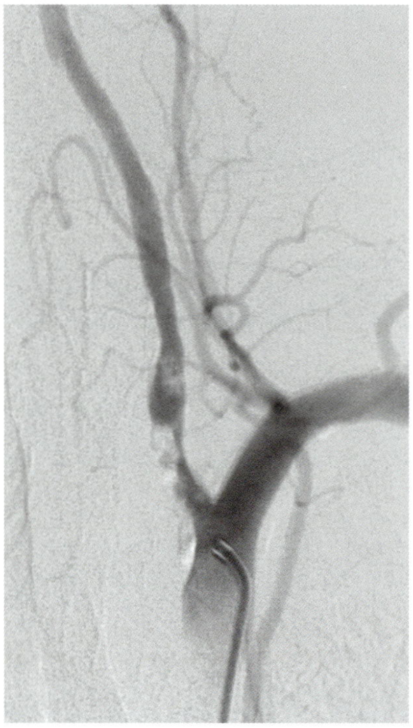

Fig. 15.1a Angiogram of a 56-year-old man who developed VA insufficiency shows occlusion of his right VA and severe stenosis of his left VA.

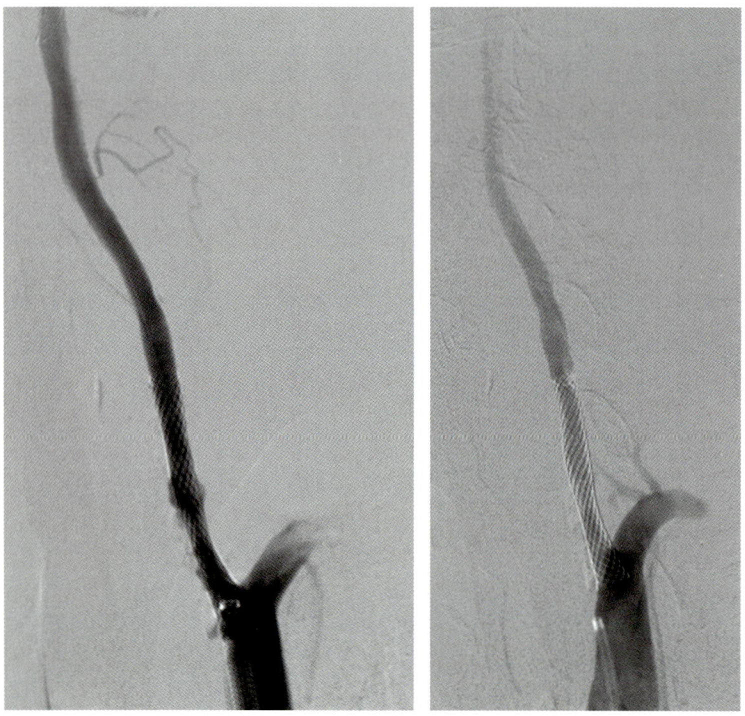

b,c

Fig. 15.1b, c Angioplasty was performed, followed by stenting, and his symptoms resolved.

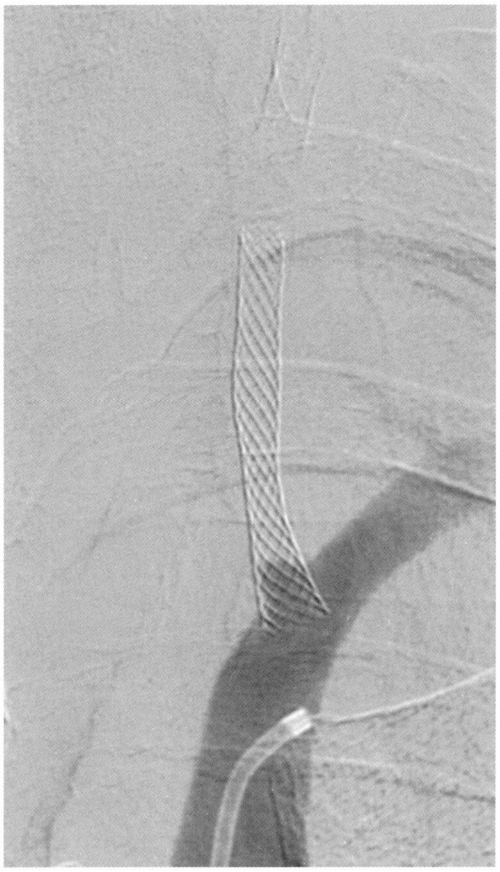

Fig. 15.1d After a new onset of VA insufficiency, a repeat angiogram showed occlusion of the VA.

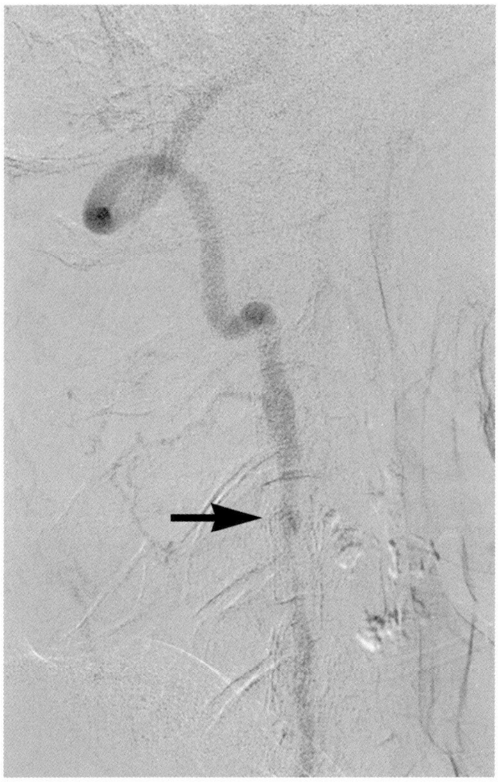

Fig. 15.1e Late-phase angiogram showing flow in distal VA after the VA was reconstituted (*arrow*) through small branches from the ECA.

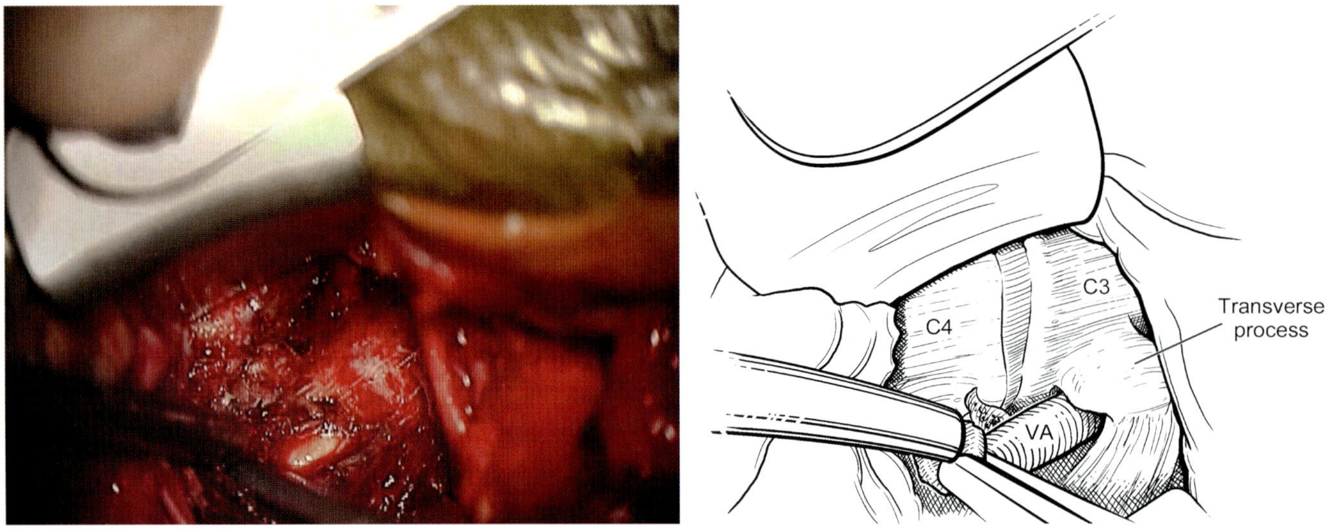

Fig. 15.1f The left VA is exposed in the transverse foramen at the level of C3-C4.

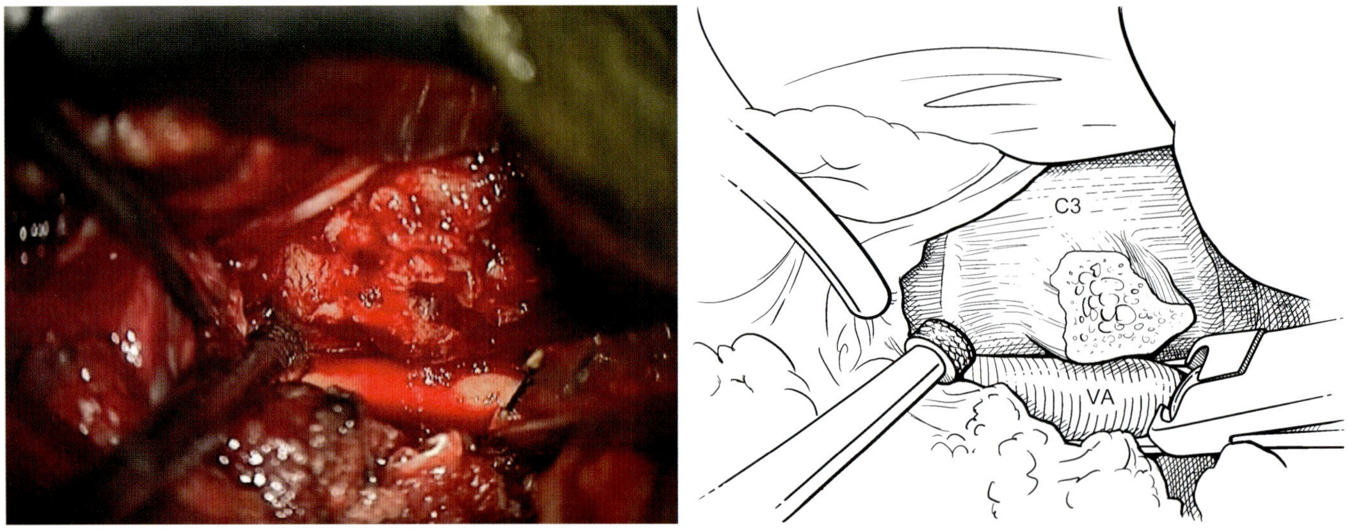

Fig. 15.1g The exposure of the VA is extended and a temporary clip is placed on the superior end of the segment.

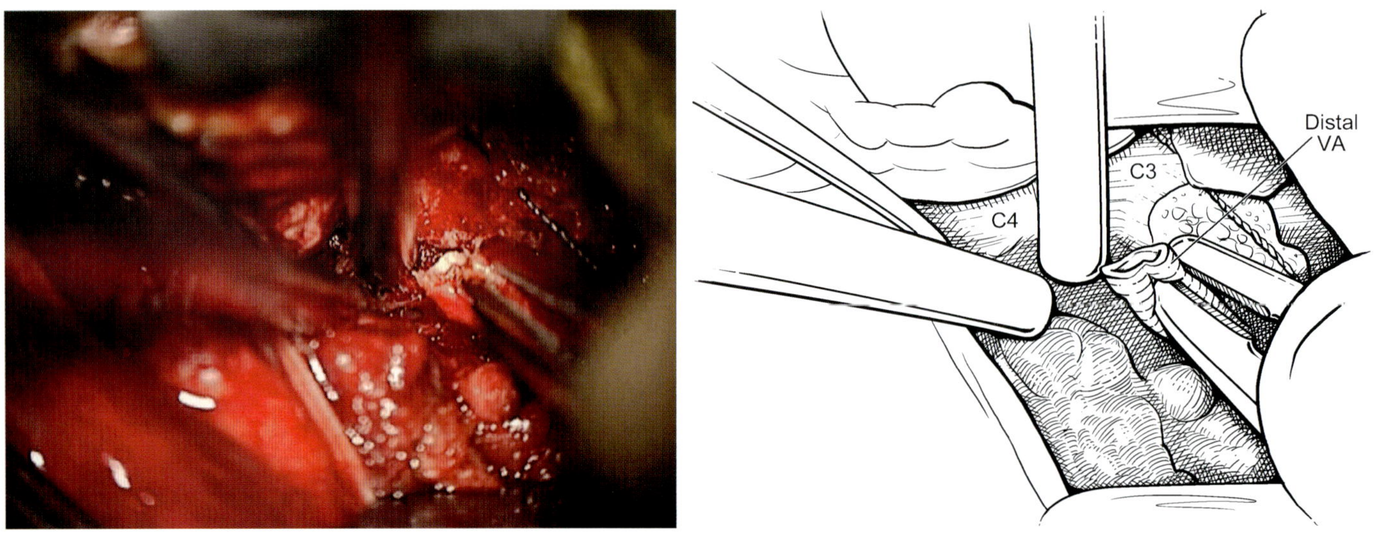

Fig. 15.1h The VA is divided at the inferior end of the exposure.

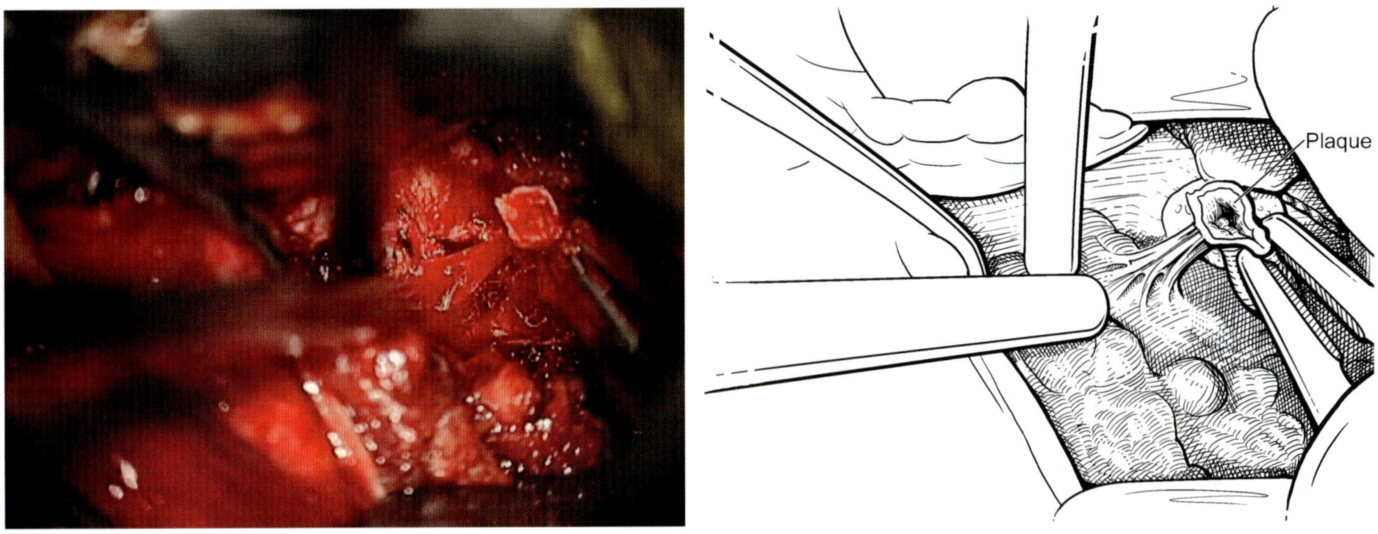

Fig. 15.1i The VA is mobilized superiorly. Plaque limits backflow.

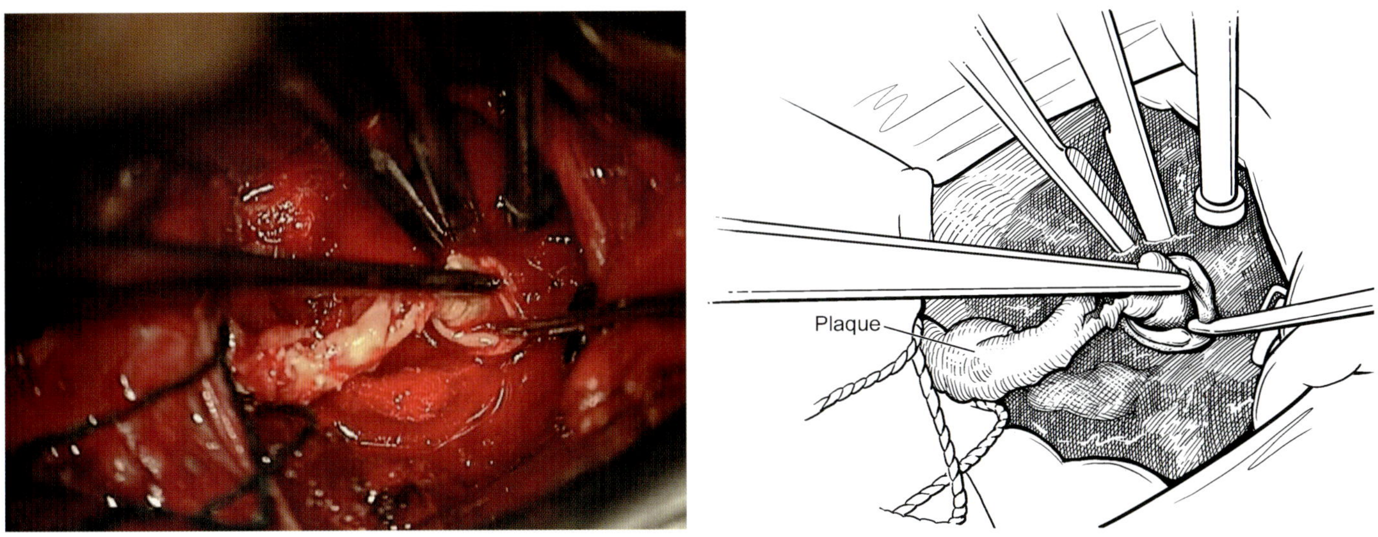

Fig. 15.1j An endarterectomy is performed.

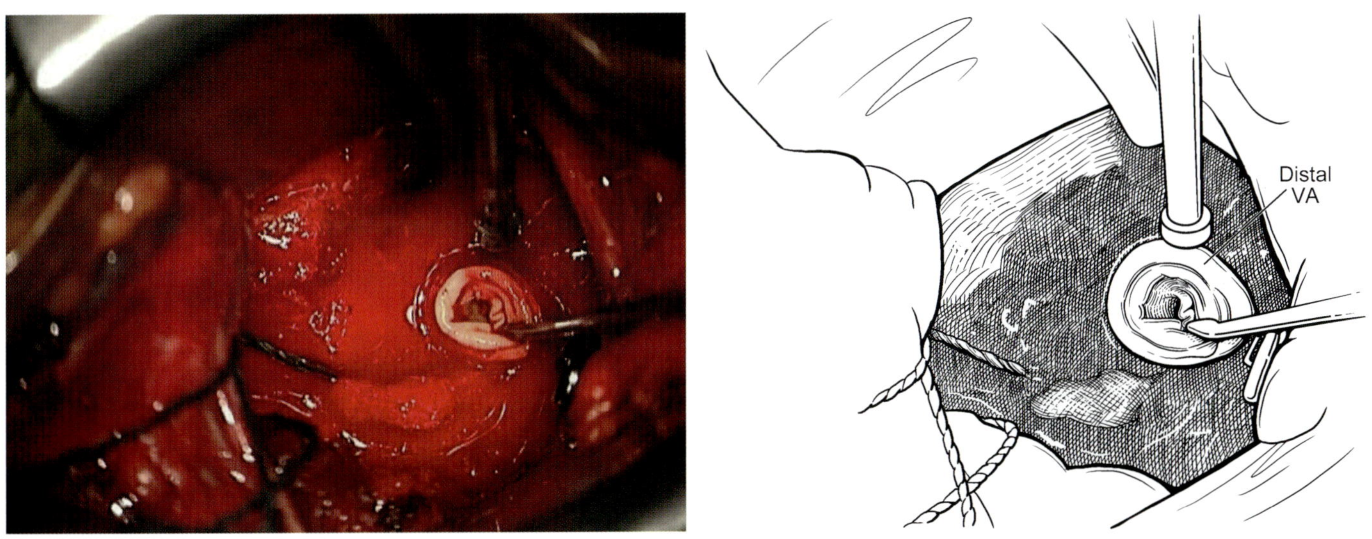

Fig. 15.1k After the endarterectomy is performed, the cut end of the VA is visible. Blood now backflows freely.

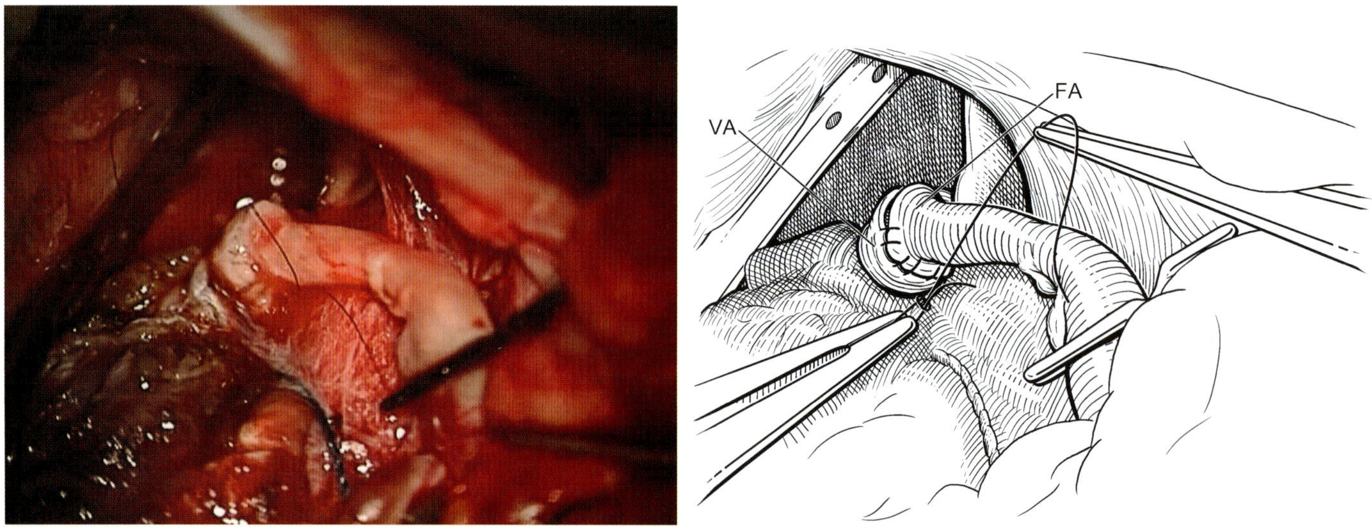

Fig. 15.1l The left facial artery was identified at its origin on the ECA, clipped distally, and cut. It was anastomosed directly to the distal portion of the VA.

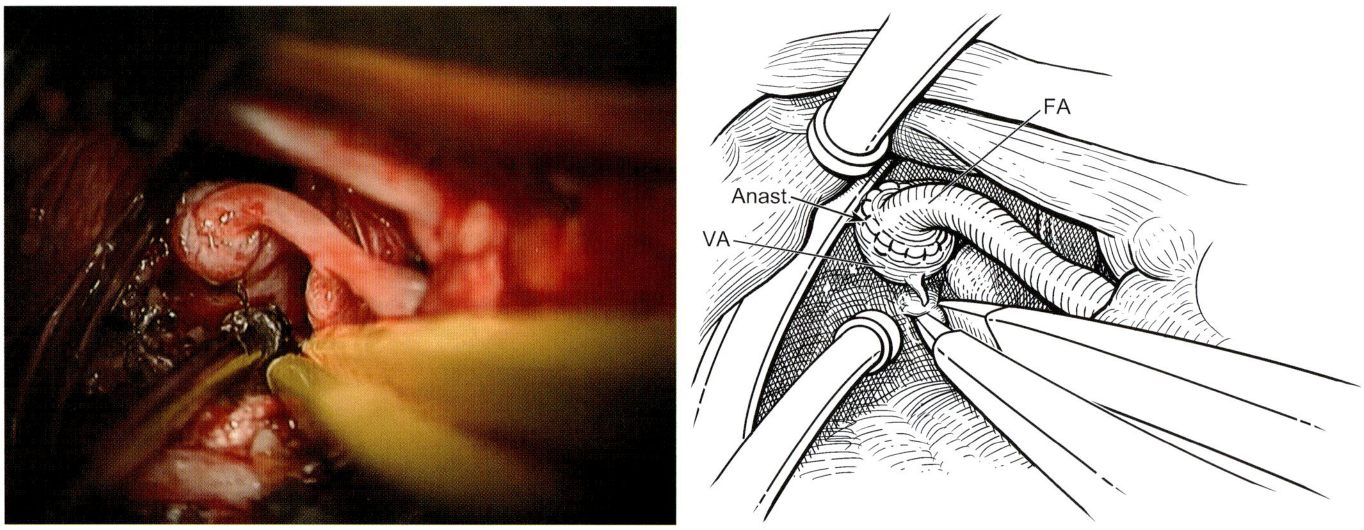

Fig. 15.1m The anastomosis is complete.

n

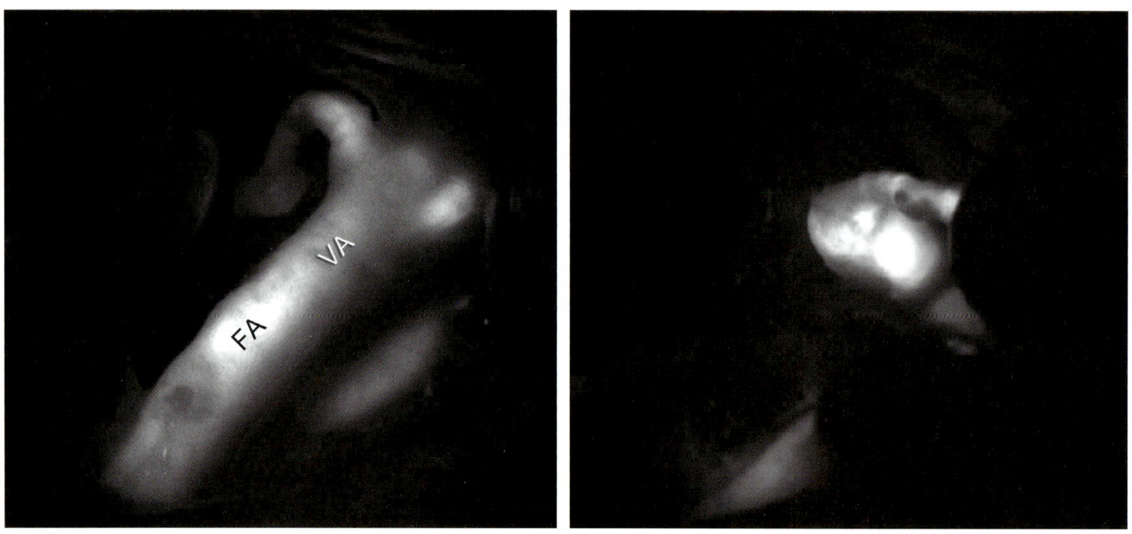

o

Fig. 15.1n, o Intraoperative ICG angiograms confirm the patency of the facial artery-to-VA anastomosis.

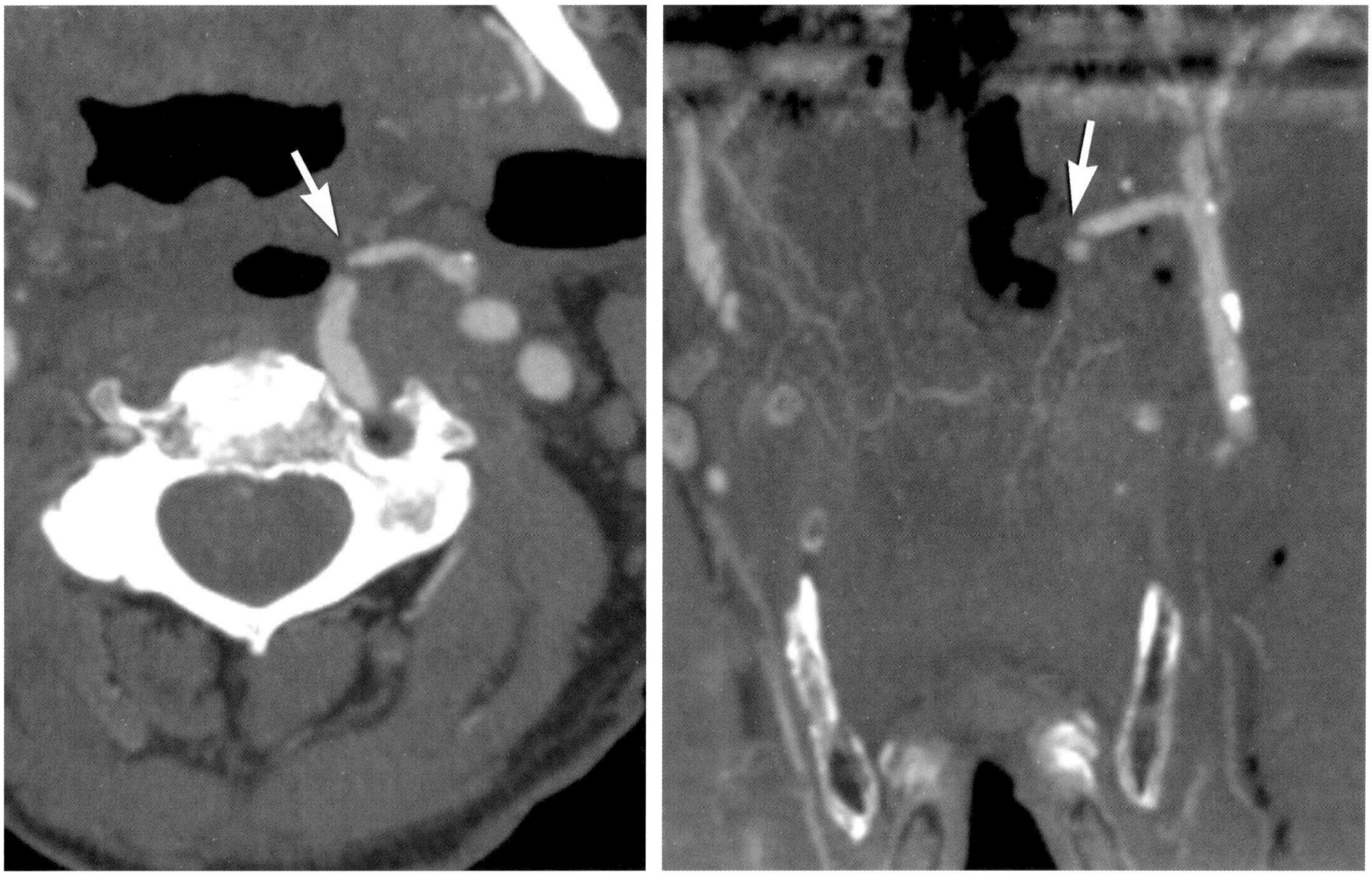

p q

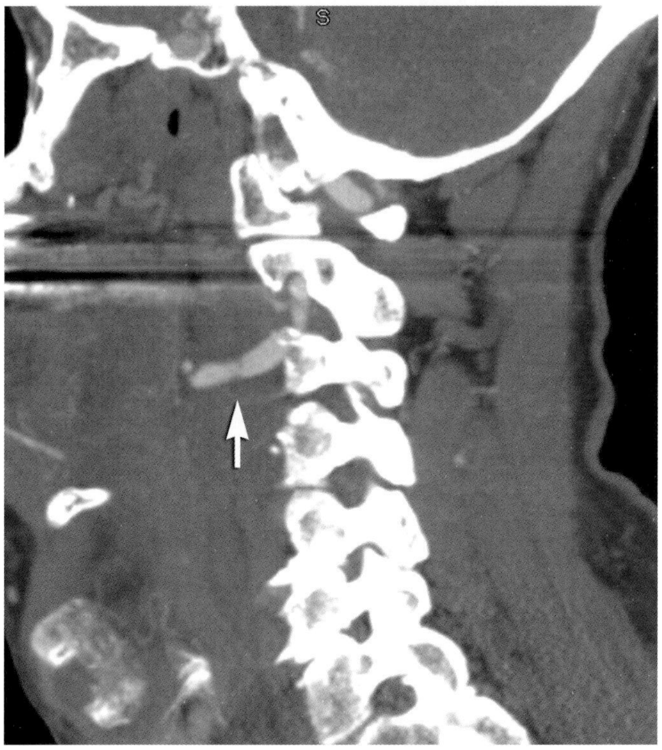

r

Fig. 15.1p–r CT angiograms at different phases confirm patency of the bypass (*arrows*).

16 VA Reconstruction and VA-to-CCA Transposition

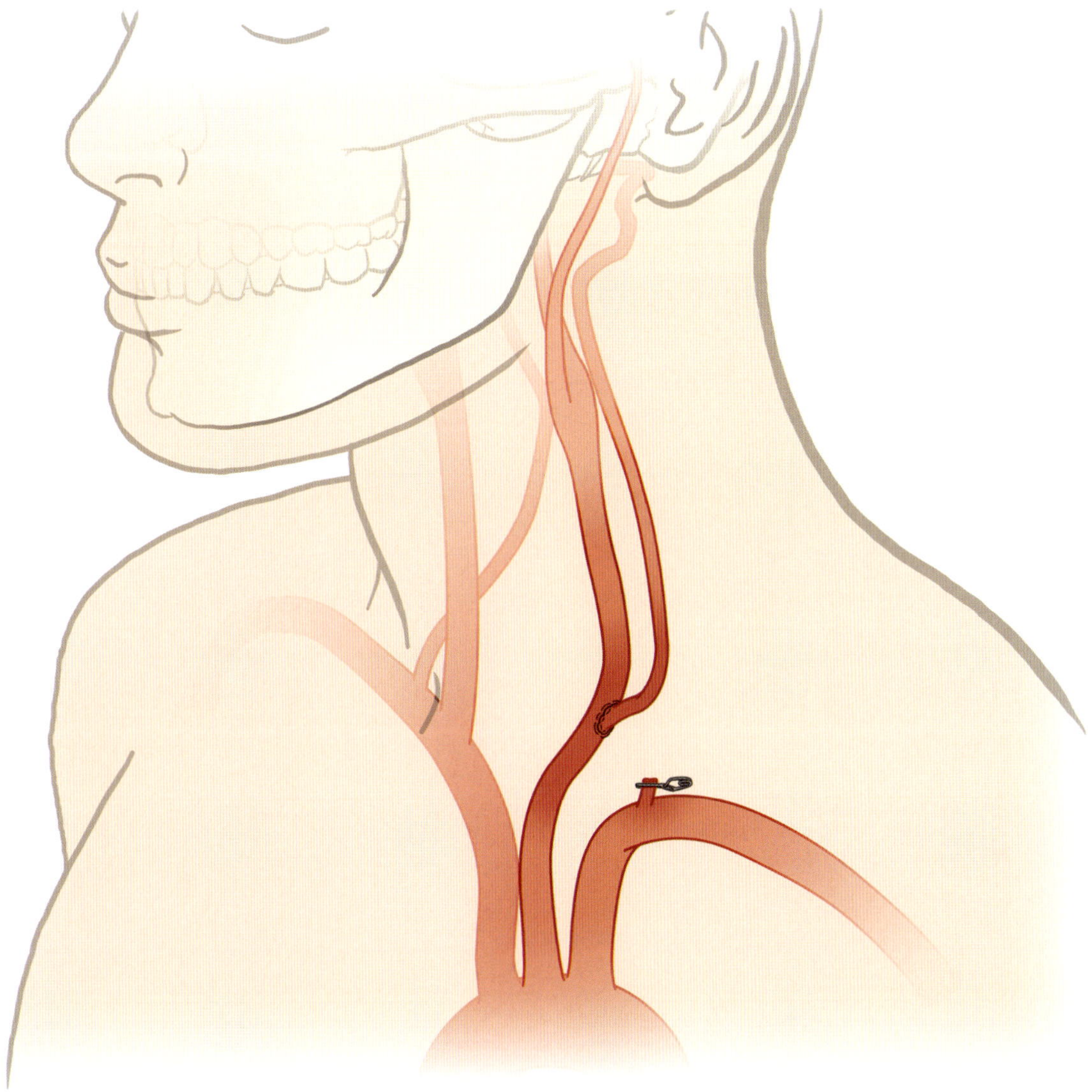

A VA-to-CCA transposition is an excellent way to achieve blood flow in a VA with significant stenosis at its origin or in an occluded but patent VA. Almost the only time a patient has symptoms related to VA insufficiency is when the contralateral VA is vestigial entering the PICA or is occluded. The insufficiency can be exacerbated by rotation of the head, which compromises blood flow at C2-C1 and the skull base.

The subclavian artery is exposed through a transverse supraclavicular incision with a longitudinal extension along the CCA. If further length is needed, the VA is exposed and freed from its bony canal. After the CCA is occluded proximally and distally, the artery is opened with a vascular punch. An end-to-side anastomosis is created with the VA using 6–0 or 7–0 suture.

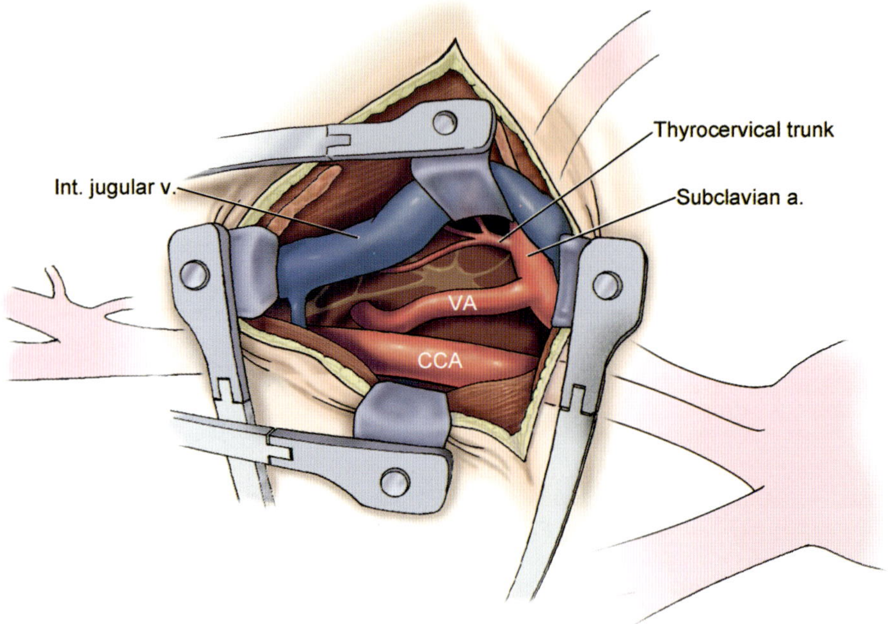

Fig. 16.0a Schematic representation of a supraclavicular exposure shows the CCA and VA along with the subclavian artery and its branches.

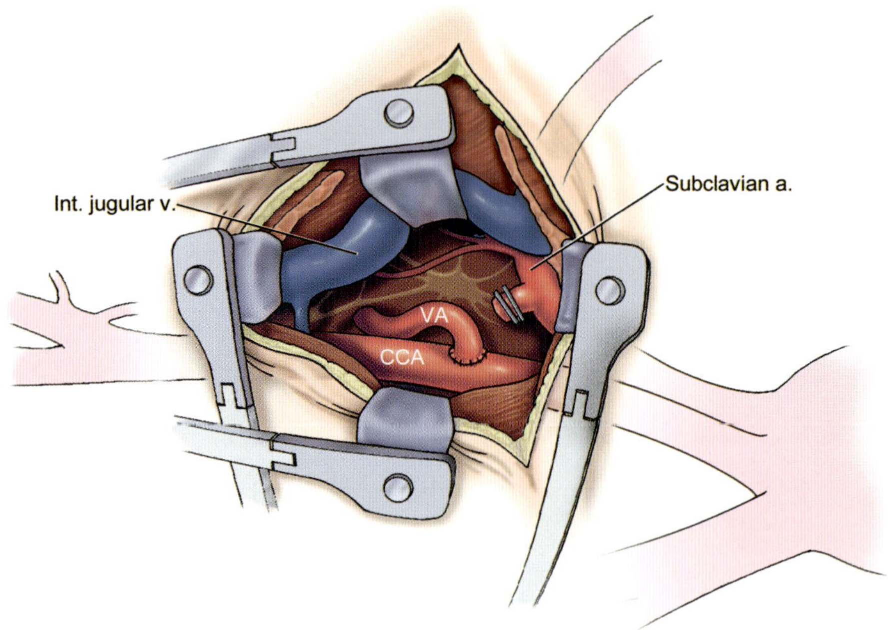

Fig. 16.0b Schematic representation of the completed VA-to-CCA transposition. (Used with permission from *Journal of Neurosurgery*.)

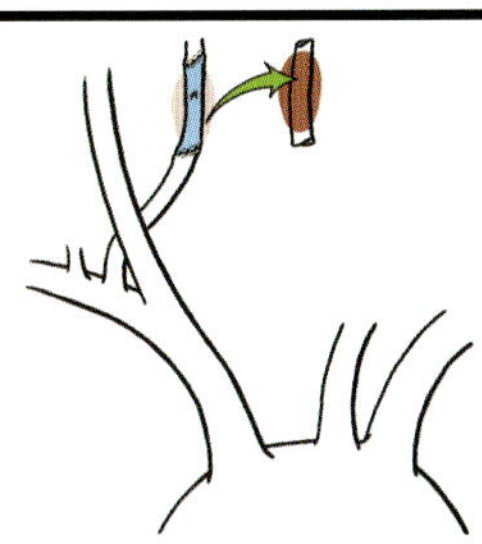

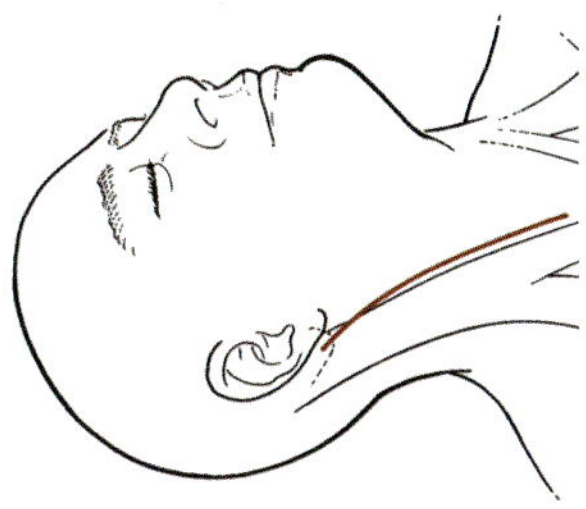

Case 16-1

Diagnosis: Traumatic dissection of right VA at C6

Bypass: Direct VA reconstruction with saphenous vein graft

Approach: Right anterior cervical

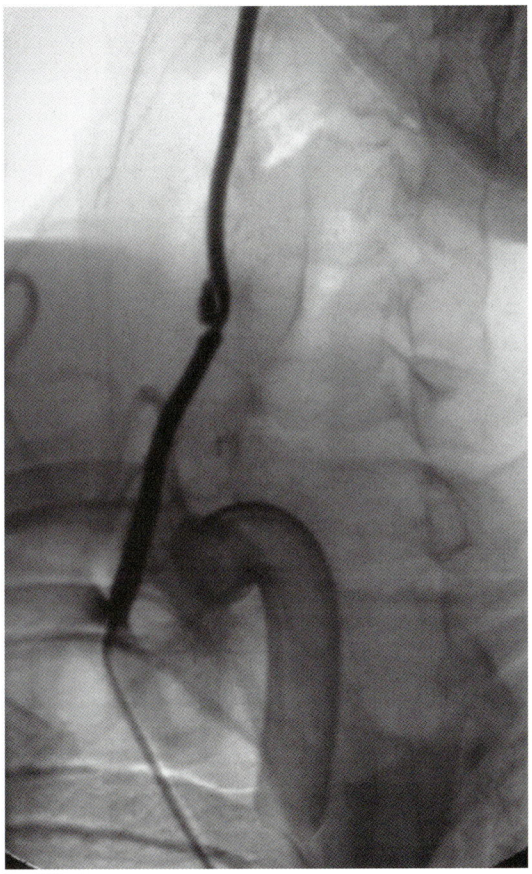

Fig. 16.1a Selective angiographic injection of the right VA shows a dissecting pseudoaneurysm at C6.

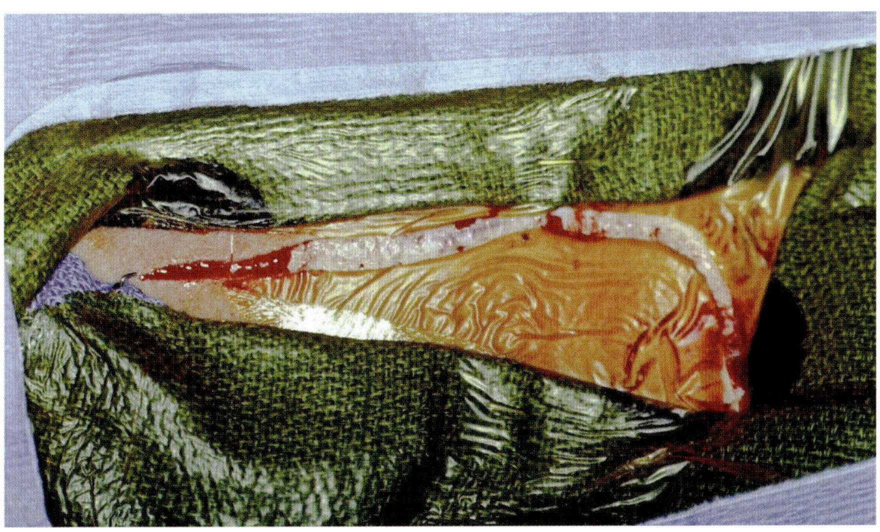

Fig. 16.1b A vertical incision is made along the anterior border of the SCM muscle.

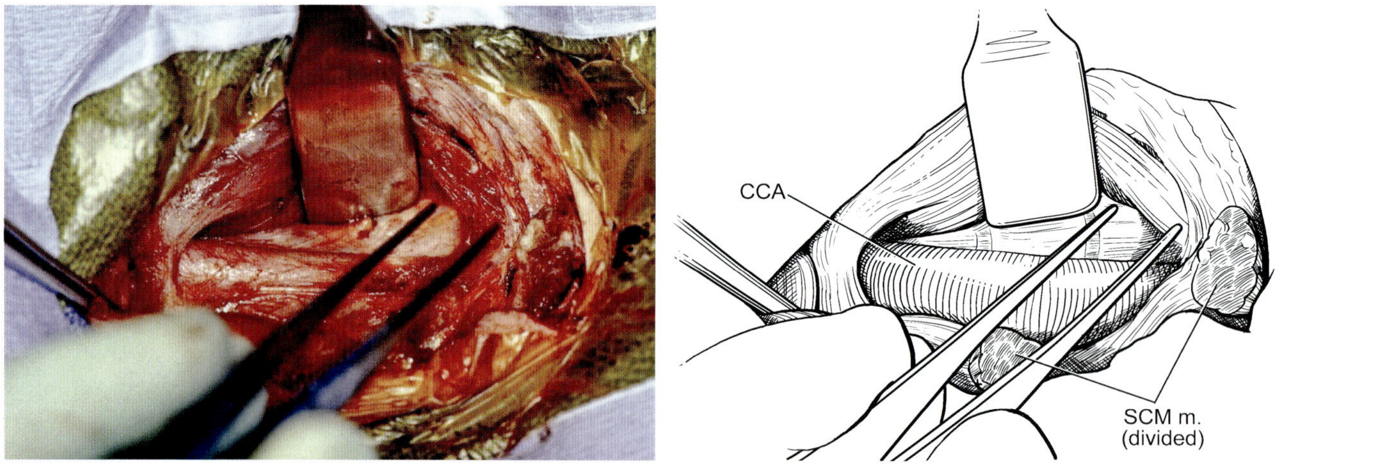

Fig. 16.1c The sternal head of the SCM muscle is divided between suture ligatures. Next, the omohyoid muscle is sectioned. The SCM muscle and carotid sheath are pushed laterally, and the esophagus and trachea are retracted medially.

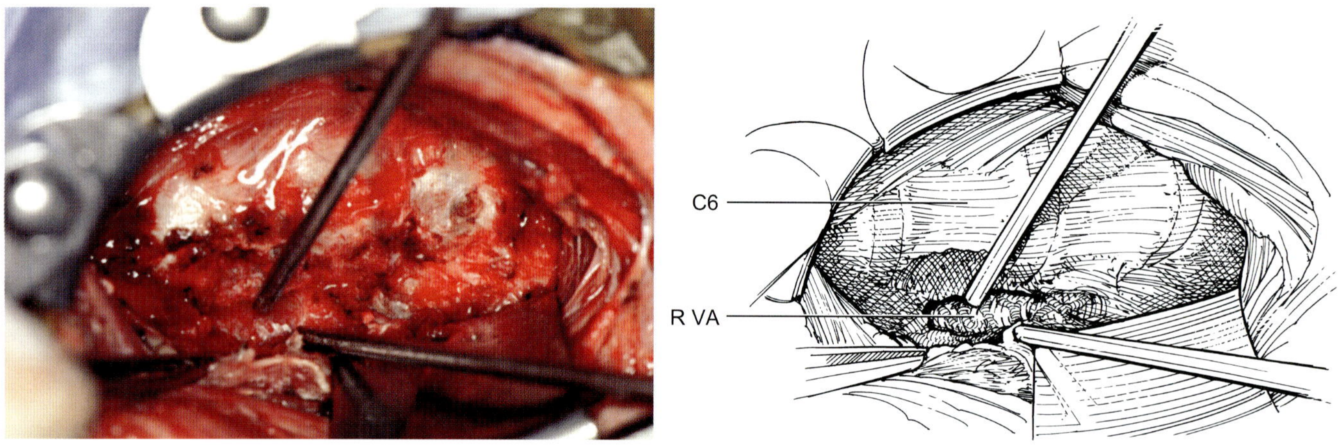

Fig. 16.1d The longus colli muscles are completely dissected from the transverse processes and the transverse foramina are drilled away. A venous plexus often surrounds the VA.

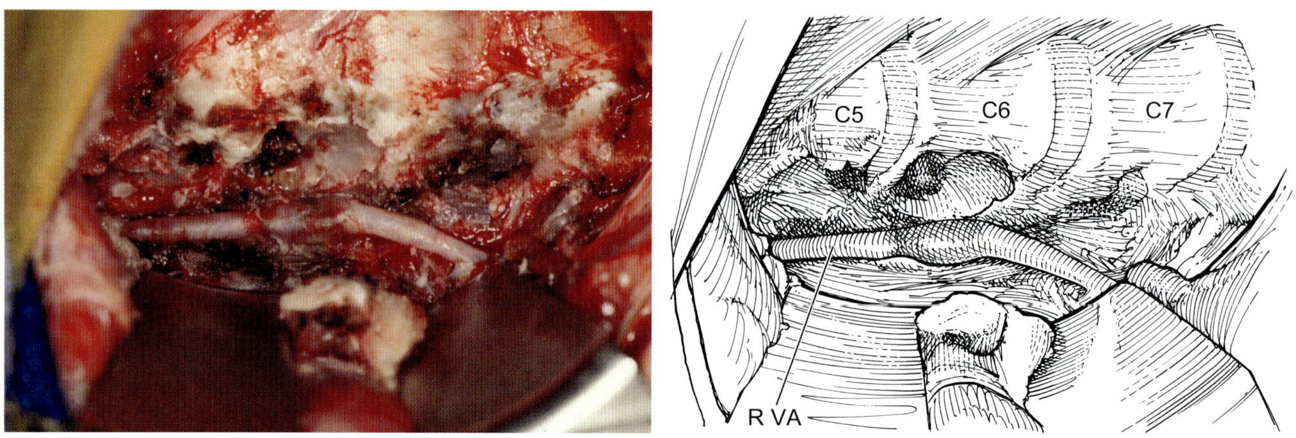

Fig. 16.1e The venous plexus is removed, exposing the VA above and below the area of injury.

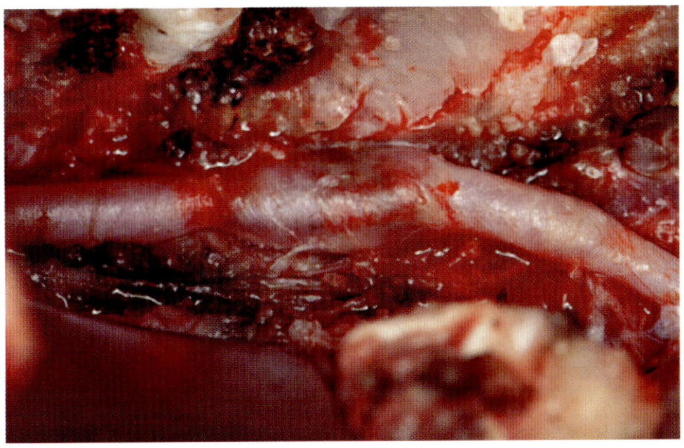

Fig. 16.1f High magnification view of the injured segment of the VA shows evidence of dissection and hemorrhage into the vessel wall.

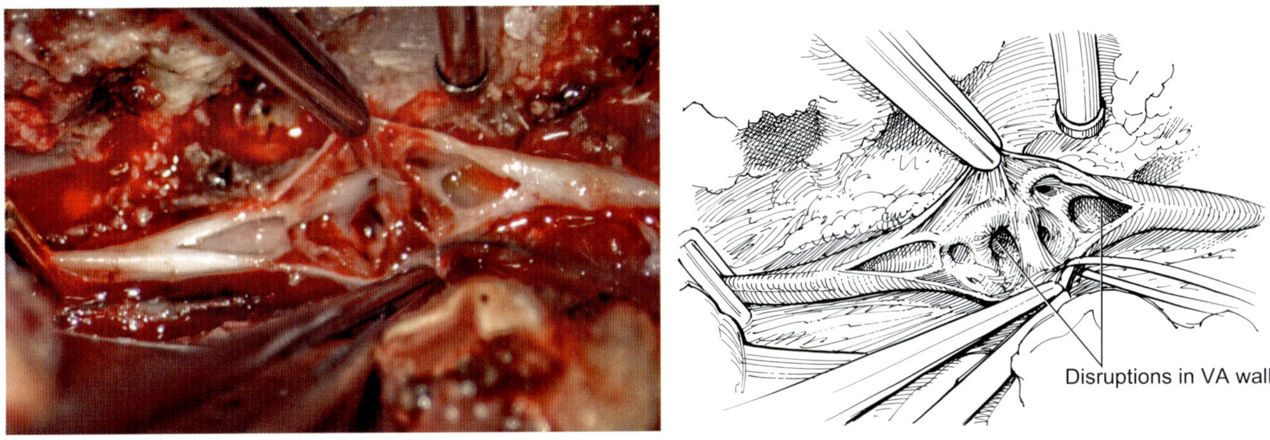

Fig. 16.1g The vessel is open through the area of injury, demonstrating the intimal dissection with associated hemorrhage into the wall and marked narrowing of the lumen.

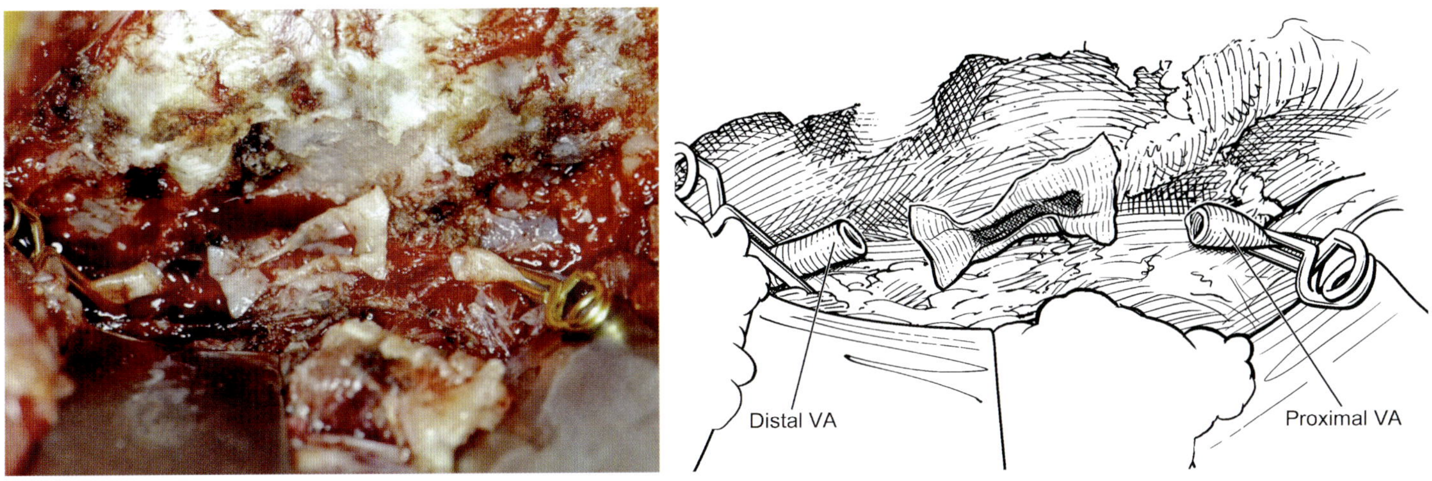

Fig. 16.1h The VA is endarterectomized and the pseudoaneurysm is removed. Temporary aneurysm clips secure the two cut ends of the VA.

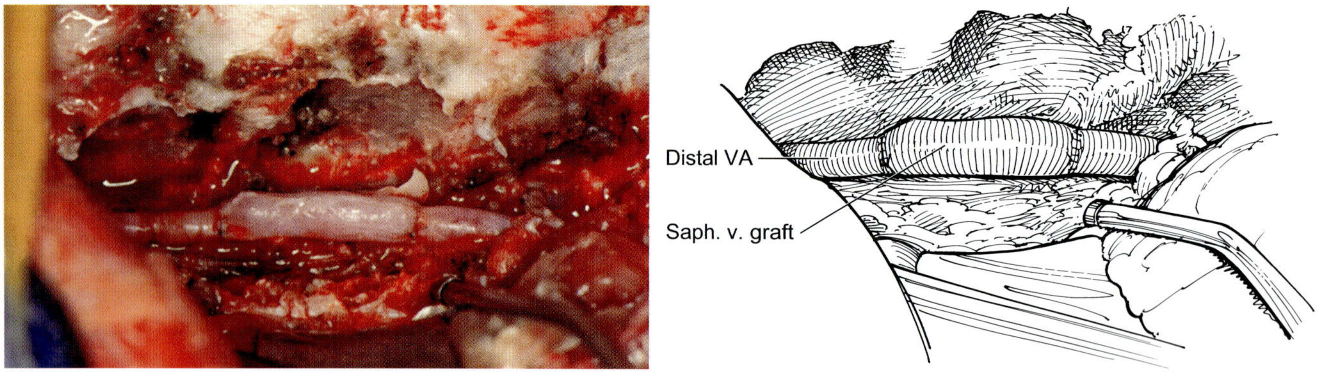

Fig. 16.1i A saphenous vein interposition graft reconstructs the VA, thereby preserving it.

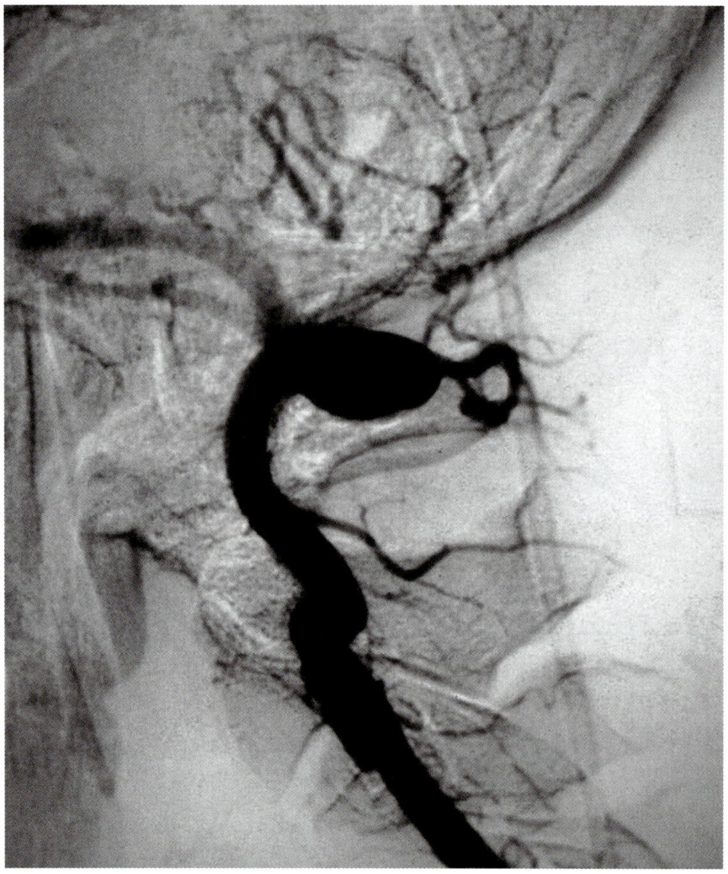

Fig. 16.1j Postoperative lateral VA angiogram confirms good flow in the artery.

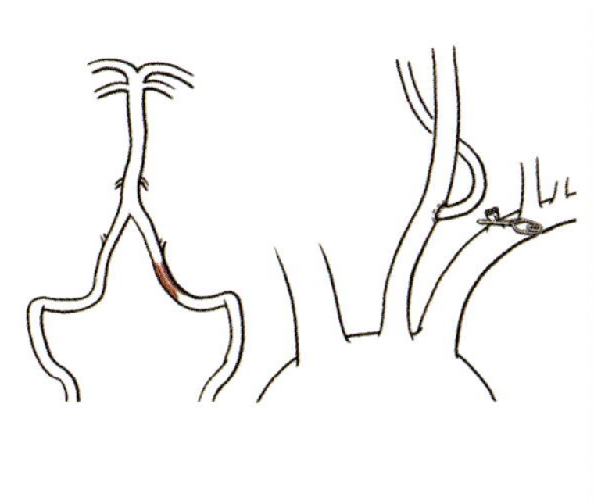

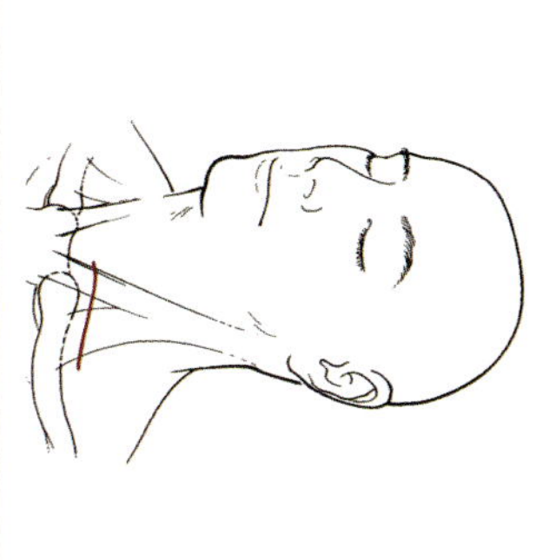

Case 16-2

Diagnosis: Left VA stenosis

Bypass: VA-to-CCA transposition with 17 years of follow-up

Approach: Left transverse supraclavicular

Video

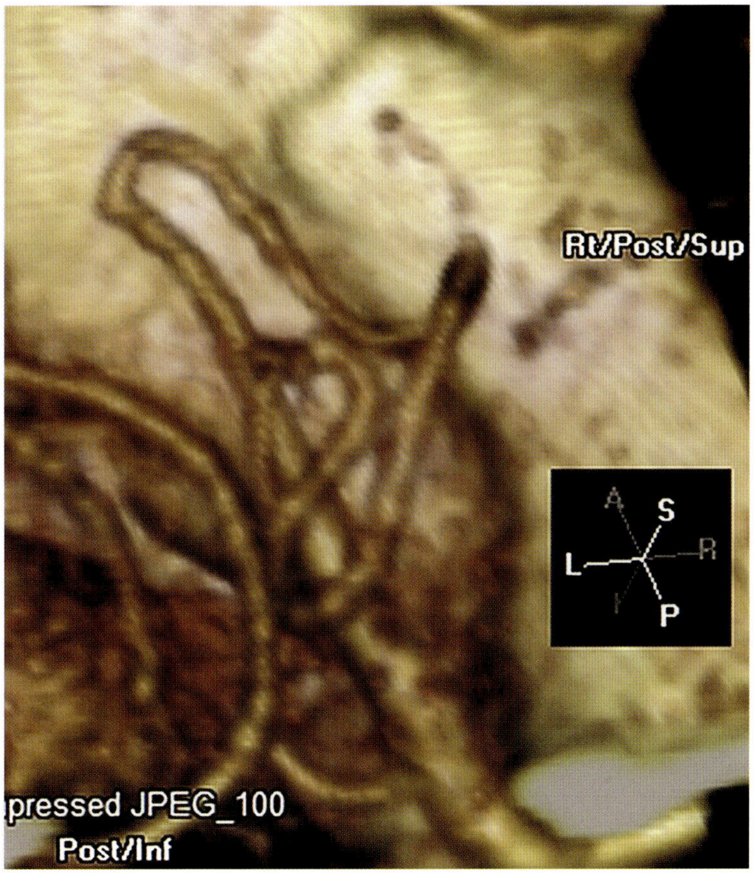

Fig. 16.2a Three-dimensional MR angiographic reconstruction of the right VA shows that it terminates in the PICA. In 1988, the patient had presented with severe symptoms referable to the BA, which was treated with a left VA-to-CCA transposition. He returned 17 years later with a new BA ischemic event that led to an angiographic injection of the VA.

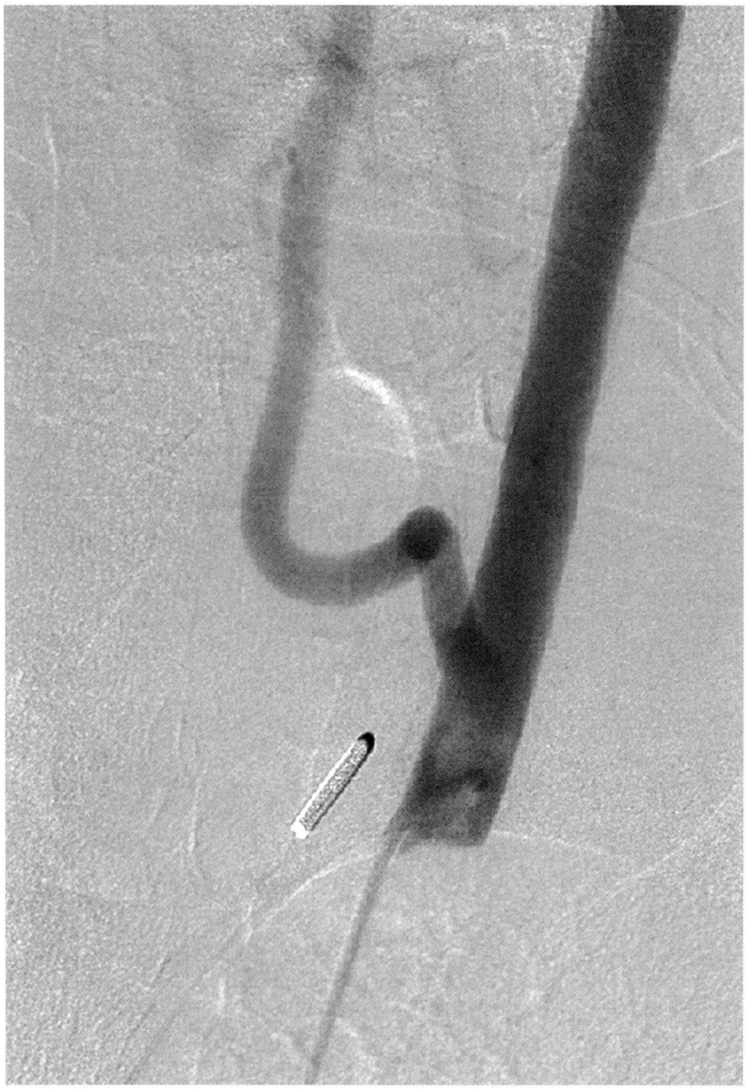

Fig. 16.2b The repeat VA angiogram shows the fully patent VA-to-CCA transposition.

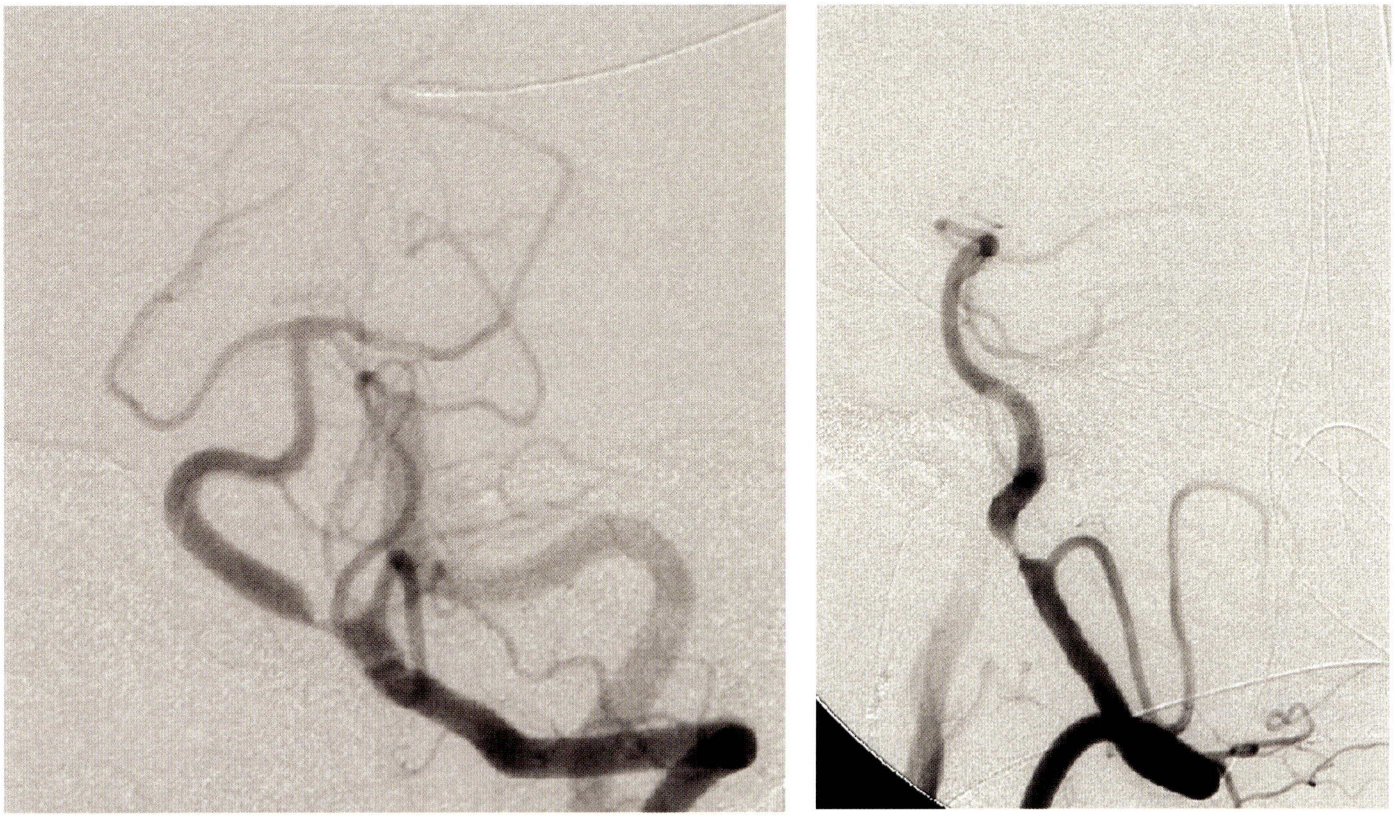

c d

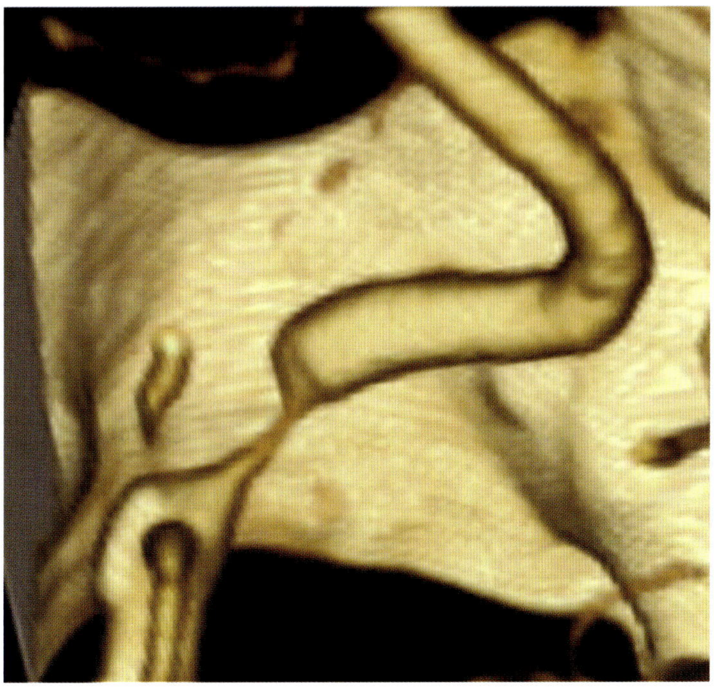

e

Fig. 16.2c–e Anteroposterior (**c**), lateral (**d**), and three-dimensional (**e**) reconstruction angiograms show new severe intracranial stenosis of the left VA.

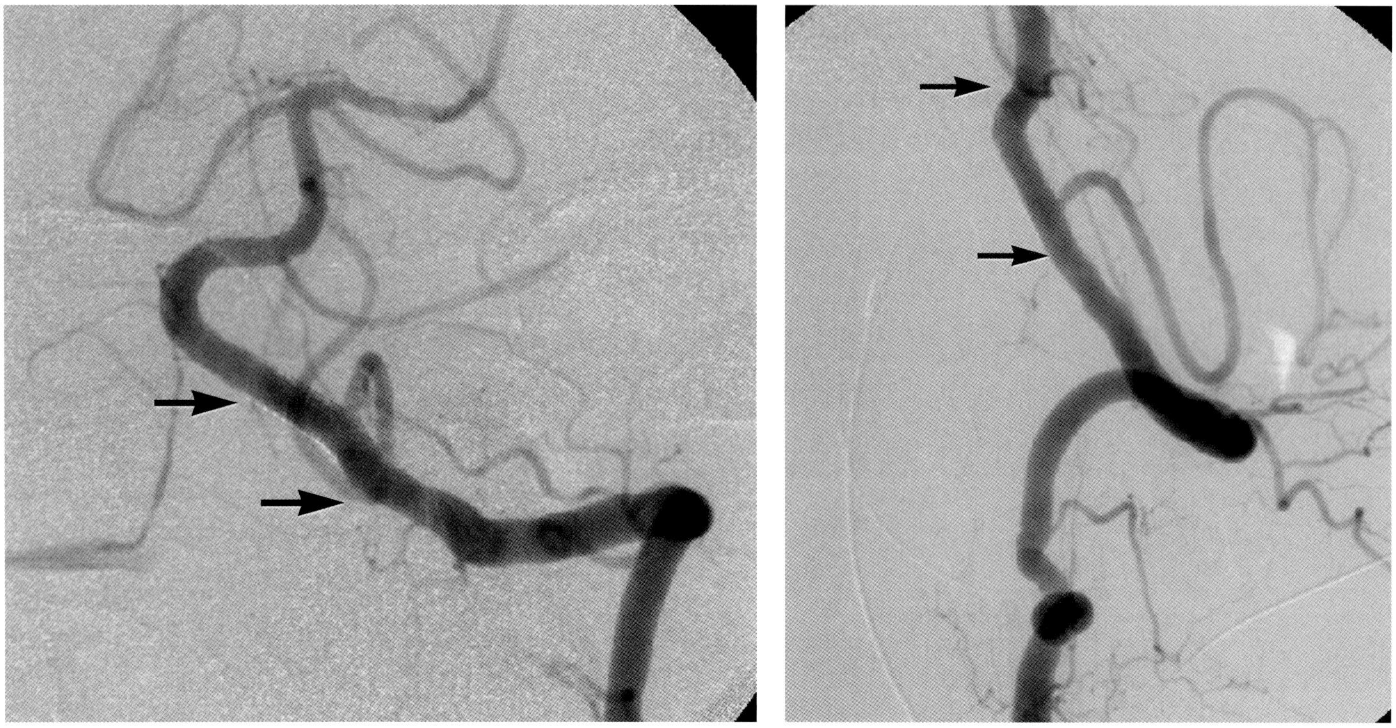

f g

Fig. 16.2f, g Angiograms show that placement of the stent (*arrows*) through the transposition dilates the narrowing. The patient's symptoms ceased. This case demonstrates the longevity of a VA-to-CCA transposition.

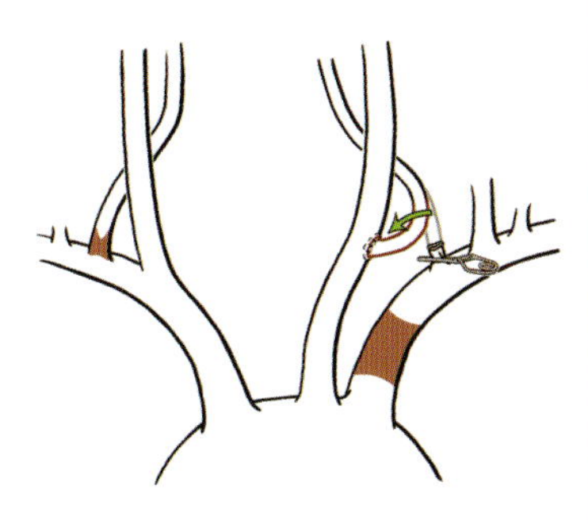

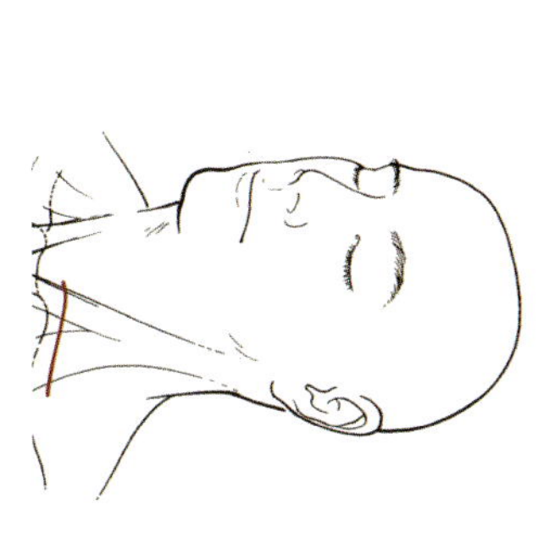

Case 16-3

Diagnosis: Posterior fossa TIAs, right VA occlusion, and left VA stenosis

Bypass: VA-to-CCA transposition

Approach: Left transverse supraclavicular

Video

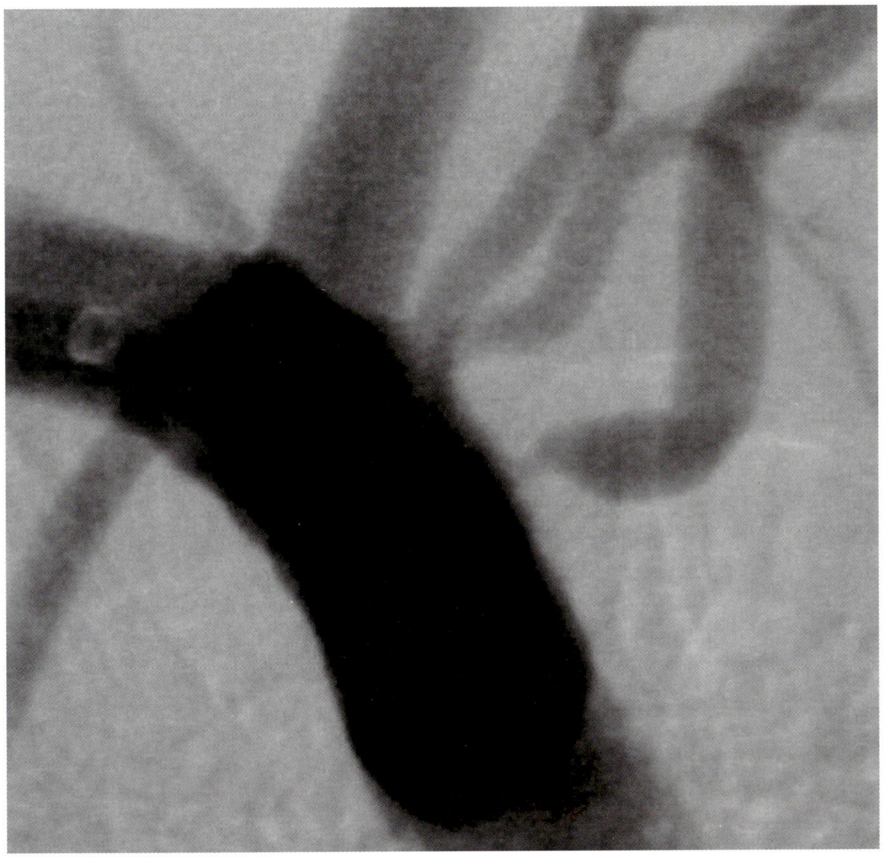

Fig. 16.3a Subclavian arch injection shows severe stenosis of the left VA in a patient with posterior fossa TIAs and right VA occlusion.

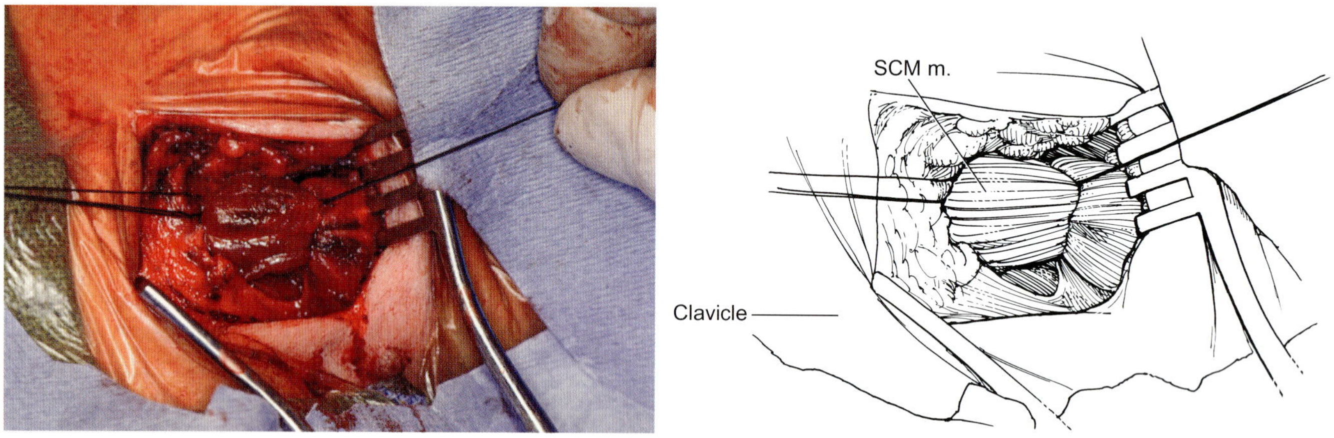

Fig. 16.3b The SCM is identified in the left supraclavicular exposure and the medial two-thirds of the muscle are cut.

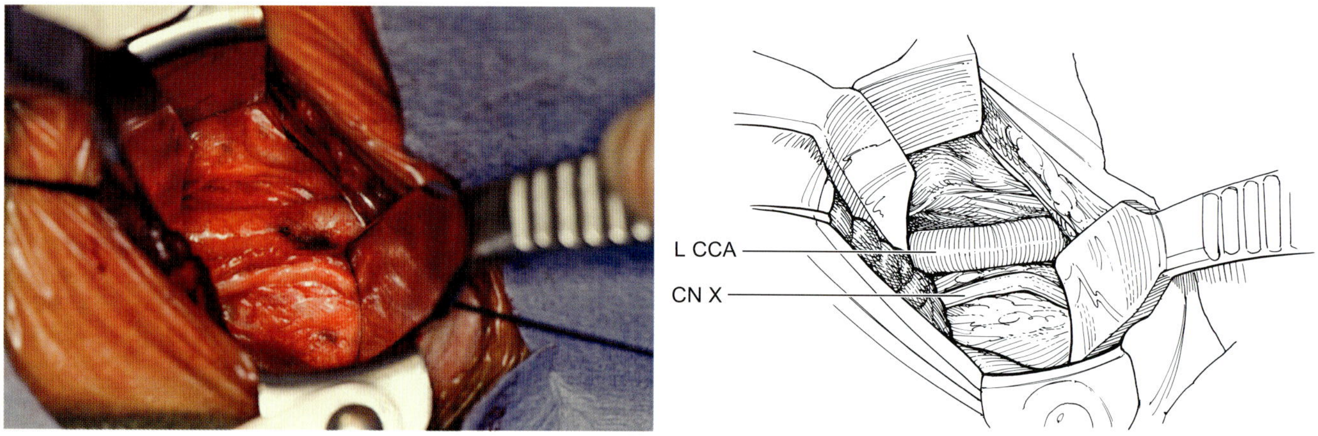

Fig. 16.3c The left CCA and CN X are identified.

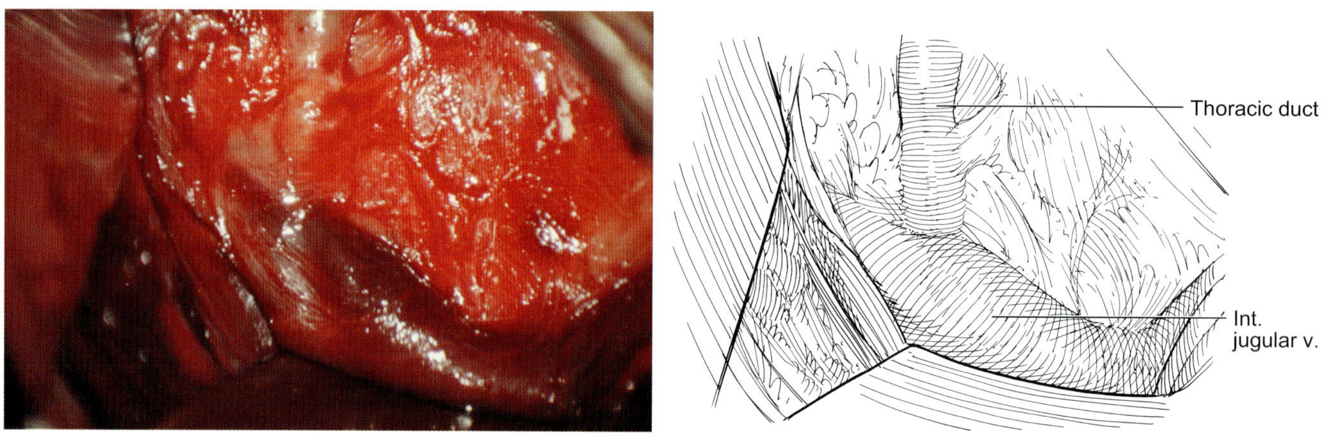

Fig. 16.3d The thoracic duct is visible as it enters the internal jugular vein. It is important to keep the thoracic duct and its branches intact so they can be ligated securely to avoid a chylous accumulation.

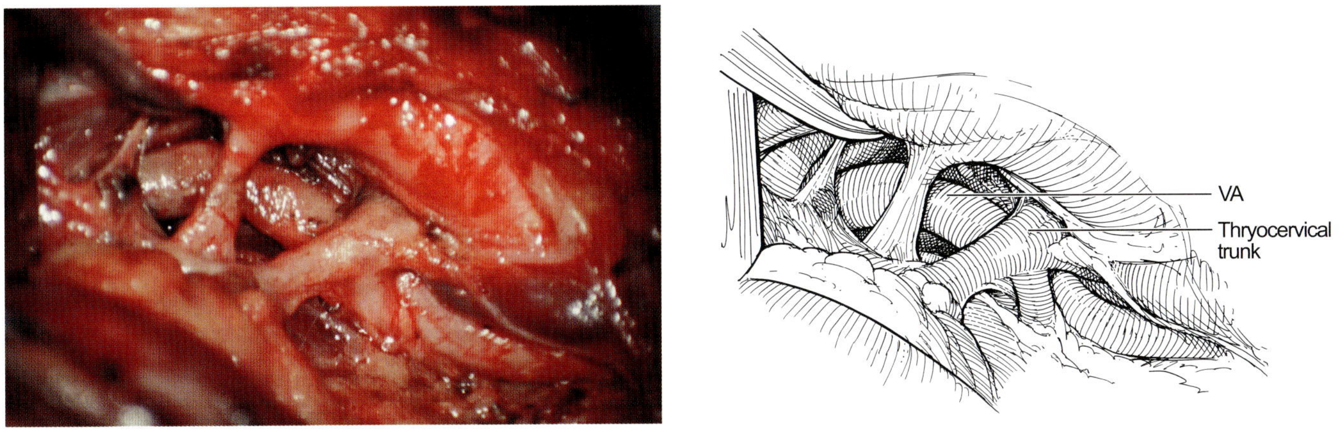

Fig. 16.3e The left VA is exposed just deep to the branches of the thyrocervical trunk.

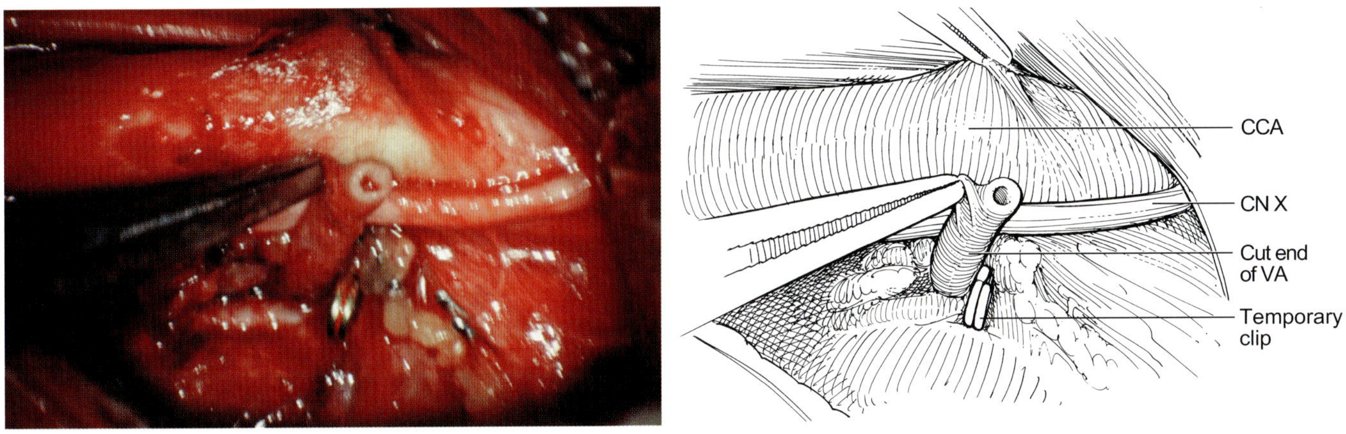

Fig. 16.3f The VA is divided at its origin from the subclavian artery. The stump is apposed to the CCA to determine if sufficient length has been mobilized to allow an end-to-side anastomosis. If necessary, further length can be obtained by opening the transverse foramen of C6. In this figure, a temporary aneurysm clip occludes the VA where it enters the left C6 transverse foramen.

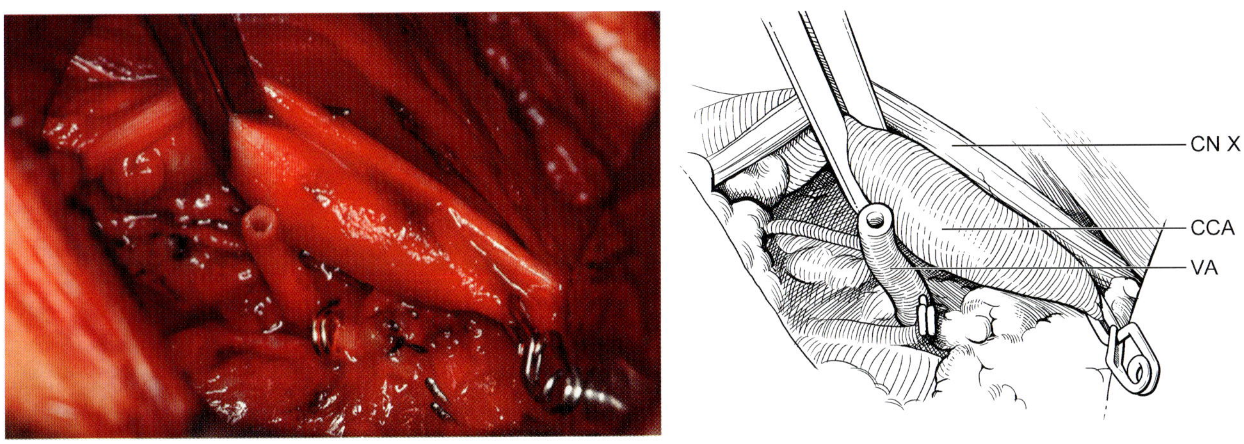

Fig. 16.3g A segment of the CCA is isolated between vascular clamps. The clamps are applied from the lateral side and then rotated 90 degrees medially to bring the posterolateral wall into view. The anastomosis is completed on this surface. When the clamps are released, the bypass enters from a more natural posterolateral direction. CN X has been displaced medially and superiorly to the carotid artery so that it does not interfere with the anastomosis.

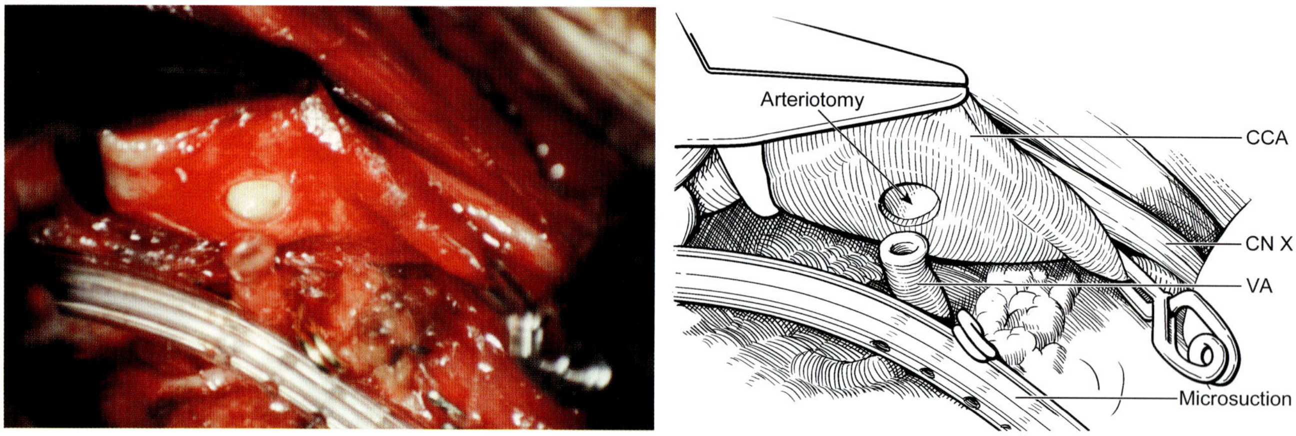

Fig. 16.3h An arteriotomy made with a 4-mm punch is inspected. Punches are available in 1-mm increments to match the size of the graft vessel. The 4-mm punch is used most often.

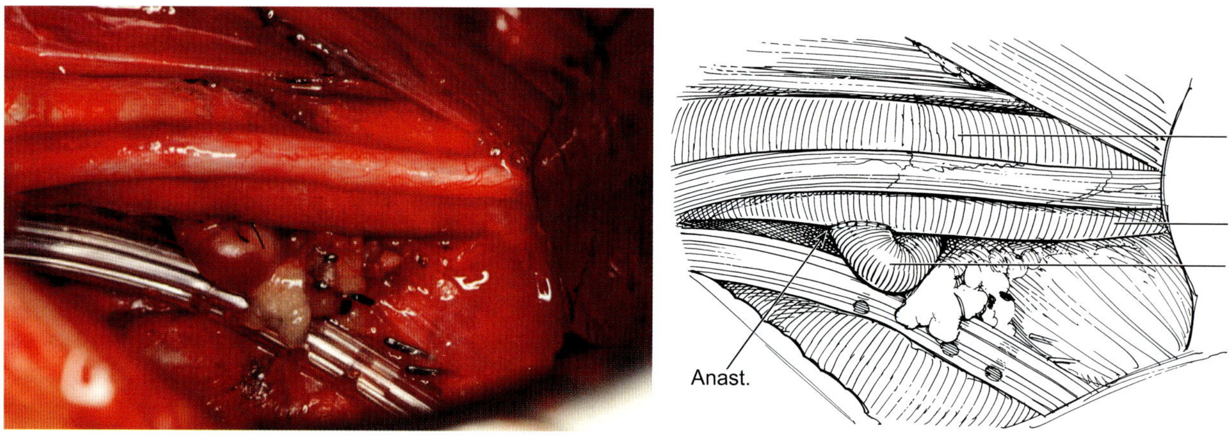

Fig. 16.3i The anastomosis is completed with 6–0 suture and inspected for hemostasis.

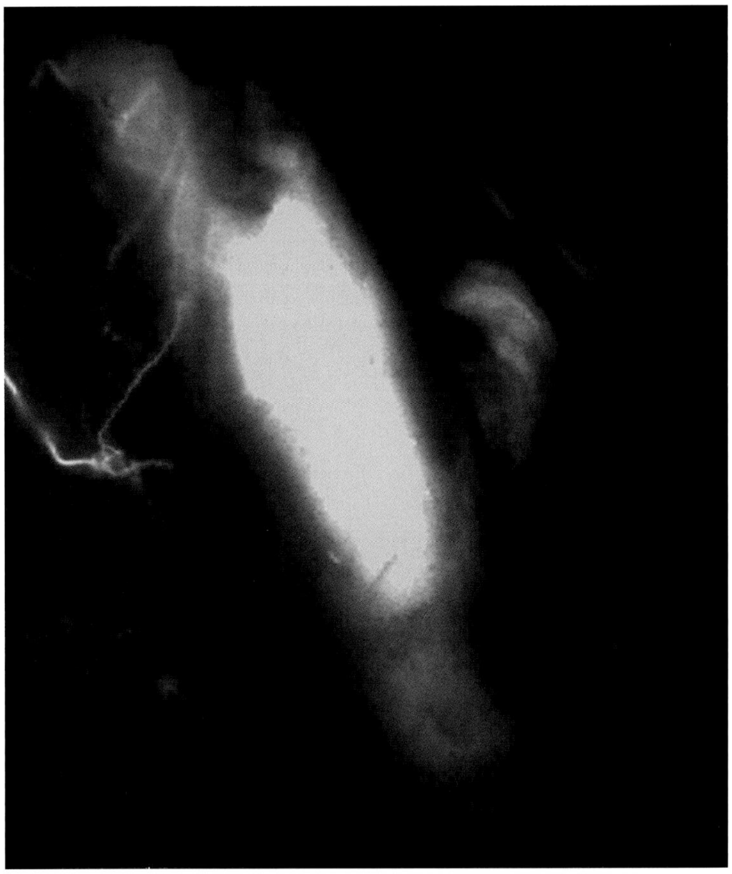

Fig. 16.3j Intraoperative ICG angiogram confirms patency of the transposition.

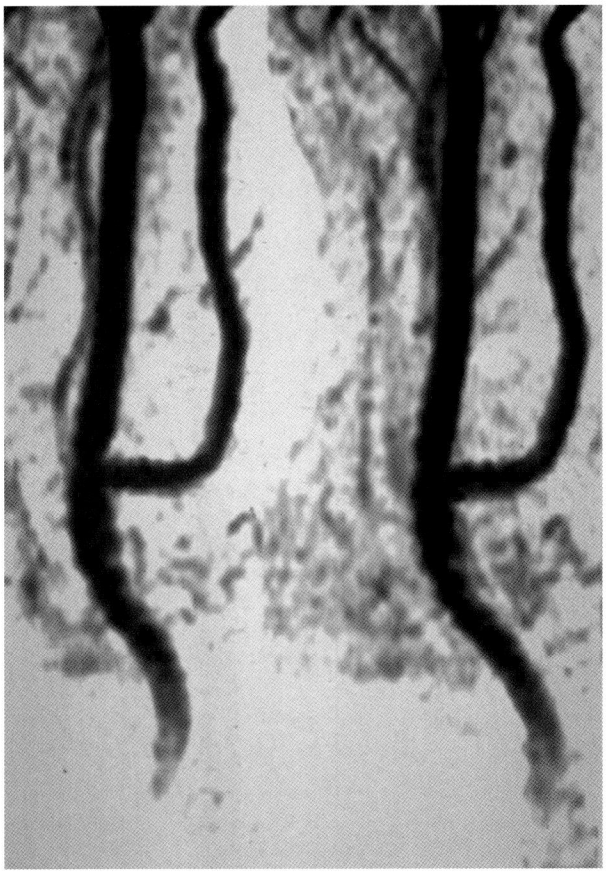

Fig. 16.3k Postoperative left CCA MR angiograms show a widely patent VA-to-CCA transposition with antegrade flow in both vessels. The visualization of vessels with retrograde flow, such as the deep draining veins, is blocked in this sequence by the application of saturation pulses along the field of view.

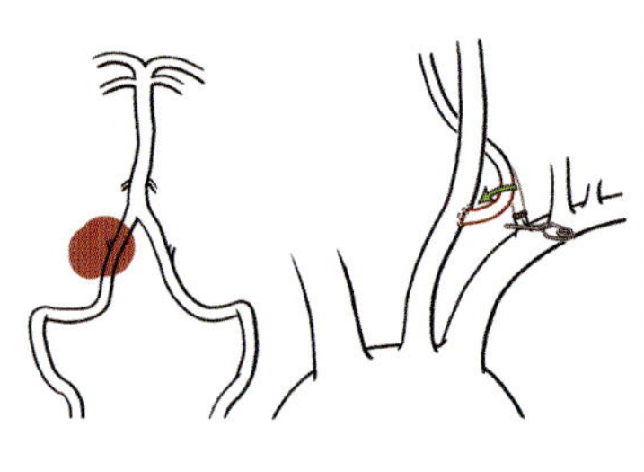

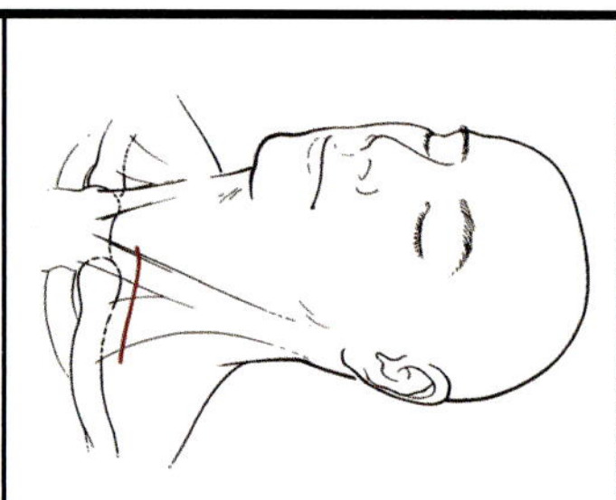

Case 16-4

Diagnosis: Subclavian steal, right to left, with recurrent VA aneurysm

Bypass: VA-to-CCA transposition

Approach: Left transverse supraclavicular

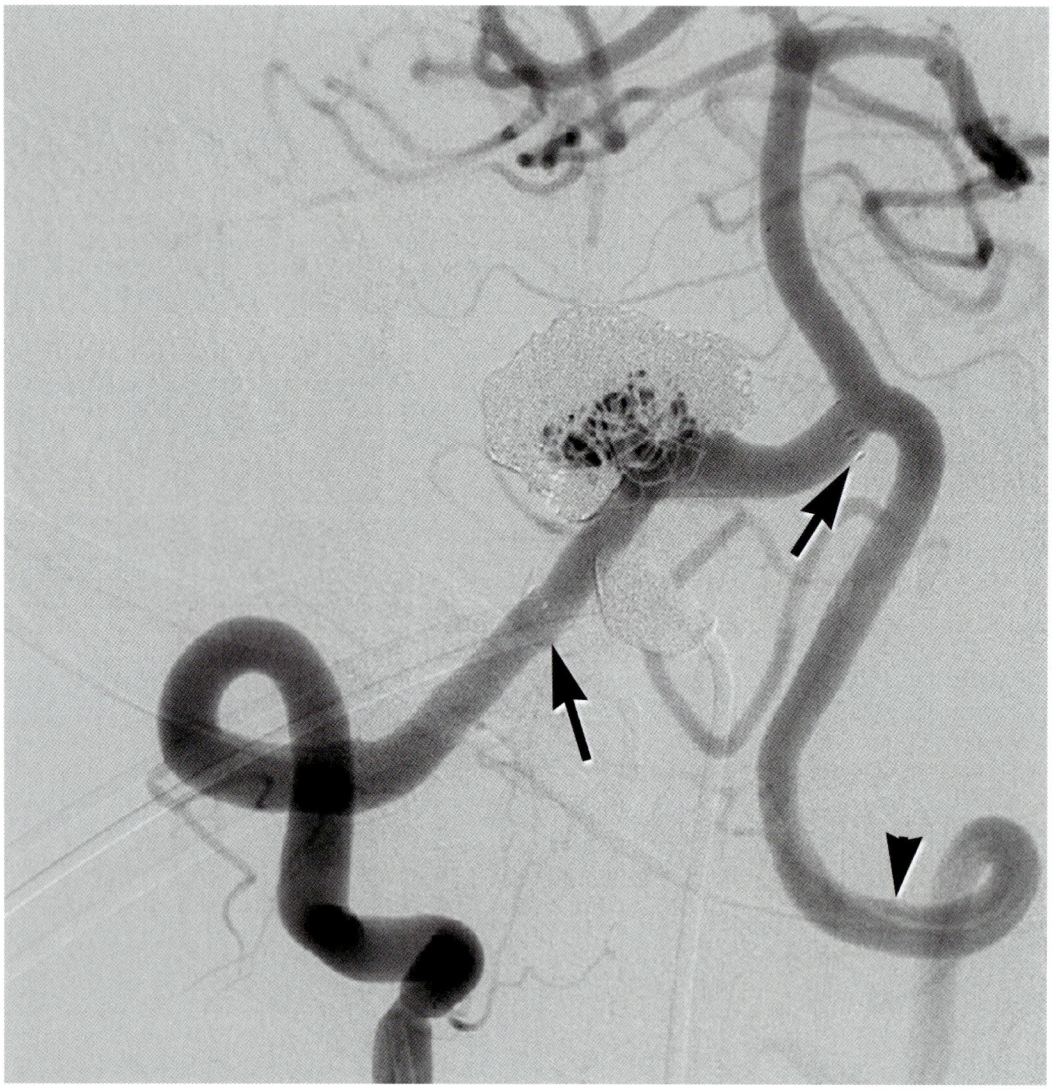

Fig. 16.4a Anteroposterior angiogram of the right VA shows a recurrent VA aneurysm, despite the presence of a stent (*arrows*). Note the presence of subclavian steal (*arrowhead*.)

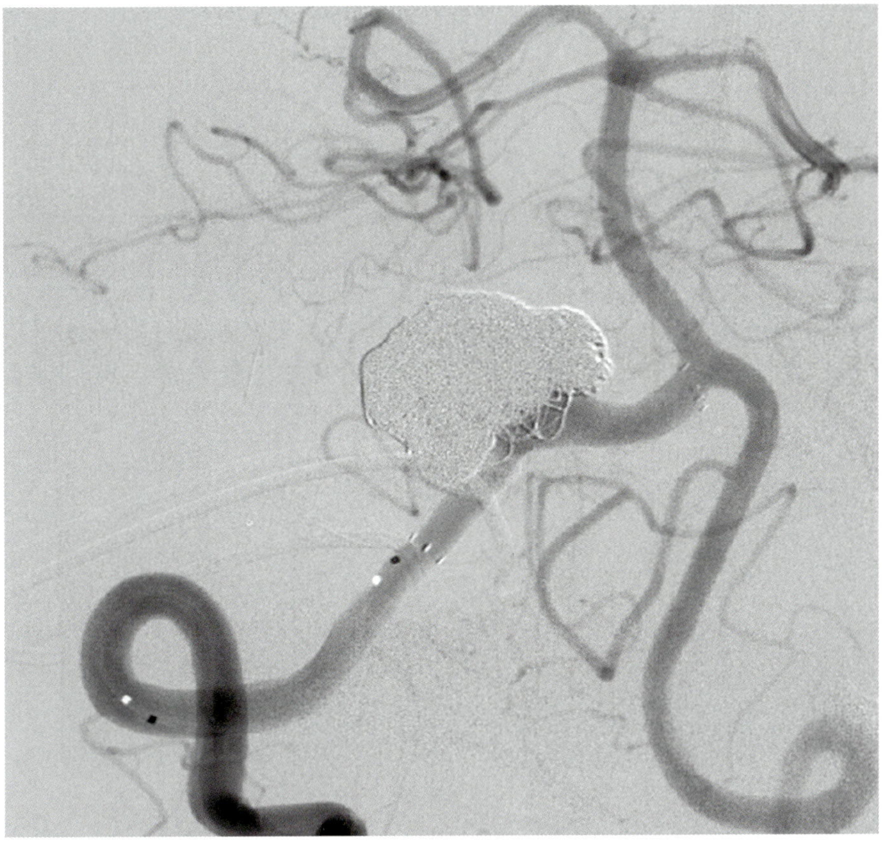

Fig. 16.4b The aneurysm is recoiled, but in the presence of the subclavian steal, fear that the large amount of blood flow at the base of the aneurysm would cause a recurrence motivated a plan to treat the subclavian steal with a left VA-to-CCA transposition. The transposition would greatly diminish the flow in the right VA and base of the aneurysm.

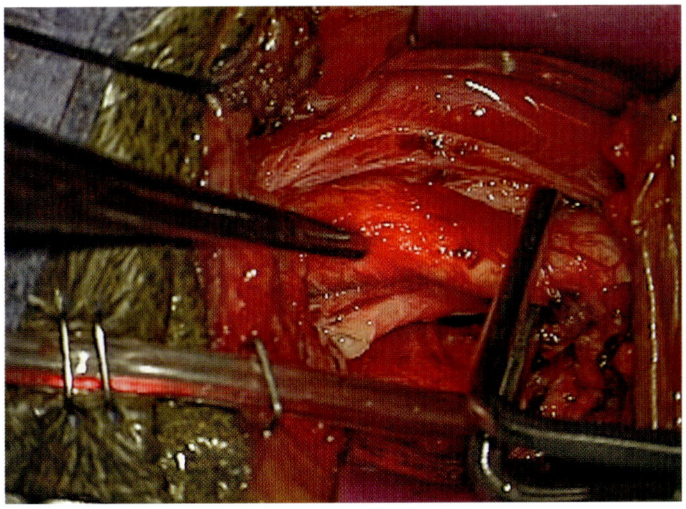

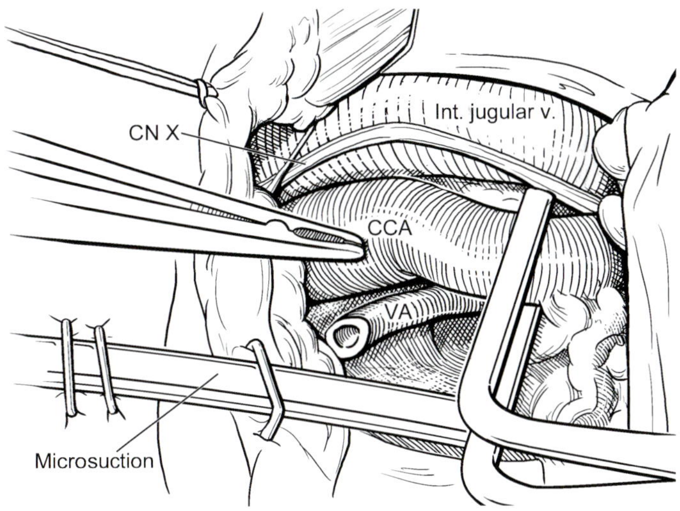

Fig. 16.4c The VA has been cut and prepared for anastomosis to the CCA. A malleable microsuction device has been placed in the surgical field so that constant irrigation fluid can be evacuated.

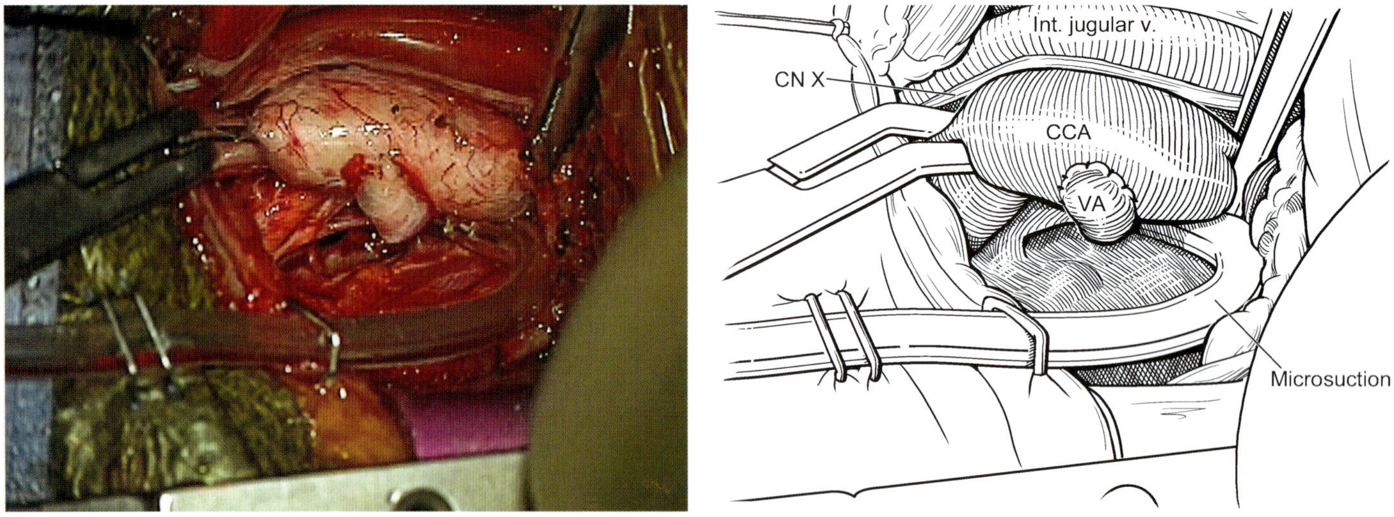

Fig. 16.4d The transposition is completed. The vascular clamps are still in place. Their release will allow the CCA to rotate so that the anastomosis is located in the back wall of the vessel.

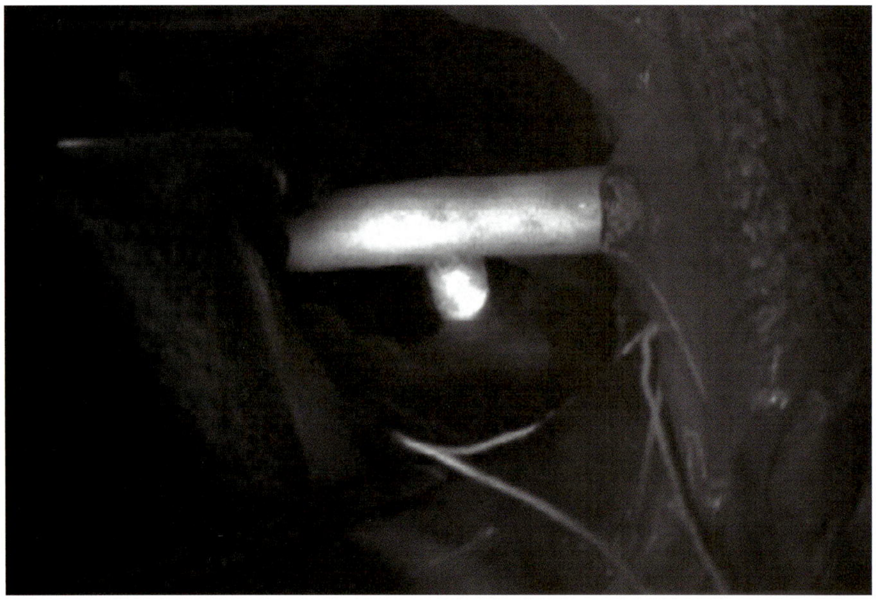

Fig. 16.4e ICG angiography demonstrates the bypass.

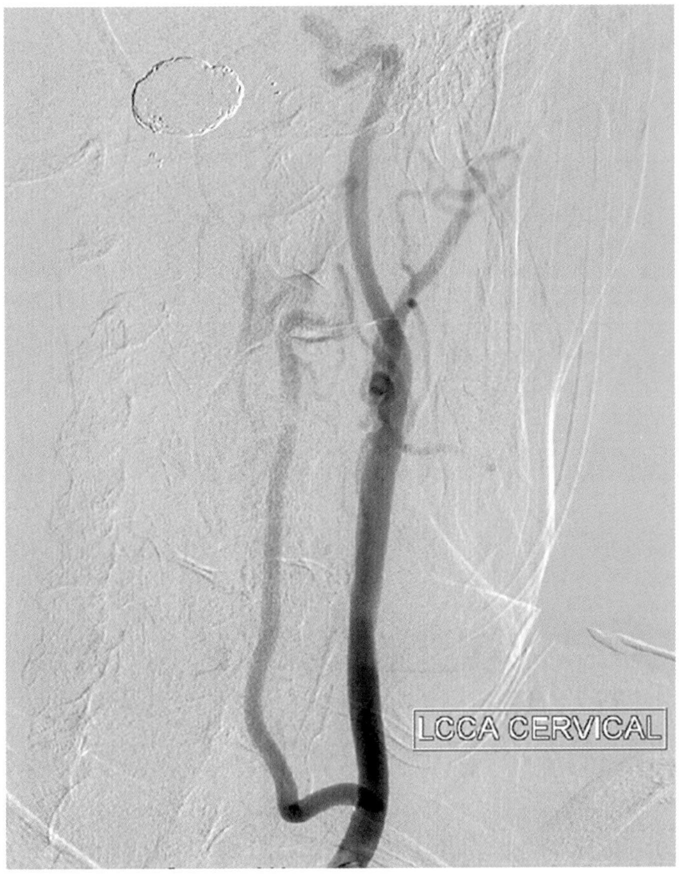

Fig. 16.4f Lateral CCA angiographic injection shows the VA transposition.

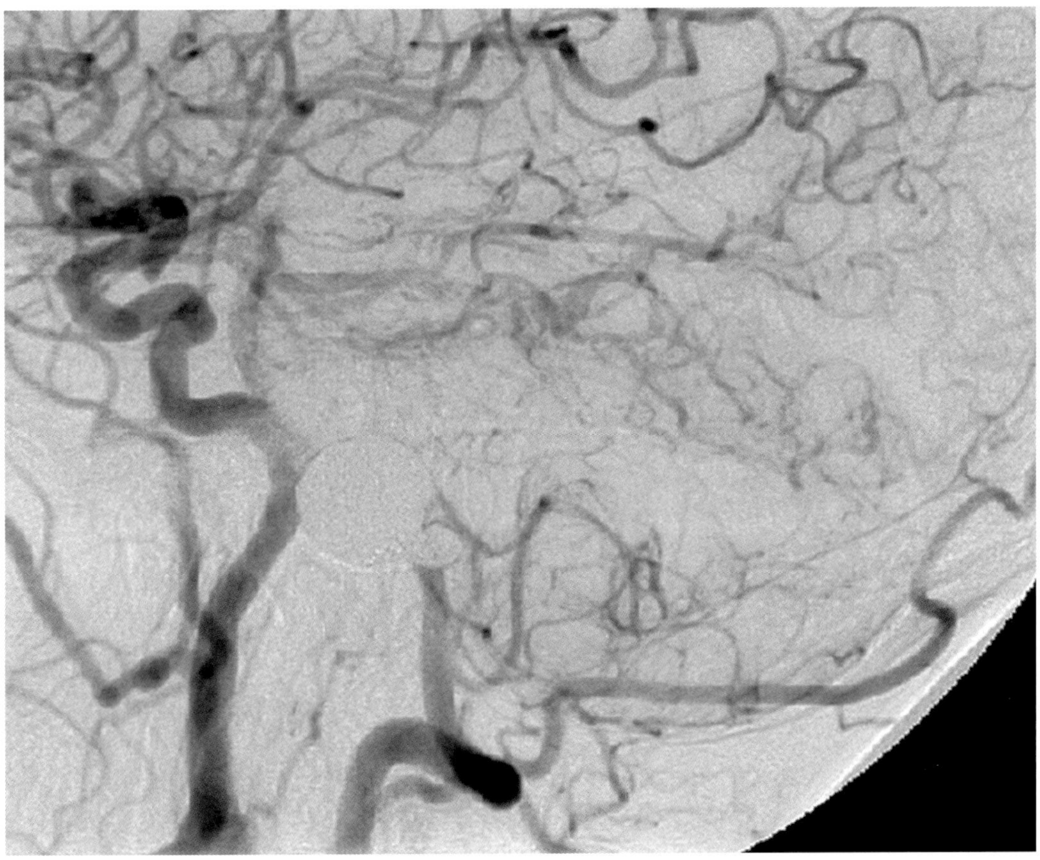

Fig. 16.4g High magnification view of a left CCA angiographic injection shows that the posterior fossa is filled through the transposition, dramatically decreasing blood flow through the right VA and the neck of the aneurysm.

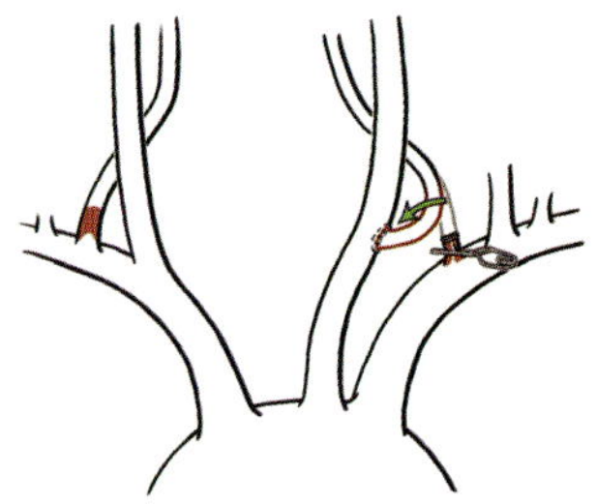

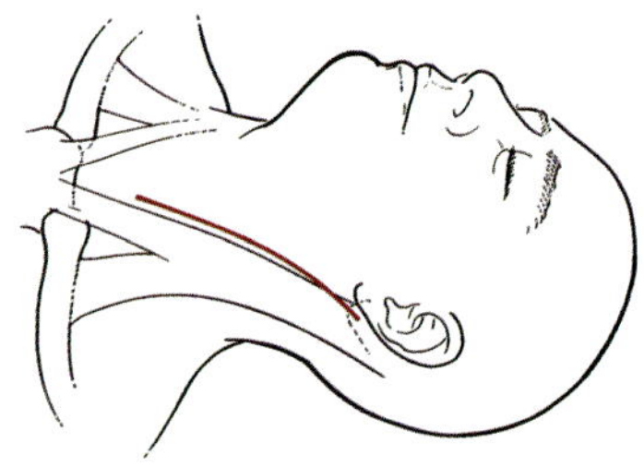

Case 16-5

Diagnosis: Posterior fossa TIAs

Bypass: VA-to-CCA transposition

Approach: Left Anterior cervical

Video

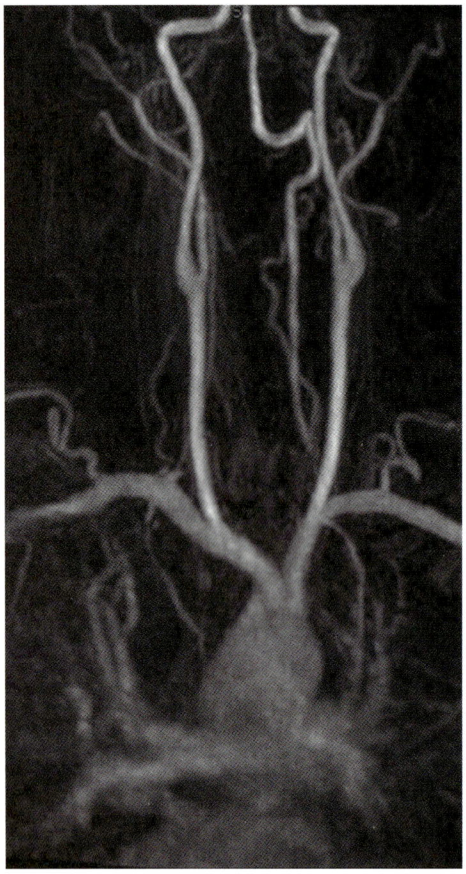

Fig. 16.5a MR angiogram demonstrates a right VA occlusion and severe left VA stenosis in a 48-year-old physician.

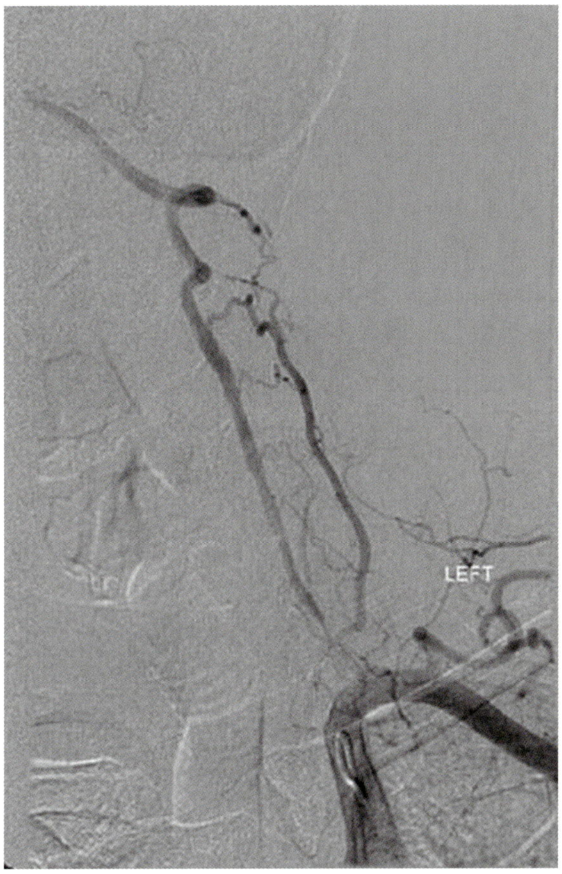

Fig. 16.5b Angiogram shows severe left VA stenosis with collaterals from the cervical trunk.

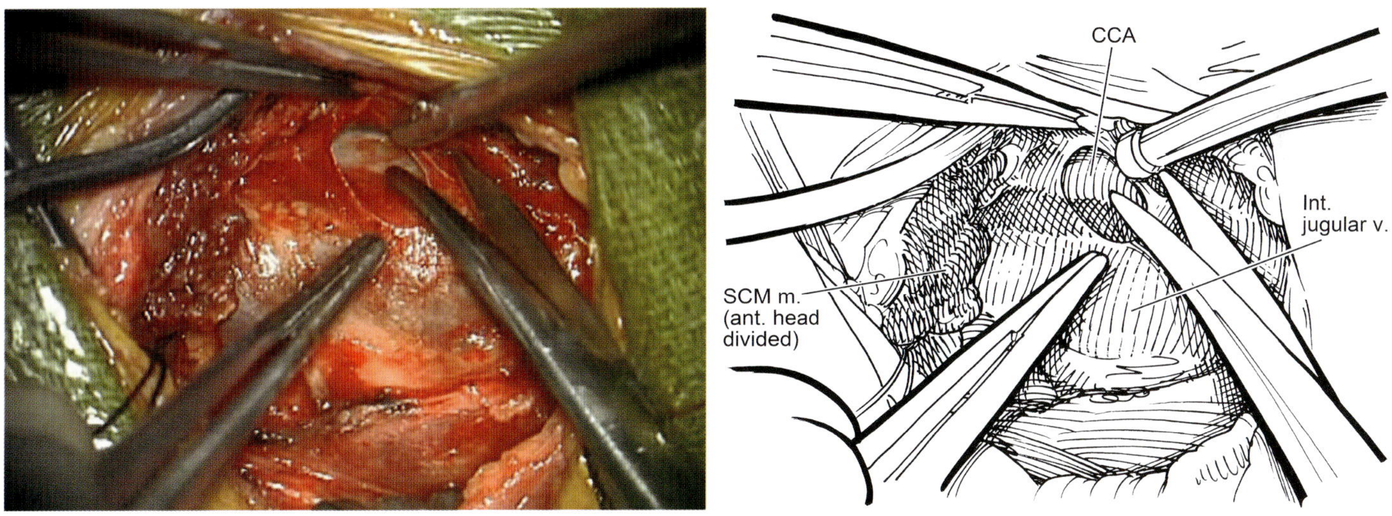

Fig. 16.5c With part of the SCM muscle cut as it inserts along the clavicle, the internal jugular vein is exposed.

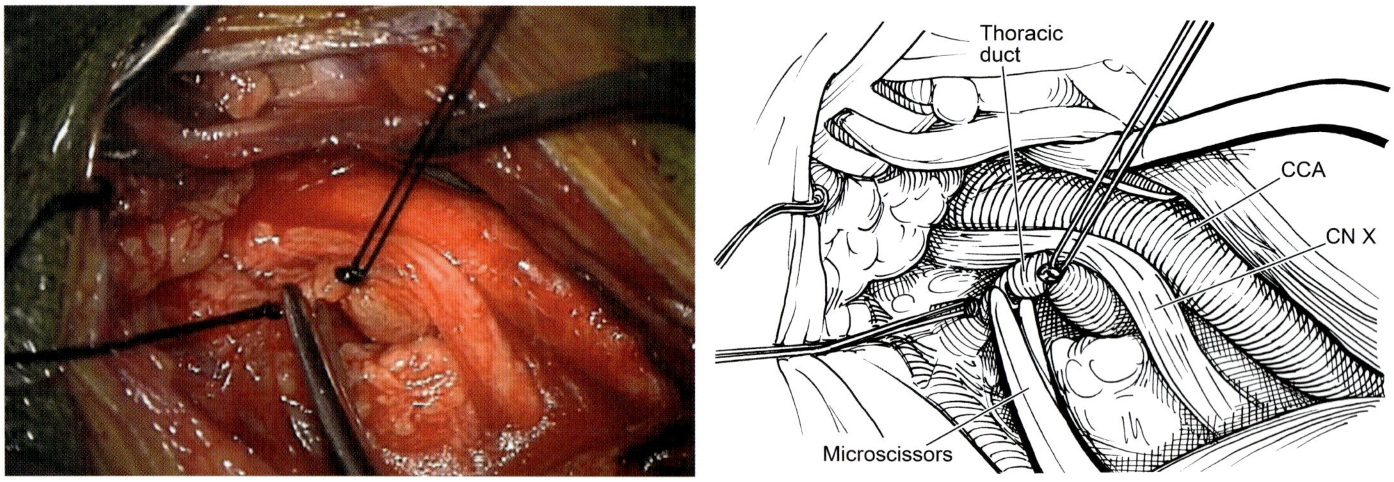

Fig. 16.5d The thoracic duct is identified and ligated.

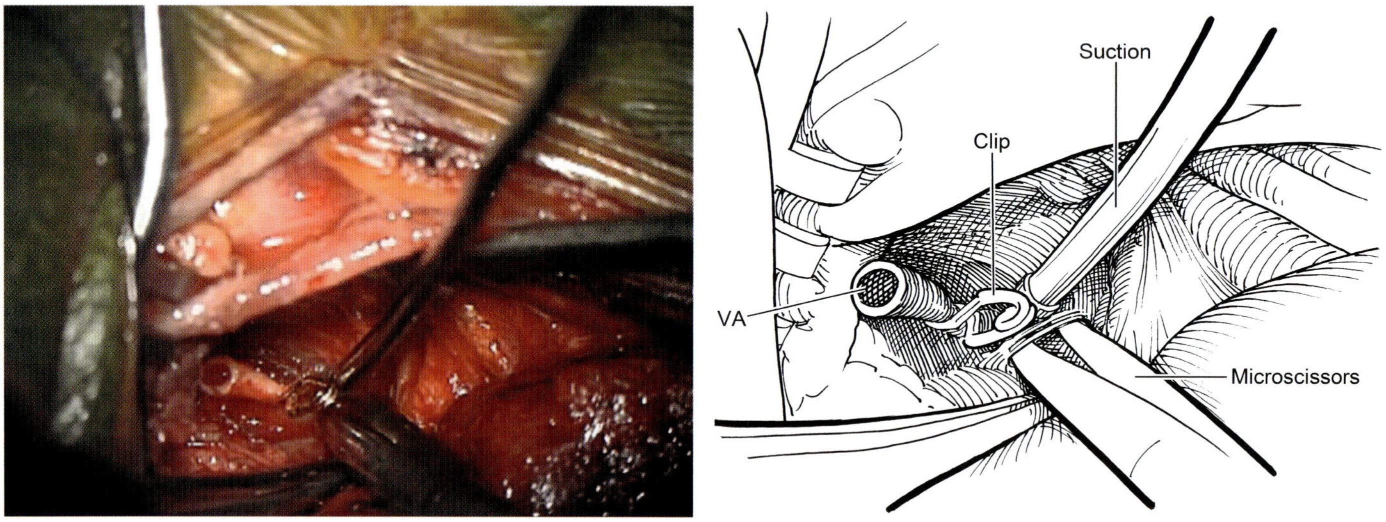

Fig. 16.5e The VA is cut.

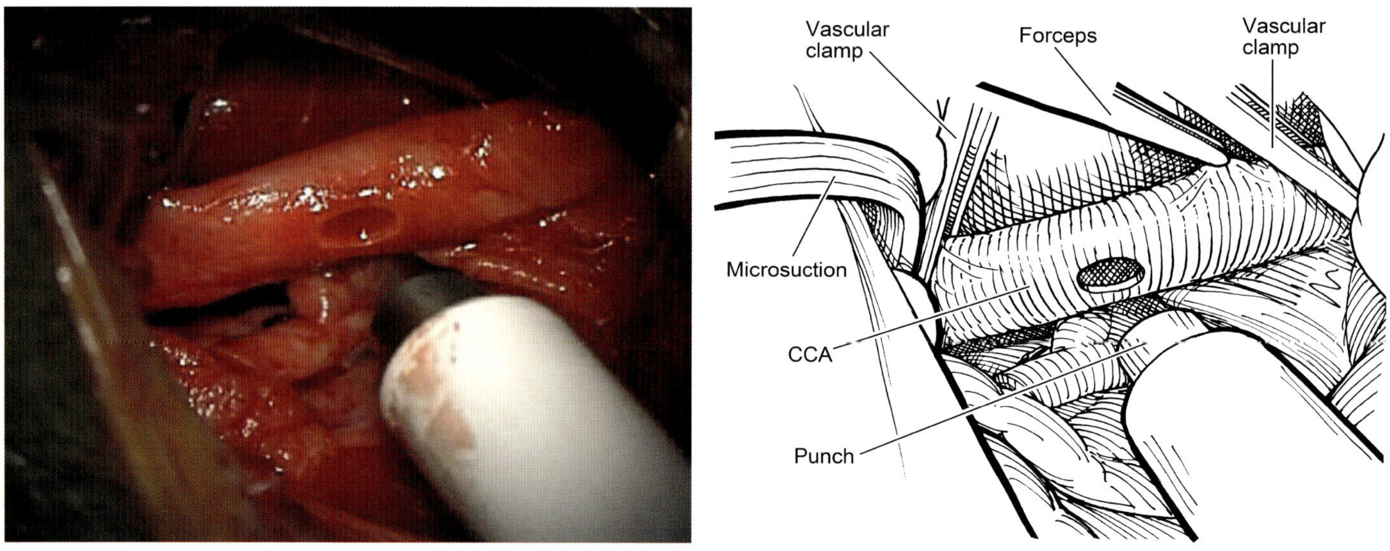

Fig. 16.5f A hole is placed in the CCA with a 4-mm aortic punch.

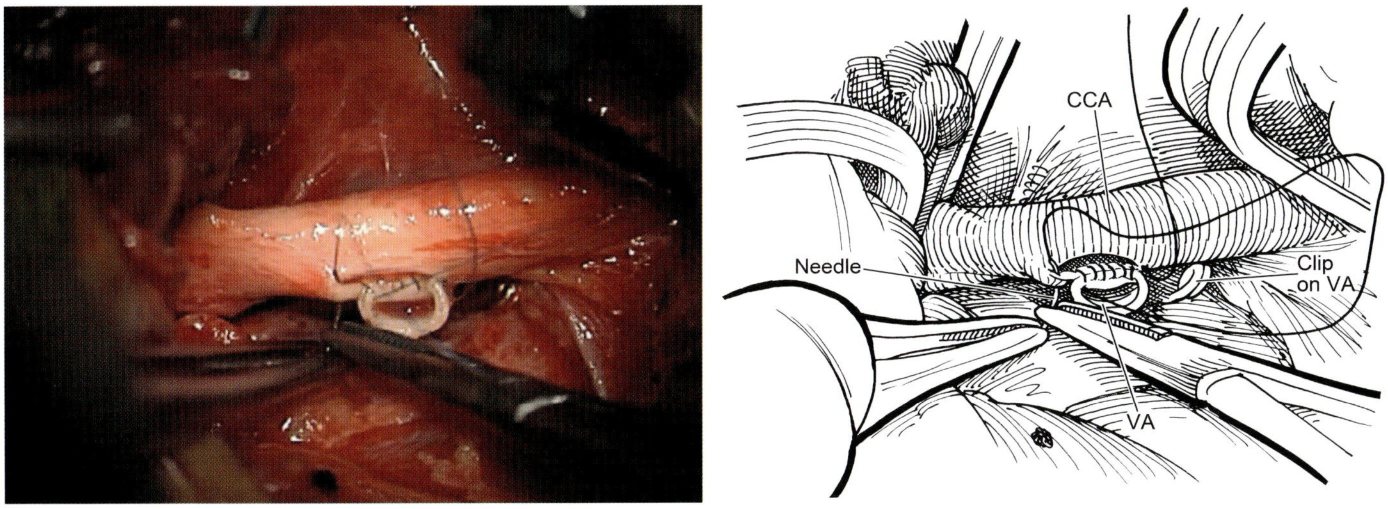

Fig. 16.5g The back wall of the transposition is performed.

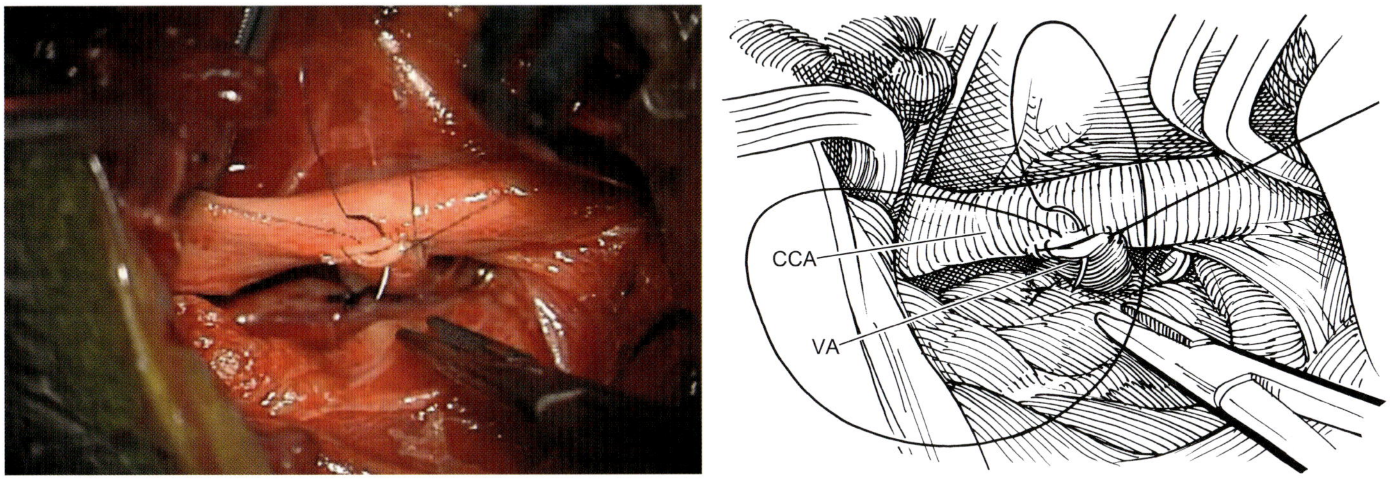

Fig. 16.5h The front wall is sutured.

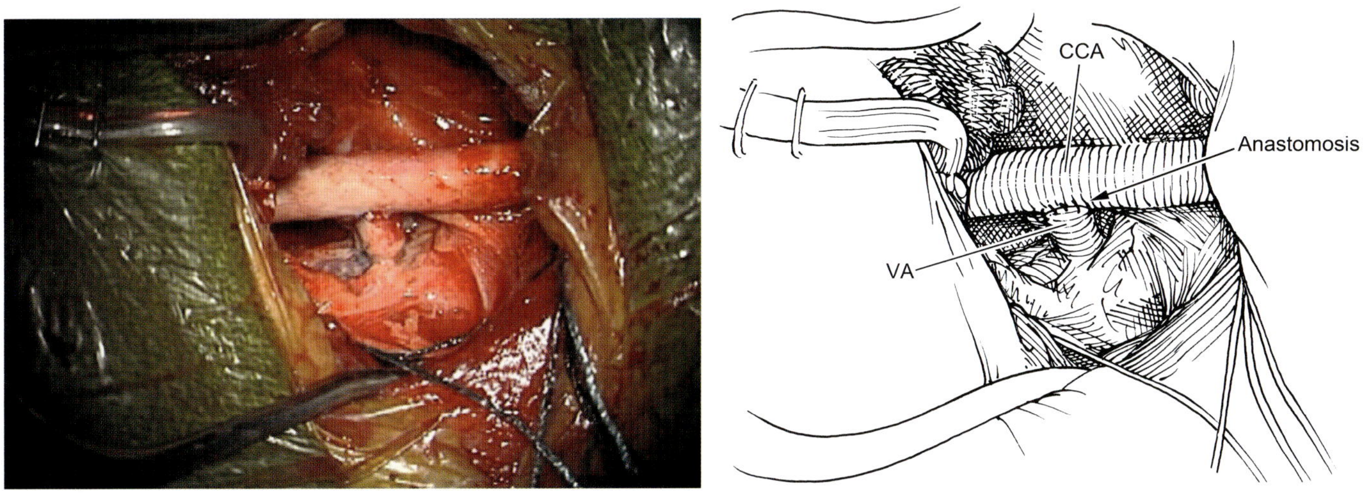

Fig. 16.5i The anastomosis is completed.

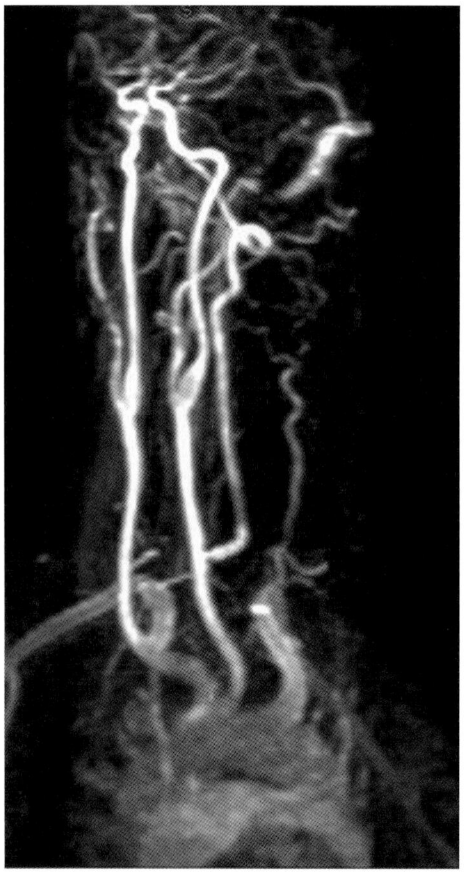

Fig. 16.5j Postoperative MR angiogram demonstrating the patent transposition. The patient's TIAs ceased, allowing him to return to his practice.

Index